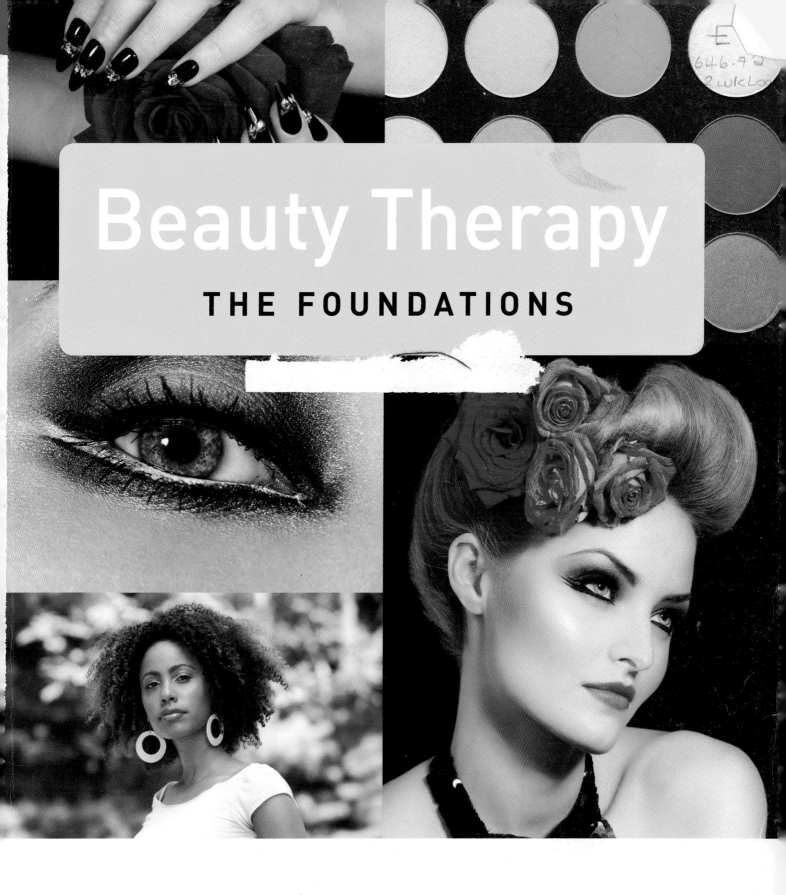

Beauty Therapy

THE FOUNDATIONS

HABIA SERIES LIST

Hairdressing

Student textbooks

Begin Hairdressing: The Official Guide to Level 1 1e *Martin Green*

Hairdressing – The Foundations: The Official Guide to Level 2 6e *Leo Palladino and Martin Green*

Professional Hairdressing: The Official Guide to Level 3 5e *Martin Green and Leo Palladino*

The Official Guide to the City & Guilds Certificate in Salon Service 1e *John Armstrong with Anita Crosland, Martin Green and Lorraine Nordmann*

The Colour Book: The Official Guide to Colour for NVQ Levels 2 & 3 1e *Tracey Lloyd with Christine McMillan-Bodell*

eXtensions: The Official Guide to Hair Extensions 1e *Theresa Bullock*

Salon Management *Martin Green*

Men's Hairdressing: Traditional and Modern Barbering 2e *Maurice Lister*

African-Caribbean Hairdressing 2e *Sandra Gittens*

The World of Hair Colour 1e *John Gray*

The Cutting Book: The Official Guide to Cutting at S/NVQ Levels 2 and 3 *Jane Goldsbro and Elaine White*

Professional Hairdressing titles

Trevor Sorbie: The Bridal Hair Book 1e *Trevor Sorbie and Jacki Wadeson*

The Art of Dressing Long Hair 1e *Guy Kremer and Jacki Wadeson*

Patrick Cameron: Dressing Long Hair 1e *Patrick Cameron and Jacki Wadeson*

Patrick Cameron: Dressing Long Hair 2 1e *Patrick Cameron and Jacki Wadeson*

Bridal Hair 1e *Pat Dixon and Jacki Wadeson*

Professional Men's Hairdressing: The art of cutting and styling 1e *Guy Kremer and Jacki Wadeson*

Essensuals, the Next GenerationToni and Guy:Step by Step 1e *Sacha Mascolo, Christian Mascolo and Stuart Wesson*

Mahogany Hairdressing: Step to Cutting, Colouring and Finishing Hair 1e *Martin Gannon and Richard Thompson*

Mahogany Hairdressing: Advanced Looks 1e *Martin Gannon and Richard Thompson*

The Total Look: The Style Guide for Hair and Make-up Professional 1e *Ian Mistlin*

Trevor Sorbie: Visions in Hair 1e *Trevor Sorbie, Kris Sorbie and Jacki Wadeson*

The Art of Hair Colouring 1e *David Adams and Jacki Wadeson*

Beauty therapy

Beauty Basics: The Official Guide to Level 1 3e *Lorraine Nordmann*

Beauty Therapy – The Foundations: The Official Guide to Level 2 5e *Lorraine Nordmann*

Professional Beauty Therapy – The Official Guide to Level 3 4e *Lorraine Nordmann*

The Official Guide to the City & Guilds Certificate in Salon Services 1e *John Armstrong with Anita Crosland, Martin Green and Lorraine Nordmann*

The Complete Guide to Make-Up 1e *Suzanne Le Quesne*

The Encyclopedia of Nails 1e *Jacqui Jefford and Anne Swain*

The Art of Nails: A Comprehensive Style Guide to Nail Treatments and Nail Art 1e *Jacqui Jefford*

Nail Artistry 1e *Jacqui Jefford*

The Complete Nail Technician 2e *Marian Newman*

Manicure, Pedicure and Advanced Nail Techniques 1e *Elaine Almond*

The Official Guide to Body Massage 2e *Adele O'Keefe*

An Holistic Guide to Massage 1e *Tina Parsons*

Indian Head Massage 2e *Muriel Burnham-Airey and Adele O'Keefe*

Aromatherapy for the Beauty Therapist 1e *Valerie Worwood*

An Holistic Guide to Reflexology 1e *Tina Parsons*

An Holistic Guide to Anatomy and Physiology 1e *Tina Parsons*

The Essential Guide to Holistic and Complementary Therapy 1e *Helen Beckmann and Suzanne Le Quesne*

The Spa Book 1e *Jane Crebbin-Bailey, Dr John Harcup, and John Harrington*

SPA: The Official Guide to Spa Therapy at Levels 2 and 3, *Joan Scott and Andrea Harrison*

Nutrition: A Practical Approach 1e *Suzanne Le Quesne*

Hands on Sports Therapy 1e *Keith Ward*

Encyclopedia of Hair Removal: A Complete Reference to Methods, Techniques and Career Opportunities, *Gill Morris and Janice Brown*

The Anatomy and Physiology Workbook: For Beauty and Holistic Therapies Levels 1–3. *Tina Parsons*

The Anatomy and Physiology CD-Rom.

Beautiful Selling: The Complete Guide to Sales Success in the Salon *Rath Langley*

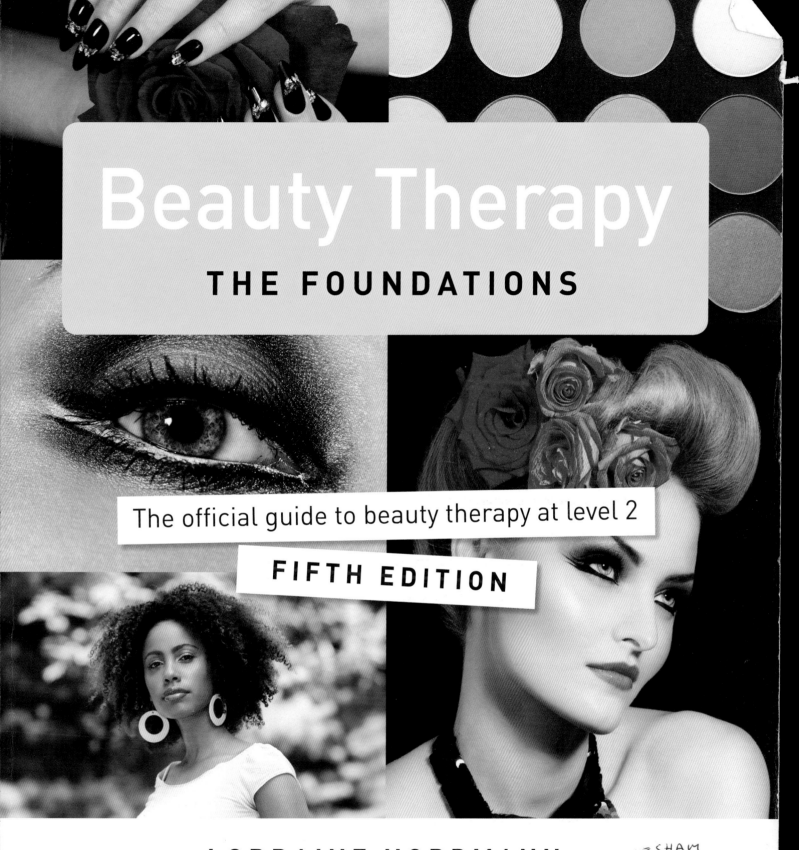

Beauty Therapy

THE FOUNDATIONS

The official guide to beauty therapy at level 2

FIFTH EDITION

LORRAINE NORDMANN

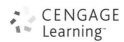

CENGAGE
Learning™

Australia • Brazil • Japan • Korea • Mexico • Singapore • Spain • United Kingdom • United States

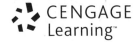

Beauty Therapy – The Foundations
Fifth Edition
Lorraine Nordmann

Publishing Director: Linden Harris

Publisher: Melody Dawes

Development Editor: Lucy Mills

Content Project Editor: Lucy Arthy

Production Controller: Eyvett Davis

Marketing Executive: Lauren Redwood

Typesetter: MPS Limited, A Macmillan Company

Cover design: HCT Creative

Text design: Design Deluxe

For product information and technology assistance,
contact **emea.info@cengage.com**.
For permission to use material from this text or product,
and for permission queries,
email **clsuk.permissions@cengage.com**.

British Library Cataloguing-in-Publication Data
A catalogue record for this book is available from the British Library.

ISBN: 978-1-4080-1936-8

Cengage Learning EMEA
Cheriton House, North Way, Andover, Hampshire SP10 5BE
United Kingdom

Cengage Learning products are represented in Canada by Nelson Education Ltd.

For your lifelong learning solutions, visit **www.cengage.co.uk**

Purchase your next print book, e-book or e-chapter at
www.CengageBrain.co.uk

Printed by Cambrian Printers, Wales
3 4 5 6 7 8 9 10 11 – 12 11 10

Contents

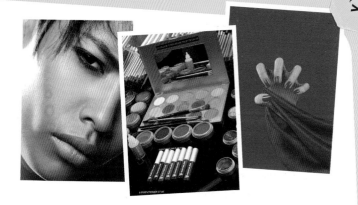

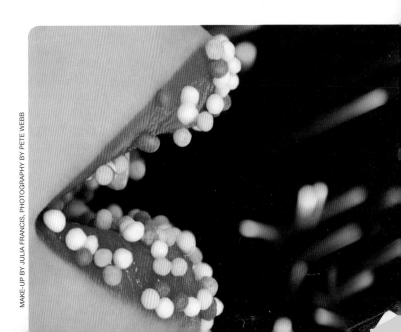

MAKE-UP BY JULIA FRANCIS. PHOTOGRAPHY BY PETE WEBB

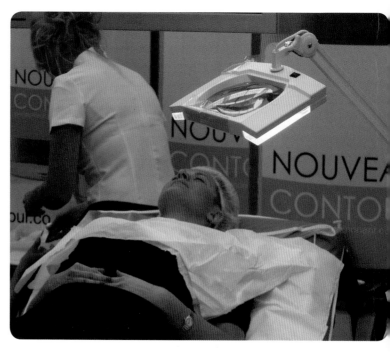

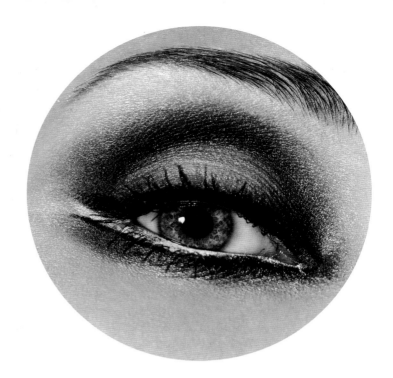

12 Manicure Services (N2) 367

13 Pedicure Services (N3) 407

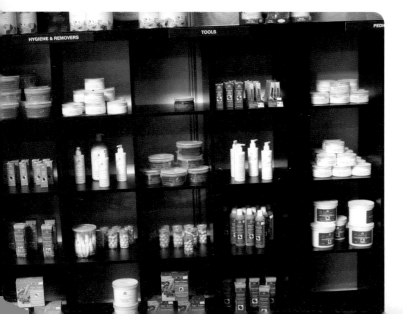

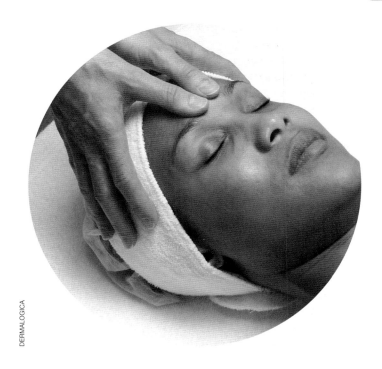

DERMALOGICA

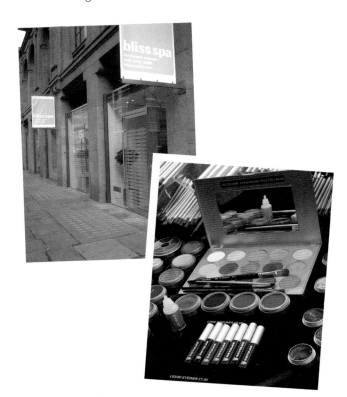

Foreword

I can scarcely believe that it has been 15 years since I wrote the foreword for the second edition of Lorraine Nordmann's excellent book *Beauty Therapy – The Foundations: The Official Guide to Level 2.*

Since then, the beauty industry has gone from strength to strength, advancing in professionalism, technology and capability. The new national occupational standards incorporate all that has been achieved in the industry since the millennium and there have been many exciting changes over this time. I have also seen a real shift in the way that consumers of both genders invest in their appearance and well-being.

UK standards are widely considered the best in the world and I am certain that Lorraine has played a huge role in pushing the development of beauty therapy to the quality we now see. With her dedication, expertise and passion, she has helped to make the industry the success it is today.

If you've never had the opportunity of meeting Lorraine, her passion for the industry and keeping her skills up to date is overwhelming. She is also a good straight talker and knows exactly what is needed from a trainer, college or salon perspective.

The fact that the fifth edition has now been published is testament to the popularity of her books and the depth and knowledge that they provide to year after year of students. Her commitment to the development and introduction of innovative learning support and guidance is clearly reflected in her work.

Without doubt, *Beauty Therapy – The Foundations, Fifth Edition,* is the most informative book to cover the Level 2 Beauty Therapy Standards as laid down by Habia.

Alan Goldsbro
Chief Executive Officer, Habia

About this book

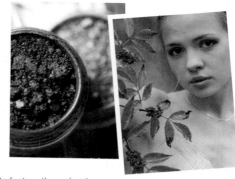

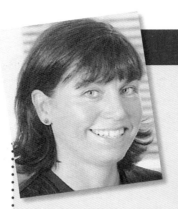

ROLE MODEL

Janice Brown
*Director of HOF Beauty
(House of Famuir Ltd)*

> My career journey has taken me from working in and later managing a group of salons, through, sales, teaching, training, research and development and I am currently director of HOF Beauty Ltd. Along the way I have specialized in electrolysis and hair removal. I am the co-author of *The Encyclopedia of Hair Removal* along with Gill Morris. I am proud to say that I have been able to make a real difference to people's lives by helping to correct skin, body and hair growth issues. I hope I have also been able to inspire and encourage fellow beauty therapists through the training I have provided. In the course of my career I have been fortunate enough to travel the world and work with wonderful people. Beauty therapy for me is not only a career but is a true passion.

Industry Role Models feature throughout the book and are your insight into the exciting beauty industry. Their profile is included at the start of the chapter and they provide subject specific tips that are both practical and inspiring.

ACTIVITY

List some examples of what being courteous means to you, when dealing with a client. Consider the scenarios below and state how you would deal with each in a courteous manner:

- A client arriving at reception when you are already busy with another client
- A client arriving late for a service
- A client receiving a service for the first time

Activity boxes feature within all chapters and provide additional tasks for you to further your understanding.

> Selling is a vital part of the role of a therapist. It is important that the client gets the right service and products in order to get the results they are after. Clients do not buy our services or products, they buy the benefits and results. It is your job to help them imagine how using the products and services will make them look and feel. Remember that we all hate to be sold to but love to buy; so practice and perfect your selling skills.
>
> **Janice Brown**

Role Model quotes are included throughout a number of core chapters. Each quote provides valuable insight into the world of work, providing helpful and practical advice about working in such a varied and innovative industry.

A & P icon

A & P icons highlight essential anatomy and physiology knowledge needed for the unit

Anatomy and physiology essential knowledge for unit

B4	Provide facial skincare treatments
B6	Carry out waxing services
B7	Carry out ear piercing
N2	Provide manicure services
N3	Provide pedicure services
B8	Provide make-up services

BEST PRACTICE

All staff should be aware of any promotions that their business is offering so that they can build on a client's initial interest in a product or service and turn it into a sale.

Best Practice boxes suggest good working practice and help you develop your skills and awareness during your training.

ALWAYS REMEMBER

Psoriasis

With the skin disorder psoriasis, cell division occurs much more quickly, resulting in clusters of dead skin cells appearing on the skin's surface.

Always Remember boxes draw your attention to key information or helpful hints that will help you prepare for assessment.

TOP TIP

Whilst training at your work placements it is vital to improve your confidence and practical skills 'on the job'. This will increase your CV and as a make-up artists help you to build an impressive portfolio.

Top Tips share the author's experience and provide positive suggestions to improve knowledge and skills for each unit.

EQUIPMENT AND MATERIAL LIST

Clean, dampened and clean, dry cotton wool
With sit-up and lie-down positions and an easy-to-clean surface

Cotton wool eye pads (2) pre-shaped, round and dampened

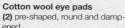

Scissors
To cut cotton wool eye pads (if cotton wool discs are not used)

YOU WILL ALSO NEED:

Disposable tissue roll Such as bedroll

Towels (2) Freshly laundered for each client

Flat mask brushes (3) Disinfected

Trolley To display all facial treatment products to be used in the facial service

Client's record card To record all the details relevant to the client's service

Facial toning lotions (a selection) To suit various types of skin

Equipment Lists help you prepare for each practical treatment and show you the tools, materials and products required.

HEALTH & SAFETY

Skin protection

Although the skin is structured to avoid penetration of harmful substances by absorption, certain chemicals can be absorbed through the skin. Always protect the skin when using potentially harmful substances, and wear gloves when using harsh chemical cleaning agents.

Health & Safety boxes draw your attention to related health and safety information essential for each technical skill.

Sample client record card

Date	Beauty therapist name	
Client name		Date of birth (Identifying client age group)
Home address		Postcode
Landline phone number	Mobile phone number	Email address
Name of doctor	Doctor's address and phone number	
Related medical history (Conditions that may restrict or prohibit service application.)		
Are you taking any medication? (This may affect the condition of the skin or skin sensitivity.)		

Client record cards illustrate what you need to assess and gain from the client at consultation and also provide guidance on information following a treatment.

Step-by-step: Deep cleansing

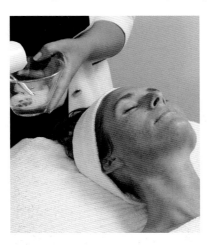

1 Select a cleansing medium to suit your client's skin type. The procedure for application is the same as that for the superficial cleanse.

Step-by-step sequences demonstrate the featured practical skills using colour photographs to enhance your understanding.

ASSESSMENT OF KNOWLEDGE AND UNDERSTANDING

Having covered the learning objectives for **making sure your own actions reduce risks to health and safety**, test what you need to know and understand by answering the following short questions below.

Actions to avoid health and safety risks

1 What are your main legal responsibilities under the Health and Safety at Work Act (1974)?

2 Name four different pieces of legislation relating to health and safety in the workplace.

3 What is the purpose of a salon health and safety policy? What sort of information does it include?

4 What is the importance of personal presentation in respect of your salon workplace policy?

5 Why is your personal conduct important to maintain the health and safety of yourself, colleagues and clients?

6 Why must regular health and safety checks be carried out in the workplace?

Assessment of knowledge and understanding questions are provided at the end of all core chapters. You can use the questions to prepare for oral and written assessments and help test your own knowledge throughout. Seek guidance from your supervisor/assessor if there are areas you are unsure of.

Beauty Therapy
E-Teaching Website

E-Teaching website

A **new E-Teaching website for trainers** accompanies this textbook. This resource includes **handouts, PowerPoint™ slides, interactive assessments, an image bank and videoclips** – all carefully designed to help trainers make classroom delivery more interactive and to provide extra materials for lesson planning.

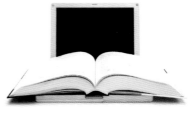

Please visit **www.eteachbeautytherapy.co.uk** for more information or contact your Cengage Learning sales representative at emea.info@cengage.com.

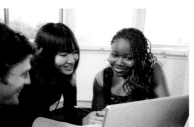

Students! Access your FREE online resources by following the Level 2 student links on **www.eteachbeautytherapy.co.uk** and entering your password 'bronzing'.

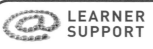

TUTOR SUPPORT

Links to the E-Teach resources are flagged throughout the text. If your trainer subscribes to one E-Teaching website, they will be able to download these and use them in class.

LEARNER SUPPORT

Free online Student Resources are available wherever you see this red symbol.

About the author

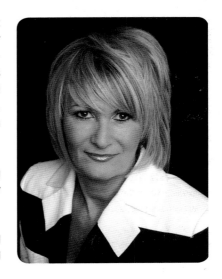

I am proud to have worked in beauty therapy for the past 30 years and am amazed at the technological advances that have been made. The beauty therapy industry is never boring, offers immense job satisfaction, clear progression opportunities and is increasingly diverse allowing you to specialize in what has effectively become micro-industries within what was traditionally termed beauty therapy, i.e. nails, make-up, massage and spa. This allows you to excel in the area of the industry that you feel passionate about, which ultimately raises the profile of our industry. Industry role models feature in each chapter to share their experiences offering practical advice throughout.

The revisions to *Beauty Therapy – The Foundations: Fifth edition* will support you attaining your qualification and develop the skills and attributes needed to meet current industry requirements whichever your training route.

Possibilities are infinite of what can be achieved and the content of the 2010 national occupational standards reflects this – setting the scene for the new decade where we will continue to see exciting developments in this increasingly respected profession.

Enjoy your training and I wish you great success in the industry.

Lorraine Nordmann

About the Contributor

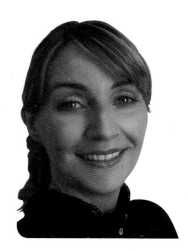

Following a career in nursing I entered the beauty industry in 1995. After many years as a therapist and salon owner I decided to follow my passion for education and began to lecture at a further education college in Surrey.

In the following six years I gained further professional skills and qualifications including writing examination questions for CIBTAC (Confederation of International Beauty Therapy and Cosmetology), achieving the Cert.Ed. teaching qualification and embarking on training to become a beauty therapy Examiner.

I set up my first training company The National School of Threading in 2006 in response to a growing demand for experienced threading teachers and have since performed many demonstrations and exhibitions in London and will be giving a lecture at the World Skills Championships this year.

I have been privileged to work alongside some high profile businesses to provide both training and consultative work including Nails Inc - trade testing, training and launching their 'Get Lashed' brand and GMTTEC Training Education Consultancy.

Since 2007 I have been working closely with the ASA (Asian Style Awards) to assist the regulation of South Asian treatments and training, in particular threading, with a view to raising standards and protect other businesses and our consumers. I was selected to judge at their 2008 awards ceremony in London and will be writing a feature in their trade journal.

More recently I have been working with Habia – the government recognised body which sets the National Occupational Standards for hair and beauty – to develop Threading standards for a new industry qualification in threading which will be introduced in September 2010.

My plan for 2010 is to begin recruiting students at my new school established in September 2009 in Surrey – The Surrey school of Beauty & Complementary Health – and to expand my Threading expertise into Europe where the skill is still relatively unknown.

Lorraine Onorato

Acknowledgements

The author and publishers would like to thank the following:

For providing the cover image:

Make-up by Julia Francis, www.juliafrancis.co.uk and photography by Pete Webb, www.petewebb.com.

For providing pictures for the book:

Absolute Aesthetics www.absoluteaesthetics.co.uk

Alamy

Aquadome Ireland, www.aquadome.ie

Aqua Sana, Centre Parcs www.aquasana.co.uk

Australian Bodycare

Babor

Beauty Express Ltd

Bliss Spa, www.blisslondon.co.uk

Caflon Ltd, www.caflon.com

Caress, www.caressmanufacturing.co.uk,

Corbis

Covermark, Farmeco www.farmeco.com

Daylight Company Ltd

Dermalogica, The International Dermal Institute www.dermalinstitute.co.uk

Dorling Kindersley Ltd

Dr A L Wright

Dr John Gray, *The World of Skincare*

Dr M H Beck

Ellisons

Everlash

Gloss Communications

Gorgeous PR

Guinot

Habia

Health and Safety Executive

Helinova Ltd

House of Famuir, www.hofbeauty.co.uk

Intercontinental Hotel Group, Holiday Inn Hotel, Newton-le-Willows, Spirit Health Club http://www.spirit-fit.com/clubs/haydock

Istock photo

Jane Iredale, www.janeiredaleuk.eu

Jessica Cosmetics, www.jessicacosmetics.co.uk

Korres Natural Products, www.korres.com

Mavala

Mediscan

Moom waxing, www.moom-uk.com

Wellcome Photo Library

Naissance, www.enaissance.co.uk

National Cancer Institute

NHF inspire, photography by Simon Powell

Salon Iris, www.saloniris.co.uk

Simon Jersey Ltd, www.simonjersey.com

Sister PR

Studex UK Ltd, www.studex.com

The Colour Wheel Company www.colourwheelco.com

Thalgo UK Ltd, www.thalgo.com

The Beauty Lounge

The Sanctuary at Covent Garden Ltd, www.thesanctuary.co.uk

Unilever

www.shavata.co.uk

World of Beauty by Katy, Park Road, London

For their help with the photoshoot:

Mike Turner, www.miketurner-photography.co.uk

For their contribution as industry role models:

Jacqui Jefford
Jade Rogers
Janice Brown
Julia Francis
Lorraine Onorato
Pamela Linforth
Ruth Langley
Sally Biles
Sally Penford
Sally-Anne Braithwaite
Shavata Singh
Vicky Kennedy
Wendy Turner

For providing the student case study:

Kaylie Carter

For their help with the review process:

Debbie Le Grave, Newham College London
Joanne Mackinnon, London College of Beauty Therapy
Anita Crosland, Product Manager for Beauty, Nails Services, Spa and Complementary Therapies, City & Guilds

Every effort has been made to trace the copyright holders, but if any have been inadvertently overlooked the publisher will be pleased to make the necessary arrangements at the first opportunity. Please contact the publisher directly.

The author would personally like to thank:

Kathryn Leach
Shane Noden – Personal Trainer, Club Manager for Spirit Health Club, Holiday Inn Hotel, Newton-le-Willows, Spirit Health Club
Clare Kirkman
Christine Berry
Mike Turner – Photographer
Helen Eastwood
Chloe Eastwood
Gemma Hanlon
Vicky Kennedy: salon owner and beauty therapist, New Woman, New Man and Evolve, Westhoughton
Jacqueline Davi

1 Introduction

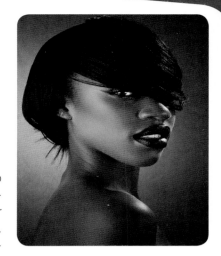

This book covers the practical skills and essential knowledge and understanding required to become a beauty therapist or make-up artist qualified at Diploma Level 2 (S/NVQ), a work-related, competency-based qualification. It may also, however, be used as a reference text for non-S/NVQ qualifications, such as Diploma Level 2 Vocationally Related Qualifications (VRQ). An S/NVQ qualification in beauty therapy or make-up may be attained through different government-approved awarding bodies. Examples are provided below with their website addresses:

- City & Guilds – www.cityandguilds.com
- Edexcel – www.edexcel.com
- ITEC – www.itecworld.co.uk
- VTCT – www.vtct.org.uk

You can also complete CIBTAC and CIDESCO qualifications, which are internationally recognized like City & Guilds.

Each awarding organization is required to cover the same standards, referred to as National Occupational Standards (NOS) in the design of their qualification. The Standards are provided by the government-approved standards setting body for hairdressing, beauty therapy, nails and spa therapy, Habia (Hairdressing and Beauty Therapy Industry Authority). This ensures an employer can be confident of the skills an employee will be able to perform competently in accordance with what S/NVQ level they have achieved, whichever awarding body has accredited it. The certificate you receive when successfully qualified will bear the logo of the awarding body you registered and qualified with, as well as the Habia logo to show it approves it.

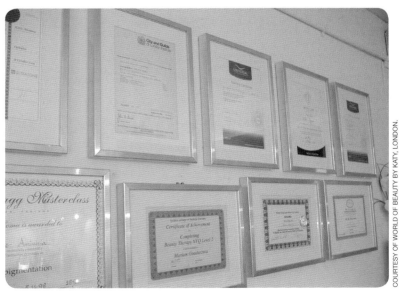

COURTESY OF WORLD OF BEAUTY BY KATY, LONDON.

Beauty therapy qualification certificates

The Habia website provides a list of the qualifications that can be studied on their website www.habia.org.

Your choice of how to study towards your qualification may be either in a college or employed in a beauty therapy or make-up business while training. A list of approved training centres can be found on the Habia website.

NVQs/SVQs

National Vocational Qualifications (NVQs) and Scottish Vocational Qualifications (SVQs) are nationally recognized qualifications with a common structure and design. They follow a similar format for all occupational and vocational sectors. The award of an NVQ/SVQ demonstrates that the person has the competence (sufficient skill and knowledge) to perform job roles/tasks effectively in their occupational area. An NVQ at Level 2 covers a wide range of varied real work activities, some of which are complex and will require you to use your initiative and make decisions.

Each NVQ/SVQ is structured in the same way and is made up of a number of units and outcomes.

A **unit** relates to a specific task or skill area of work. It is the smallest part of a qualification, and carries its own credit value, which you can build up to achieve a qualification.

An **outcome** describes in detail the skill and knowledge components of the unit.

An example of a unit and its outcome from NVQ Level 2 Beauty Therapy (General and Make-up Route) is shown below.

The title of the unit is: **Unit B5 Enhance the appearance of eyebrows and eyelashes.**

The outcomes for the unit detail the practical skills and knowledge requirements essential to provide eyelash and eyebrow services.

The *outcomes* which detail the *unit* components include:

Outcome 3: Shape eyebrows

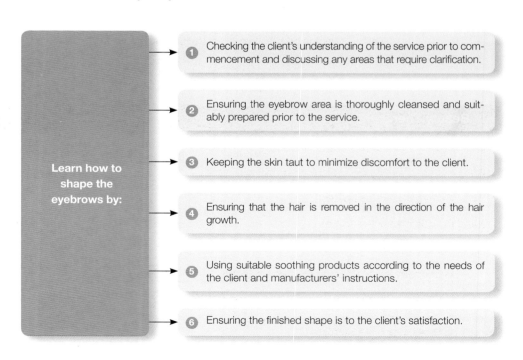

Learn how to shape the eyebrows by:

1. Checking the client's understanding of the service prior to commencement and discussing any areas that require clarification.

2. Ensuring the eyebrow area is thoroughly cleansed and suitably prepared prior to the service.

3. Keeping the skin taut to minimize discomfort to the client.

4. Ensuring that the hair is removed in the direction of the hair growth.

5. Using suitable soothing products according to the needs of the client and manufacturers' instructions.

6. Ensuring the finished shape is to the client's satisfaction.

Units and outcomes

For each unit, when all competence evidence requirements have been achieved, a unit of certification may be awarded, such as Unit B5 Enhance the appearance of eyebrows and eyelashes.

Each NVQ/SVQ qualification is made up of a specific number of units required for the occupational area. Some of the units are termed mandatory (compulsory) and some are termed optional (not compulsory).

Mandatory units must be competently achieved to gain the NVQ/SVQ qualification.

Optional units must be selected to study in addition to the mandatory units to attain the qualification.

The NVQ/SVQ will state the mandatory units required to achieve the qualification plus the number of optional units, which must be completed in order to achieve the full NVQ/SVQ qualification.

The **core mandatory** units are essential units to be achieved. These are as follows:

- G20 Make sure your own actions reduce risks to health and safety
- G8 Develop and maintain your effectiveness at work
- G18 Promote additional services or products to clients

The Level 2 NVQ/SVQ qualifications structure is shown in the following table.

National Occupational Standards: Level 2 Beauty Therapy NVQ/ SVQ Qualification Structure
Candidates will need to achieve the 'core' mandatory units plus the mandatory units from one of the two routes and the specified number of optional units for that route.

'Core' Manadatory Units (all units must be achieved)
G20 Make sure your own actions reduce risks to health and safety (ENTO Unit HSS1)
G18 Promote additional services or products to clients (ICS Unit 10)
G8 Develop and maintain your effectiveness at work

Beauty Therapy General (mandatory units)	Beauty Therapy Make-up (mandatory units)
B4 Provide facial skincare treatments	**B4** Provide facial skincare service
B5 Enhance the appearance of eyebrows and lashes	**B5** Enhance the appearance of eyebrows and lashes
B6 Carry out waxing services	**B8** Provide make-up services
N2 Provide manicure services	**B9** Instruct clients in the use and application of skincare products and make-up
N3 Provide pedicure services	
Plus **one** optional unit (see the following page)	*Plus* **one** optional unit (see the following page)

ENTO   Employment National Training Organisation
ICS   Institute of Customer Services

Optional Units (the relevant number of optional units must be achieved)

G4	Fulfil salon reception duties
B7	Carry out ear piercing
B8	Provide make-up services
B10	Enhance appearance using skin camouflage
S1	Assist with spa operations
B34	Provide threading services

Note: Where units are achieved as mandatory units in either of the two routes, these do not count as optional units as well.

Performance criteria – what you must do

The performance criteria appears as a list of the necessary actions or what you must do to complete a task competently (demonstrating sufficient practical skill, confidence and experience to the assessor).

It is necessary that you are able to meet the expected standard for all the performance criteria listed for each outcome that makes up the unit to be assessed as competent.

Range – what you must cover

Range statements are often identified for each outcome. The assessment range relates to what you must cover and the different conditions under which a skill must be competently demonstrated for the outcome.

For example, for the **range** assessment requirements for Unit B5 Outcome 4, Tint eyebrows and lashes, your performance must cover the following situations:

Range: Your performance must cover the following occasions:	
a	Fair
b	Red
c	Dark
d	White

It is not sufficient to be able to only practically perform the task – you must know and understand why you are doing it, and be able to transfer your knowledge to a variety of situations. This is referred to as your *knowledge and understanding*. Further assessment of your knowledge and understanding of the skill, the knowledge specification, may be assessed through written tests, assignments and oral questioning.

What often occurs is that the same knowledge and understanding may be necessary for similar units. This can be seen, for example, in the knowledge and understanding for **Organizational and Legal Requirements**. This duplication is necessary as some units may be studied and accredited as an individual skill, e.g. Unit B7 Carry out ear piercing.

Where evidence has been achieved, this is cross-referenced (directed) in the portfolio (a place where you store your evidence of competence) to where the evidence can be found.

To achieve unit competence, all performance criteria, range, and knowledge and understanding requirements must have been met and evidence presented as necessary. Evidence is usually provided in your assessment book and portfolio. These may be paper-based or electronic.

Where there is evidence of previous experience and achievement, this may be presented to the assessor for consideration for accreditation. This is called Accreditation of Prior Learning (APL).

Beauty Therapy – The Foundations follows the Beauty Therapy NVQ/SVQ Beauty Therapy General and Beauty Therapy Make-up Level 2 practical and theoretical requirements for both the mandatory and optional units.

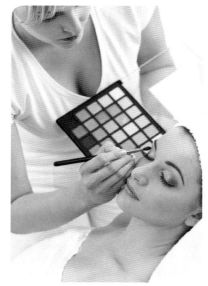

Professional beauty therapist/make-up artist

VRQs

In addition to the NVQ/SVQ termed job-ready qualifications, there has been a review of qualifications to meet the priority for industry. You may be studying towards an Award, Certificate or Diploma Vocational Related Qualification (VRQ) termed preparation for work qualification. *Beauty Therapy – The Foundations* provides essential knowledge and understanding requirements whichever your qualification.

Job-ready (competence based) means that you are ready for work when qualified. All awarding bodies will use the same assessment criteria for job ready qualifications they offer. Preparation for work qualifications provide knowledge, understanding and capability but without the ability to be immediately ready for work.

A successful career in beauty therapy and make-up

To gain employment within the industry, as well as having received the necessary training and qualifications you must also have good employability skills. An employer regards these as being just as important as your qualification.

An employer would expect you to be at all times:

Professional – presenting a consistent good image of yourself and the workplace, completing services to the best of your ability and following all relevant legislation, codes of practice and work-related policies and procedures.

Courteous – clients should be treated with respect in all communication and contact, both verbal and non-verbal and during each stage of service delivery.

ACTIVITY

Why is employee image important to a business?

Give examples of professional best practice in your work role as a Level 2 beauty therapist/ make-up artist

ACTIVITY

List some examples of what being courteous means to you, when dealing with a client. Consider the scenarios below and state how you would deal with each in a courteous manner:

- A client arriving at reception when you are already busy with another client
- A client arriving late for a service
- A client receiving a service for the first time

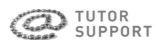

TUTOR SUPPORT

Activity 1: Professional
appearance poster

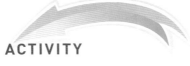

ACTIVITY

Write a list of the personal strengths you feel you have that would make you successful as
a beauty therapist/make-up artist employee.

Write a list of any weaknesses you have e.g. poor punctuality, which need improvement to
improve your personal employability skills?

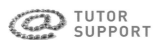

TUTOR SUPPORT

Activity 2: Professional
approach report

ACTIVITY

If a client could not receive a service because she had a skin disorder that could not be
treated, how would you deal with this discreetly?

Discreet – you must be careful and tactful in how you communicate and express yourself
at all times in the working environment. Certain conversation topics may not be suitable
and cause embarrassment. Always 'think before you speak'. Avoid passing on personal
opinions which may cause offence. In compliance with the legislation of the Data Protection Act 1998 never pass on client or staff information unless agreement has been given.

Personable – a successful business requires employees who are personable or pleasant
and have people skills. These would mean having a positive attitude, being able to work
well, co-operate and communicate with others – a team player.

Enthusiastic – employers want employees to have high aspirations and be willing to work
hard to achieve them.

Responsible – your employer will expect you to think carefully when performing any tasks
to avoid unnecessary error. Self discipline is a good attribute to ensure all tasks are completed competently and meet the required deadline.

When you have successfully completed your N/SVQ in Beauty Therapy or Make-up at
Level 2 you can gain employment or progress your training, gaining a further or higher
qualification.

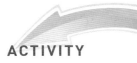

ACTIVITY

List further employability skills
you think are important and
explain why.

Employment opportunities

Beauty Therapy:

- Business owner

- Freelance working for yourself

- Junior therapist in a salon

- Retail in cosmetics and skincare, referred to as a make-up consultant

TOP TIP

While training, completing work placements, voluntary or paid, is vital
to improve your confidence and practical skills 'on the job'. This will increase
your CV and as a make-up artist help you to build an impressive portfolio.

- Specializing in a particular area of beauty therapy such as skincare or waxing hair removal
- Employment in a spa or leisure centre providing beauty therapy services.

Make-up:

- Business owner
- Freelance working for yourself
- Retail in cosmetics and skincare, referred to as a make-up consultant
- Junior make-up artist
- Modelling agency make-up artist
- Make-up promotional work.

Progression opportunities

- Business owner
- Level 3 beauty therapy or make-up
- Other associated industry qualifications in hairdressing, nails, massage or spa
- Further training to gain advanced practical techniques to maintain Continuous Professional Development (CPD). CPD is important to keep yourself up to date and meet the emerging trends of the industry.
- On achievement of Level 3 qualifications you may find employment dependent upon your training route as a:
  - ○ college lecturer and assessor
  - ○ salon trainer and assessor
  - ○ technician for a manufacturer providing training on products, equipment and services
  - ○ salon manager
  - ○ senior therapist or make-up artist
  - ○ sales and marketing manager
  - ○ cruise ship or airline beauty therapist
- Other routes include:
  - ○ working in the media – magazines, advertisements and television
  - ○ specializing in a particular area such as electrology or photographic make-up
  - ○ working as a make-up artist working on film sets, in television studio, theatre, music videos and fashion providing fashion runway make-up

Again when you achieve your Level 3 qualification in beauty therapy or make-up you can continue to update and advance your skills as relevant to your career path/goals.

The following Employability Skills table highlights many of the skills and attributes required to make a successful employee

TOP TIP

Visiting trade shows provide an excellent opportunity to keep up to date with new products, equipment and services as well as subscribing to professional trade magazines.

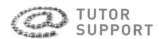

TUTOR SUPPORT

Activity 3: Employability skills and recruitment

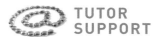

TUTOR SUPPORT

Activity 4: Personal development plan

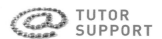

TUTOR SUPPORT

Activity 5: Beauty sector roles research

Employability Skills table, extracted from the Companion Document for the Diploma in Hair and Beauty Studies, and published by Habia

Willingness to learn	Teamwork	Flexible working	Customer care	Positive attitude	Personal and professional ethics	Self management	Creativity	Communica-tion skills	Leadership
Drive and commitment	Respect and consideration for others	Ability to multitask	Tolerant nature	Drive and commitment	Honest	Overcome difficulties and set backs	Innovative	Good social skills	Problem solving
Actively seeks to improve	Adaptability	Adaptability	Respect and consideration for others	Patient	Awareness of Timekeeping	Ability to self-assess	Actively seeks new challenges	Listening skills	Obtaining feedback
Enquiring and curious mind	Empathy towards others		Social sensitivity and awareness	Good sense of humor	Social sensitivity and awareness	Copes with pressure and stress	Ability to inspire others	Verbal communication skills	Giving feedback
Good work ethic	Able to take constructive criticism		Empathy towards others	Overcome difficulties and set backs	Good work ethic	Organised		Non-verbal communication skills	Set objectives
Study skills	Problem solving		Problem solving	Able to take constructive criticism		Sets own standards		Obtaining feedback	Can influence and persuade others
Researching	Giving feedback		Obtaining feedback			Can manage own learning		Giving feedback	Actively seeks new challenges
Actively seeks new challenges	Obtaining feedback		Giving feedback			Prioritising own activities		Network with others	Helps and supports others
Dedication to continued learning	Helps and supports others		Managing conflict			Evalution skills			Willingness to recognise achievements of others
Setting objectives	Works cooperatively with others		Negotiation skills			Monitoring and review of own work			Network with others

Employability Skills table, extracted from the Companion Document for the Diploma in Hair and Beauty Studies, and published by Habia (continued)

Willingness to learn	Teamwork	Flexible working	Customer care	Positive attitude	Personal and professional ethics	Self management	Creativity	Communica-tion skills	Leadership
	Motivating others					Managing time			Ability to inspire others
	Negotiation skills					Planning skills			Dedication to continued learning
						Problem solving			Motivating others
						Obtaining feedback			Team building
						Set objectives			Delegation
						Career management			Thinking strategically
						Managing conflict			Managing conflict
									Negotiation skills
									Analysis finding gaps

STUDENT CASE STUDY

Name: Kaylie Carter

Title of Qualification:
NVQ Level 2 Beauty Therapy, NVQ Level 3 Beauty Therapy
(nearly completed Level 3)

What did you enjoy most about studying, and what did you find most challenging?

I really enjoyed being able to work in the salon environment and study at the same time as it enabled me to gain the experience in a salon and build up my own clientele. Luckily I haven't come across many challenges during my course as I have my co-workers and teachers who are always really helpful, although carrying out new treatments can feel a little awkward at first.

What are your next steps in your career development, and where would you like to see yourself in the future?

I am due to finish my NVQ Level 3 in Beauty Therapy in the next couple of months. Once this has been completed, I look forward to working in the salon and building my skills up further. In the future I would like to speciallize in make-up and dermatology.

Please describe your work experience so far.

When I started my beauty therapy course, I was offered a job at Matisse Beauty Clinic as an apprentice. My job role included cleaning the work areas, setting up treatment rooms for my colleagues, client care and taking telephone bookings. I was very lucky to work at this particular salon as my colleagues always made sure that I was shown the various treatments and techniques to increase my knowledge and help me become a good therapist. I have now worked at Matisse for 3 years and have worked my way up as a beauty therapist, building a substantial clientele along the way. I have also been Clarins-trained in London meaning I get to carry out relaxing Clarins facials along with various other treatments on a day-to-day basis. My job is always interesting as I get to meet new people every day and there are so many treatments to learn.

What is your job role and where do you work?

I work at Matisse Beauty Clinic in Christchurch where I work as a busy beauty therapist. My job role is to have excellent client care and to carry out all the treatments I am qualified to do, in the correct and professional way. We are also encouraged to work as a team to keep the salon tidy and hygienic.

What do you find rewarding about your current job and what do you find challenging about your job?

Some clients who come into the salon just want someone to talk to or they are unconfident. It is so nice when they tell you that you have made them feel so much better and they come in again to see you. I also really enjoy the relationships that build-up between the beauty therapists and the clients as it becomes a really fun environment to work in.

What do you think makes a good beauty therapist?

I think to be good beauty therapist you need to be polite and professional with your clients, and also be able to show empathy where necessary. The hygiene and appearance of the therapist is also extremely important.

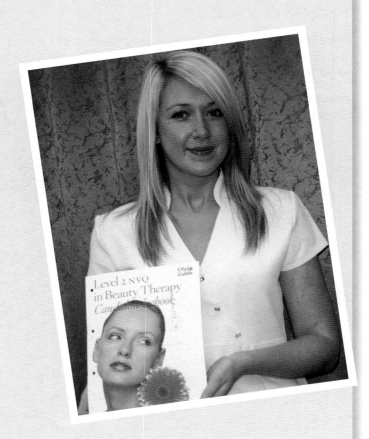

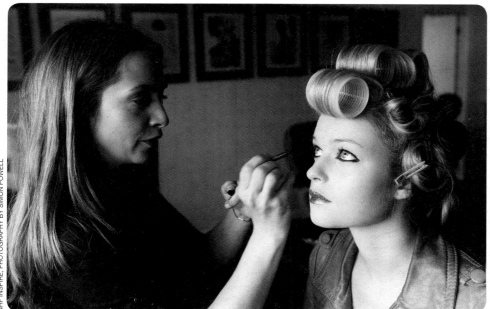

NHF INSPIRE, PHOTOGRAPHY BY SIMON POWELL

Fashion photo shoot

ACTIVITY

Consider what would be your 'dream job'. Using professional journals/magazines or online job advertisements search for a vacancy and obtain a job description so you can see the qualifications, experience and personal attributes that you will need to have. You can then draw up a plan of what you will need to achieve when and how to gain the necessary evidence and experience. This is your career path, the journey required to achieve your career goal.

Industry role models

In the beauty therapy and make-up industry there are many role models who have extensive experience which has helped raise the industry profile, and a passion for their work which is inspirational to our beauty therapists and make-up artists of the future.

Industry role models have contributed 'tips of the trade' in this book sharing their expertise and valued knowledge. These include:

TOP TIP

Beauty therapy is one of the UK's 20 happiest sectors to work in, according to City & Guilds scoring 8 out of 10.

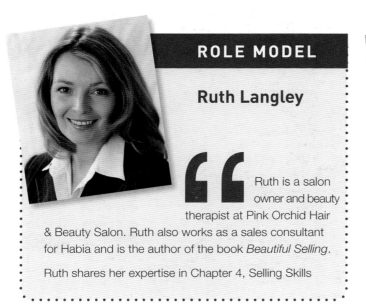

ROLE MODEL

Ruth Langley

Ruth is a salon owner and beauty therapist at Pink Orchid Hair & Beauty Salon. Ruth also works as a sales consultant for Habia and is the author of the book *Beautiful Selling*.

Ruth shares her expertise in Chapter 4, Selling Skills

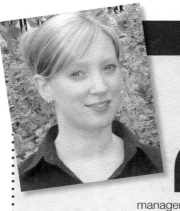

ROLE MODEL

Sally-Anne Braithwaite

Sally-Anne is front of house manager at Oxley's at Ambleside – Blue Fish Spa. Sally-Anne's responsibilities include running reception, meeting and greeting customers, product sales and helping with marketing and accounts.

Sally-Anne shares her expertise in Chapter 6, Salon Reception

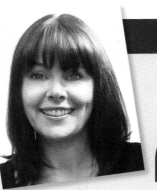

ROLE MODEL

Sally Penford

" As Education Manager for the International Dermal Institute in the United Kingdom, Sally Penford is responsible for training and development of a highly specialized team of lecturers, along with overall operations for the education division in training centres located across the country.

Sally shares her expertise in Chapter 7, Facial Skincare

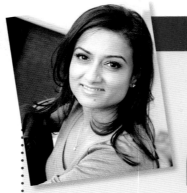

ROLE MODEL

Shavata Singh

" Shavata Singh is Brand Director Shavata UK (encompassing Shavata Brow Studio and LASH LOUNGE by Shavata).

Shavata shares her expertise in Chapter 8, Eyebrows and Eyelashes Services

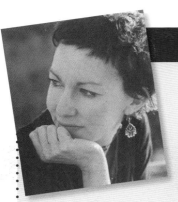

ROLE MODEL

Julia Francis

" Julia is a professional make-up artist and body painter. Julia is also an experienced teacher and make-up consultant and has been conducting workshops for many years.

Julia shares her expertise in Chapter 9, Make-up Services

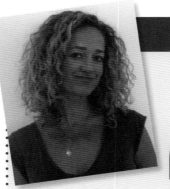

ROLE MODEL

Wendy Turner

" Wendy is a hair and make-up stylist and has worked for a number of professional photographers and best-selling magazines. Wendy is a stylist on television shows and has a number of celebrity clients.

Wendy shares her expertise in Chapter 10, Instruction and Application of Skincare Products and make-up

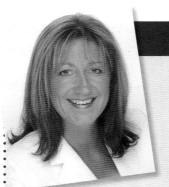

ROLE MODEL

Jacqui Jefford

" Jacqui has been in the nail and beauty industry for over 25 years, and is one of the leading figures in the industry in the UK and internationally. Her work has taken her to many countries as a consultant in education, competitions (winning, designing and judging them), taking educational seminars and working in PR, TV and with the consumer press. Jacqui has her own salon, school and distribution company, and continues to work with many FE colleges as a tutor, assessor and internal verifier. Jacqui has also worked at London and Paris Fashion Weeks as well as decorating the covers of top magazines such as Vogue. Her passion has always been good education and she has worked alongside Habia on many projects over the last ten years. Jacqui is author to four successful books and five DVDs.

Jacqui shares her expertise in Chapter 12, Manicure Services

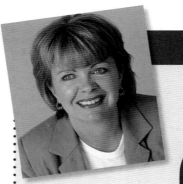

ROLE MODEL

Pamela Linforth

" Pamela's career has moved through working in a salon, electrolysis clinic, spa and into teaching. Pamela has worked in the FE sector and industry and is now Head of Human Resources at Ellisons, suppliers to the professional hair and beauty industry.

Pamela shares her expertise in Chapter 11, Skin Camouflage

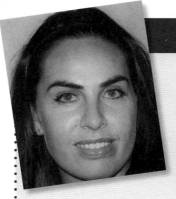

ROLE MODEL

Vicky Kennedy

" Vicky is a paramedical skin practitioner and beauty therapist and has been the principle owner of a very successful beauty therapy salon since 1991.

Vicky shares her expertise in Chapter 13, Pedicure Services

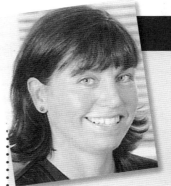

ROLE MODEL

Janice Brown

" Janice is Director of Beauty (House of Famuir Ltd). Her career journey has taken her from working in and later managing a group of salons, through sales, teaching, training, research and development. Janice is the co-author of the *Encyclopaedia of hair removal* along with Gill Morris.

Janice shares her expertise in Chapter 14, Waxing Services

ROLE MODEL

Jade Rogers

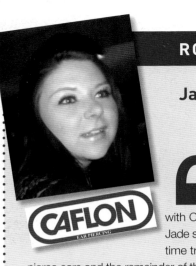

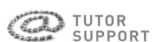

"Jade is a Sales Technician with Caflon Ltd within the UK. Jade spends 70 per cent of her time training people in how to pierce ears and the remainder of the time she visits Caflon customers throughout the UK. Jade's customers come from the world of hair and beauty, others from the medical field and a core of clients from the jewellery industry.

Jade shares her expertise in Chapter 15, Ear-Piercing

ROLE MODEL

Sally Biles

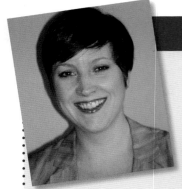

"Sally has worked in the beauty industry for over 18 years. Over the years, Sally has worked as a therapist, spa manager, college lecturer and trainer, gaining experience and knowledge. Sally is currently working at the Sanctuary in Covent Garden and is responsible for training and service development.

Sally shares her expertise in Chapter 16, Spa Operations

TUTOR SUPPORT

Activity 6: Develop a professional CV

ROLE MODEL

Lorraine Onorato

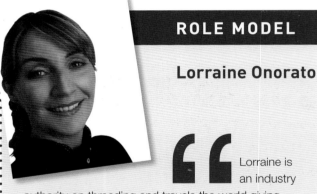

"Lorraine is an industry authority on threading and travels the world giving demonstrations and lectures. As Principal of The Surrey School of Beauty & Complementary Health, Lorraine is working with Habia to develop threading standards for a new industry qualification in threading which will be introduced in September 2010.

Lorraine shares her her expertise in Chapter 17, Threading Services.

On successful completion of your level 2 qualification you will be able to work in a rewarding job full of variety with career possibilities that are endless!

2 Anatomy and Physiology

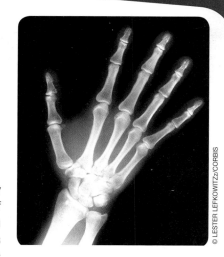

As a beauty therapist it is important that you have a good understanding of anatomy and physiology, as many of your services aim to improve the particular functioning of systems of the body. For example, a facial massage will improve blood and lymph circulation locally as you massage the skin's surface, and increase cellular renewal as you improve nutrition to the living cells, while removing dead skin cells. The result is healthier looking skin.

Anatomy and physiology knowledge and understanding requirements

It is necessary for you to know and understand anatomy and physiology as relevant to each beauty therapy unit. You may be assessed through oral or written questions, or assignments. To guide you in your studies the essential anatomy and physiology you need to know and understand for each unit has been identified with an A & P symbol. Look for the A & P symbol to remind you to check back here for your essential anatomy and physiology knowledge!

Anatomy and physiology essential knowledge for unit	
The beauty therapy units with essential anatomy and physiology knowledge requirements are:	
B4 Provide facial skincare treatment	Chapter 7
B6 Carry out waxing services	Chapter 14
B7 Carry out ear piercing	Chapter 15
N2 Provide manicure services	Chapter 12
N3 Provide pedicure services	Chapter 13
B8 Provide make-up services	Chapter 9
B10 Enhance appearance using skin camouflage	Chapter 11
B34 Provide threading Services	Chapter 17

Anatomy and physiology knowledge and understanding is located in this chapter, but it can also be found within each of the beauty therapy chapters where essential anatomy and physiology knowledge assessment requirements are identified as above.

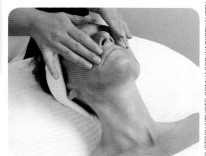

Facial massage being performed

Anatomy and physiology essential knowledge for unit

UNIT	B4	B6	B7	B8	B10	N2	N3	B34
Skin structure and function	✓	✓		✓	✓	✓	✓	✓
Factors affecting skin condition and skin characteristics	✓	✓		✓	✓	✓	✓	✓
Structure of hair and types of hair growth			✓					✓
Hair growth cycle			✓					✓
Nail structure and function						✓	✓	
Nail growth						✓	✓	
Muscle groups in parts of the body, position and action	✓					✓	✓	
Muscle tone	✓							
Bones in parts of the body, position, structure and function	✓					✓	✓	
Composition and function of blood and lymph	✓							
Blood and lymphatic system	✓					✓	✓	
External ear structure (see Chapter 14)			✓					

Anatomical terminology

Anatomical terminology is used to describe the location, function and description of a body part. It is useful to know these terms, as it will assist your anatomy understanding. As you read through this chapter you will notice those terms.

Anterior	Front (usually refers to front of the body)	**Superficial**	Near the surface
Posterior	Back (usually refers to the back of the body)	**Superior**	Above
Proximal	Nearest to	**Inferior**	Below
Medial	Middle	**Plantar**	Front surface
Distal	Furthest away	**Dorsal**	Back surface
Lateral	Side		

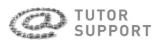

TUTOR SUPPORT

Activity 1: Anatomical terms handout

The skin

The skin varies in appearance according to our race, gender and age. It also alters from season to season and from year to year, and reflects our general health, lifestyle and diet.

The outer layer of the epidermis, the stratum corneum is up to 20 per cent thicker in men than women. Male skin also contains more collagen, a skin protein providing strength. Collagen production in females slows at the menopause which can result in sudden skin ageing. As such, skin ageing appears faster in females than males. Males produce more of the skin's natural oil sebum making it appear oilier and have less sweat glands.

More information on how race, gender and age affects skins appearance can be found in Chapter 7, pages 176–179.

At puberty the chemical substances (**hormones**) that control many of our bodies' activities become very active. Among other effects, this activity causes the skin to become more oily, and often blemishes appear on the skin's surface. Seven out of ten teenagers find that their skin becomes blemished with blackheads (**comedones**), inflamed angry spots (**pustules** and **papules**) and even scars at this time: a skin disorder called **acne vulgaris.**

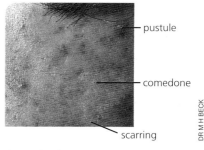

pustule

comedone

scarring

DR M H BECK

Acne vulgaris

During our twenties our skin should look its best; any hormonal imbalance that occurred at puberty should by now have stabilized. As we grow older, the skin ages too. In our late twenties and early thirties we will see fine lines appearing on the skin's surface, especially around the eyes where the skin is thinner and gradually becomes drier as the production of the skin's natural oil, sebum, slows.

At around the age of 40, hormone activity in the body becomes slower and the skin begins to lose its strength and elasticity. The skin becomes increasingly drier, and lines and wrinkles appear on the surface. In our late fifties brown patches of discoloured skin (**lentigines**) may appear: these are commonly seen at the temple region of the face and on the backs of the hands and are caused by ultra-violet light damage.

Fortunately help is at hand to care for the skin: there is an ever-increasing number of skin-care products from a vast and highly profitable cosmetics industry, and there are the skill and expertise of the qualified beauty therapist.

If it is your intention to become a qualified beauty professional, you need to learn about skin types and construction, its function, and how and why skin is changed by both internal and external influences.

Cells

The human body consists of many trillions of microscopic cells. Each cell contains a chemical substance called **protoplasm**, which contains various specialized structures whose activities are essential to our health. If cells are unable to function properly, a disorder results.

Surrounding the cell is the **cell membrane**. This forms a boundary between the cell contents and their environment. The membrane has a porous surface which permits food to enter and waste materials to leave.

In the centre of the cell is the **nucleus**, which contains the **chromosomes**. On these are the genes we have inherited from our parents. The **genes** are ultimately responsible for cell reproduction and cell functioning.

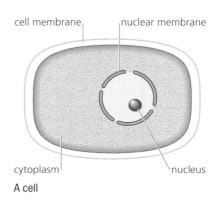

cell membrane

nuclear membrane

cytoplasm

nucleus

A cell

The liquid within the cell membrane and surrounding the nucleus is called **cytoplasm**. Scattered throughout this are other small bodies, the **organelles** or 'little organs'; each has a specific function within the cell.

Cells in the body tend to specialize in carrying out particular functions. Groups of cells which share function, shape, size or structure are called tissues.

Tissues

If the tissues are damaged, for example if the skin is accidentally broken, the tissue cells divide to repair the damage – called **regeneration**. The body is composed of four basic tissues. These are described below.

Types of tissue and general functions

Name of tissue	Examples	General functions
Epithelial	Epidermis outer layer of skin.	Forms surface and linings for protection.
Connective	Dermis layer of skin. Collagen fibres. Bone. Ligaments. Tendons.	A structural tissue that supports, surrounds and connects different parts of the body.
Muscular	Voluntary or skeletal, muscle tissue.	Contracts and shortens producing movement. Skeletal muscle tissue moves the body and maintains posture.
	Involuntary or smooth muscle tissue.	Smooth muscle tissue moves substances through the body.
Nervous	Neurones (nerve cells).	Forms a communication system between different parts of the body, controlling and co-ordinating most body processes.

nucleus   muscle fibres

spindle-shaped cell
nucleus

cells separated from each other

Tissues may be grouped to form the larger functional and structural units we know as **organs**, such as the heart.

Functions of the skin

The human skin is an organ – the largest of the body. It provides a tough, flexible covering, with many different important functions. The main functions are listed below.

Protection

The skin protects the body from potentially harmful substances and conditions.

- The outer surface is **bactericidal**, helping to prevent the multiplication of harmful microorganisms. It also prevents the absorption of many substances (unless the surface is broken), because of the construction of the cells on its outer surface, which form a chemical and physical barrier.

- The skin cushions the underlying structures from physical injury.

- The skin provides a **waterproof coating**. Its natural oil, sebum, prevents the skin from losing vital water, and thus prevents skin dehydration.

- The skin contains a pigment called melanin. This absorbs harmful rays of ultra-violet light.

Heat regulation

Humans maintain a normal body temperature of 36.8–37°C. Body **temperature** is controlled in part by heat loss through the skin and by sweating. If the temperature of the body is increased by 0.25–0.5°C, the sweat glands secrete sweat on to the skin's surface. The body is cooled by the loss of heat used to evaporate the sweat from the skin's surface. If the body becomes too warm there is an increase in blood flow into the blood capillaries in the skin. The blood capillaries widen (dilate) and heat is lost from the skin. Hair limits heat loss from the scalp.

Excretion

Small amounts of certain **waste products**, such as urea, water and salt, are removed from the body in sweat by excretion from sweat glands through the surface of the skin from the skin's pores.

Warning

The skin affords a warning system against outside invasion. **Redness** and **irritation** of the skin indicate that the skin is intolerant to something, either external or internal.

Sensitivity

The skin is a sensory organ and the sensations of **touch, pressure, pain, heat** and **cold** are identified by sensory nerves and receptors in the skin. It also allows us to recognize objects by their feel and shape.

HEALTH & SAFETY

Skin protection
Although the skin is structured to avoid penetration of harmful substances by absorption, certain chemicals can be absorbed through the skin. Always protect the skin when using potentially harmful substances, and wear gloves when using harsh chemical cleaning agents.

TOP TIP

Did you know?
Although the skin has a waterproof property it allows approximately 500ml of water to be lost from the tissues through evaporation every day.

TOP TIP

Functions of the skin
By remembering the word *SHAPES* this will help you remember the functions of the skin:

Sensation
Heat regulation
Absorption
Protection
Excretion
Secretion

HEALTH & SAFETY

If the external temperature becomes low, blood flow nearer the skin's surface is decreased and the blood capillaries narrow (constrict), preventing heat loss and conserving heat.

ALWAYS REMEMBER

The skin's correct functioning is essential to life. It becomes darker to protect against excessive UV exposure but can also produce vitamin D. A fatty substance in the skin is converted to vitamin D with UV light from the sun. This circulates in the blood and with the mineral salts calcium and phosphorus helps the formation and maintenance of the health of the body's bones. Lack of vitamin D can lead to bone softening disease.

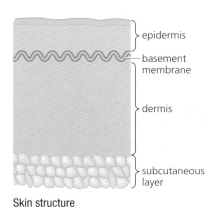

Skin structure

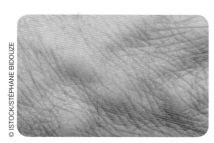

Surface of the skin (epidermis)

© ISTOCK/STÉPHANE BIDOUZE

Nutrition

The skin provides storage for fat, which provides an energy reserve. It is also responsible for producing a significant proportion of our vitamin D, which is created by a chemical reaction when sunlight is in contact with the skin.

Moisture control

The skin controls the movement of moisture from within the deeper layers of the skin.

The structure of the skin

If we looked within the skin using a microscope, we would be able to see two distinct layers: the epidermis and the dermis. Between these layers is a specialized layer which acts like a 'glue', sticking the two layers together: this is the **basement membrane**. If the epidermis and dermis become separated, body fluids fill the space, creating a **blister**.

Situated below the epidermis and dermis is a further layer, the subcutaneous layer or fat layer. The fat layer consists of cells containing fatty deposits, called adipose cells. The thickness of the subcutaneous layer varies according to the body area, and is, for example, very thin around the eyes.

The epidermis

The epidermis is located directly above the dermis. It is composed of five layers, with the surface layer forming the outer skin – what we can see and touch. The main function of the epidermis is to protect the deeper living structures from invasion and harm from the external environment.

There is no blood supply in the epidermis. Nourishment of the epidermis, essential for growth is received from a liquid called the **interstitial fluid** formed from blood plasma. This acts as a link between the blood and cells.

Each layer of the epidermis can be recognized by its shape and by the function of its cells. The main type of cell found in the epidermis is the **keratinocyte**, which produces the protein keratin. It is keratin that makes the skin tough and that reduces the passage of substances into or out of the body.

Over a period of about four weeks, cells move from the bottom layer of the epidermis to the top layer, the skin's surface, changing in shape and structure as they progress. The process of cellular change takes place in stages:

- *The cell is formed* – by division of an earlier cell. This type of cell division is called mitosis.

- *The cell matures* – it changes structure and moves upwards and outwards.

- *The cell dies* – it moves upwards and becomes an empty shell, which is eventually shed.

The layers of the epidermis There are five layers or **strata** that makeup the epidermis. The thickness of these layers varies over the body's surface. Each layer is found either in the germinative zone or keratinization zone. This is illustrated and described below:

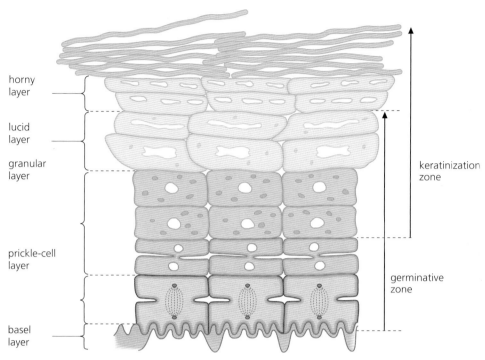

horny layer

lucid layer

granular layer

keratinization zone

prickle-cell layer

germinative zone

basel layer

The layers of the epidermis

ALWAYS REMEMBER

Psoriasis
With the skin disorder psoriasis, cell division occurs much more quickly, resulting in clusters of dead skin cells appearing on the skin's surface.

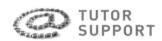

TUTOR SUPPORT

Activity 2: Epidermis label the diagram

The germinative zone In the **germinative zone** the cells of the epidermis layers are living cells. The germinative zone layers of the epidermis are the **stratum germinativum, stratum spinosum** and **stratum granulosum.**

Stratum germinativum The **stratum germinativum**, or **basal layer**, is the lowermost layer of the epidermis. It is formed from a single layer of column-shaped cells joined to the basement membrane. These cells divide continuously and produce new epidermal cells (keratinocytes), a process known as mitosis.

Stratum spinosum The **stratum spinosum**, or **prickle-cell layer**, is formed from two to six rows of elongated cells; these have a surface of spiky spines which connect to surrounding cells. Each cell has a large nucleus and is filled with fluid.

Two other important cells are found in the germinative zone of the epidermis: langerhan cells and melanocyte cells.

ALWAYS REMEMBER

When the epidermis cell dies and is eventually shed from the skin's surface this is termed desquamation by the beauty therapist.

Langerhan cells

Special defence cells absorb and remove foreign bodies that enter the skin. They then move from the epidermis to the dermis below, and finally enter the lymph system (the body's waste-transport system) where the foreign bodies are made safe by neutralizing them.

ALWAYS REMEMBER

Stratum is the Latin word for *layer.*

Melanocyte cells

Produce the skin pigment **melanin**, which contributes to our skin colour. About one in every ten germinative cells is a melanocyte. Melanocytes are stimulated to produce melanin by ultra-violet rays, and their main function is to protect the other epidermal cells in this way from the harmful effects of ultra-violet.

The quantity and distribution of melanocytes differs according to race. In a white Caucasian person the melanin tends to be destroyed when it reaches the granular layer. With stimulation from artificial or natural ultra-violet light, however, melanin will also be present in the upper epidermis.

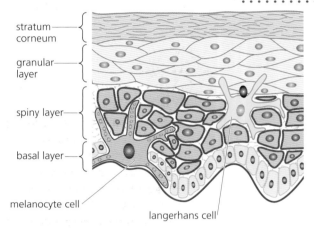

stratum corneum
granular layer
spiny layer
basal layer
melanocyte cell
langerhans cell

Melanocyte and langerhan cells in the skin

In contrast a black skin has melanin present in larger quantities throughout *all* the epidermal layers, a level of protection that has evolved to deal with bright ultra-violet light. This increased protection allows less ultra-violet to penetrate the dermis below, reducing the possibility of premature ageing from exposure to ultra-violet light. The more even quality and distribution of melanin also means that people with dark skins are less at risk of developing skin cancer.

Another pigment, **carotene**, which is yellowish, also occurs in epidermal cells. Its contribution to skin colour lessens in importance as the amount of melanin in the skin increases.

Skin colour also increases when the skin becomes warm. This is because the **blood capillaries** at the surface dilate, bringing blood nearer to the surface so that heat can be lost – this is called vaso-dilation. If the temperature is cold the blood capillaries become narrower so less blood is brought to the skin's surface to conserve heat – this is called vaso-constriction and the skin will lose colour.

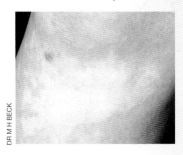
Stratum granulosum

The **stratum granulosum**, or **granular layer**, is composed of one, two or three layers of cells that have become much flatter. The nucleus of the cell has begun to break up, creating what appear to be granules within the cell cytoplasm. These are known as **keratohyaline granules** and later form keratin. At this stage the cells form a new, combined layer.

The keratinization zone
The **keratinization zone**, or **cornified zone**, is where the cells begin to die and where finally they will be shed from the skin. The cells at this stage become progressively flatter, and the cell cytoplasm is replaced with the hard protein keratin.

Stratum lucidum

The **stratum lucidum**, **clear layer** or **lucid layer**, is only seen in non-hairy areas of the skin such as the palms of the hands and the soles of the feet. The cells here lack a nucleus and are filled with a clear substance called eledin produced at a further stage of keratinization.

Stratum corneum

The **stratum corneum**, **cornified** or **horny layer**, is formed from several layers of flattened, scale-like overlapping cells, composed mainly of keratin. These help to reflect ultra-violet light from the skin's surface; black skin, which evolved to withstand strong ultra-violet, has a thicker stratum corneum than does Caucasian skin.

It takes about three weeks for the epidermal cells to reach the stratum corneum from the stratum germinativum. The cells are then shed, a process called **desquamation**.

The dermis

The dermis is the inner portion of the skin, situated underneath the epidermis and composed of dense **connective tissue** containing other structures such as the lymphatic system, blood vessels and nerves. It is much thicker than the epidermis.

HEALTH & SAFETY

Sunburn

If the skin becomes red on exposure to sunlight, this indicates that the skin has been over-exposed to ultra-violet. It will often blister and shed itself. A harmful effect of UVL.

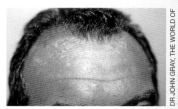

DR JOHN GRAY, THE WORLD OF SKINCARE

TOP TIP

Calluses

The skin will become much thicker in response to friction. A client with a manual occupation may therefore develop hard skin (calluses) on their hands. The skin condition can be treated with an emollient preparation, which will moisturise and soften the dry skin.

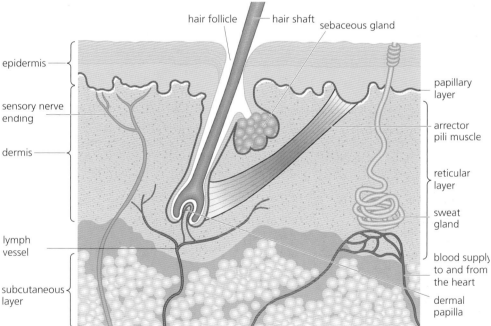

The skin

Labels: epidermis, sensory nerve ending, dermis, lymph vessel, subcutaneous layer, hair follicle, hair shaft, sebaceous gland, papillary layer, arrector pili muscle, reticular layer, sweat gland, blood supply to and from the heart, dermal papilla

TUTOR SUPPORT

Activity 3: Label cross section of the skin

TOP TIP

The formation of the papillae ridges in the dermis are unique to each individual, and this provides our fingerprint.

The papillary layer Near the surface of the dermis are tiny projections called **papillae**; these contain both nerve endings and blood capillaries. This part of the dermis is known as the **papillary layer**, and it also supplies the upper epidermis with its nutrition.

The reticular layer The dermis contains a dense network of protein fibres called the reticular layer. These fibres allow the skin to expand, to contract, and to perform intricate, supple movements.

HEALTH & SAFETY

Sunbathing

When sunbathing, always protect the skin with an appropriate protective sunscreen product, and always use an emollient aftersun preparation to minimize the cumulative effects of premature ageing, by rehydrating and soothing the skin.

ALWAYS REMEMBER

Sensory nerve endings

Sensory nerve endings are most numerous in sensitive parts of the skin, such as the finger tips and the lips.

This network is composed of two sorts of protein fibre: yellow **elastin** fibres and white **collagen** fibres. Elastin fibres give the skin its elasticity, and collagen fibres give it its strength. The fibres are produced by specialized cells called **fibroblasts**, and are held in a gel called the **ground substance**.

While this network is strong, the skin will appear youthful and firm. As the fibres harden and fragment, however, the network begins to collapse, losing its elasticity. The skin then begins to show visible signs of ageing.

A major cause of damage to this network is unprotected exposure of the skin to ultra-violet light and to weather. Sometimes, too, the skin loses its elasticity because of a sudden increase in body weight, for example at puberty or pregnancy. This results in the appearance of **stretch marks**, streaks of thin skin are a different colour from the surrounding skin: on white skin they appear as thin reddish streaks; on black skin they appear slightly lighter than the surrounding skin. The lost elasticity cannot be restored. Cosmetic services can be applied to improve their appearance.

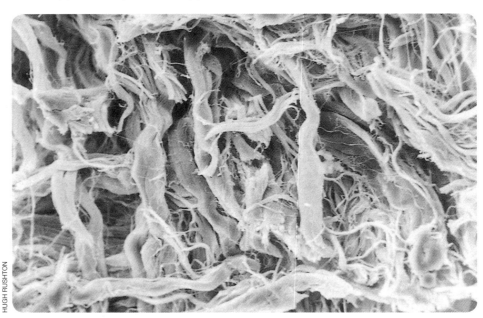

HUGH RUSHTON

Collagen and elastin fibres in the dermis

Nerve endings The dermis contains different types of sensory nerve endings, which register the sensations of touch, pressure, pain and temperature. These send messages to the central nervous system and the brain, informing us about the outside world and what is happening on the skin's surface. The appearance of each of these nerve endings is quite varied. The sensory nerve endings in the skin cause us to have a reflex action to unpleasant stimuli protecting the skin from injury.

Growth and repair The body's blood system of arteries and veins continually brings blood to the capillary networks in the skin and takes it away again. The blood carries the nutrients and oxygen essential for the skin's health, maintenance and growth, and takes away waste products.

Defence Within the dermis are the structures responsible for protecting the skin from harmful foreign bodies and irritants.

One set of cells, the **mast cells**, burst when stimulated during inflammation or allergic reactions, and release a chemical substance called **histamine**. This causes the blood

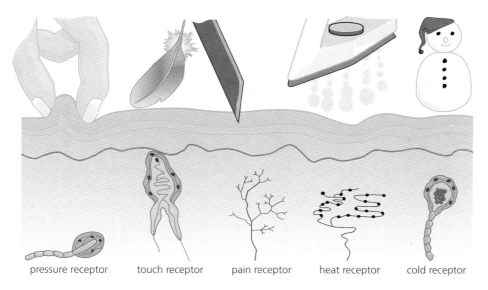

pressure receptor touch receptor pain receptor heat receptor cold receptor

Sensory nerves

vessels nearby to enlarge, thereby bringing more blood to the site of the irritation to limit skin damage and begin repair.

In the blood, and also in the lymph and the connective tissue, are another group of cells: the **macrophages** or 'big eaters'. These destroy microorganisms and engulf dead cells and other unwanted particles. When necessary, they travel to an area where they are needed, for example, the site of an infection. They form a role in the immune system that protects the body from disease-causing microorganisms.

Collecting Waste Lymph vessels in the skin carry a fluid called **lymph**, a straw-coloured fluid similar in composition to blood plasma. Plasma is the liquid part of the blood that disperses from the blood capillaries into the tissue spaces. Lymph is composed of water, lymphocytes (a type of white blood cell that plays a key role in the immune system), oxygen, nutrients, hormones, salts and waste products. The waste products are eliminated and usable protein is recycled for further use by the body. It acts as a link between the blood and the cells.

Control of skin functioning **Hormones** are chemical messengers transported in the blood. They control the activity of many organs in the body, including the cells and glands in the skin. These include **melanosomes**, which produce skin pigment, and the sweat glands and sebaceous glands.

Hormone imbalance at different times of our life may disturb the normal functioning of these cells and structures, causing various **skin disorders**.

Skin appendages Within the dermis are structures called skin appendages. These include:

- sweat glands
- sebaceous glands
- hair follicles, which produce **hair**
- nails

HEALTH & SAFETY

Moisture balance
Excessive sweating, which can occur through exposure to high temperatures or during illness, can lead to *skin dehydration* – insufficient water content. Fluid intake must be increased to rebalance the body fluids.

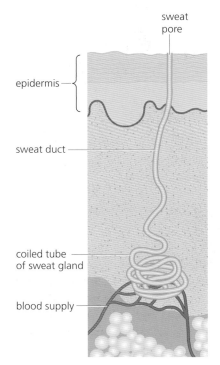

An eccrine sweat gland

labels:
- sweat pore
- epidermis
- sweat duct
- coiled tube of sweat gland
- blood supply

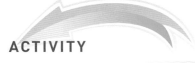

ACTIVITY

Preventing body odour
Produce a checklist that should be followed daily to reduce the possibility of body odour.

Sweat glands

Sweat glands or **sudoriferous glands** are composed of **epithelial tissue**, a specialized lining tissue which extends from the epidermis into the dermis. These glands are found all over the body, but are particularly abundant on the palms of the hands and the soles of the feet. Their function is to regulate body temperature through the evaporation of sweat from the surface of the skin. Fluid loss and control of body temperature are important to prevent the body overheating, especially in hot, humid climates. For this reason, perhaps, sweat glands are larger and more abundant in black skins than white skins.

There are two types of sweat glands: *eccrine glands* and *apocrine glands*. **Eccrine glands** are simple sweat-producing glands, found over most of the body, appearing as tiny tubes (**ducts**). The eccrine glands are responsive to heat. They are straight in the epidermis, and coiled in the dermis. The duct opens directly onto the surface of the skin through an opening called a **pore**.

Eccrine glands continuously secrete small amounts of sweat, even when we appear not to be perspiring. In this way they maintain the body temperature at a constant 36.8–37°C.

Apocrine glands are found in the underarm, the nipples and the groin area. This kind of gland is larger than the eccrine gland, and is attached to a hair follicle. Apocrine glands are controlled by hormones, becoming active at puberty. They also increase in activity when we are excited, nervous or stressed. The fluid they secrete is thicker than that from the eccrine glands, and may contain urea, fats, sugars and small amounts of protein. Also present are traces of aromatic molecules called **pheromones**, which are thought to cause sexual attraction between individuals.

An unpleasant smell – **body odour** – develops when apocrine sweat is broken down by skin bacteria. Good habits of personal hygiene will prevent this.

Cosmetic perspiration control

To extend hygiene protection during the day, apply either a deodorant or an antiperspirant. **Antiperspirants** reduce the amount of sweat that reaches the skin's surface: they have an astringent action which closes the pores. **Deodorants** contain an active antiseptic ingredient which reduces the skin's bacterial activity, thereby reducing the risk of odour from stale sweat.

Sebaceous glands

The **sebaceous gland** appears as a minute sac-like organ. Usually it is associated with the hair follicle with which it forms the **pilosebaceous unit,** but the two can appear independently.

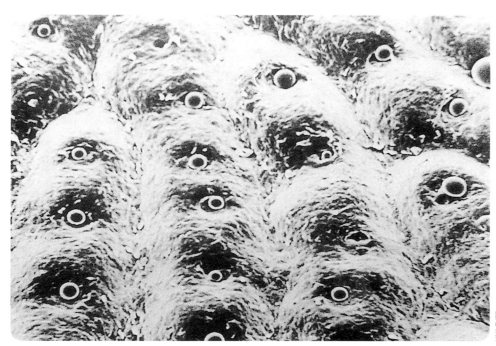

Sweat pores on the skin's surface

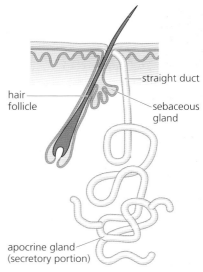

straight duct

hair follicle

sebaceous gland

apocrine gland (secretory portion)

Apocrine gland

UNILEVER

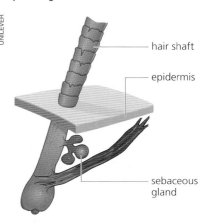

hair shaft

epidermis

sebaceous gland

Sebaceous gland

HEALTH & SAFETY

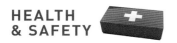

Antiperspirants

The active ingredient in most antiperspirant products is aluminium chlorohydrate. This is known to cause contact dermatitis in some people, especially if the skin has been damaged by recent removal of unwanted hair. Bear this in mind if you are performing an under arm depilatory wax service. (See the aftercare instructions, pages 463–464.)

Sebaceous glands are found all over the body, except on the palms of the hands and the soles of the feet. They are particularly numerous on the scalp, the forehead, and in the back and chest region. The cells of the glands decompose, producing the skin's natural oil, **sebum**. This empties directly into the hair follicle.

The activity of the sebaceous gland increases at puberty, when stimulated by the male hormone **androgen**. In adults, activity of the sebaceous gland gradually decreases again. Men secrete slightly more sebum than women; and on black skin the sebaceous glands are larger and more numerous than on white skin.

TOP TIP

Moisturisers
Cosmetic moisturisers mimic sebum in providing an oily covering for the skin's surface to reduce moisture loss.

HEALTH & SAFETY

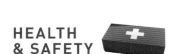

Skin problems are common at puberty when changes in hormone levels cause sebaceous glands to produce excess sebum and the skin's surface becomes oily. Growth of skin bacteria can increase in the sebum causing inflammation of the surrounding tissues. This can lead to the skin disorder acne vulgaris see page 15. The skin should always be kept clean and handled with clean hands.

HEALTH & SAFETY

The lips

Sebaceous glands are not present on the surface of the lips. For this reason the lips should be protected with a lip emollient preparation to prevent them from becoming dry and chapped.

HEALTH & SAFETY

Using alkaline products

Because the skin has an acid pH, if alkaline products are used on it the acid mantle will be disturbed. It will take several hours for this protective film to be restored; during this time, the skin will be irritated and sensitive.

Sebum is composed of fatty acids and waxes. These have **bactericidal** and **fungicidal** properties, and so discourage the multiplication of microorganisms on the surface of the skin. Sebum also reduces the evaporation of moisture from the skin, and so prevents the skin from drying out.

Acid mantle Sweat and sebum combine on the skin's surface, creating an acid film. This is known as the **acid mantle** and discourages the growth of bacteria and fungi.

Acidity and alkalinity are measured by a number called the pH. An *acidic solution* has a pH of 0–6.9; a *neutral solution* has a pH of 7; and an *alkaline solution* has a pH of 7.1–14. The acid mantle of the skin has a pH of 5.5–5.6.

Subcutaneous layer Beneath the dermis lies the subcutaneous layer made up of adipose (fat) tissue. It is supplied with a network of arteries that run parallel to the skin's surface. Fat cells are called adipocytes and contain droplets of fat.

The fatty layer has a protective function and:

- acts as an insulator to conserve body heat

- cushions muscles and bones below from injury

- acts as an energy source, as excess fat is stored in this layer.

TOP TIP

Liposuction

Liposuction is a cosmetic surgery service that involves the removal of fat cells by suction from any area of the body. Tiny incisions are made where the fat removal is required. Fat is then removed through a hollow surgical tube. The tube is moved around in the skin, breaking up the fat, which is then sucked out.

A new service uses ultrasound waves applied to the skin's surface to liquefy fat. The fat is then naturally excreted from the body.

The hair

The structure and function of hair and the surrounding tissues

A hair is a long, slender structure which grows out of, and is part of, the skin. Each hair is made up of dead skin cells, which contain the protein called keratin. Hairs cover the whole body, except for the palms of the hands, the soles of the feet, the lips, and parts of the sex organs.

Hair has many functions:

- *scalp hair* insulates the head against cold, protects it from the sun, and cushions it against bumps

- *eyebrows* cushion the brow bone from bumps, and prevent sweat from running into the eyes

- *eyelashes* help to prevent foreign particles entering the eyes

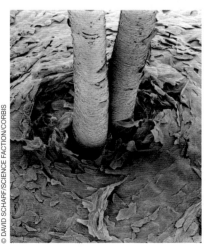

Hair extending from the scalp

- *nostril hair* traps dust particles inhaled with the air

- *ear hair* helps to protect the ear canal

- *body hair* helps to provide an insulating cover (though this function is almost obsolete in humans), has a valuable sensory function, and is linked with the secretion of sebum onto the surface of the skin.

Hair also plays a role in social communication.

The structure of hair

Most **hairs** are made up of three layers of different types of epithelial cells: the *medulla*, the *cortex* and the *cuticle*.

The **medulla** is the central core of the hair. The cells of the medulla contain soft keratin, and sometimes some pigment granules. The medulla only exists in medium to coarser hair – there is usually no medulla in thinner hair.

The **cortex** is the thickest layer of the hair, and is made up of several layers of closely packed, elongated cells. These contain pigment granules and hard keratin.

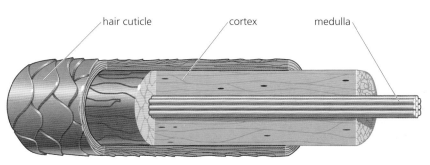

Cross-section of the hair

It is the **pigment** in the cortex that gives hair its colour. When this pigment is no longer made, the hair appears white. As the proportion of white hairs rises, the hair seems to go 'grey'; in fact, however, each individual hair is either coloured as before, or white.

The **cuticle** is the protective outer layer of the hair, and is composed of a layer of thin, unpigmented, flat, scale-like cells. These contain hard keratin, and overlap each other from the base to the tip of the hair.

The parts of the hair and related skin

Each **hair** is recognized by three parts: the **root**, the **bulb** and the **shaft**:

- the **root** is the part of the hair that is in the follicle

- the **bulb** is the enlarged base of the root

- the **shaft** is the part of the hair that can be seen above the skin's surface

Each hair grows out of a tube-like indentation in the epidermis, the **hair follicle**. The walls of the follicle are a continuation of the epidermal layer of the skin.

The **arrector pili muscle** is attached at an angle to the base of the follicle. Cold, aggression or fright stimulates this muscle to contract, pulling the follicle and the hair upright.

TOP TIP

Did you know?
There are approximately 100 000 hairs on the scalp.

TOP TIP

Did you know?
A strand of hair is stronger than an equivalent strand of nylon or copper.

ACTIVITY

The function of hair
Humans are not very hairy but their hairs sometimes stand on end! How does the appearance of skin change? What is the purpose of hair standing on end?

TOP TIP

Eyelash perm lotion and the eyelash/eyebrow tint mixed with hydrogen peroxide swell and penetrate the cuticle so that the products can enter the cortex. The coarser the hair the more resistant it is! Eyelash and eyebrow tints and perming make the permanent chemical changes to the hair's natural appearance in the cortex.

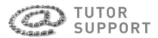

TUTOR SUPPORT

Activity 4: Label the hair follicle

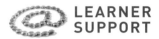

LEARNER SUPPORT

Label the hair follicle

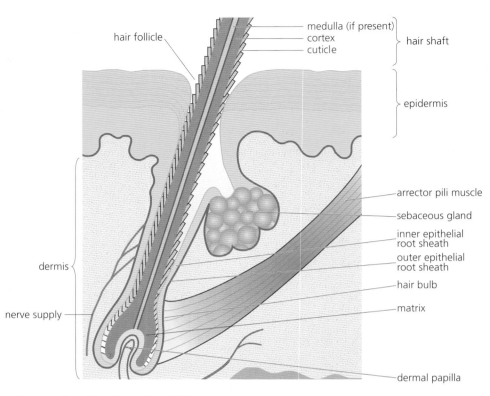

Cross-section of the skin and hair follicle

The **sebaceous gland** is attached to the upper part of the follicle; from it, a duct enters directly into the hair follicle. The gland produces an oily substance, **sebum**, which is secreted into the follicle. Sebum waterproofs, lubricates and softens the hair and the surface of the skin; it also protects the skin against bacterial and fungal infections. The contraction of the arrector pili muscle aids the secretion of sebum.

The dermal papilla, a connective tissue sheath, is surrounded by the hair bulb. It has an excellent blood supply, necessary for the growth of the hair. It is not itself part of the follicle, but a separate tiny organ which serves the follicle.

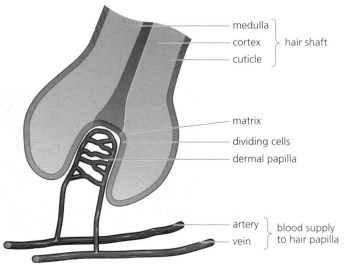

The hair bulb

The **bulb** is the expanded base of the hair root. A gap at the base leads to a cavity inside, which houses the papilla. The bulb contains in its lower part the dividing cells that create the hair. The hair continues to develop as it passes through the regions of the upper bulb and the root.

The **matrix** is the name given to the lower part of the bulb, which comprises actively dividing cells from which the hair is formed.

The hair follicle The hair follicle extends into the dermis, and is made up of three sheaths: the *inner epithelial root sheath*, the *outer epithelial root sheath* and the surrounding *connective-tissue sheath*.

The **inner epithelial root sheath** grows from the bottom of the follicle at the papilla; both the hair and the inner root sheath grow upwards together. The inner surface of this sheath is covered with cuticle cells, in the same way as the outer surface of the hair: these cells lock together, anchoring the hair firmly in place. The inner root sheath ceases to grow when level with the sebaceous gland.

The **outer epithelial root sheath** forms the follicle wall. This does not grow up with the hair, but is stationary. It is a continuation of the growing layer of the epidermis of the skin.

The **connective-tissue sheath** surrounds both the follicle and the sebaceous gland, providing both a sensory supply and a blood supply. The connective-tissue sheath includes, and is a continuation of, the papilla.

The *shape* of the hairs is determined by the shape of the hair follicle – an angled or bent follicle will produce an oval or flat hair, whereas a straight follicle will produce a round hair. Flat hairs are curly, oval hairs are wavy, and round hairs are straight. As a general rule, during waxing curly hairs break off more easily than straight hairs.

TOP TIP

Broken hairs

When hairs break off due to incorrect waxing technique, they will break at the level at which they are locked into the follicle by the cells of the inner root sheath.

TOP TIP

An angled follicle may cause the hair to be broken off at the angle during waxing, instead of being completely pulled out with its root. If this happens, broken hairs will appear at the skin's surface within a few days.

By causing damage to the follicle and changing its shape, waxing can cause the regrowth of hairs to be frizzy or curled where previously the hairs have been straight.

Curly	Wavy	Straight
Flat ribbon-like	Less oval	Round

Hair shapes

The nerve supply The number, size and type of nerve endings associated with hair follicles is related to the size and type of follicle. The follicles of vellus hairs (see page 32) have the fewest nerve endings; those of terminal hairs have the most.

The nerve endings surrounding hair follicles respond mainly to rapid movements when the hair is moved. Nerve endings that respond to touch can also be found around the surface openings of some hair follicles, as well as just below the epidermis.

The three types of hair

There are three main types of hair: *lanugo*, *vellus* and *terminal*.

Lanugo hairs are found on the body prior to birth. They are fine and soft, do not have a medulla, and are often unpigmented. They grow from around the third to the fifth month of pregnancy, and are shed to be replaced by the secondary vellus hairs around the seventh to the eighth month of pregnancy. Lanugo hairs on the scalp, eyebrows and eyelashes are replaced by terminal hairs.

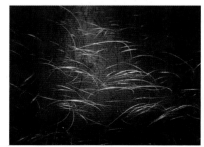

© NEVIT DILMAN

lanugo hairs

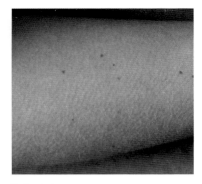

Vellus hairs

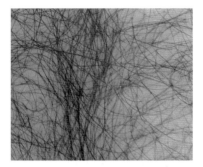

Terminal hairs

Vellus hairs are fine, downy and soft, and are found on the face and body. They are often unpigmented, rarely longer than 20mm, and do not have a medulla or a well-formed bulb. The base of these hairs is very close to the skin's surface. If stimulated, the shallow follicle of a vellus hair can grow downwards and become a follicle that produces terminal hairs.

Terminal hairs are longer and coarser than vellus hairs, and most are pigmented. They vary greatly in shape, in diameter and length, and in colour and texture. The follicles from which they grow are set deeply in the dermis and have well-defined bulbs. Terminal hair is the coarse hair of the scalp, eyebrows, eyelashes, pubic and underarm regions. It is also present on the face, chest and sometimes the back of males.

ALWAYS REMEMBER

Waxing terminal hair

Some areas of the body – for example, the bikini line and underarm areas – often have terminal hairs with very deep follicles. When these hairs are removed, the resulting tissue damage may cause minor bleeding from the entrance of the follicle. Removal of these deep-seated hairs is obviously more uncomfortable than the removal of shallower hairs.

Hair growth

All hair has a **cyclical pattern of growth**, which can be divided into three phases: *anagen, catagen and telogen.*

Anagen is the actively growing stage of the hair – the follicle has re-formed; the hair bulb is developing, surrounding the life-giving dermal papilla; and a new hair forms, growing from the matrix in the bulb.

Catagen is the changing stage when the hair separates from the papilla. Over a few days it is carried by the movement of the inner root sheath, up the follicle to the base of the sebaceous gland. Here it stays until it either falls out or is pushed out by a new hair growing up behind it.

This stage can be very rapid, with a new hair growing straight away; or slower, with the papilla and the follicle below the sebaceous gland degenerating and entering a resting stage, telogen.

Telogen is a resting stage. Many hair follicles do not undergo this stage, but start to produce a new hair immediately. During resting phases, hairs may still be loosely inserted in the shallow follicles.

TOP TIP

Vellus hairs

Vellus hairs grow slowly and take two to three months to return after waxing. They can remain dormant in the follicle for six to eight months before shedding.

TOP TIP

A hair pulled out at the anagen stage will be surrounded by the inner and outer root sheaths and have a properly formed bulb.

TOP TIP

A hair pulled out at the catagen or telogen stage can be recognized by the brush-like appearance of the root.

TOP TIP

Because of the cyclical nature of hair growth, the follicles are always at different stages of their growth cycle. When the hair is removed, therefore, the hair will not all grow back at the same time. For this reason, waxing or threading can appear to reduce the quantity of hair growth. This is not so; given time, all the hair would regrow. Waxing and threading are classed as a temporary means of hair removal.

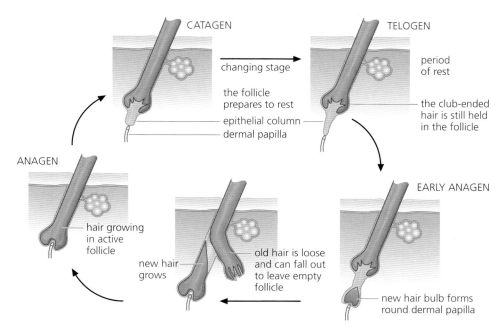

CATAGEN

TELOGEN

changing stage

the follicle
prepares to rest

period
of rest

the club-ended
hair is still held
in the follicle

epithelial column
dermal papilla

ANAGEN

EARLY ANAGEN

hair growing
in active
follicle

new hair
grows

old hair is loose
and can fall out
to leave empty
follicle

new hair bulb forms
round dermal papilla

The hair growth cycle

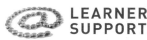

**LEARNER
SUPPORT**

Skin and hair true or false?

Speed of growth The anagen, catagen and telogen stages last for different lengths of time in different hair types and in different parts of the body:

- *scalp hair* grows for two to seven years, and has a resting stage of three to four months

- *eyebrow hair* grows for one to two months, and has a resting stage of three to four months

- *eyelashes* grow for three to six weeks, and have a resting stage of three to four months.

After a waxing service, body hair will take approximately six to eight weeks to return.

Because hair growth cycles are not all in synchronization, we always have hair present at any given time. On the scalp, at any one time for example, 85 per cent of hairs may be in the anagen phase. This is why hair growth after waxing starts within a few days: what is seen is the appearance of hairs that were already developing in the follicle at the time of waxing.

**TOP
TIP**
**Male facial hair grows
at a rate of approximately
10mm a month.**

Types of hair growth **Hirsutism** is a term used to describe a pattern of hair growth that is abnormal for that person's sex, such as when a woman's hair growth follows a man's hair-growth pattern. The hair growth is usually terminal when it should be of a vellus type.

Hypertrichosis is an abnormal growth of excess hair for a person's sex, age and race. It is usually due to abnormal conditions brought about by disease or injury.

Superfluous hair (excess hair) is perfectly normal at certain periods in a woman's life, such as during puberty or pregnancy. Terminal hairs formed at these times usually disappear once the normal hormonal balance has returned. Those newly formed during the menopause are often permanent unless treated with a permanent method of hair removal, such as electrical epilation or laser service.

ALWAYS REMEMBER

Alopecia
This is often caused by a nervous disorder and is where there are round patches of smooth scalp as the hair follicles are not producing new hairs.

HEALTH & SAFETY

African-Caribbean clients
The body hair of African-Caribbean clients is prone to breaking during waxing, and to ingrowing after waxing. Skin damage can result in the loss of pigmentation (hypopigmentation).

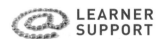

LEARNER SUPPORT

Nails true or false?

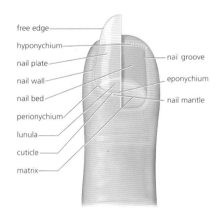

free edge
hyponychium
nail plate
nail wall
nail bed
perionychium
lunula
cuticle
matrix
nail groove
eponychium
nail mantle

The structure of the nail

ALWAYS REMEMBER

Dark streaks caused by pigmentation are common on the nail plate of black-skinned clients. These tend to increase with age.

Factors affecting the growth rate and quantity of hair
Hair does not always grow uniformly:

- *Time of day* – Hair grows faster at night than during the day.
- *Weather* – Hairs grow faster in warm weather than in cold.
- *Pregnancy* – In women, hairs grow faster and during mid-pregnancy.
- *Age* – Hairs grow faster between the ages of 16 and 24. The rate of hair growth slows down with age. In women, however, facial hair growth continues to increase in old age, while trunk and limb hair increases into middle age and then decreases.
- *Colour* – Hairs of different colour grow at different speeds – for example, coarse black hair grows more quickly than fine blonde hair.
- *Part of the body* – Hair in different areas of the body grows at different rates, as do different types and thicknesses of hair. The weekly growth rate varies from approximately 1.5mm (fine hair) to 2.8mm (coarse hair), when actively growing.
- *Heredity* – Members of a family may have inherited growth patterns, such as excess hair that starts to grow at puberty and increases until the age of 20–25.
- *Health and diet* – Health and a varied, balanced diet are crucial in the rate of hair growth and appearance.
- *Stress* – Emotional stress can cause a temporary hormonal imbalance within the body, which may lead to a temporary growth of excess hair.
- *Medical conditions* – A sudden unexplained increase of body hair growth may indicate a more serious medical problem, such as malfunction of the ovaries, or result from the taking of certain drugs, such as corticosteroids and certain birth control and high blood pressure medications.

The quantity as well as the type of hair present may vary with race:

- *People of Latin extraction* tend to possess heavier body, facial and scalp hair, which is relatively coarse and straight.
- *People of East Asian extraction* tend to possess very little or no body and facial hair growth, and usually their scalp hair growth is relatively coarse and straight. This gives the appearance of greater hair density by they actually have a lower hair density than Caucasian and Latin African-Caribbean people.
- *People of Northern European and Caucasian extraction* tend to have light to medium body and facial hair growth, with their scalp hair growth being wavy, loosely curled or straight.
- *People of African-Caribbean extraction* tend to have little body and facial hair growth, but usually their scalp hair growth is relatively coarse and tightly curled.

The nails

The structure and function of the nail

Nails grow from the ends of the fingers and toes and serve as a form of protection. They also help when picking up small objects. The different components of the nails and surrounding tissues are discussed below.

The nail plate

The **nail plate** is composed of compact translucent layers of keratinized epidermal cells: it is this that makes up the main body of the nail. The layers of cells are packed very closely together, with fat but very little moisture.

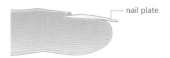
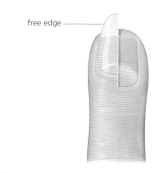

The nail plate

The nail gradually grows forward over the nail bed, until finally it becomes the free edge. The underside of the nail plate is grooved by longitudinal ridges and furrows, which help to keep it in place.

In normal health the plate curves in two directions:

● **transversely** – from side to side across the nail

● **longitudinally** – from the base of the nail to the free edge

There are no blood vessels or nerves in the nail plate: this is why the nails, like hair, can be cut without pain or bleeding. The pink colour of the nail plate derives from the blood vessels that pass beneath it – the nail bed.

Function: To protect the living nail bed of the fingers and toes.

The free edge

The free edge

The **free edge** is the part of the nail that extends beyond the fingertip; this is the part that is filed. It appears white as there is no nail bed underneath.

Function: To protect the tip of the fingers and toes and the hyponychium (see page 34).

The matrix

The **matrix**, sometimes called the nail root, is the growing area of the nail. It is formed by the division of cells in this area, called mitosis, and is part of the stratum germinativum layer of the epidermis. It lies under the eponychium (see page 35), at the base of the nail. The process of keratinization takes place in the epidermal cells of the matrix, forming the hardened tissue of the nail plate.

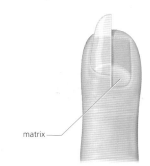

The matrix

Function: To produce new nail cells.

The nail bed

The **nail bed** is the portion of skin upon which the nail plate rests. It has a pattern of grooves and furrows corresponding to those found on the underside of the nail plate; these interlock, keeping the nail in place, but separate at the end of the nail to form the free edge. The nail bed is liberally supplied with blood vessels, which provide the nourishment necessary for continued growth; and sensory nerves, for protection.

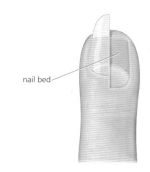

Function: To supply nourishment and protection.

The nail mantle

The **nail mantle** is the layer of epidermis at the base of the nail above the matrix, before the cuticle. It appears as a deep fold of skin.

The nail bed

Function: To protect the matrix from physical damage.

The lunula

The crescent-shaped **lunula** is located at the base of the nail. These cells gradually harden through keratinization. It is white, relative to the rest of the nail, and there are two theories to account for this:

● newly formed nail plates may be more opaque than mature nail plates

● the lunula may indicate the extent of the underlying matrix – the matrix is thicker than the epidermis of the nail bed, and the capillaries beneath it would not show through as well.

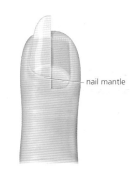

Function: None.

The nail mantle

ALWAYS REMEMBER

If the nail bed is pink this means the blood circulation to the nail bed is good. Poor health disorders such as respiratory illness and anaemia can affect the appearance of the nail colour called 'blue nail'.

TOP TIP

Did you know?
Fingernails grow more quickly than toenails. Fingernails grow about 0.1mm each day, 3–4mm per month (4cm per year), and grow faster in summer than in winter.

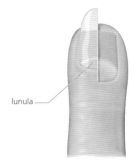

Lunula

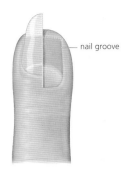

Hyponychium

Nail grooves

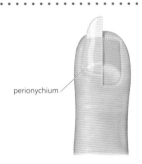

Perionychium

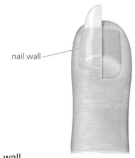

Nail wall

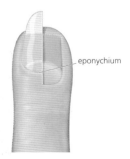

Eponychium

The hyponychium The **hyponychium** is part of the epidermis under the free edge of the nail.

Function: To protect the nail bed from infection by preventing dirt and bacteria gathering underneath the nail plate by forming a waterproof barrier.

The nail grooves The **nail grooves** run alongside the edge of the nail plate.

Function: To guide the body of the nail plate as it grows forward over the nail bed.

The perionychium The **perionychium** is the collective name given to the cuticle at the sides of the nail.

Function: To protect the nail bed from infection by preventing dirt and bacteria getting underneath the nail plate by forming a waterproof barrier.

The nail walls The **nail walls** are the folds of skin overlapping the sides of the nails.

Function: To cushion and protect the nail plate and grooves from damage.

The eponychium The **eponychium** is the extension of the cuticle at the base of the nail plate, under which the nail plate emerges from the matrix.

Function: To protect the matrix from infection by preventing dirt and bacteria getting underneath the nail plate by forming a waterproof barrier.

The cuticle The **cuticle** is the overlapping epidermis around and extending onto the base of the nail, developing from the stratum corneum. When in good condition, it is soft and loose.

Function: To protect the matrix and nail bed from infection by preventing dirt and bacteria getting underneath the nail plate by forming a waterproof barrier.

Nail growth

When **nail growth** occurs the cells divide in the matrix and the nail grows forward over the nail bed, guided by the nail grooves, until it reaches the end of the finger or toe, where it becomes the free edge. As they first emerge from the matrix the translucent cells are plump and soft, but they get harder and flatter as they move toward the free edge. The top two layers of the epidermis form the nail plate; the remaining three form the nail bed.

The nails' cells die in a process called keratinization where the cells become filled with a protein called keratin.

The nail bed has a pattern of grooves and furrows corresponding to those found on the underside of the nail plate: the two surfaces interlock, holding the nail in place.

Fingernails grow at approximately twice the speed of toenails. It takes about six months for a fingernail to grow from cuticle to free edge, but about 12 months for a toenail to do so.

The nervous system

The **nervous system** transmits messages between the brain and other parts of the body and is vast and complex. It controls everything that the body does with another body system, the endocrine system. The nervous system is made up of a network of nerve cells, called neurones. They transmit messages to and from the central nervous system (CNS) in the form of impulses. The nervous system of the body has two main divisions:

1 The central nervous system.

2 The autonomic nervous system.

The central nervous system

The central nervous system (CNS) is composed of the brain and spinal cord. The CNS co-ordinates the activities of the entire body.

The brain transmits impulses to all parts of the body in order to stimulate other organs to act and is protected by the bones of the cranium. The spinal cord runs along inside the vertebral column and is protected by the bones (vertebrae) of the spinal column. The brain is composed of several parts, each of which performs special functions.

Nerves

A nerve is a whitish bundle of fibres made up of neurones (nerve cells) that transmits impulses of sensations between the brain or spinal cord and other parts of the body. Nerve cells are long, narrow and delicate. They are made up of a cell body containing a large central nucleus and nerve fibres that transmit messages to other neurones.

Kinds of nerves There are two types of nerve: *sensory nerves* and *motor nerves*. Both are composed of white fibres enclosed in a sheath.

- **Sensory or afferent nerves** These receive information from receptors in the sense organs and relay it to the brain and spinal cord. They are found near to the skin's surface and respond to touch, pressure, temperature and pain.

- **Motor or efferent nerves** These are situated in muscle tissue and act on information received from the brain or spinal cord to a muscle or gland, causing a particular response, typically muscle movement.

All nerves emerge from the CNS. Sensory (receptor) nerves are linked to sensory receptors, while motor (effector) nerves end in a muscle or gland. Twelve pairs of cranial nerves emerge from the brain; 31 pairs of spinal nerves emerge from between the vertebrae of the spinal column.

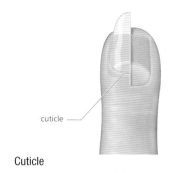

cuticle

Cuticle

ACTIVITY

Recognizing nail structure
With a colleague, try to identify the structural parts of each other's nails. Write down both the parts that you can see and the parts that you cannot see.

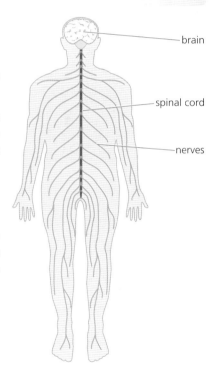

brain

spinal cord

nerves

Central nervous system

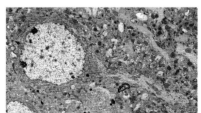

A nerve cell

HEALTH & SAFETY

Nerve damage
Nerve cells do not reproduce; when damaged, only a limited repair occurs.

TOP TIP

Massage
Appropriate massage manipulations, when applied to the skin, produce a stimulating or relaxing effect on nerves.

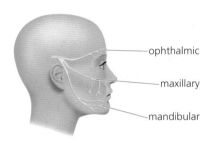

5th cranial nerve

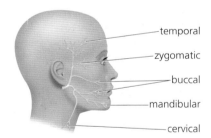

7th cranial nerve

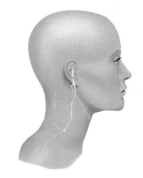

11th cranial nerve

Nerves of the face and neck These nerves link the brain with the muscles of the head, face and neck.

Cranial nerves control muscles in the head and neck region, or carry nerve impulses from sense organs to the brain. Those of concern to the beauty therapist when performing a facial service are as follows:

- the 5th cranial nerve, or **trigeminal** controls the muscles involved in mastication (chewing) and passes on sensory information from the face such as the eyes
- the 7th cranial nerve, or **facial** controls the muscles involved in facial expression
- the 11th cranial nerve, or **accessory** controls muscles involved in moving the head, the sternocleidomastoid and trapezius muscle.

5th cranial nerve This nerve carries messages to the brain from the sensory nerves of the skin, the teeth, the nose and the mouth. It also stimulates the motor nerve to create the chewing action when eating. The 5th cranial nerve has three branches:

- the **ophthalmic nerve** serves the tear glands of the eye, the skin of the forehead, and the upper cheeks
- the **maxillary nerve** serves the upper jaw and the mouth
- the **mandibular nerve** serves the lower jaw muscle, the teeth and the muscle involved with chewing.

7th cranial nerve This nerve passes through the temporal bone and behind the ear, and then divides. It serves the ear muscle and the muscles of facial expression, the tongue and the palate.

The 7th cranial nerve has five branches:

- the **temporal nerve** serves the orbicularis oculi and the frontalis muscles
- the **zygomatic nerve** serves the eye muscles
- the **buccal nerve** serves the upper lip and the sides of the nose
- the **mandibular nerve** serves the lower lip and the mentalis muscle of the chin
- the **cervical nerve** serves the platysma muscle of the neck

11th cranial nerve This nerve serves the sternomastoid and trapezius muscles of the neck, and its function is to move the head and shoulders.

Nerve impulses The CNS transmits instructions to organs through nerve impulses – tiny electrical signals – that pass along a neurone. Each nerve consists of a nerve cell and its parts, axons and dendrites. Axons carry nerve impulses away from the cell; dendrites carry impulses towards the cell.

When an impulse reaches the end of a nerve fibre, a chemical called a *neurotransmitter substance* is released. This chemical passes across a tiny gap called a *synapse* and is taken up by an adjacent neurone, generating an electrical impulse in the neurone.

When neuro-transmitters land at their receptor sites they can stimulate or inhibit the receiving cell. Both responses are important to relay the correct message through the nervous system.

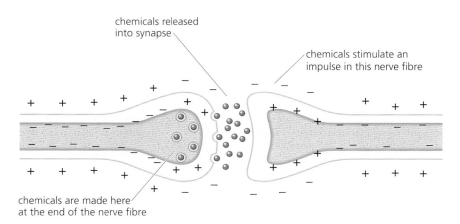

chemicals released into synapse

chemicals stimulate an impulse in this nerve fibre

chemicals are made here at the end of the nerve fibre

Passage of an impulse across a synapse

Neurones can stimulate muscle fibres to contract. The *motor point* is where a motor nerve enters a muscle. When stimulated by a motor nerve, muscle contraction occurs.

The autonomic nervous system

The other nervous system division is the autonomic nervous system. The main function being to maintain constant conditions within the body called *homeostasis*.

The autonomic nervous system controls those body structures over which there is no conscious control – the involuntary activities. It regulates the functioning of organs such as the heart, the stomach, the lungs and the secretion of most glands. There are two divisions of the autonomic nervous system – the *sympathetic* and *parasympathetic nervous systems*.

Many organs receive a supply from each division. Fibres from one division stimulate the organ while fibres from the other division inhibit it, thus ensuring balance in the body.

The sympathetic nervous system is stimulated in periods of stress or danger and prepares the body for physical activity. Fibres of the sympathetic division increase blood flow by causing the heart to beat faster and the blood vessels in the muscles to widen. Activities that are not essential in this stressful situation are inhibited.

The parasympathetic nervous system is associated with resting and causes the blood flow to slow by causing the heart to beat slower and the blood vessels in the muscles to contract (go smaller). Fibres of this division stimulate digestion and absorption of food.

The nervous system therefore co-ordinates the activities of the body by responding to stimuli received by sense organs, including the nose, tongue, eyes, ears and skin.

TOP TIP

Botox® botulinum toxin A

Botox® has been developed as a cosmetic service from its previous use medically to treat eye spasms and disorders of the central nervous system. A purified protein called botulinum toxin A is injected into the face where it binds to the nerve endings, which prevent the release of the neuro-transmitter substance that stimulates the muscle fibres to contract. The result is a paralysis of the muscle preventing expressions that may lead to visible expression lines on the face, such as frown lines.

TOP TIP

Lifestyle factors affect the nervous system

Caffeine is a stimulant and will increase the release of the neurotransmitter chemical across the synapse between adjacent neurones.

Alcohol is a sedative and will slow the release of the neurotransmitter chemical across the synapse between adjacent neurones.

Can you think of other substances that affect the nervous system?

TOP TIP

Memory aid

The sympathetic division is associated with stress. The parasympathetic system is associated with peace.

sympathetic = stress
parasympathetic = peace

The muscular system

Muscles are responsible for the movement of body parts. Each is made up of a bundle of elastic fibres bound together in a sheath, the **fascia**. Muscular tissue contracts (shortens) and produces movement. Muscles never completely relax – there are always a few contracted fibres in every muscle. These make the muscles slightly tense and this tension is called **muscle tone**.

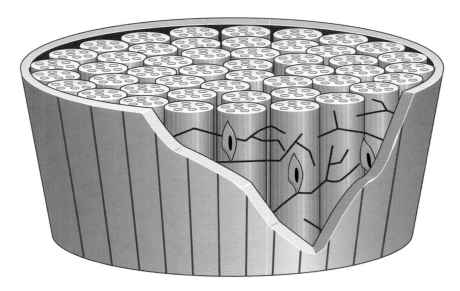

Muscle tissue

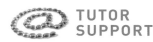

TUTOR SUPPORT

Activity 10: Label the muscles that move the head

Muscle tissue has the following properties:

- it has the ability to contract

- it is extensible (when the extensor muscle in a joint contracts the corresponding flexor muscle will be stretched or lengthened)

- it is elastic – following contraction or extension it returns to its original length

- it is responsive – it contracts in response to nerve stimulation

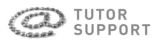

TUTOR SUPPORT

Activity 11: Label the muscles of the face and neck

A muscle is usually anchored by a strong tendon to one bone: the point of attachment is known as the muscle's **origin**. The muscle is likewise joined to a second bone: the attachment in this case is called the muscle's **insertion**. It is this second bone that is moved: the muscle contracts, pulling the two bones towards each other. (A different muscle, on the other side of the bone, has the contrary effect.) Not all muscles attach to bones, however: some insert into an adjacent muscle, or into the skin itself. The muscles with which we are concerned here are those of the face, the neck and the shoulders.

Facial muscles

Many of the muscles located in the face are very small and are attached to (insert into) another small muscle or the facial skin. When the muscles contract, they pull the facial skin in a particular way; this creates facial expressions.

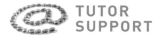

TUTOR SUPPORT

Activity 12: Facial muscles handout

With age, the facial expressions that we make every day produce lines on the skin – frown lines. The amount of tension, or **tone**, also decreases with age. When performing facial massage, the aim is to improve the general tone of the facial muscles.

TOP TIP

Terminology for action

Flexor – bends a joint   *Extensor* – straightens a joint

If a muscle has 'flexor' or 'extensor' in front of the muscle name you will know what the action of the muscle is!

Abduction – 'move away'   *Adduction* – 'move towards'

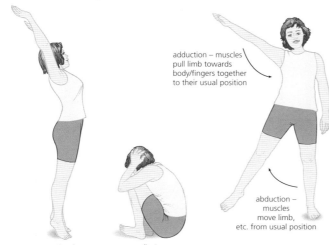

adduction – muscles pull limb towards body/fingers together to their usual position

abduction – muscles move limb, etc. from usual position

extension   flexion

ALWAYS REMEMBER

Nerves of the face
Almost all facial muscles are controlled by the 7th cranial or facial nerve.

TUTOR SUPPORT

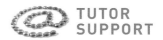

Activity 18: Label the 5th and 7th cranial nerves

Muscles of facial expression

Muscle	Expression	Location	Action
Frontalis	Surprise	The forehead.	Raises the eyebrows, causes wrinkling across forehead.
Corrugator	Frowning	Between the eyebrows.	Draws the eyebrows down and together.
Orbicularis oculi	Winking	Surrounds the eyes.	Closes the eyelid.

corrugator

orbicularis oculi

Muscle	Expression	Location	Action
Risorius	Smiling, grinning	Extends diagonally from the masseter muscle to the corners of the mouth.	Draws mouth corners outwards and backwards.
Buccinator	Blowing	Inside the cheeks, between upper jaw and lower jaw.	Compresses the cheeks.
Zygomaticus (made up of major and minor muscles)	Smiling, laughing	Extend diagonally from the zygomatic (cheek bone) to the corners of the mouth.	Lifts the corners of the mouth backwards and upwards.
Procerus	Distaste	Covers the bridge of the nose.	Draws down eyebrows and wrinkles the skin over the bridge of the nose.
Nasalis (made up of several small muscles)	Anger	Covers the front of the nose and surrounds nostrils.	Opens and closes the nasal openings.
Levator labii	Distaste	Surrounds the upper lip.	Raises and draws back the upper lips and nostrils.

Muscle	Expression	Location	Action
Depressor labii	Sulking	Surrounds the lower lip.	Pulls down the lower lip and draws it slightly to one side.
Orbicularis oris	Pout, kiss, doubt	Surrounds the mouth.	Purses the lip (as in blowing), closes the mouth.
Triangularis	Sadness	The corner of the lower lip extends over the chin.	Draws down the mouth's corners.
Mentalis	Doubt	Covers the front of the chin.	Raises the lower lip, causing the chin to wrinkle.
Platysma	Fear, horror	The sides of the neck and chin.	Draws the mouth's corners downwards and backwards.

Crow's feet

To avoid the premature formation of 'crow's feet':

- avoid squinting in bright sunlight – wear sunglasses

- have your eyes tested regularly

- if you use a visual display unit, ensure that you take regular breaks, and have a protective filter screen to remove glare

ACTIVITY

Facial expressions

In front of a mirror, move the muscles of your face to create the expressions that you might form each day.

What expressions can you make? Which part or parts of the face are moving? Which facial muscles do you think have contracted to create these expressions?

To balance and move the head and facial features the muscles of the head, face and neck work together.

Muscles of mastication The muscles responsible for the movement of the lower jawbone (the **mandible**) when chewing are called the **muscles of mastication**.

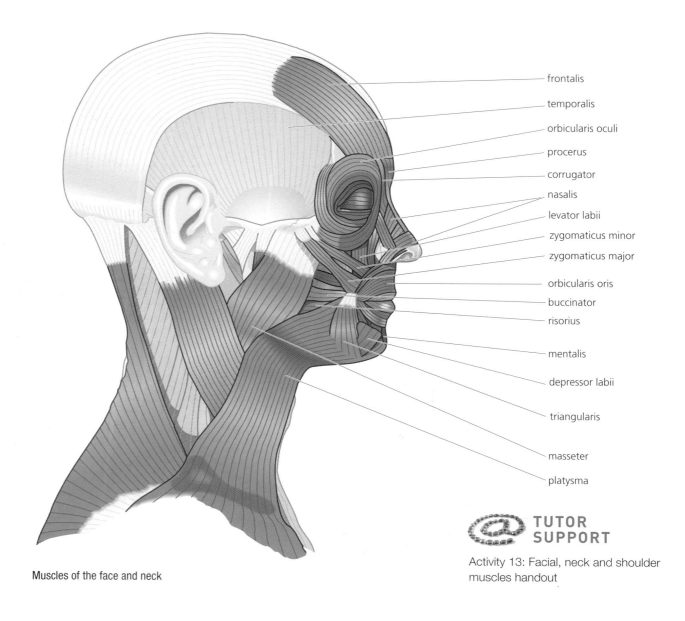

frontalis
temporalis
orbicularis oculi
procerus
corrugator
nasalis
levator labii
zygomaticus minor
zygomaticus major
orbicularis oris
buccinator
risorius
mentalis
depressor labii
triangularis
masseter
platysma

Muscles of the face and neck

TUTOR SUPPORT

Activity 13: Facial, neck and shoulder muscles handout

Muscle	Location	Action
Masseter	The cheek area: extends from the zygomatic bone to the mandible.	Clenches the teeth; raises the lower jaw and closes the mouth.
Temporalis	Extends from the temple region at the side of the head to the mandible.	Raises the jaw and draws it backwards, as in chewing.

Muscles that move the head

Muscle	Location	Action
Sterno-cleido-mastoid	Runs from the sternum to the clavicle bone and the temporal bone.	Flexes the neck; rotates and bows the head.
Trapezius	A large kite-shaped muscle, covering the back of the neck and the upper back.	Draws the head backwards and allows movement at the shoulder.
Occipitalis	Covers the back of the head.	Draws scalp backwards.

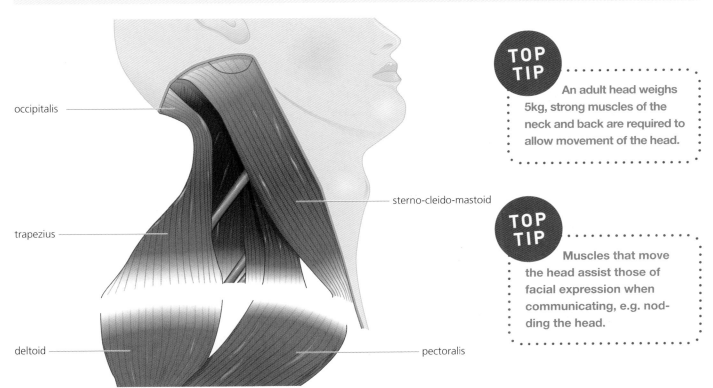

occipitalis

trapezius

deltoid

sterno-cleido-mastoid

pectoralis

TOP TIP

An adult head weighs 5kg, strong muscles of the neck and back are required to allow movement of the head.

TOP TIP

Muscles that move the head assist those of facial expression when communicating, e.g. nodding the head.

Muscles that move the head and muscles of the upper body

Muscles of the upper body
When massaging the shoulder area you will cover the following muscles of the upper body.

Muscle	Location	Action
Pectoralis major	The front of the chest.	Moves the arm towards the upper body.
Deltoid	A thick triangular muscle, covering the shoulder.	Takes the arm away from the side of the body.

The muscles of the hand and arm

The hand and fingers are moved primarily by muscles and tendons in the forearm. These muscles contract, pulling the tendons, and thereby move the fingers much as a puppet is moved by strings.

The muscles of the hand and arm that bend the wrist, drawing it towards the forearm, are **flexors**; other muscles, **extensors**, straighten the wrist and the hand.

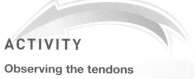

ACTIVITY

Observing the tendons
Tendons are made of strong connective tissue and attach muscle to bone. Hold your palm face upwards, with your sleeve pulled back so that you can see your forearm. Move the fingers individually towards the palm. Can you see the tendons moving?

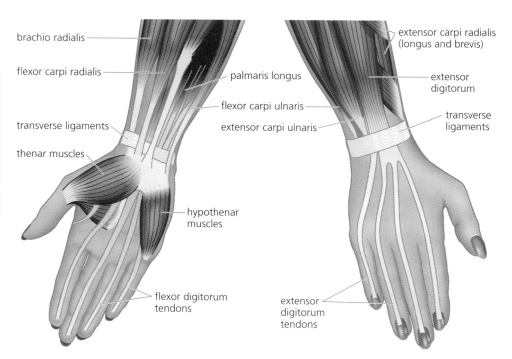

brachio radialis

flexor carpi radialis

transverse ligaments

thenar muscles

palmaris longus

flexor carpi ulnaris

extensor carpi ulnaris

hypothenar muscles

flexor digitorum tendons

extensor carpi radialis (longus and brevis)

extensor digitorum

transverse ligaments

extensor digitorum tendons

Muscles of the arm and hand

Muscle	Location	Action
Brachio radialis	On the outer (thumb side) of the forearm.	Flexes arm at the elbow.
Flexor carpi radialis	Middle of the forearm.	Flexes and abducts the wrist.
Extensor carpi radialis (longus and brevis)	Thumb side of the forearm.	Extends and abducts the hand and wrist.

Muscle	Location	Action
Flexor carpi ulnaris	Front of the forearm.	Muscle that flexes and adducts the wrist joint in towards the body.
Extensor carpi ulnaris	Back of the forearm.	Extends and adducts the wrist.
Palmaris longus	Middle of the front of the forearm.	Flexes the wrist and tenses the palm of the hand.
Hypothenar muscle	In the palm of the hand, below the little finger.	Flexes the little finger and moves it outwards and inwards.
Thenar muscle	In the palm of the hand, below the thumb.	Flexes the thumb and moves it outwards and inwards.
Flexor digitorum tendons	Front of fingers.	Flexes the fingers when contracted.
Extensor digitorum tendons	Back of fingers.	Extends the fingers when contracted.

The muscles of the foot and lower leg

The **muscles of the foot** work together to help move the body when walking and running. In a similar way to the movement of the hand, the foot is moved primarily by **muscles in the lower leg**; these pull on tendons, which in turn move the feet and toes.

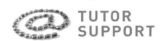

TUTOR SUPPORT

Activity 14: Muscles of the leg and foot handout

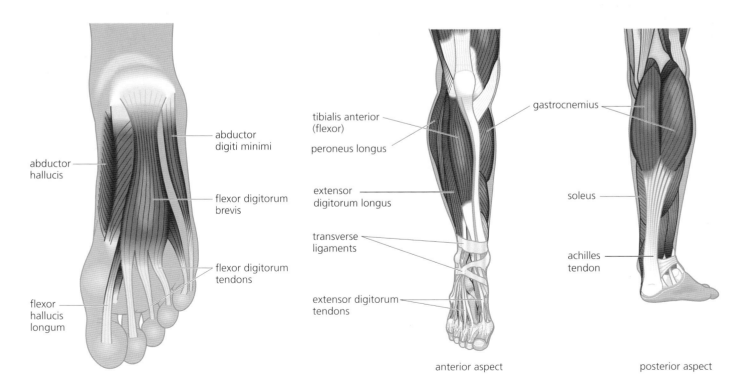

Muscles and tendons of the foot

Muscles of the lower leg

Muscles and tendons of the lower leg and foot

Muscle	Location	Action
Gastrocnemius	Calf of the leg, inserts through the Achilles tendon into the heel.	Flexes the lower leg; plantar flexes the foot (extends and points the toes down).
Tibialis anterior	Front of the lower leg.	Inverts the foot (turns sole inwards) dorsi flexes the foot (flexes and points the toes up); rotates foot outwards. Supports the medial longitudinal arch of the foot when running or walking.
Soleus	Calf of the leg, situated below the gastrocnemius muscle. Inserts through the Achilles tendon into the heel.	Plantar flexes the foot (flexes and points toes down). Assists forward motion when walking or running.
Peroneus longus	Lateral side of the lower leg.	Plantar flexes the foot and everts (turns sole outwards). Supports the foot arches.
Extensor digitorum longus	Lateral side of the front of the lower leg.	Dorsi flexes the foot up at the ankle and extends the toes.
Flexor digitorum longus	Front of lower leg to the toes.	Plantar flexes foot downwards and inverts the foot. Helps the toes to grip. Supports the lateral longitudinal arch of the foot.
Achilles tendon	Attached to the soleus and gastrocnemius down to the heel.	Raises the foot when related muscle contracts.
Extensor digitorum tendons	Tops of toes.	Straightens the toes when related muscle contracts.
Flexor digitorum tendons	Underneath the toes.	Bends the toes when related muscle contracts.

The bones

When carrying out a massage to the face, hands and feet, you will feel below your hands the underlying bones. **Bone** is the hardest structure in the body: it protects the underlying structures, gives shape to the body and provides an attachment point for our muscles, thereby allowing movement.

The skeleton is made up of many bones. The average skeleton has 206 bones. Each bone is connected to its neighbour by *connective tissue,* a structural tissue that supports, surrounds and links different parts of the body. Fibrous connective tissue is used for immovable joints such as those of the cranium. *Fibro-cartilage* is used for semi-immovable joints such as those between the bones of the vertebrae. The most common joints – *synovial joints* – are freely moveable and are loosely held together by a form of connective tissue called a *ligament.*

Bones have different shapes, according to their function.

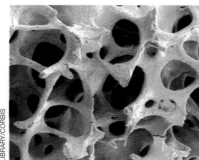

Bone tissue

flat bone, as the parietal bone found in the skull

short bone, as the phalange bone found in the finger

irregular as vertebral bones found in the spinal column.

long bone, as the femur found in the leg

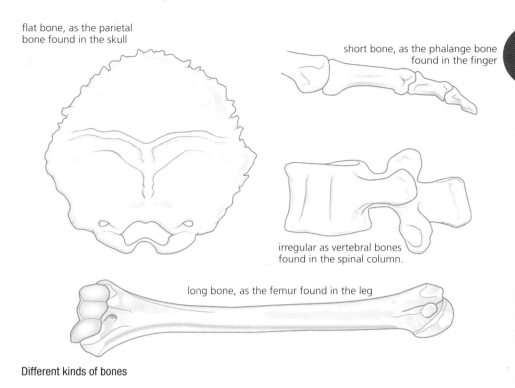

Different kinds of bones

TOP TIP

Bone acts as a reservoir for important minerals such as calcium and phosphorus and also makes new cells for the blood in certain bones in tissue called bone marrow.

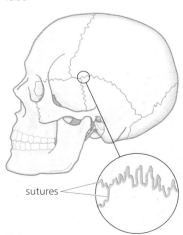

Ball and socket joint, as in the shoulder

Bones of the head, neck, chest and shoulders

The bones which form the head are collectively known as the **skull**. The skull can be divided into two parts, the face and the cranium, which together are made up of 22 bones:

● the fourteen **facial bones** form the face

● the eight cranial bones form the rest of the head

As well as forming our facial features, the facial bones support other structures such as the eyes and the teeth. Some of these bones, such as the nasal bone, are made from **cartilage**, connective tissue, a softer tissue than bone.

The cranium surrounds and protects the brain. The bones are thin and slightly curved, and are held together by connective tissue. After childhood, the joints become immovable, and are called **sutures** appearing as wavy lines.

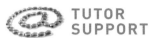

TUTOR SUPPORT

Activity 7: Label the bones of the neck, chest and shoulder

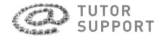

TUTOR SUPPORT

Activity 6: Label the bones of the face

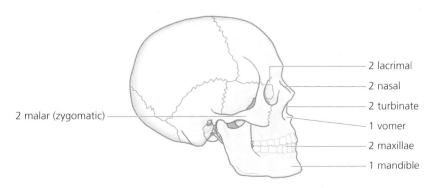

2 malar (zygomatic)

2 lacrimal
2 nasal
2 turbinate
1 vomer
2 maxillae
1 mandible

Bones of the face (14 in total)

sutures

Sutures

Facial bones

Bone	Number	Location	Function
Nasal	2	The nose.	Form the bridge of the nose.
Vomer	1	The nose.	Forms the dividing bony wall of the nose.
Palatine	2	The nose.	Form the floor and wall of the nose and the roof of the mouth.
Turbinate	2	The nose.	Form the outer walls of the nose.
Lacrimal	2	The eye sockets.	Form the inner walls of the eye sockets; contain a small groove for the tear duct.
Malar (zygomatic)	2	The cheek.	Form the cheekbones.
Maxillae	2	The upper jaw.	Fused together, to form the upper jaw, which holds the upper teeth.
Mandible	1	The lower jaw.	The largest and strongest of the facial bones; holds the lower teeth.

Cranial bones

Bone	Number	Location	Function
Occipital	1	The lower back of the cranium.	Contains a large hole called the *foramen magnum:* through this pass the spinal cord, the nerves and blood vessels.
Parietal	2	The sides of the cranium.	Fused together to form the sides and top of the head (the 'crown').
Frontal	1	The forehead.	Forms the forehead and the upper walls of the eye sockets.
Temporal	2	The sides of the head.	Provide two muscle attachment points: the mastoid process and the zygomatic process.
Ethmoid	1	Between the eye sockets.	Forms part of the nasal cavities.
Sphenoid	1	The base of the cranium, the back of the eye sockets.	A bat-shaped bone that joins together all the bones of the cranium.

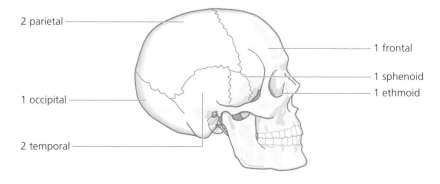

Bones of the cranium (8 in total)

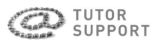

TUTOR SUPPORT

Activity 5: Label the bones of the cranium

Bones of the neck, chest and shoulder

Bone	Number	Location	Function
Cervical vertebra	7	The neck.	These vertebrae form the top of the spinal column: the *atlas* is the first vertebra, which supports the skull; the *axis* is the second vertebra, which allows rotation of the head.
Hyoid	1	A U-shaped bone at the front of the neck.	Supports the tongue.
Clavicle	2	Slender long bones at the base of the neck.	Commonly called the *collar bones*, these form a joint with the sternum and the scapula bones, allowing movement at the shoulder.
Scapula	2	Triangular bones in the upper back.	Commonly called the *shoulder blades*, the scapulae provide attachment for muscles which move the arms. The shoulder girdle, which allows movement at the shoulder, is composed of the clavicles and the scapulae.
Humerus	2	The upper bones of the arms.	Form ball-and-socket joints with the scapulae: these joints allow movement in any direction.
Sternum	1	The breastbone.	Protects the inner organs; provides a surface for muscle attachment and supports muscle movement.

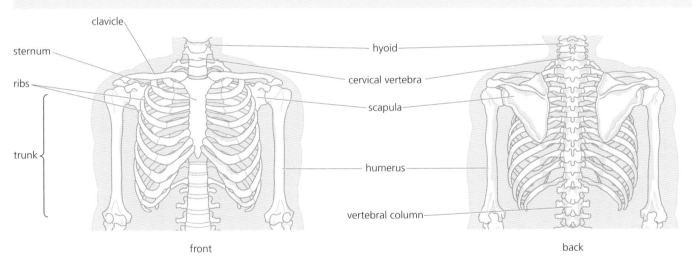

Bones of the neck, chest and shoulder

The hand and the forearm

The bones of the hand There are 27 bones of the hand. The wrist consists of eight small **carpal** bones, which glide over one another to allow movement. This is called a **condyloid** or **gliding joint**.

There are then five **metacarpal** bones that make up the palm of the hand.

The fingers are made up of 14 individual bones called **phalanges** – two in the thumb, and three in each of the fingers.

The bones of the arm The bones of the arm are three long bones: the **humerus** is the bone of the upper arm, from the shoulder to the elbow; the **radius** and **ulna** lie side by side in the lower arm, from the elbow to the wrist.

ACTIVITY

Identifying bones in the hand
Look very closely at your hand. Can you identify where the bones are? Try feeling the bones with your other hand. How many can you feel?

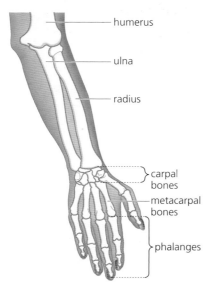

Bones of the arm

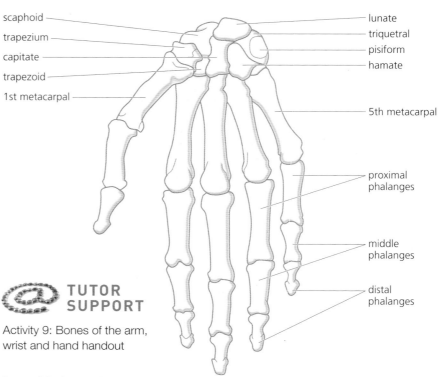

TUTOR SUPPORT

Activity 9: Bones of the arm, wrist and hand handout

Bones of the hand and wrist

Having two bones in the lower arm makes it easier for your wrist to rotate. This movement that causes the palm to face downwards is called **pronation**; the movement that causes it to face upwards is called **supination**.

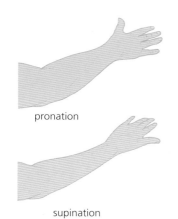

Pronation and supination

The foot and the lower leg

The bones of the foot There are 26 bones of the foot. They are seven **tarsal** (ankle) bones, five **metatarsal** (ball of foot) bones, and 14 **phalanges** (toes). These bones

Arches

Footprints made by bare feet show that only part of the foot touches the ground. Weight transfers from the heel to the ball to the big toe when walking. Feet with reduced arches are referred to as 'flat feet', caused by weak ligaments and tendons.

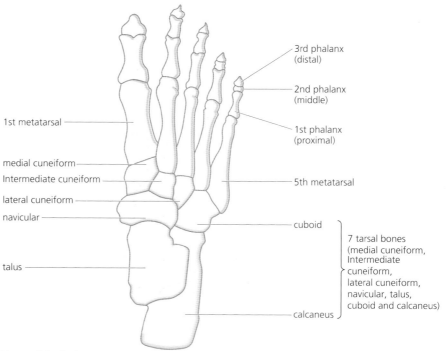

Bones of the foot

fit together to form arches, which help to support the foot and to absorb the impact when we walk, run and jump.

The arches of the foot

The **arches** of the foot are created by the formation of the bones and joints, and supported by ligaments. These arches support the weight of the body and help to preserve balance when we walk on even surfaces.

The longitudinal arch runs longitudinally from the calcaneus to the metatarsals. The arch on the inside aspect of the foot is the medial longitudinal arch, on the outside aspect it is the lateral longitudinal arch. The transverse arch lies perpendicular to this in the metatarsal area, as shown below.

ALWAYS REMEMBER

Anatomical definitions

Medal: towards the midline (middle) of the body

Lateral: away from the median line (middle) line of the body. The outer side of the body.

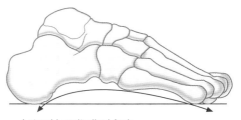
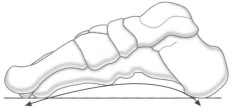

Medial Longitudinal Arch   Lateral Longitudinal Arch   Transverse Arch

The bones of the lower leg

The bones of the lower leg are two long bones, the **tibia** and the **fibula**. These bones have joints with the upper leg (at the knee) and with the foot (at the ankle). Having two bones in the lower leg – as with the forearm – allows a greater range of movement to be achieved at the ankle.

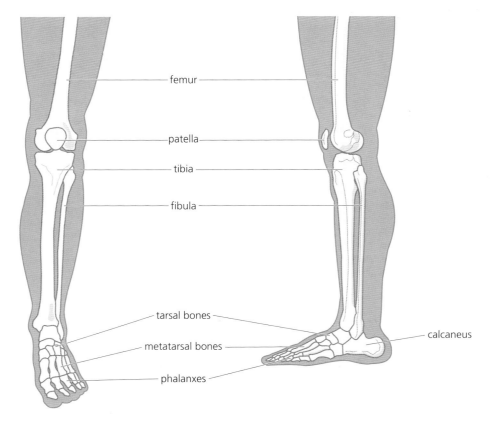

Bones of the lower leg

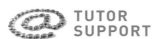

TUTOR SUPPORT

Activity 8: Bones of the leg, ankle and foot handout

The blood

Composition and function of blood

Blood is a collection of specialized cells suspended in a liquid called plasma supplying the needs of the body's cells keeping the body healthy. It is transported around the body by a network of vessels with a length of 90 000 miles.

Blood transports various substances around the body:

- It carries oxygen from our lungs, and nutrients from our digested food to supply energy – these allow the cells to develop and divide, and the muscles to function.

- It carries waste products and carbon dioxide from the cells and tissues away for elimination from the body.

- It carries various cells and substances which allow the body to prevent or fight disease and heal injuries.

- Transports hormones, the body's chemical messengers to their target tissue to cause a particular response.

The main constituents of blood

Blood consists of the following:

- **Plasma** This constitutes 50 per cent of blood and is a straw-coloured liquid: mainly water (90 per cent), with foods and carbon dioxide.

- **Red blood cells (erythrocytes)** These constitute 40–50 per cent of blood. These cells appear red because they contain **haemoglobin** a protein responsible for their colour. It is this that carries oxygen from the lungs to the body cells.

- **White blood cells (leucocytes)** There are several types of white blood cells. Their main role is to protect the body destroying foreign bodies and dead cells, and carrying away the debris (a process known as **phagocytosis**).

- **Platelets (thrombocytes)** When blood is exposed to air, as happens when the skin is injured, these cells bind together to form a clot. White blood cells and platelets constitute 1–2 per cent of blood.

- **Other chemicals** Hormones also are transported in the blood – 'chemical messengers' to target tissues.

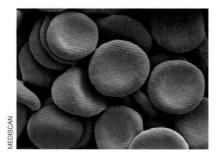

MEDISCAN

Blood cells

The circulation

The circulation of blood is under the control of the **heart**, a powerful muscular organ, the size of a clenched fist, which pumps the blood around the body. The heart requires a constant supply of oxygen and energy from blood.

Blood leaving the heart is carried in large, elastic tubes called **arteries**. The blood to the head arrives via the **carotid arteries**, which are connected via other main arteries to the heart. There are two main carotid arteries, one on each side of the neck.

These arteries divide into smaller branches, the *internal carotid* and the *external carotid*. The **internal carotid artery** passes the temporal bone and enters the head, taking blood to the brain. The **external carotid artery** stays outside the skull, and divides into branches:

● the **occipital branch** supplies the back of the head and the scalp

● the **temporal branch** supplies the sides of the face, the head, the scalp and the skin

● the **facial branch** supplies the muscles and tissues of the face

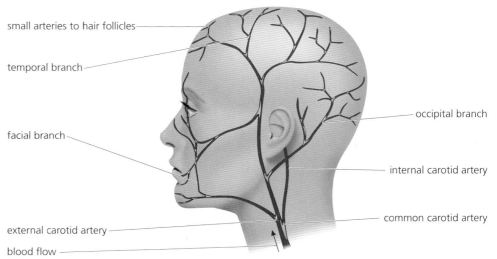

small arteries to hair follicles

temporal branch

facial branch

external carotid artery

blood flow

occipital branch

internal carotid artery

common carotid artery

The blood supply to the head

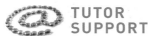

TOP TIP

Pulse rate

The pumping of the blood under pressure through the carotid arteries can be felt as a pulse in the neck. Press gently on the neck just inside the position of the sternomastoid muscle.

Pulse rate relates to the speed of the heartbeat. The strength of the pulse is affected by the pressure of the blood flow leaving the heart. The heart on average beats 70 times per minute.

Blood pressure increases during activity and decreases during rest.

Relaxing services such as facial massage lower blood pressure.

TUTOR SUPPORT

Activity 17: Label the blood supply to and from the head

These arteries also divide repeatedly, successive vessels becoming smaller and smaller until they form tiny blood **capillaries**. These vessels are just one cell thick, allowing substances carried in the blood to pass through them into the **tissue fluid** which bathes and nourishes the cells of the various body tissues.

The blood capillaries begin to join up again, forming first small vessels called **venules**, then larger vessels called **veins**. These return the blood to the heart.

Veins are less elastic than arteries, and are closer to the skin's surface. Along their course are **valves**, which prevent the backflow of blood.

The main veins are the external and internal jugular veins. The **internal jugular vein** and its main branch, the **facial vein**, carry blood from the face and head. The **external jugular vein** carries blood from the scalp and has two branches: the **occipital branch** and the **temporal branch**. The jugular veins join to enter the **subclavian vein**, which lies above the clavicle.

Blood returns to the heart, which pumps it to the lungs, where the red blood cells take on fresh oxygen, and where carbon dioxide is expelled from the blood. The blood returns to the heart, and begins its next journey round the body.

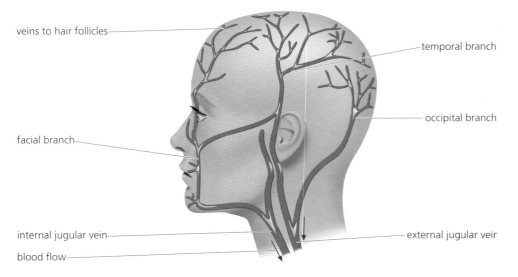

veins to hair follicles

temporal branch

occipital branch

facial branch

internal jugular vein

external jugular vein

blood flow

The blood supply from the head

The arteries of the arm and hand

The arm and hand are nourished by a system of arteries that carry oxygen-rich blood to the tissues. You can see the colour of the blood from the capillaries beneath the nail: it is these that give the nail bed its pink colour.

The brachial artery supplies blood to the upper arm. This branches into the ulnar and radial artery which supply the forearm and fingers. The radial and ulnar arteries are connected across the palm by the superficial and deep palmar arches. These arteries divide to form the metacarpal and digital arteries, which supply the palm and fingers.

The veins of the arms and hands Veins deliver deoxygenated blood back to the heart. Blood which has had oxygen removed appears blue. Veins often pass through muscles. Each time muscles contract, veins are squeezed and the blood is pushed along. Massage is particularly beneficial to help this process.

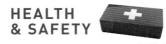

HEALTH & SAFETY

Capillaries
The strength and elasticity of the capillary walls can be damaged, for example by a blow to the tissues. Broken capillaries are capillaries whose elasticity is damaged and they remain constantly dilated with blood.

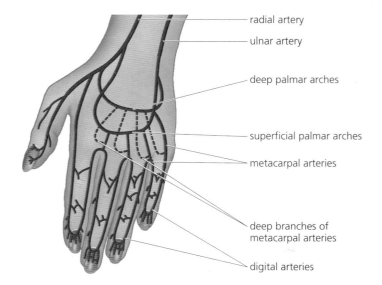

radial artery

ulnar artery

deep palmar arches

superficial palmar arches

metacarpal arteries

deep branches of metacarpal arteries

digital arteries

Arteries of the hand

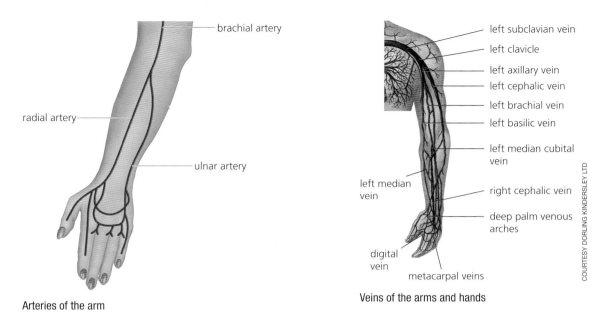

Arteries of the arm

Veins of the arms and hands

Blood in the digital veins drains blood from the fingers. The palmar venous arches drains blood from the hands. The cephalic and basilic veins drain blood from the forearm.

The arteries of the foot and lower leg

The lower leg and feet are nourished by a system of arteries that carry oxygen rich blood to the tissues.

The anterior and tibial artery supplies blood to the lower leg and foot. The peroneal artery branches off the posterior tibial artery. At the ankle the anterior tibial artery becomes the dorsalis pedis artery. The posterior tibial artery divides at the ankle to form the medial and lateral plantar arteries. The plantar and dorsalis pedis arteries supply the digital arteries of the toes.

When it is cold, and when the circulation is poor, insufficient blood reaches the feet and they feel cold. Severe circulation problems in the feet may lead to **chilblains**.

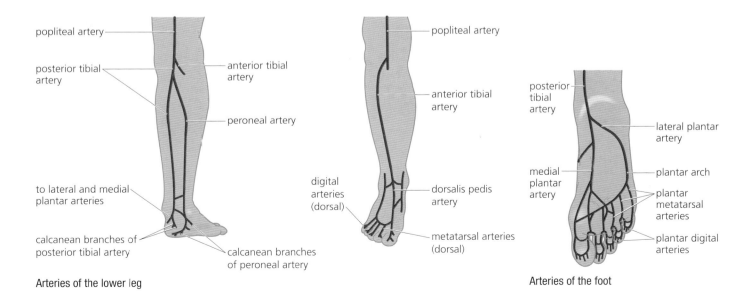

Arteries of the lower leg

Arteries of the foot

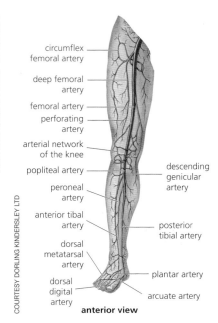

COURTESY DORLING KINDERSLEY LTD

circumflex femoral artery
deep femoral artery
femoral artery
perforating artery
arterial network of the knee
popliteal artery
peroneal artery
anterior tibal artery
dorsal metatarsal artery
dorsal digital artery
descending genicular artery
posterior tibial artery
plantar artery
arcuate artery

anterior view

Veins of the foot and lower leg

The veins of the foot and lower leg The digital veins from the toes drain into the plantar and dorsal venous arch. The dorsalis pedis veins drain to the saphenous vein. The following deep veins drain the lower leg: the posterior tibial vein at the back of the leg and the peroneal vein, and the anterior tibial vein at the front of the leg. The deep tibial veins join to form the popliteal vein.

The lymphatic system

The lymphatic system is closely connected to the blood system, and can be considered as supplementing it. Its primary function is defensive: to remove bacteria and foreign materials, thereby preventing infection. It also drains away excess fluids for elimination from the body.

The lymphatic system consists of the fluid lymph, the lymph vessels and the **lymph nodes** (or glands). You may have experienced swelling of the lymph nodes in the neck when you have been ill.

Unlike the blood circulation, the lymphatic system has no muscular pump equivalent to the heart. Instead, the lymph moves through the vessels and around the body because of movements such as contractions of large muscles. Contractions of the body muscles push the lymph through a series of one-way valves. Massage can play an important part in assisting this flow of lymph fluid, thereby encouraging the improved removal of the waste products transported in the lymph.

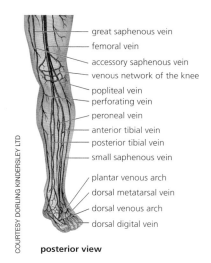

COURTESY DORLING KINDERSLEY LTD

great saphenous vein
femoral vein
accessory saphenous vein
venous network of the knee
popliteal vein
perforating vein
peroneal vein
anterior tibial vein
posterior tibial vein
small saphenous vein
plantar venous arch
dorsal metatarsal vein
dorsal venous arch
dorsal digital vein

posterior view

Veins of the foot and lower leg

Lymph

Lymph is a straw-coloured fluid, derived from blood plasma, which has filtered through the walls of the capillaries. Lymph drains into a network of lymph capillaries and then into larger vessels known as lymphatics which contain special filters called nodes or glands. The composition of lymph is similar to that of blood, though less oxygen and fewer nutrients are available. In the spaces between the cells where there are no blood capillaries, lymph provides nourishment. It also carries **lymphocytes** (a type of white blood cell), which play an important role in the immune system. They can destroy dangerous cells and disease-causing bacteria and viruses directly before they return to the bloodstream.

Lymph travels only in one direction: from body tissues back towards the heart.

Lymph vessels

Lymph vessels often run very close to veins, forming an extensive network throughout the body. The lymph moves quite slowly, and the valves along the lymph vessels prevent backflow of the lymph.

The lymph vessels join to form larger lymph vessels, which eventually flow into one or other of two large lymphatic vessels: the **thoracic duct** (or **left lymphatic duct**) and the **right lymphatic duct**. The thoracic duct receives lymph from the left side of the head, neck, chest, abdomen and lower body; the right lymphatic duct receives lymph from the right side of the head and upper body.

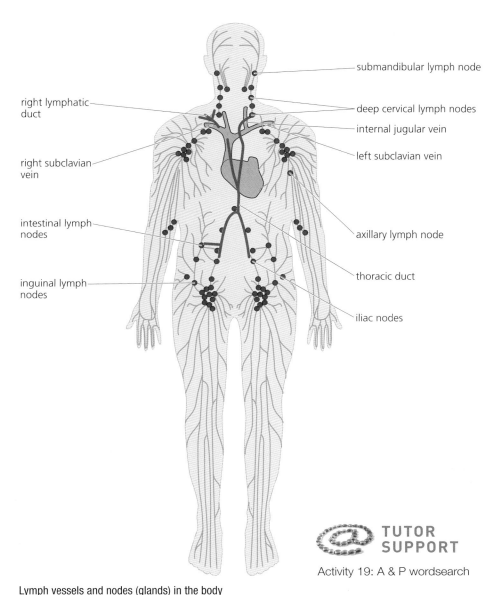

submandibular lymph node

deep cervical lymph nodes

internal jugular vein

left subclavian vein

axillary lymph node

thoracic duct

iliac nodes

right lymphatic duct

right subclavian vein

intestinal lymph nodes

inguinal lymph nodes

Lymph vessels and nodes (glands) in the body

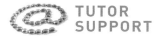

TUTOR SUPPORT

Activity 16: Label lymph nodes of the body

TUTOR SUPPORT

Activity 19: A & P wordsearch

These principal lymphatic vessels then empty their contents into a vein at the base of the neck, which in turn empties into the **vena cava**. The lymph is mixed into the venous blood as it is returned to the heart.

Lymph nodes

Lymph nodes or **glands** are tiny oval structures made from lymphatic tissue encased in a fibrous capsule which filters the lymph, extracting poisons, pus and bacteria, and thus defending the body against infection by destroying harmful organisms. They are located along the routes of the principal lymphatic vessels. **Lymphocytes** and macrophages, found in the lymph glands, are special cells which produce **antibodies** which enable us to resist invasion by microorganisms, preventing disease.

Lymph filters through at least one lymph node before returning to the bloodstream.

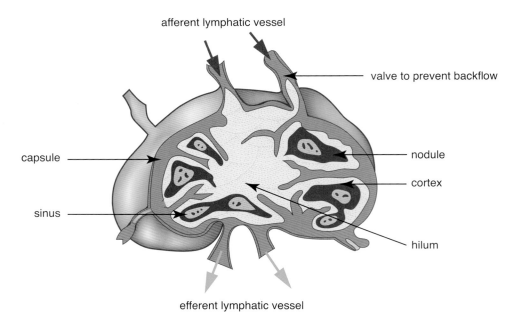

Lymph Node Structure

afferent lymphatic vessel

valve to prevent backflow

capsule

nodule

cortex

sinus

hilum

efferent lymphatic vessel

Lymph node

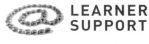

LEARNER SUPPORT

A & P mini crossword

When performing massage, the hands should be used to apply pressure to direct the lymph towards the nearest lymph node: this encourages the speedy removal of waste products. Various groups of lymph nodes drain the lymph of the head and neck.

Lymph nodes of the head

- The buccal group drains the eyelids, the nose and the skin of the face.

- The mandibular group drains the chin, the lips, the nose and the cheeks.

- The **mastoid group** drains the skin of the ear and the temple area.

- The **occipital group** drains the back of the scalp and the upper neck.

- The **submental group** drains the chin and the lower lip.

- The **parotid group** drains the nose, eyelids and ears.

Lymph nodes of the neck

- The **superficial cervical group** drains the back of the head and the neck.

- The **lower deep cervical group** drains the back area of the scalp and the neck.

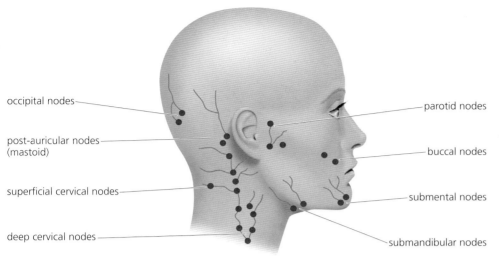

occipital nodes

post-auricular nodes (mastoid)

superficial cervical nodes

deep cervical nodes

parotid nodes

buccal nodes

submental nodes

submandibular nodes

Lymph nodes of the head and neck

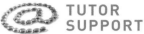

TUTOR SUPPORT

Activity 15: Label lymph nodes of the head

Lymph nodes of the chest and arms
The nodes of the armpit area drain various regions of the arms and chest.

TOP TIP

Frontal–Temporal–Parietal–Occipital–Mandible (mandibular)–Cervical

Learn and remember these names of the main regions of the head and neck. Not only will this assist you in recalling the names and locations of the bones, it will also help you greatly with the names and locations of muscles, arteries, veins, nerves and lymph nodes.

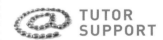

TUTOR SUPPORT

Activity 20: Multiple choice quiz

GLOSSARY OF KEY WORDS

Anagen the active growth stage of the hair growth cycle.

Apocrine gland sweat gland found in the armpit, nipple and groin area. Larger than the eccrine sweat gland and attached to the hair follicle. These sweat glands are controlled by hormones and become active at puberty.

Arrector pili muscle a small muscle attached to the hair follicle and base of the epidermis. When the muscle contracts (shortens) it causes the hair to stand upright in the hair follicle.

Blood nutritive liquid circulating through the blood vessels. It transports essential nutrients to the cells and removes waste

products. It also transports other important substances such as oxygen and hormones.

Blood vessel transports blood through the body in either an artery or a vein. An artery transports blood away from the heart at high pressure, the vein returns blood to the heart at low pressure.

Bone the hardest structure in the body. It protects the underlying structures, gives shape to the body and provides an attachment point for muscles.

Bones of the neck a type of connective tissue that supports the skull and includes the cervical vertebrae.

Bones of the chest a type of connective tissue that protects the inner organs, and provides a surface for muscle attachment that allows movement and includes the sternum.

Bones of foot and lower leg a type of connective tissue that provides a surface for muscle attachment. These include in the foot the tarsals, metatarsal and phalanxes. In the lower leg the tibia and fibula.

Bones of lower arm and hand a type of connective tissue that provide a surface for muscle attachment. These include in the lower arm the radius and ulna. In the hand the carpals, metacarpals and phalanges.

Catagen the stage of the hair growth cycle where the hair becomes detached from its source of nourishment, the dermal papilla, and stops growing.

Cell basic units of life which specialize in carrying out particular functions in the body. Groups of cells which share function, shape, size or structure are called tissues. The human body consists of trillions of cells.

Circulatory system transports material around the body.

Collagen protein fibre found in the dermis of the skin that gives the skin its strength.

Cortex the thickest layer of the hair structure.

Cyclical pattern of growth the hair growth cycle, which can be divided into three phases: anagen, catagen and telegen.

Dermal papilla an organ that provides the hair with blood, necessary for hair growth.

Dermis the inner portion of skin situated underneath the epidermis.

Eccrine gland simple sweat producing gland responsive to heat, appearing as tiny tubes which are straight in the epidermis, and coiled in the dermis. Its function is to maintain the body temperature by sweating.

Elastin protein fibre found in the dermis of the skin which gives the skin its elasticity.

Epidermis the outer layer of the skin.

External ear structure funnels sound waves into the ear to enable hearing. It comprises the pinna, lobe, cartilage and cartilaginous tissue.

Facial bones a type of connective tissue forming a hard structure that forms the face and forms an attachment point for muscles. These include the zygomatic, mandible, maxilla, nasal, vomer, turbinate, lacrimal and palatine.

Hair a long slender structure that grows out of, and is part of the skin. Each hair is made up of dead skin cells, which contain the protein called keratin.

Hair follicle an appendage (structure) in the skin formed from epidermal tissue. Cells move up the hair follicle from the bottom (the hair bulb), changing in structure, to form the hair.

Keratin a protein produced by cells in the epidermis called keratinocytes. Keratin makes the skin tough and reduces the passage of substances into our bodies. Each hair and nail contains keratin.

Lymph a clear, straw-coloured liquid circulating in the lymph vessels and lymphatics of the body, filtered out of the blood plasma.

Lymphatic system closely connected to the blood system. Its primary function is defensive: to remove bacteria and foreign materials to prevent infection.

Lymph vessel referred to as lymphatics. They transport lymph a watery fluid that flows through the lymphatic system from the tissues to the blood.

Melanin a pigment in the skin and hair that contributes to skin and hair colour.

Melanocytes cells that produce the skin pigment melanin that contributes to skin colour.

Muscle contractile tissue responsible for movement of the body.

Muscle tone the normal degree of tension in healthy muscle.

Muscles that move the neck these include sternocleido mastoid, platysma, trapezius.

Muscles of facial expression muscles which when contracted, pull the facial skin in a particular way and create facial expressions. These include the frontalis, corrugators, temporalis, orbicularis oculi, levator labii, orbicularis oris, buccinators, risorius, mentalis, zygomaticus, masseter, depressor labii.

Muscles of foot and lower leg the muscles of the foot work together to help move the body. The foot is moved by muscles in the lower leg which pull on tendons that attach the muscle to the bone.

Muscle of lower arm and hand the hands and fingers are moved by muscles and tendons. The muscles that bend the

wrist in towards the forearm are flexors; the extensors straighten the wrist and hand.

Muscles of the upper body these move the arm and include pectoralis and deltoid.

Nail growth cells divide in the matrix and the nails grow forward over the nail bed until they reach the end of the finger. The nail cells harden as they grow through a process called keratinization.

Nail structure composed for protection the nail is made up of the following parts: nail plate, nail bed, matrix, cuticle, lunula, hyponychium, eponychium, nail wall, free edge, lateral nail fold.

Nails hard, horny, epidermal cells that protect the living nail bed of the fingers and toes.

Nerve a collection of single neurones surrounded by a protective sheath through which impulses are transmitted between the brain or spinal cord and another part of the body.

Neurones nerve cells which make up nervous tissue.

Nervous system co-ordinates the activities of the body by responding to stimuli received by sense organs.

Pigment the skin's and hair's colour, called melanin. The amount of pigment varies for each client, resulting in different skin/hair colour.

Sebaceous gland a minute sac-like organ usually associated with the hair follicle. The cells of the gland decompose and produce the skin's natural oil sebum. Found all over the body, except for the soles of the feet and the palms of the hands.

Sebum the skin's natural oil which keeps the skin supple.

Sensory nerve endings these nerves receive information and relay this to the brain. They are found near the skin's surface and respond to touch, pressure, temperature and pain.

(Hair) Shaft the part of the hair that can be seen above the skin's surface, extending from the hair follicle.

Shoulder girdle bones a type of connective tissue that provides attachment for the muscles which move the arms, and includes the clavicle and scapula.

Skin appendages structures within the skin including sweat glands (that excrete sweat), hair follicles (that produce hair), sebaceous glands (produce the skin's natural oil, sebum) and nails (a horny substance that protects the ends of the fingers/toes).

Skin characteristics while looking at the skin type, the skin additional characteristics may be seen. These include skin that may be sensitive, dehydrated, moist or oedematous (puffy).

Sweat gland or sudoriferous glands are composed of a specialized lining tissue called epithelial tissue. Their function is

to control body temperature through the evaporation of sweat from the surface of the skin.

Skin type the different physiological functioning of each person's skin dictates their skin type. There are four main skin types: normal (balanced), dry (lacking in oil), oily (excessive oil) and combination (a mixture of two skin types, e.g., dry and oily).

Skull bones a type of connective tissue forming a hard structure. It surrounds and protects the brain and forms an attachment point for muscles. These include the occipital, frontal, parietal, temporal, sphenoid and ethmoid.

Subcutaneous layer a layer of fatty tissue situated below the epidermis and dermis.

Telogen the resting stage of the hair growth cycle, when the hair is finally shed.

Terminal hair deep-rooted, thick, course, pigmented hair found on the scalp, underarms, pubic region, eyelash and brow areas.

Tissues cells in the body which specialize in carrying out particular functions. These include epithelial, connective, muscular and nervous tissue.

Vellus hair fine, downy and soft hair – found on the face and body.

Vitamin D a fatty substance in the skin converted to vitamin D with UV light from the sun. This circulates in the blood and with the mineral salts calcium and phosphorus helps the formation and maintenance of the health of the body's bones.

ASSESSMENT OF KNOWLEDGE AND UNDERSTANDING

You have now learnt about the related anatomy and physiology for the beauty therapy units with an essential knowledge requirement.

To test your level of knowledge, answer the following short questions. These will prepare you for your summative (final) assessment.

Skin structure and function

1 Referring to the cross section of the skin, name and briefly describe the function of the structures shown in 1–4.

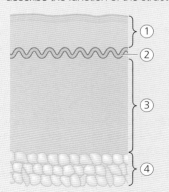

2 Name six functions of the skin.

3 Name the layers of the epidermis shown in 1–5. Which layer is continuously being shed?

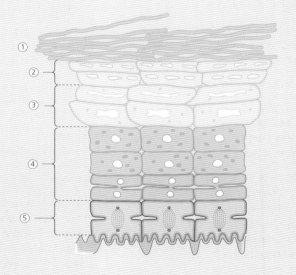

4 What are tissues? Name three types of body tissues.

5 Describe the structure of the dermis and label the illustration of the dermis shown below.

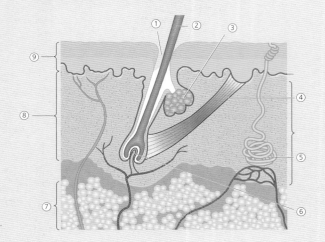

6 What is the function of the sensory nerves in the skin?

7 How is the temperature of the body regulated?

8 What gives the skin its colour? How does the skin become tanned on exposure to ultra-violet light?

9 Name two appendages of the skin and describe their function.

10 Name two protein fibres found in the reticular layer of the skin and describe their functions.

Structure of hair

1 Referring to the cross section of the hair follicle, briefly describe the name and function of each numbered area.

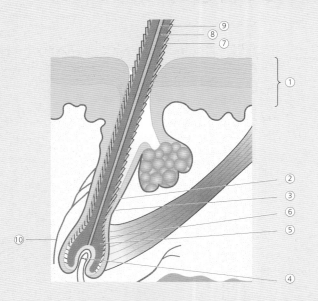

2 What is the soft downy hair on the face called?

3 What is coarse pigmented hair called?

4 What is the name of the protein found in skin cells?

5 What is the function of the dermal papilla in relation to the hair and the hair growth cycle?

Hair growth cycle

1 What are the different stages of the hair growth cycle called?

2 What happens to the hair at each stage?

3 What relevance has the hair growth cycle for a wax depilation service?

4 What is the difference in the time between the hair growth cycle anagen to telogen for scalp hair and eyebrow hair?

Nail structure and function

1 Referring to the cross section of the nail, briefly describe the name and function of each of the numbered areas.

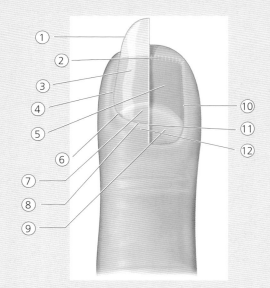

2 Why does the nail bed appear pink?

3 Why does the nail bed contain nerve endings?

Nail growth

1 In which part of the nail structure do the cells divide to form the nail?

2 As the nail cells grow forward they harden; what is this process called?

3 How long does it take for a fingernail to grow from cuticle to free edge?

4 When do nails grow faster – in summer or winter?

5 What is the difference in growth rate between finger-nails and toenails?

6 Why does localized massage to the hand and foot encourage healthy nail growth?

7 What other factors affect nail growth?

Muscle groups in parts of the body: position, structure and function

1 What happens when muscles contract?

2 What structure attaches a muscle to a bone?

3 On the diagram of the muscles of the face, name muscles 1–6. What are the actions of these muscles?

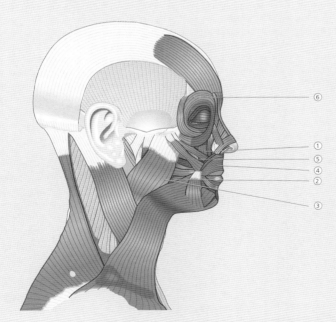

4 On the diagram of muscles that move the head and neck, name muscles 1–5. What are the actions of these muscles?

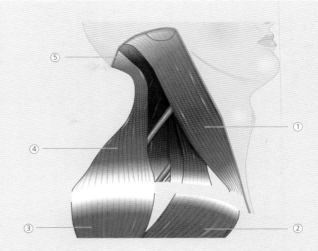

5 What is the collective name for the group of muscles that bend the wrist, drawing it towards the forearm?

6 What is the collective name for the group of muscles that straighten the wrist and the hand?

Muscle tone

1 What is muscle tone?

2 Name four properties of muscle tissue.

3 With age, the facial expressions that we make every day produce lines on the skin – frown lines. What happens to the tone of the muscles with age?

4 What effect does massage have on the tone of muscles?

Bones in parts of the body: position, structure and function

1 What is the function of bone?

2 Bones have different shapes according to their function. Name three shapes of bones and where they are found.

3 What attaches bones to different parts of the body?

4 On the diagram of the cranium name the bones numbered 1–8.

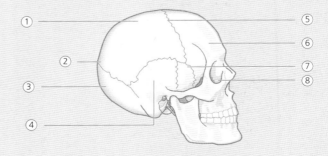

5 Name three facial bones to which you may apply contouring products during make-up.

6 Which of the bones form the:

- face?
- cranium?

7 Name the bone or bones that form the:

- forehead
- cheekbones
- jawbone

8 On the diagram of the bones of the neck, chest and shoulder name the bones and their functions (items 1–7).

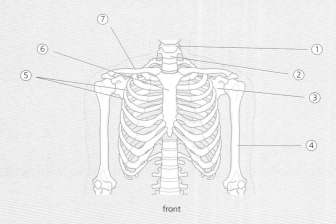

front

9 The wrist is made up of eight small carpal bones, which glide over one another to allow movement. Name them.

10 What type of joint is found in the wrist?

11 How do the fingers move?

12 Name and discuss the function of the arches of the foot.

13 Name the bones that form the ankle.

Composition and function of blood and lymph

1 What are the main constituents of blood?

2 What are the main constituents of lymph?

3 What does blood transport around the body?

4 What is the difference in function in the body between blood and lymph?

5 What is the function of lymph nodes or glands?

6 On the diagram of the head, name the lymph nodes numbered 1–5.

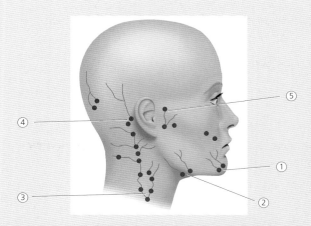

7 Blood helps to maintain body temperature. What is normal body temperature?

8 How does massage affect the circulation of lymph?

Blood flow and pulse rate

1 The circulation of the blood is under the control of the heart, which pumps blood around the body. On the illustration below label the arteries that transport blood to the head and veins that return blood from the head.

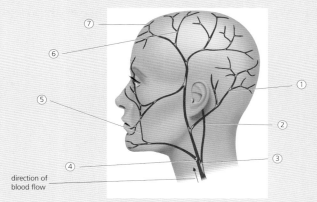

direction of blood flow

Blood supply to the head

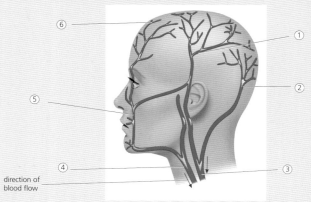

direction of blood flow

Blood supply from the head

2 How does the pressure of blood leaving the heart affect pulse rate?

3 How does activity affect blood pressure?

4 How does massage affect blood flow and pulse rate?

Central nervous system and autonomic nervous system

1 The neurological system transmits messages between the brain and other parts of the body. There are two main divisions. What are they called?

2 What is the central nervous system composed of?

3 What is the difference between sensory nerves and motor nerves?

4 To what are the main sensory nerve endings in the skin receptive?

5 How do nerve impulses pass along nerve fibres?

6 How do nerves stimulate muscles to contract?

7 What is meant by the autonomic nervous system?

8 How many pairs of cranial nerves emerge from the brain?

9 Those of concern to the beauty therapist when performing facial massage are the 5th, 7th and 11th cranial nerves.

What is the function of the:

- 5th, known as trigeminal nerve?
- 7th, known as the facial nerve?
- 11th, known as the accessory nerve?

10 Name the main branches of the 7th cranial facial nerve, items 1–5 in the diagram.

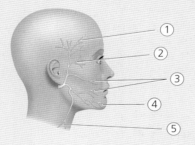

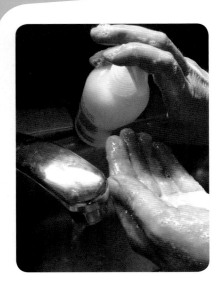

3 Health and Safety (G20)

Taking care of all in the workplace

When working in a service industry, you are legally obliged to provide a **safe and hygienic environment**. This applies wherever you are working: in a hotel, a spa, a department store or a beauty salon. Even when operating a freelance beauty therapy service, you must pay careful attention to clients' homes: it is essential to follow the normal health and safety guidelines, just as you would when working in a salon.

This chapter is for everyone at work whatever their status.

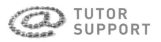

TUTOR SUPPORT

Activity 6: Health and safety wordsearch

Outcome 1: Identify the hazards and evaluate the risks in your workplace

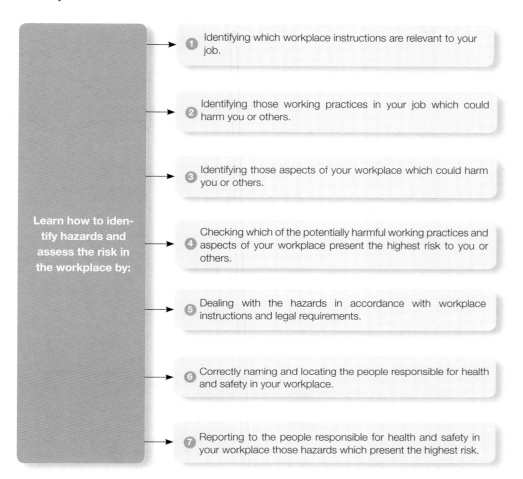

Learn how to identify hazards and assess the risk in the workplace by:

1 Identifying which workplace instructions are relevant to your job.

2 Identifying those working practices in your job which could harm you or others.

3 Identifying those aspects of your workplace which could harm you or others.

4 Checking which of the potentially harmful working practices and aspects of your workplace present the highest risk to you or others.

5 Dealing with the hazards in accordance with workplace instructions and legal requirements.

6 Correctly naming and locating the people responsible for health and safety in your workplace.

7 Reporting to the people responsible for health and safety in your workplace those hazards which present the highest risk.

Legal responsibilities

If you cause harm to your client, or put a client at risk, you will be held responsible and you will be liable for **prosecution**, with the possibility of being fined.

There is a good deal of legislation relating to health and safety. You will need to know the laws relating to beauty therapy. Details are widely available and you must be aware of your responsibilities and your rights. It is important that you obtain and read all relevant publications from your local Health and Safety Executive (HSE) offices. The HSE provides guidance and information on all aspects of health and safety legislation.

In addition, as the standards-setting body for beauty therapy, the hair and beauty industry authority Habia provide health and safety working guidelines and legislative requirements. **Codes of practice** are available from Habia sharing best and mandatory working practice approved by both industry experts and health and safety advisors. Approved codes of practice are recognized by the HSE.

Outcome 2: Reduce the risks to health and safety in your workplace

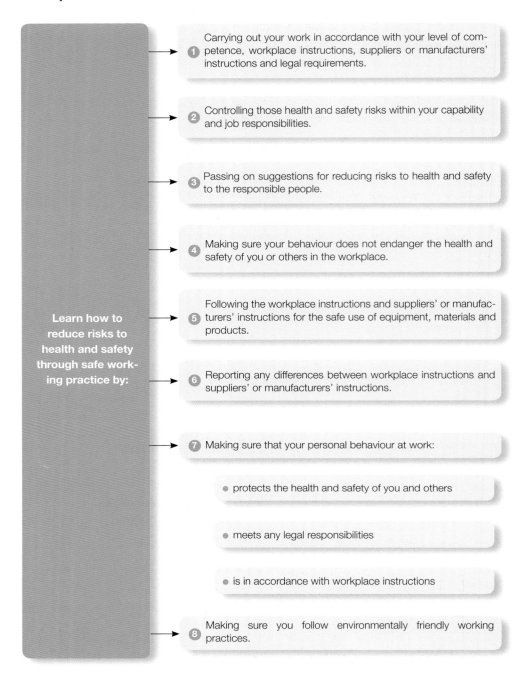

Learn how to reduce risks to health and safety through safe working practice by:

1. Carrying out your work in accordance with your level of competence, workplace instructions, suppliers or manufacturers' instructions and legal requirements.

2. Controlling those health and safety risks within your capability and job responsibilities.

3. Passing on suggestions for reducing risks to health and safety to the responsible people.

4. Making sure your behaviour does not endanger the health and safety of you or others in the workplace.

5. Following the workplace instructions and suppliers' or manufacturers' instructions for the safe use of equipment, materials and products.

6. Reporting any differences between workplace instructions and suppliers' or manufacturers' instructions.

7. Making sure that your personal behaviour at work:

   - protects the health and safety of you and others

   - meets any legal responsibilities

   - is in accordance with workplace instructions

8. Making sure you follow environmentally friendly working practices.

The Health and Safety at Work Act (1974) (HASAWA) The Health and Safety at Work Act (1974) is continually reviewed and is the main piece of legislation affecting these issues. It was developed from experience gained over 150 years and incorporates earlier legislation, including the Offices, Shops and Railway Premises Act (1963) and the Fire Precautions Act (1971). It lays down the minimum standards of health, safety and welfare required in each area of the workplace. For example, it requires business premises and equipment to be safe and in good repair. It is the employer's legal responsibility to implement the Act and to ensure, so far as is reasonably practicable, the health and safety at work of the people for whom they are responsible and those who may be affected by the work they do.

The Local Authority Environmental Health Department appoints inspectors called Environmental Health Officers (EHOs) to enforce health and safety law by visiting the workplace to check compliance is being met with all relevant health and safety legislation. Workplace Contract Officers (WCOs) are available to provide advice and guidance and gather relevant data in relation to health and safety of your business.

The Health and Safety (Information for Employees) Regulations (1989) (HSIER) were amended in April 2009, making changes to Health and Safety Law posters.

Each employer of more than five employees must formulate a written **health and safety policy** for their business. The health and safety policy identifies how health and safety is managed for that business, who does what, when and why. The policy must be issued and discussed with each employee at induction and should outline the health and safety responsibilities they should undertake. It should also include items such as:

- details of the storage of chemical substances
- details of the stock cupboard or dispensary
- details and records of the checks made by a qualified electrician on specialist electrical equipment
- names and addresses of key holders
- escape routes and emergency evacuation procedures
- whom to report emergencies and significant risks to

The health and safety policy should be reviewed regularly to ensure it meets all relevant legislation guidelines including updates. Health and safety training should also be carried out and recorded. Regular health and safety checks should be made and procedures reviewed to ensure that safety is being satisfactorily maintained.

Employees must cooperate with their employer to provide a safe and healthy workplace. As soon as an employee observes a **hazard** (anything that has potential to cause harm) this must be reported to the designated authority so that the problem can be put right. Hazards include:

- obstructions to corridors, stairways and fire exits (an obstruction is anything that blocks the traffic route in the salon work environment)
- spillages and breakages

Deal with low risk hazards within your responsibility, following **workplace policy** and legal requirements.

If there are fewer than five employees, appropriate health and safety arrangements and procedures should be in place. In 1992, European Union (EU) directives updated the legislation on health and safety management. Current legislation (at the time of writing – 2009) is outlined below.

The Health and Safety at Work Act covers many other smaller regulations also which are discussed.

Health and safety rules and regulations and examples of compliance to be displayed include:

- the fire evacuation procedures
- Public Liability insurance certificate

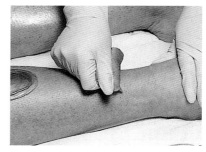

Ensure you follow health and safety guidelines when carrying out services such as removing hot wax

ACTIVITY

Health and safety rules
Discuss the rules which apply to you in your workplace's health and safety policy. The health and safety policy identifies how health and safety is managed: who does what, when and why.

HEALTH & SAFETY

Health and safety law notice
Every employer is obliged by law to display a health and safety law poster in the workplace. This explains the responsibilities of employers and also employees, what action to take if a health and safety problem arises and employment rights. A leaflet is available called 'Your health and safety – a guide for workers'. Both poster and leaflets are available from the HSE.

HEALTH & SAFETY

Lone workers
If you are self employed and work alone, consider your safety. Guidance is provided in the information 'Working alone in safety – controlling the risks of solitary work' INDG73 (rev2).

HEALTH & SAFETY

Non-smoking legislation
An example of the need to be responsive to safe working conditions and practices is the non-smoking legislation in the workplace, introduced 1 July 2007.

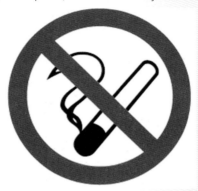

No smoking sign.

HEALTH & SAFETY

Five steps to risk assessment
This is an HSE publication providing guidance on risk assessment.

HEALTH & SAFETY

Protective equipment: gloves
If you are to come into contact with body tissue fluids or with chemicals, wear protective disposable surgical gloves. Latex gloves can cause allergic reactions and in some cases the development of asthma, and are not recommended.
An alternative glove that provides adequate protection from contamination should be used, e.g. nitrile or PVC formulation.

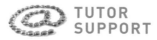

TUTOR SUPPORT

Activity 3: Risk assessment form

- Health and Safety (Information for Employees) Regulations (1989) poster updated April 2009. The previous poster can continue to be displayed until 2014
- health and safety policy (dependent upon employee numbers)
- risk assessment records and guidance.

The Management of Health and Safety at Work Regulations (1999)
These require employers to make formal arrangements for maintaining and improving safe working conditions and practices under the Health and Safety at Work Act. This includes training for employees to ensure competency and to monitor risk in the workplace (including product use), known as risk assessment. Employers with five or more employees need to record important risk assessment findings. Employers need to:

- identify potential hazards
- assess the potential risks associated with the hazard
- identify who is at risk from the hazard
- identify how the risk is to be minimized or eliminated
- set up emergency procedures
- train staff to identify and control risk
- regularly review the risk assessment process

The Personal Protective Equipment (PPE) at Work Regulations (2002)
The Personal Protective Equipment (PPE) at Work Regulations (1992) require employers to identify – through a **risk assessment** – those activities or processes which require special protective clothing or equipment to be worn. This clothing and equipment must then be made available, and must be suitable and in adequate supplies. Employees must wear the protective clothing and use the protective equipment provided, and make employers aware of any shortage so that supplies can be maintained.

Training should be provided on the correct use and application of PPE and its use should be monitored. If not used the reason should be investigated as this becomes a risk.

PPE should be 'CE' marked – that it complies with the Personal Protective Equipment at Work Regulations 1992, and satisfies basic safety requirements.

The Workplace (Health, Safety and Welfare) Regulations (1992)
The Workplace (Health, Safety and Welfare) Regulations (1992) cover a broad range of basic health, safety and welfare issues and require all that work to maintain a safe, healthy and secure working environment. These regulations aim to ensure the workplace meets the health, safety and welfare needs of all the employees including those with disabilities, and accessibility should be made where practicable. The regulations include legal requirements in relation to the following aspects of the working environment:

- Maintenance of the workplace and equipment
- Ventilation to ensure the air is changed regularly and fumes or strong smells are removed. Fresh air should be drawn from outside the workplace.
- Working temperature

- Lighting adequate to enable people to move safely and perform tasks competently

- Cleanliness of furniture, equipment, furnishing and fittings and correct handling and disposal of waste materials

- Safe salon layout, dimensions adequate for traffic flow (pedestrian traffic) and nature of the work

- Safety: falls and falling objects, objects should be stored safely

- Windows, doors, gates and walls should be safe and fit for purpose

- Safe floor and traffic routes

- Escalators and moving walkways should operate safely and have appropriate safety mechanisms

- Sanitary conveniences for all staff and clients: suitable and sufficient

- Washing facilities: hot and cold running water should be available with soap and a means of drying hands

- Drinking water: adequate supply

- Facilities for changing and storage of clothing should be adequate and secure

- Facilities for staff to rest and eat meals should be suitable

- Fire exits and fire fighting equipment

Manual Handling Operations Regulations (1992) The Manual Handling Operations Regulations (1992) apply in all occupations where manual lifting occurs, the aim being to prevent skeletal and muscular disorders and repetitive strain disorders due to poor working practice. The employer is required to carry out a risk assessment of all activities undertaken which involve manual lifting.

The risk assessment should provide evidence that the following have been considered:

- risk of injury

- the manual movement involved in performing the activity

- the physical constraint the load incurs

- the environmental constraints imposed by the workplace

- workers' individual capabilities

- action taken to minimize potential risks

Manual lifting and handling Always take care of yourself when moving goods around the salon. Assess the risk. Do not struggle or be impatient: get someone else to help. When **lifting**, reduce the risk; lift from the knees, not the back. When **carrying**, balance weights evenly in both hands and carry the heaviest part nearest to your body.

Provision and Use of Work Equipment Regulations (PUWER) (1998) The Provision and Use of Work Equipment Regulations (PUWER) (1998) lay down the important health and safety controls on the provision and use of work equipment. They state the duties for employers and for users, including the self-employed.

ACTIVITY

PPE Risk assessment
Carry out your own risk assessment on risks of cross-infection by contamination. List the potentially hazardous substances that you may be required to handle. What protective clothing should be available?

ACTIVITY

Moving objects in the salon
What equipment or objects may you be required to move in the salon? Think of three examples and how best they should be lifted and handled.

BEST PRACTICE

Broken goods
When you unpack a delivery, make sure the product packaging is undamaged, to avoid possible personal injury from broken goods.

ACTIVITY

European directives
As a result of directives adopted in 1992 by the European Union, health and safety legislation has been updated.

1 Obtain a copy of the eight directives. *Workplace (Health & Safety & Welfare) Regulations 1992.*

2 Look through the publication, and make notes on any information relevant to you in the workplace.

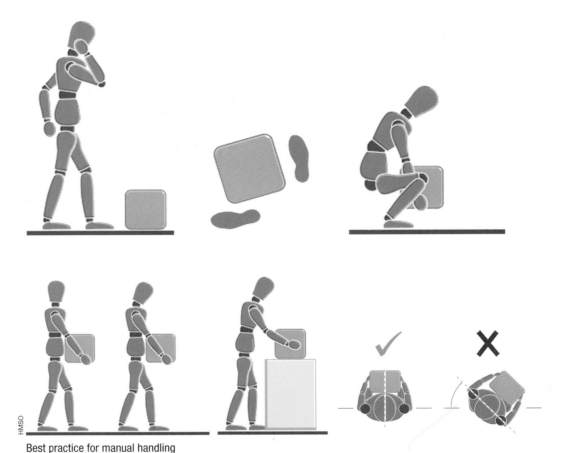

Best practice for manual handling

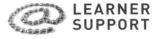

LEARNER SUPPORT

Health & safety fill-in-the-blanks

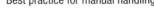

ALWAYS REMEMBER

Temperature and lighting

The salon temperature should be a minimum of 16°C within one hour of employees arriving for work. The salon should be well ventilated, or carbon dioxide levels will increase, which can cause nausea. Many substances used in the salon can become hazardous without adequate ventilation. If the working environment is too warm this can cause heat stress, a condition that is recognized by the HSE. Lighting should be adequate to ensure that services can be carried out safely and competently, with the minimum risk of accident.

They affect both old and new equipment. They identify the requirements in selecting suitable equipment and in maintaining it. They also discuss the information provided by equipment manufacturers, and instruction and training in the safe use of equipment. Specific regulations address the dangers and potential risks of injury that could occur during operation of the equipment.

Health and Safety (Display Screen Equipment) Regulations (1992) The **Health and Safety (Display Screen Equipment) Regulations (1992)** cover the use of display screen equipment and computer screens. They specify acceptable levels of radiation emissions from the screen and identify correct posture, seating position, permitted working heights and rest periods. Employers have a responsibility to comply with this regulation to ensure the welfare of their employees in avoiding the potential risks of eyestrain, mental stress and muscle fatigue.

Control of Substances Hazardous to Health (COSHH) Regulations (2002) The **Control of Substances Hazardous to Health (COSHH) Regulations (2002)** were designed to make employers consider the substances used in their workplace and assess the possible risks to health. Many substances that seem quite harmless can prove to be hazardous if used or stored incorrectly. Hazardous substances are anything that can harm your health.

Employers are responsible for assessing the risks from hazardous substances and controlling exposure to them to prevent ill health. Any hazardous substances identified must

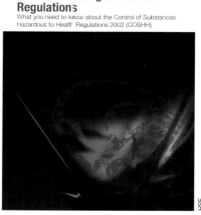

COSHH information packs available from beauty suppliers

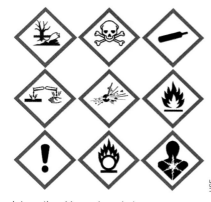

COSHH regulations

International hazard symbols

be formally recorded in writing. Safety precaution procedures should then be implemented and training given to employees to ensure that the procedures are understood and will be followed correctly. Employers must control substances that can harm employees' health.

Hazardous substances are identified by the use of known symbols, examples of which are shown below. Any substance in the workplace that is hazardous to health must be identified on the packaging and stored and handled correctly.

Hazardous substances can enter the body via the:

- eyes
- skin
- nose (**inhalation**)
- mouth (**ingestion**)

Each beauty product supplier is legally required to make guidelines available on how materials should be used and stored. These are called material safety data sheets (MSDSs) and will be supplied on request.

Cosmetic Products (Safety) Regulations (2008) The Cosmetic Products (Safety) Regulations (2008) consolidates earlier regulations and incorporates current European directives. Part of consumer protective legislation, it requires that cosmetics and toiletries are safe in their formulation and are safe for use for their intended purpose as a cosmetic before being placed on the market and comply with labelling requirements.

Electricity at Work Regulations (1989) The Electricity at Work Regulations (1989) state that every piece of electrical equipment in the workplace must be

HEALTH & SAFETY

COSHH assessment
All hazardous substances must be identified when completing the risk assessment. This includes cleaning agents such as a wax equipment cleaner.

High-risk products should, where possible, be replaced with lower risk products.

COSHH assessments should be reviewed on a regular basis and updated to include any new products.

HEALTH & SAFETY

Hazardous substances
Potentially hazardous substances include:

- aerosols
- disinfectants
- water treatment chemicals used in spa pools

ACTIVITY

Identifying hazards
Make a list of potential electrical hazards in the workplace e.g. damaged plugs. Who should these be reported to?

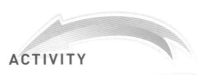

ACTIVITY

COSHH assessment
Carry out a COSHH assessment on selected service products used in the salon. Consider nail services, waxing and facial and eye services.

TOP TIP

COSHH essential information for beauticians is available on the HSE website in a section called, COSHH and your industry. How does COSHH affect you?

HEALTH & SAFETY

Breakages and spillages
When dealing with hazardous breakages and spillages, the hands should always be protected with gloves. To avoid injury to others, broken glass should be put in a secure container prior to disposing of it in a waste bin, in compliance with waste disposal regulations.

TUTOR SUPPORT

Activity 4: Salon manager report form

tested every 12 months by a qualified electrician. This is called portable appliance testing or (PAT). A written record of testing must be retained and made available for inspection. A list of all salon electrical equipment should be available with its unique serial number and date of purchase/disposal.

In addition to annual testing, a trained member of staff should regularly check all electrical equipment for safety. This is recommended every three months. Report to your supervisor if you see any of these potential hazards:

- exposed wires in flexes
- cracked plugs or broken sockets
- worn cables
- overloaded sockets

Although it is the employer's responsibility to ensure all equipment is safe to use, it is also the responsibility of the employee to check that equipment is safe before use, and never to use it if it is faulty. This complies with the requirements of public liability insurance. Failure to do so could lead to an accident which would be considered negligent.

Any pieces of equipment that appear faulty must be checked immediately and, if necessary, repaired before use. If faulty they must be labelled to ensure that they are not used by accident.

Accidents

Accidents in the workplace usually occur through negligence by employees or unsafe working conditions.

Any accidents occurring the workplace must be recorded on a **report form**, and entered into an **accident book**. Incidents in the accident book should be reviewed regularly to see where improvements to working practice can be made. The **accident form** requires more details than the accident book. You must note:

- the date and time of the accident
- the date of entry into the accident book
- the name of the person or people involved
- the accident details
- the injuries sustained
- the action taken
- the signature of the person making the entry

In the instance of an accident, first aid should only be administered by employees qualified to do so.

Breakages and spillage Accidents can damage stock, resulting in breakage of containers and spillage of contents. Breakage of glass can cause cuts; spillages can cause somebody to slip and fall. Any breakages or spillages should therefore be dealt with immediately and in the correct way.

You must determine whether the spillage is a potential hazard to health and what action is necessary. To whom should you report it? What equipment is required to remove the spillage? How should the materials be disposed of? Always consider your COSHH data and check to see how the product should be handled and disposed of.

Reporting of Injuries, Diseases and Dangerous Occurrences Regulations (RIDDOR) (1995)

The Reporting of Injuries, Diseases and Dangerous Occurrences Regulations (RIDDOR) (1995) requires employers, the self-employed and those in a position of control for the workplace to report workplace cases to the HSE Incident Contact Centre where employees or trainees suffer personal injury at work.

These cases include loss of sight, amputation, fracture and electric shock. When an occurrence results in death, major injury or more than 24 hours in hospital and incapacity to work for more than three calendar days, it can be reported via telephone, fax or the internet. In all cases where personal injury occurs, an entry must be made in the workplace accident book. Where visitors to the work premises are injured this must be reported also. A record of any reportable injury, disease or dangerous occurrence must be kept for three years after the date it happened or until the injured person is eighteen years old. This information assists the HSE in investigation of serious accidents.

First aid

The Health and Safety (First Aid) Regulations (1981) state that workplaces must have first aid provision. Employers must have appropriate and adequate first aid arrangements in the event of an accident or illness occurring. It is recommended that at least one person holds an HSE-approved basic first aid qualification.

All employees should be informed of the first aid procedures, including:

- where to find the first aid box
- who is responsible for the maintenance of the first aid box
- which member of staff to inform in the event of an accident or illness occurring
- the staff member to inform in the event of an accident or emergency

An adequately stocked first aid box that complies with health and safety first aid for your workplace needs should be available.

Basic items include:

- basic first aid guidance leaflet (1)
- assorted individually wrapped sterile adhesive dressings (20)
- individually wrapped sterile triangular bandages (6)
- safety pins (6)
- sterile eye pads, with attachments (2)
- medium-sized individually wrapped sterile unmedicated wound dressings, 10 cm x 8 cm (6)
- large individually wrapped sterile unmedicated wound dressings 13 cm x 9 cm (2)

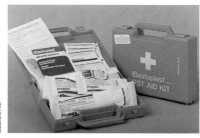

First aid kits

- extra large sterile individually wrapped medicated wound dressings 28 cm x 17.5 cm (3)
- individually wrapped medical wipes

Where clean tap water is not readily available, sterile water should be stored in sealed containers for bathing eyes.

Examples of first aid procedures

Problem	Action to be taken
Casualty is not breathing	1 Place the casualty on their back. Open and clear their mouth. Shout for help. 2 Tilt head backwards to open airway (maintain this position throughout). Support the jaw. 3 Kneel beside casualty, while keeping head backwards. Open mouth and pinch nose. 4 Open your mouth and take a deep breath. Seal mouth with yours and breathe firmly into it. Casualty's chest should rise. Remove your mouth and let their chest fall. If chest does not rise, check head is tilted sufficiently. Repeat at a rate of ten times a minute until the casualty is breathing alone. 5 Place them in the recovery position. 6 If not breathing normally call 999.
Unconscious	Place into recovery position.
Severe bleeding	Control by direct pressure using fingers and thumb on the bleeding point. Apply a dressing. Raising the bleeding limb (unless it is broken) will reduce the flow of blood.
Suspected broken bones	Do not move the casualty unless they are in a position which exposes them to immediate danger. Gain expert help.
Burns and scalds (due to heat)	Do not remove clothing sticking to the burns or scalds. Do not burst any blisters. If burns and scalds are small, flush them with plenty of clean, cool water for ten minutes before applying a sterilized dressing. If burns and scalds are large or deep, wash your hands, apply a dry sterilized dressing and send the casualty to hospital.
Burns (chemicals)	Avoid contaminating yourself with the chemical. Remove any contaminated clothing that is not stuck to skin. Flush with plenty of cool water for 10–15 minutes. Apply a sterilized dressing and send to hospital.
Foreign body in eye	Wash out eye with clean cool water or sterile fluid in a sealed container. A person with an eye injury should be sent to hospital with the eye covered by an eye pad. Never attempt to remove the foreign body.
Chemicals in eyes	Wash out the open eye continuously with clean, cool water for 10–15 minutes gently holding the eye lid open. A person with an eye injury should be sent to hospital with the eye covered with an eye pad.
Electric shock	Don't touch the casualty until the current is switched off. If the current cannot be switched off, stand on some dry insulating material and use a wooden or plastic implement to free the casualty from the electrical source. If breathing has stopped start mouth-to-mouth breathing and continue until the casualty starts to breathe by themselves or until professional help arrives.
Gassing	Use suitable protective equipment. Move casualty to fresh air. If breathing has stopped start mouth-to-mouth breathing and continue until the casualty is breathing by themself or until professional help arrives. Send to hospital with a note of the gas involved.
Minor injuries	Casualties with minor injuries of a nature they would normally attend to themselves may wash their hands and apply a small sterilized dressing from the first aid box. Keep wounds clean and dry.

Disposal of waste

Waste should be disposed of in an enclosed waste bin fitted with a polythene bin liner that is durable enough not to tear. The bin should be regularly disinfected in a well-ventilated area: wear protective gloves while doing this. Hazardous waste must be disposed of following the COSHH procedures and training by the employer.

Clinical (contaminated) waste is waste derived from human tissues. This includes blood and tissue fluids. **Clinical waste**, such as wax strips, should be disposed of as recommended by the Environment Agency in accordance with the **Controlled Waste (Amendment) Regulations (1993)**. Items which have been used to pierce the skin, such as disposable milia extractors, should be safely discarded in a disposable **sharps container**. Contact your local environment health department to check on disposal arrangements.

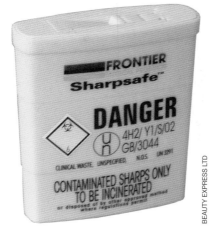

Sharps container

Inspection and registration of premises

Inspectors from the HSE or your local authority enforce Health and Safety law. They visit the workplace to ensure compliance with government legislation is being met.

If the inspector identifies any area of danger, it is the responsibility of the employer to remove this danger within a designated period of time. The inspector issues an **improvement notice**. Failure to comply with the notice will lead to prosecution. The inspector also has the authority to close a business or stop a particular activity until they are satisfied that all danger to employees and public has been removed. Such closure involves the issuing of a **prohibition notice**.

TUTOR SUPPORT

Activity 2: Accident report form

Certain services carried out in beauty therapy, such as ear piercing, pose additional risk because they might produce blood and body tissue fluid. Inspection of the premises is necessary before such services can be offered to the public. The inspector will visit to make sure that the guidelines listed in the **Local Government (Miscellaneous Provisions) Act (1982)** relating to this area are being complied with in terms of levels of hygiene and training. Good infection control systems are essential and the working environment must be suitable. When the inspector is satisfied, a certificate of registration will be awarded.

Fire

The **Regulatory Reform (Fire Safety) Order (2005)** replaces all previous legislation relating to fire, including fire certificates which no longer have any validity. This law is applicable to England and Wales only. Northern Ireland and Scotland have their own similar legislation.

The Regulatory Reform (Fire Safety) Order (2005) places responsibility for fire safety onto the 'responsible person' which is usually the employer. The 'responsible person' will have a duty to ensure the safety of everyone who uses their premises and those in the immediate vicinity who may be at risk if there is a fire. The 'responsible person' must carry out a fire safety risk assessment.

Fire risk assessments will include:

● Identifying and removing any obstacles that may hinder fire evacuation

● Ensuring that suitable fire detection equipment is in place, such as a **smoke alarm**

Fire alarm

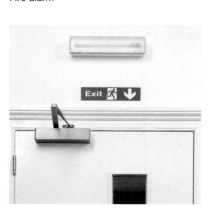

Fire exit door

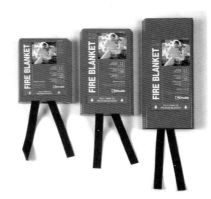

Fire blankets

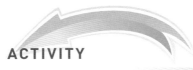

ACTIVITY

Fire drill

Each workplace should have a fire drill regularly. This enables staff to practise so that they know what to do in the event of a real fire. What is the fire drill procedure in your workplace?

HEALTH & SAFETY

Fire!

If there is a fire, never use a lift. A fire quickly becomes out of control. You do not have very long to act!

Fire drill notices should be visible to show people to the emergency exit route.

HEALTH & SAFETY

Fire exits

Fire-exit doors must be clearly marked, remain unlocked during working hours and be free from obstruction.

- Making sure that all escape routes are clearly marked and free from obstacles

- Testing fire alarm systems regularly to ensure they are in full operational condition

All staff must be trained in fire and emergency evacuation procedures for their workplace. The **emergency exit route** will be the easiest route by which staff and clients can leave the building safely. Fire action plans should be prominently displayed to show the emergency exit route. Fire-fighting equipment should be available and maintained, to be used only by those trained to use it.

Fire-fighting equipment Fire-fighting equipment must be available, located in a specified area. The equipment includes fire extinguishers, blankets, sand buckets and water hoses. Fire-fighting equipment should be used only when the cause of the fire has been identified – using the *wrong* fire extinguisher could make the fire worse.

Fire classifications include class A, B and C. Symbols are used to identify these classifications and choice of fire extinguisher as shown below:

Class D Fires involve metals.

Never use fire-fighting equipment unless you are trained in its use.

Class A Fire – Carbonaceous materials such as paper and wood.

Class B Fire – Flammable liquids such as petrol, oil and paints.

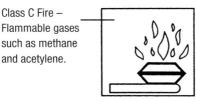

Class C Fire – Flammable gases such as methane and acetylene.

Electrical hazard symbol – For extinguisher products safe on electrical fires.

Fire extinguisher symbols

Fire extinguishers Fire extinguishers are available to tackle different types of fire. These should be located in a set place known to all employees. It is important that these are checked and maintained as required.

Fire blankets are used to smother a small, localized fire or if a person's clothing is on fire. **Sand** is used to soak up liquids if these are the source of the fire, and to smother the fire. **Water hoses** are used to extinguish large fires caused by paper materials and the like – buckets of water can be used to extinguish a small fire. *Remember turn off the electricity at the mains first!*

Never put yourself at risk – fires can spread quickly. Leave the building at once if in danger and raise the alarm by telephoning the emergency services on the emergency telephone numbers, **999** or **112**.

KNOW YOUR FIRE EXTINGUISHER COLOUR CODE

Cylinder Colour Coding and Contents

Classification of Fire Risk	WATER	FOAM	CO₂ CARBON DIOXIDE	DRY POWDER	VAPOURISING LIQUIDS
	Unsafe all voltages Wood, Paper Textiles etc.	Unsafe all voltages Flammable liquids	Safe all voltages Flammable liquids	Safe all voltages Flammable liquids	Safe all voltages Flammable liquids
A Paper, Wood, Textile and Fabric	✓	✓		✓	✓
B Flammable Liquids		✓	✓	✓	✓
C Flammable Gases			✓	✓	✓
Electrical Hazards			✓	✓	✓
Vehicle Protection		✓		✓	✓

COLOUR CODING IN ACCORDANCE WITH BS EN3: 1996 - PORTABLE FIRE EXTINGUISHERS FLAMMABLE GAS FIRES MUST BE EXTINGUISHED BY THE EMERGENCY SERVICES ONLY

Fire extinguisher label colour code

Cause of fire and choice of fire extinguisher

Cause	Extinguisher type	Lable colour code
Electrical fire	Carbon dioxide (CO_2) extinguisher.	Black.
Solid material fire (paper, wood, etc.)	Water extinguisher.	Red.
Flammable liquids	Foam extinguisher.	Cream/yellow.
Electrical Fire	Dry-powder extinguisher.	Blue.
Flammable metal fires	Vapourizing liquid.	Green.

Other emergencies

Other possible emergencies that could occur relate to fumes and flooding. Learn where the water and gas stopcocks are located. In the event of a gas leak or a flood, the stopcocks should be switched off and the appropriate emergency service contacted.

ALWAYS REMEMBER

Fire extinguishers
Label colour and symbols indicate the use of particular fire extinguishers. Make sure you know the meaning of each of the colours and symbols.

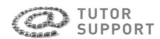

TUTOR SUPPORT

Activity 1: Firefighting equipment handout

HEALTH & SAFETY

Using fire extinguishers
The vapours emitted when using vapourizing liquid extinguishers 'starve' a fire of oxygen. They are therefore dangerous when used in confined spaces, as people need oxygen too!

ACTIVITY

Health and Safety awareness

Where can you find the following in your workplace:

1   fire extinguisher(s)?

2   information sheets stating how products should be stored/used. MSDS (Material Safety Data Sheets)?

3   health and safety workplace information?

4   first aid kit?

5   sterilization/disinfection equipment?

6   personal protective equipment (PPE)?

7   the fire exit/s?

8   accident book?

9   sharps box and waste bags for contaminated waste?

ACTIVITY

Noise levels

Assess the noise level at your workplace. Are there any intrusive noise levels preventing normal communication i.e., do voices need to be raised?

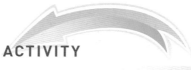

ACTIVITY

Causes of fires

Can you think of several potential causes of fire in the salon? How could each of these be prevented?

In the event of a bomb alert staff must be trained in the appropriate emergency procedures. This will involve recognition of a suspect package, how to deal with a bomb threat, evacuation of staff and clients and contacting the emergency services. Your local Crime Prevention Officer (CPO) will advise on bomb security.

Environmentally friendly working practices

Reflect on how you work, use and dispose of products within your work. Are you always environmentally friendly? Consider the following changes:

● use biodegradable packaging for disposal of non-contaminated waste

● for hospitality drinks rather than use disposable plastic cups revert back to cups and glasses that can be washed

● dispose of chemicals safely, not down the sinks

● use wooden spatulas from sustainable wood sources

● use recycled consumable materials where possible, e.g. bed-roll, tissues and cleaning products

● use light bulbs that minimize energy use

● switch off lights in rooms not being used and also equipment when not in use – if safe to do so

● turn down the heating thermostat rather than opening windows, this will save money too

● buy in bulk, reducing trips to the wholesaler, and buy locally

● recycle your waste and packaging where possible, use colour-coded waste bags that are of course made from recycled materials

● recycle used printer cartridges

● some beauty companies will provide a free product on the return of a used product packaging

Small steps can make a big difference.

Control of Noise at Work Regulations (2005)

Loud noise can damage hearing. Noise is measured in decibels (db). A-weighting is sometimes written as 'dB(A)' which is average noise level. C-weighting is 'dB(C)' – noise which is at its highest point, i.e., explosives.

As an employer a safe working environment should be provided with noise levels kept within safe levels. This does not include low-level noise. As in all workplace practices, noise levels can be classified as a risk. If a risk is identified, action should be taken to correct it. This could be a PPE hearing protection. Information, instruction and training must be provided which is monitored.

Insurance

Public Liability Insurance protects employers and employees against the consequences of death or injury to a third party while on the premises. Professional indemnity insurance extends public liability insurance to cover named employees against claims.

Product and **Treatment Liability Insurance** is usually included with your public liability insurance but should be checked with the insurance company. Product Liability Insurance covers you for risks which might occur as a result of the products you are using and/or selling.

It is a legal requirement under the Employer's Liability (Compulsory Insurance) Act (1969) that every employer must have **Employer's Liability Insurance**. This provides financial compensation to an employee should they be injured as a result of an accident in the workplace. This certificate must be displayed indicating that a policy of insurance has been obtained.

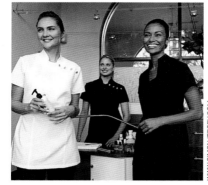

WWW.SIMONJERSEY.COM

Beauty uniforms

Personal health, hygiene and presentation

Your appearance enables the client to make an initial judgement about both you and the salon, so make sure that you create the correct impression! Employees in the workplace should always reflect the desired image of the profession that they work in.

Personal presentation

Assistant beauty therapist The assistant beauty therapist qualified to Level 1 will be required to wear a clean protective overall as they will be preparing the working area for client services and may be involved in preparing clients and performing basic skills in facial, nail and make-up services.

Beauty therapist Due to the nature of many of the services offered, the beauty therapist must wear protective, hygienic work wear. The cotton overall is ideal; air can circulate, allowing perspiration to evaporate and discouraging body odour. The use of a colour such as white immediately shows the client that you are clean. A cotton overall might comprise a dress, in a length suited to a work role, a jumpsuit or a tunic top, with coordinating trousers. Overalls should be laundered regularly and a fresh, clean overall worn each day.

Receptionist If receptionists are employed solely to carry out reception duties, they may wear a different salon dress/uniform, complementary to those worn by the practising therapists. As the receptionist will not be as active, it may be appropriate for them to wear a smart jacket or cardigan. If on the other hand they are also carrying out services, the standard salon overall must be worn.

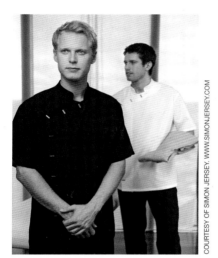

COURTESY OF SIMON JERSEY. WWW.SIMONJERSEY.COM

HEALTH & SAFETY

Aprons and the Personal Protective Equipment (PPE) at Work Regulations (1992)
For certain services, such as spa services, it is necessary to wear a protective apron over the overall. Assistant beauty therapists may also wear an apron while preparing and cleaning the working area, to protect the overall and keep it clean.

General rules for employees

Make-up Wear attractive make-up, and use the correct skincare cosmetics to suit your skin type. A healthy complexion will be a positive advertisements for your work. First impressions count!

Jewellery Keep jewellery to a minimum, such as a wedding ring, a fob watch and small stud earrings.

Nails Nails should be short, neatly manicured and free of nail polish unless the employee's main duties involve nail services or reception duties. Nail polish contains ingredients which can cause an allergic response in some people.

HEALTH & SAFETY

Workplace policy
Employers will advise you on personal presentation requirements in relation to facial piercings.

ACTIVITY

Personal appearance

1 Collect pictures from various suppliers of overalls. Select those that you feel would be most practical for a Level 2 beauty therapist, make-up artist or receptionist. Briefly describe why you feel these are the most suitable.

2 Design various hairstyles, or collect pictures from magazines, to show how the hair could be smartly worn by a therapist with medium-length to long hair.

ACTIVITY

Staying healthy

Ask your tutor for guidelines before beginning this activity.

1 Write down all the foods and drinks that you most enjoy. Are they healthy? If you are unsure, ask your tutor.

2 How much exercise do you take weekly?

3 How much sleep do you regularly have each night?

4 Do you think you could improve your health and fitness levels?

ACTIVITY

Code of ethics

As a professional beauty therapist it is important that you adhere to a code of ethical practice. You may wish to join a professional organization, which will issue you with a copy of its agreed standards.

Shoes Wear flat, well-fitting, comfortable shoes that enclose the feet fully and complement the overall. Flesh-coloured tights may be worn to protect the legs. Remember that you will be on your feet for most of the day!

Ethics

Beauty therapy has a **code of ethics**. This is a code of behaviour and expected standards for the professional beauty therapist to follow, which will uphold the reputation of the industry and ensure best working practice for the safety of the industry and members of the public. Beauty therapy professional bodies produce codes of practice for their members. A business may have its own code of practice. Although not a legal requirement, this code may be used in criminal proceedings as evidence of improper practice.

Code of Ethics

1. Towards BABTAC

   a) By not bringing the profession as a whole into disrepute

   b) By protecting collective morality. Members should not professionally associate themselves with any person or premises which may be deemed to be unprofessional or disreputable, as such an Association which may put the good name of the therapist and of BABTAC at risk.

2. Towards clients (concerned with the individual therapist/client relationship)

   a) Appointments must be kept. If unforeseen circumstances arise every effort must be made to make the client aware of the treatment cancellation.

   b) Client confidentiality - personal information should be kept private and only used for the specific purpose for which it is given, namely, to enable the therapist to carry out a safe and effective treatment.

   c) Information concerning the client and views formed must be kept confidential. The member should make every effort to ensure that this same level of confidence is upheld by receptionists and assistants where applicable.

   d) Client treatment details should remain confidential. Possible exceptions are the following:

   i) The client's knowledge and written consent are obtained.

   ii) There is a necessity for the information to be given for example if the client is being referred on to another professional.

   The exceptions are:

   iii) If the therapist is required by law to disclose the information.

   iv) If the therapist considers it their duty for the protection of the public.

   If a therapist has information of a criminal nature the member is advised to take legal advice.

An excerpt from The BABTAC Handbook, code of ethics, www.babtac.com/www.babtac.com

Diet, exercise and sleep

A beauty therapist requires stamina and energy. To achieve this you need to eat a healthy, well-balanced diet, take regular exercise and have adequate sleep.

Posture

Posture is the way you hold yourself when standing, sitting and walking. *Correct* posture enables you to work longer without becoming tired, it prevents muscle fatigue, repetitive strain injury (RSI) and stiff joints, and it also improves your appearance.

Good standing posture If you are standing with good posture, these terms will describe you:

- head up, centrally balanced
- shoulders slightly back, and relaxed
- chest up and out
- abdomen flat
- hips level
- fingertips level
- bottom in
- knees level
- feet slightly apart and weight evenly distributed

Good sitting posture Sit on a suitable chair or stool with a good back support and

- sit with the lower back pressed against the chair back
- keep the chest up and the shoulders back
- distribute the body weight evenly along the thighs
- keep the feet together, and flat on the floor
- do not slouch, or sit on the edge of your seat

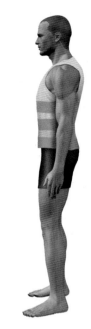

Good standing posture

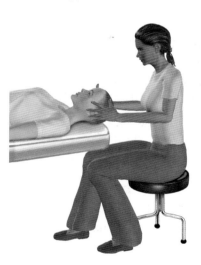

Good sitting posture

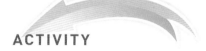

ACTIVITY

The importance of posture

1   Which services will be performed sitting, and which standing?

2   In what way do you feel your services would be affected if you were not sitting or standing correctly?

Personal hygiene

It is vital that you have a high standard of personal **hygiene**. You are going to be working in close proximity with people.

Bodily cleanliness is achieved through daily showering or bathing. This removes the stale sweat, dirt and bacteria which cause body odour. An antiperspirant or deodorant may be applied to the underarm area to reduce perspiration and thus the smell of sweat. Clean underwear should be worn each day.

Hands Your hands and everything you touch are covered with germs. Although most are harmless, some can cause ill health or disease. Wash your hands regularly, especially after you have been to the toilet and before eating food. You must also wash your hands before and after treating each client, and during a service if necessary. Washing the hands before treating a client minimizes the risk of cross-infection and presents to the client a hygienic, professional, caring image. Disinfecting hand gel may also be applied to the clean hands before services are delivered.

HEALTH & SAFETY

Repetitive strain injury (RSI)
If you do not follow correct postural positional requirements when performing services, muscle and ligaments may become overstretched and over-used resulting in repetitive strain injury (RSI). This may result in you being unable to work in the short term, and potentially long term in the occupation.

Step-by-step: How to wash your hands

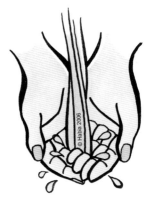

1 Wet your hands, wrists and forearms thoroughly using running water

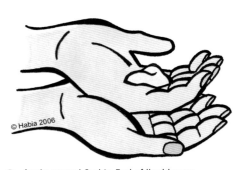

2 Apply around 3ml to 5ml of liquid soap

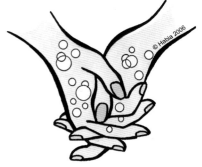

3 Start the lathering process, rubbing palm to palm

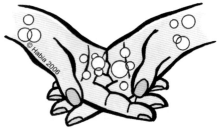

4 Interlock fingers and rub, ensuring a good lather

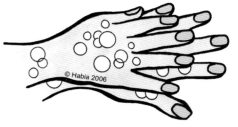

5 Rub right hand over back of left, then left over right hand

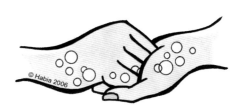

6 Rub with fingers locked in palm of hand ensuring fingertips are cleaned

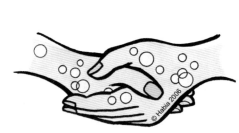

7 Lock thumbs and rotate hands

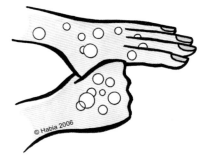

8 Grasp thumb with hand and rotate, repeat with opposite thumb

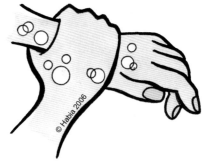

9 Rotate hand around wrist, repeat on opposite wrist

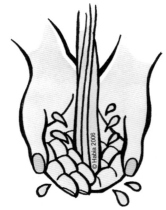

10 Rinse hands and wrists thoroughly using running water

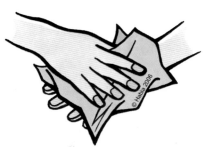

11 Dry the hands and wrists thoroughly

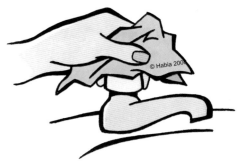

12 Turn off the tap using a paper towel

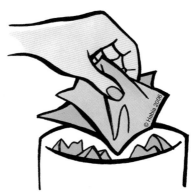

13 Dispose of paper towel without touching any part of the waste bin

ACTIVITY

Hand hygiene
What further occasions can you think of when it will be necessary to wash your hands when treating a client?

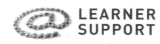

HEALTH & SAFETY

Soap and towels

Wash your hands with liquid soap from a sealed dispenser. This should take 10–20 seconds. Don't refill disposable soap dispensers when empty: if you do they will become a breeding ground for bacteria.

Disposable paper towels or warm-air hand dryers should be used to thoroughly dry the hands.

Protecting yourself

You will be wise to have the relevant inoculations, including those against tetanus and hepatitis, to protect yourself against ill health and even death.

Protecting the client

If you have any cuts or abrasions on your hands, cover them with a clean dressing to minimize the risk of secondary infection. Disposable gloves may be worn for additional protection.

Certain skin disorders are contagious. Therapists suffering from any such disorder must not work, but must seek medical advice immediately.

Face masks may be worn when working in close proximity to the client.

Feet Keep your feet fresh and healthy by washing them daily and then drying them thoroughly, especially between the toes to avoid foot disorders developing such as athlete's foot. Deodorizing foot powder may then be applied.

Oral hygiene Avoid bad breath by brushing your teeth at least twice daily and flossing the teeth frequently. Use breath fresheners and mouthwashes as required to freshen your breath. Visit the dentist regularly, to maintain healthy teeth and gums. Avoid eating strong flavoured foods which could cause offence in close proximity.

Hair Your hair should be clean and tidy. Have your hair cut regularly to maintain its appearance, and shampoo and condition your hair as often as needed.

If your hair is long, wear it off the face and taken to the crown of the head. Medium-length hair should be clipped back, away from the face, to prevent it falling forwards.

@ LEARNER SUPPORT

Health & safety true or false?

TOP TIP · · · · · · · · · · · ·
Fresh breath
When working, avoid eating strong-smelling highly spiced food.
· · · · · · · · · · · · · · · ·

HEALTH & SAFETY

Long hair
If long hair is not taken away from the face, the tendency will be to move the hair away from the face repeatedly with the hands, and this in turn will require that the hands be washed repeatedly.

Hygiene in the workplace

Infections Effective hygiene is necessary in the salon to prevent *cross-infection* and *secondary infection*. These can occur through poor practice, such as the use of implements that are not sterile. Infection can be recognized by red and inflamed skin, or the presence of pus.

Cross-infection occurs because some microorganisms are contagious – they may be transferred through personal contact or by contact with an infected instrument that has not been disinfected or sterilized.

Secondary infection can occur as a result of injury to the client during the service or, if the client already has an open cut, if bacteria penetrate the skin and cause infection. **Sterilization** and disinfection procedures (below) are used to minimize or destroy the harmful microorganisms which could cause infection – **bacteria**, **viruses** and **fungi**.

Infectious diseases that are contagious **contra-indicate** beauty service: they require medical attention. People with certain other skin disorders, even though these are not contagious, should likewise not be treated by the beauty therapist, as treatment might lead to secondary infection.

Sterilization and disinfection **Sterilization** is the total destruction of all living microorganisms in metal tools and equipment. **Disinfection** is the destruction of most living microorganisms in non-metal tools, equipment and work areas. Sterilization and disinfection techniques practised in the beauty salon involve the use of *physical* agents such as radiation and heat and *chemical* agents such as antiseptics and disinfectants.

Radiation – a quartz mercury-vapour lamp can be used as the source for ultra-violet (UV) light, which minimizes harmful microorganisms. However, UV light has limited effectiveness and cannot be relied upon for complete sterilization. A UV cabinet is a good place to store previously sterilized objects

The UV lamp must be contained within a closed cabinet. This cabinet is an ideal place for storing sterilized objects.

Heat – dry and moist heat can both be used in sterilization. One method is to use a dry **hot-air oven**. This is similar to a small oven, and heats to 150–180°C. It is seldom used in the salon.

More practical is a **glass-bead sterilizer**. This is a small, electrically heated unit that contains glass beads: these transfer heat to objects placed in contact with them. This method of sterilization is suitable for small tools such as tweezers and scissors. All objects should be cleaned before being placed in the glass-bead sterilizer to remove surface dirt and debris.

Water is boiled in an **autoclave** (similar to a pressure cooker): because of the increased pressure, the water reaches a temperature of 121–134°C. Autoclaving is the most effective method for sterilizing objects in the salon.

Disinfectants and antiseptics If an object *cannot* be sterilized, it should be placed in a chemical **disinfectant** solution. A disinfectant destroys most microorganisms,

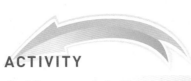

ACTIVITY

Avoiding cross-infection

1 List the different ways in which infection can be transferred in the salon.

2 How can you avoid cross-infection in the workplace?

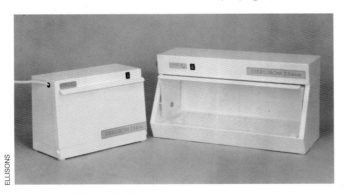

ELLISONS

An ultra-violet light cabinet

HEALTH & SAFETY

Sterilization record

Ultra-violet light is dangerous, especially to the eyes. The lamp must be switched off before opening the cabinet. A record must be kept of usage, as the effectiveness of the lamp decreases with use.

HEALTH & SAFETY

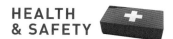

Using an autoclave

- The autoclave should only be used by those trained to do so.

- Not all objects can safely be placed in the autoclave. Before using this method, check whether the items you wish to sterilize can withstand this heating process.

- All objects should be cleaned, using an effective cleaning agent, e.g. surgical spirit, to remove surface dirt and debris before placing in the autoclave.

- To avoid damaging the autoclave, always use distilled de-ionized water.

- To avoid rusting, metal objects placed in the sterilizing unit must be of good-quality stainless steel.

- Never overload the autoclave. Follow manufacturer's instructions in its use.

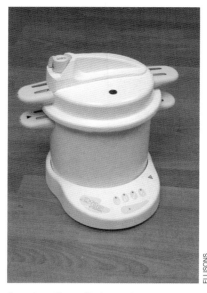

An automatic medical autoclave

but not all. Hypochlorite is a disinfectant – bleach is an example of a hypochlorite. Hypochlorite is suitable for cleaning work surfaces but is particularly corrosive and unsuitable for use with metals – use as directed by the manufacturer. Alcohol-impregnated wipes are a popular way to clean the skin using a disinfectant such as isopropyl alcohol.

An **antiseptic** prevents the multiplication of microorganisms. It has a limited action and does not kill all microorganisms.

All sterilization/disinfection techniques must be carried out safely and effectively:

1 Select the appropriate method of sterilization or disinfectant for the object. *Always* follow the manufacturer's guidelines on the use of the sterilizing or disinfecting unit or agent.

2 Clean the object in clean water and detergent to remove dirt and grease. (Dirt left on the object might prevent effective sterilization or disinfection.)

3 Dry it thoroughly with a clean, disposable paper towel.

4 Sterilize or disinfect the object, allowing sufficient time for the process to be completed.

5 Place tools that have been sterilized or disinfected in a clean, covered container.

Keep several sets of the tools you use regularly, so that you can carry out effective sterilization and disinfection.

HEALTH & SAFETY

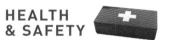

Aseptic conditions

This is the situation you should try to ensure occurs in the workplace by eliminating bacteria. All treatment procedures must be aseptic, i.e, wearing PPE, hand hygiene, correct methods of waste disposal etc.

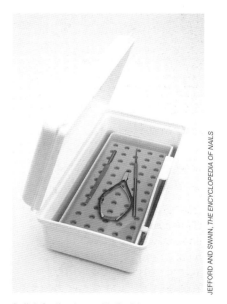

A disinfection tray with liquid

HEALTH & SAFETY

Using disinfectant

Disinfectant solutions should be changed as necessary to ensure their effectiveness. After removing the object from the disinfectant, rinse it in clean water to remove traces of the solution. (These might otherwise cause an allergic reaction on the client's skin.)

ALWAYS REMEMBER

Before sterilization, surgical spirit applied with clean cotton wool may be used to clean small objects.

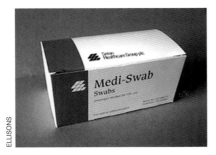

ELLISONS

Medi-swabs (sterile isopropyl tissues)

TOP TIP

HSE advice on cleaning

Advice on cleaning work surfaces and equipment can be found on the COSHH Essentials website: www .coshh-essentials.org.uk.

HEALTH & SAFETY

Cuts on the hands

Open, uncovered cuts provide an easy entry for harmful bacteria, and may therefore lead to infection. Always cover cuts.

Misuse of Drugs Act (1971)

This Act categorizes drugs into classes and details the penalties for those caught possessing them. Therefore, you are acting illegally.

TUTOR SUPPORT

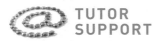

Activity 5: Workplace policies task

HEALTH & SAFETY

Damaged equipment

Any equipment in poor repair must be repaired or disposed of. Such equipment may be dangerous and may harbour germs.

Using chemical agents

Always protect your hands with gloves before immersing them in chemical cleaning agents, to minimize the risk of an allergic reaction.

Workplace policies Each workplace should have its own workplace policy to identify hygiene rules.

- *Health and safety* Follow the health and safety policies for the workplace.

- *Personal hygiene* Maintain a high standard of personal hygiene. Wash your hands with a detergent containing **chlorhexidine gluconate** which protects against a wide range of bacteria. The addition of isopropyl alcohol provides a stronger hand disinfectant removing surface bacteria and fungi.

- *Cuts on the hands* Always cover any cuts on your hands with a protective dressing.

- *Cross-infection* Take great care to avoid cross-infection in the salon. *Never* treat a client who has a contagious skin disease or disorder, or any other contra-indication. Refer the client tactfully to their GP.

- *Use hygienic tools* Never use an implement unless it has been effectively sterilized or disinfected, as appropriate.

- *Disposable applicators* Wherever possible, use disposable applicators.

- *Working surfaces* Disinfect all working surfaces (such as trolleys and couches) with a chlorine preparation, diluted to the manufacturer's instructions. Cover all working surfaces with clean, disposable paper tissue.

- *Gowns and towels* Clean gowns and towels must be provided for each client. Towels should be laundered at a temperate of 60°C.

- *Laundry* Dirty laundry should be placed in a covered container.

- *Waste* including clinical waste and non-contaminated waste, must be disposed of following the COSHH procedures and guidelines provided by the local authority and training by the employer. For contaminated waste comply with the Controlled Waste Regulations (1992). Put waste in a suitable container lined with a disposable waste bag. A yellow '**sharps' container** or heavy duty yellow bag, should be available for clinical waste contaminated with blood or tissue fluid. Protective gloves should be worn to avoid risk of contamination.

- *Eating and drinking* Never eat or drink in the service area of the salon. Not only is it unprofessional, but harmful chemicals may also be ingested.

- *Drugs and alcohol* Never carry out services in the workplace under the influence of drugs or alcohol. Your competence will be affected putting yourself, clients and possibly colleagues at risk. Any accident as a result would be termed negligent and you would be liable.

Ensure that your behaviour at work is in accordance with your workplace policies and doesn't endanger yourself or others.

Skin diseases and disorders

The beauty therapist must be able to distinguish a healthy skin from one suffering from a skin disease or disorder. Certain skin disorders and diseases **contra-indicate** a beauty service: the service would expose the therapist and other clients to the risk of cross-infection. It is therefore vital that you are familiar with the skin diseases and disorders with which you might come into contact in the workplace and those that are a risk and those that are not and the correct action to take. Relevant skin diseases and disorders are also discussed in each chapter on services. See for example the image on this page of a microscopic bacteria – streptococcus bacteria.

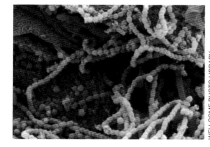

Example of a microscopic bacteria – streptococcus bacteria on the tongue

HEALTH & SAFETY

Skin problems

If you are unable to identify a skin condition with confidence, so that you are uncertain whether or not you should treat the client, don't! Tactfully refer them to their GP before proceeding with the planned service.

Bacterial infections

Bacteria are minute single-celled organisms of varied shapes. Large numbers of bacteria inhabit the surface of the skin and are harmless (**non-pathogenic**); indeed some play an important positive role in the health of the skin. Others, however, are harmful (**pathogenic**) and can cause skin diseases.

Impetigo An inflammatory disease of the surface of the skin, usually appearing on exposed areas.

Infectious? Yes.

Appearance: Initially the skin appears red and is itchy. Small thin-walled blisters appear; these burst and form into crusts. Untreated small pus-filled ulcers can occur with a dark, thick crust which can lead to scarring.

Site: The commonly affected areas are the nose, the mouth and the ears, but impetigo can occur on the scalp or the limbs.

Treatment: Medical – usually an antibiotic or an antibacterial ointment is prescribed containing corticosteroids such as hydrocortisone.

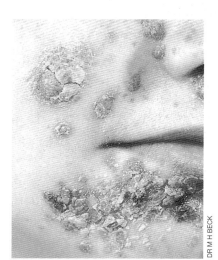

Impetigo

Conjunctivitis or pink eye Inflammation of the mucous membrane that covers the eye and lines the eyelids.

Infectious? Yes.

Appearance: The skin of the inner conjunctiva of the eye becomes inflamed and the eye becomes very red and sore. Water and pus may exude from the area leaving a sticky coating on the lashes.

Site: The eyes, either one or both, may be infected.

Treatment: Medical – usually an antibiotic lotion is prescribed. However, in some cases medical treatment will not be necessary and the infection will heal independently.

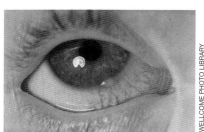

Conjunctivitis or pink eye

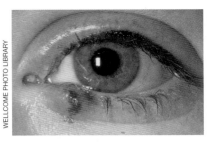

WELLCOME PHOTO LIBRARY

Hordeola or styes

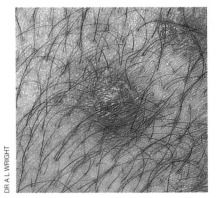

DR A L WRIGHT

Furuncle or boil

HEALTH & SAFETY

Boils

Boils occurring on the upper lip or in the nose should be referred immediately to a GP. Boils can be dangerous when near to the eyes or brain.

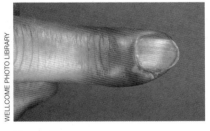

WELLCOME PHOTO LIBRARY

Paronychia

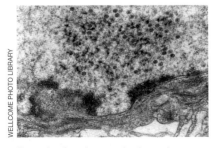

WELLCOME PHOTO LIBRARY

Example of a microscopic virus – herpes simplex virus particles (orange) in the nucleus of an epithelial cell

Hordeola or styes Infection of the sebaceous glands of eyelash hair follicles. It can be an effect of blepharitis (inflammation of the eyelids).

Infectious? Yes.

Appearance: Small red, inflamed lumps containing pus, a sign of infection.

Site: The inner rim of the eyelid.

Treatment: Medical – usually an antibiotic is prescribed.

Furuncles or boils Red, painful lumps, extending deeply into the skin.

Infectious? Yes.

Appearance: A localized red lump occurs around a hair follicle; it then develops a core or pus. Scarring of the skin often remains after the boil has healed.

Site: The back of the neck, the armpits and buttocks and thighs are common areas, but furuncles can occur anywhere.

Treatment: Medical – Antibiotics may help to control infection.

Carbuncles Infection of numerous hair follicles.

Infectious? Yes.

Appearance: A hard, round abscess, larger than a boil, which oozes pus from several points upon its surface. Scarring often occurs after the carbuncle has healed.

Site: In particular where there is friction, such as the back of the neck, or on the thighs. However, they can occur anywhere.

Treatment: Medical – usually involving incision, drainage of the pus, and a course of antibiotics.

Paronychia Infection of the skin tissue surrounding the nail (the nail fold). If left untreated, the nail bed may become infected.

Infectious? Yes.

Appearance: Swelling, redness and pus in the nail fold and the area of the nail wall.

Site: The skin surrounding the nail plate.

Treatment: Medical – usually a course of antibiotics, incision and drainage of pus is necessary if it collects next to the nail.

Viral infections

Viruses are minute entities, too small to see even under an ordinary microscope. They are considered to be **parasites**, as they require living tissue in order to survive. Viruses invade healthy body cells and multiply within the cell: in due course the cell walls break down, liberating new viral particles to attack further cells, and thus the infection spreads.

Herpes simplex This is commonly referred to as a cold sore and a recurring skin condition, appearing at times when the skin's resistance is lowered through ill health or stress. It may also be caused by exposure of the skin to extremes of temperature or to ultra-violet light.

Infectious? Yes.

Appearance: Inflammation of the skin occurs in localized areas. As well as being red, the skin becomes itchy and small vesicles appear. These are followed by a crust, which may crack and weep tissue fluid.

Site: The mucous membranes of the nose or lips; herpes can also occur on the skin generally.

Treatment: There is no specific treatment, they usually clear in 7–10 days. A proprietary brand of anti-inflammatory antiseptic drying cream is usually prescribed, which must be applied in the early stages of the condition when a tingling, itching sensation is experienced.

Herpes zoster or shingles
In this painful disease from the virus that causes chicken pox, the virus attacks the sensory nerve endings and is thought to lie dormant in the body and be triggered when the body's defences are at a low ebb.

Infectious? Yes.

Appearance: Redness of the skin occurs along a line of the affected nerves. Blisters develop and form crusts, leaving purplish-pink pigmentation.

Site: Commonly the chest and the abdomen.

Treatment: Medical – usually including anti-viral medicines. Calamine lotion can soothe the irritation. If there are complications with bacterial infection, antibiotics will be prescribed.

Verrucae or warts
Small epidermal skin growths. Warts can be raised or flat, depending upon their position. There are several types of wart: plane, common, plantar and mosaic.

Infectious? Yes.

Appearance: Warts vary in size, shape, texture and colour. Usually they have a rough surface and are raised. If a wart occurs on the sole of the foot it grows inwards, due to the pressure of body weight.

Site:

- plane wart (flat wart): the fingers, either surface of the hand, face and legs
- common wart (verruca vulgaris): the hands, elbows and knees
- plantar wart (verrucae): the sole of the foot and toes
- mosaic (palmar warts): hands and feet

Treatment: Medical – using acids, i.e. salicylic acid, solid carbon dioxide (cryotherapy) or electrocautery.

Infestations

Scabies or itch mites (sarcoptes scabiei)
A condition in which an infestation of a tiny mite parasite burrows beneath the skin and invades the hair follicles. The mite feeds on tissue and fluid as it burrows into the skin.

Infectious? Yes.

Appearance: At the onset, minute papules and wavy greyish lines appear, where dirt has entered the burrows. Secondary bacterial infection may occur as a result of scratching.

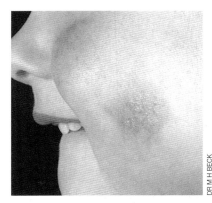
Herpes simplex

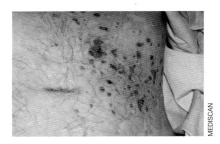
Shingles

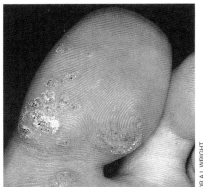
Verruca

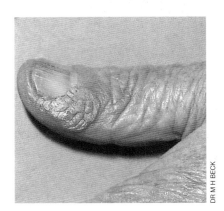
A wart

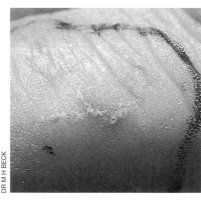

A scabies burrow

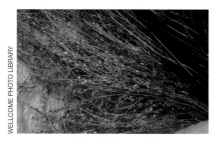

Example of a pediculosis capitis or head lice clinging to the hair

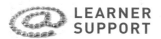

LEARNER SUPPORT

Health multiple choice quiz

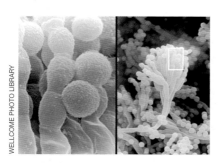

Example of a microscopic fungi – penicillium mould producing spores, plus very close up view of spore formulation

Site: Usually seen in warm areas of loose skin, such as the webs of the fingers, under the fingernails and the creases of the elbows.

Treatment: Medical – an anti-scabetic lotion containing an insecticide.

Pediculosis capitis or head lice   A condition in which small lice parasites infest scalp hair.

Infectious? Yes.

Appearance: The lice cling to the hair of the scalp. Eggs are laid, attached to the hair close to the skin. The lice bite the skin to draw nourishment from the blood; this creates irritation and itching of the skin, which may lead to secondary bacterial infection.

Site: The hair of the scalp.

Treatment: Medical – an appropriate medicated insecticide lotion or rinse.

Pediculosis pubis or pubic lice   A condition in which small lice parasites infest body hair.

Infectious? Yes.

Appearance: The lice cling to the hair of the body. Eggs are laid, attached to the hair close to the skin. The lice bite the skin to draw nourishment from the blood; this creates irritation and itching of the skin, which may lead to secondary bacterial infection.

Site: Pubic hair, eyebrows and eyelashes.

Treatment: Medical – an appropriate insecticidal lotion.

Pediculosis corporis or body lice   A condition in which small parasites live and feed on body skin.

Infectious? Yes.

Appearance: The lice cling to the hair of the body. Eggs are laid, attached to the hair close to the skin. The lice bite the skin to draw nourishment from the blood; this creates irritation and itching of the skin, which may lead to secondary bacterial infection. Where body lice bite the skin, small red marks can be seen.

Site: Body hair.

Treatment: Medical – an appropriate insecticidal lotion.

Fungal diseases

Fungi are microscopic plants. They are parasites, dependent upon a host for their existence. Fungal diseases of the skin feed off the waste products of the skin. Some fungi are found on the skin's surface; others attack the deeper tissues. Reproduction of fungi is by means of simple cell division or by the production of spores.

Tinea pedis or athlete's foot   A common fungal foot infection.

Infectious? Yes.

Appearance: Small blisters form, which later burst. The skin in the area can then become dry, giving a scaly appearance.

Site: Commonly affects the webs of skin between the toes.

Treatment: Thorough cleansing of the area. Medical application of fungicides. Untreated, infections such as bacterial infections may occur. It can also lead to infection of the toe and fingernails.

Tinea corporis or body ringworm A fungal infection of the skin.

Infectious? Yes.

Appearance: Small scaly red patches, which spread outwards and then heal from the centre, leaving a ring.

Site: The trunk of the body, the limbs and the face.

Treatment: Medical – using a fungicidal cream. Oral anti-fungal medication is necessary if there are several infection sites.

Tinea unguium or onychomycosis Ringworm infection of the fingernails.

Infectious? Yes.

Appearance: The nail plate is white and opaque. Eventually the nail plate becomes brittle and separates from the nail bed.

Site: The nail plate.

Treatment: Medical application of fungicides.

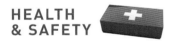

HEALTH & SAFETY

Artificial nails
Artificial nails increase the risk of developing infection due to the natural nail plate being roughened and if not maintained correctly moisture can collect between the artificial nail and the natural nail plate which provides ideal growth for fungi.

Sebaceous gland disorders

Milia Keratinization of the skin over the hair follicle occurs, causing sebum to accumulate in the hair follicle. This condition usually accompanies dry skin.

Infectious? No.

Appearance: Small, hard, pearly white cysts.

Site: The upper face or close to the eyes.

Treatment: The milium may be removed by a beauty therapist (if qualified to do so) or by a GP, depending on the location. A sterile lancet is used to pierce the skin of the overlying cuticle and thereby free the milium. Micro-dermabrasion may be used to avoid their development. Also retinoid creams may be applied which remove the outer epidermal layers.

Comedones or blackheads Excess sebum and keratinized cells block the mouth of the hair follicle.

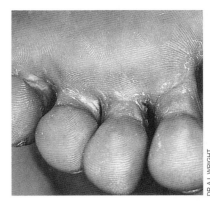
DR A L WRIGHT

Tinea pedis or athlete's foot

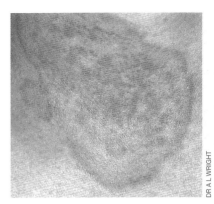
DR A L WRIGHT

Tinea corporis or body ringworm

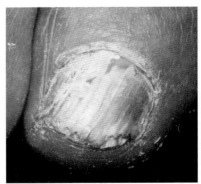
WELLCOME PHOTO LIBRARY

Tinea unguium

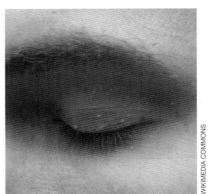
WIKIMEDIA COMMONS

Milia on the eyelid

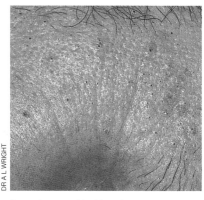

DR A L WRIGHT

Comedones or blackheads

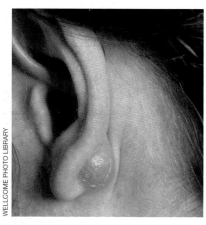

MEDISCAN

Seborrhoeic skin

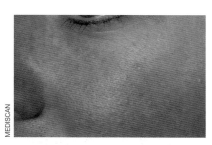

WELLCOME PHOTO LIBRARY

Sebaceous cyst

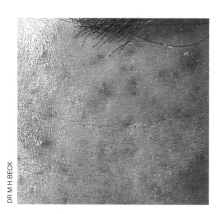

DR M H BECK

Acne vulgaris

Infectious? No.

Site: The face (the chin, nose and forehead), the upper back and chest.

Treatment: The area should be cleansed and an electrical vapour service or other pre-heating service should be given to relax the mouth of the hair follicle; a sterile comedo extractor should then be used to remove the blockage. A regular cleansing service should be recommended by the beauty therapist to limit the production of comedones.

Seborrhoea Excessive secretion of sebum from the sebaceous gland. This usually occurs during puberty, as a result of hormonal changes in the body.

Infectious? No.

Appearance: The follicle openings enlarge and excessive sebum is secreted. The skin appears coarse and oily; comedones, pustules and papules are present.

Site: The face and scalp. Seborrhoea may also affect the back and the chest.

Treatment: The area should be cleansed to remove excess oil. Medical treatment may be required – this would use locally applied steroid creams.

Steatomas, sebaceous cysts or wens Localized pockets or sacs of sebum, which form in hair follicles or under the sebaceous glands in the skin. The sebum becomes blocked, the sebaceous gland becomes distended and a lump forms.

Infectious? No.

Appearance: Semi-globular in shape, either raised or flat and hard or soft. The cysts are the same colour as the skin, or red if secondary bacterial infection occurs. A comedo can often be seen at the original mouth of the hair follicle.

Site: If the cyst appears on the upper eyelid, it is known as a **chalazion** or **meibomian cyst**.

Treatment: Medical – often a GP will remove the cyst under local anaesthetic. Small inflamed cysts can be medically treated with steroid medications or antibiotics.

Acne vulgaris Hormone imbalance in the body at puberty influences the activity of the sebaceous gland, causing an increased production of sebum. The sebum may be retained within the sebaceous ducts, causing congestion and bacterial infection of the surrounding tissues.

Infectious? No.

Appearance: Inflammation of the skin, accompanied by comedones, pustules and papules.

Site: Commonly on the face, the nose, the chin and the forehead. Acne may also occur on the chest and back.

Treatment: Medical – oral antibiotics may be prescribed, as well as medicated creams. With medical approval, regular salon services may be given to cleanse the skin deeply and also to stimulate the blood circulation.

Rosacea Excessive sebum secretion combined with a chronic inflammatory condition, caused by dilation of the blood capillaries.

Infectious? No.

Appearance: The skin becomes coarse, the pores enlarge and the cheek and nose area become inflamed, sometimes swelling and producing a butterfly pattern. Blood circulation slows in the dilated capillaries, creating a purplish appearance.

Treatment: Medical – usually including antibiotics.

Pigmentation disorders

Pigmentation of the skin varies, according to the person's genetic characteristics. In general, the darker the skin, the more pigment is present, but some abnormal changes in skin pigmentation can occur.

- **Hyperpigmentation** – increased pigment production
- **Hypopigmentation** – loss of pigmentation in the skin

Ephelides or freckles
Multiple, small hyperpigmented areas of the skin. Exposure to ultra-violet light (as in sunlight) stimulates the production of melanin, intensifying their appearance.

infectious? No.

Appearance: Small, flat, pigmented areas, darker that the surrounding skin.

Site: Commonly the nose and cheeks of fair-skinned people. Freckles may also occur on the shoulders, arms, hands and back.

Treatment: Freckles may be concealed with cosmetics if required. A sun block should be recommended, to prevent them intensifying in colour.

Lentigo (plural, lentigines)
Hyperpigmented areas of skin, slightly larger than freckles. Lentigo simplex occur in childhood. Actinic (solar) lentigines occur in middle age as a result of sun exposure.

Infectious? No.

Appearance: Brown, slightly raised, pigmented patches of skin, of variable size.

Site: The face, hands and shoulders.

Treatment: Application of cosmetic concealing products.

Chloasmata or liver spots
Hyperpigmentation in specific areas, stimulated by a skin irritant such as ultra-violet light, usually affecting women and darkly pigmented skins. The condition often occurs during pregnancy and usually disappears soon after the birth of the baby. It may also occur as a result of taking the oral contraceptive pill. The female hormone oestrogen is thought to stimulate melanin production.

Infectious? No.

Appearance: Flat, smooth, irregularly shaped, pigmented areas of skin, varying in colour from light tan to dark brown. Chloasmata are larger than ephelides, and of variable size.

Site: The back of the hands, the forearms, the upper part of the chest, the temples and the forehead.

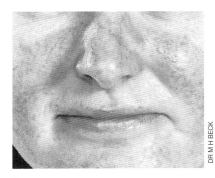

DR M H BECK

Rosacea

TOP TIP

Hypopigmentation

Hypopigmentation may result from certain skin injuries, disorders or diseases.

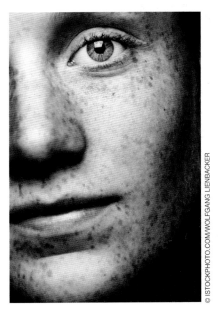

© ISTOCKPHOTO.COM/WOLFGANG LIENBACKER

Ephelides or freckles

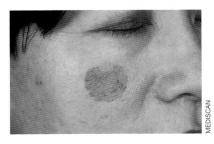

MEDISCAN

Lentigo

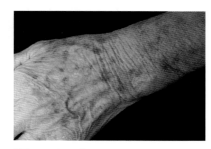

Chloasmata or liver spots

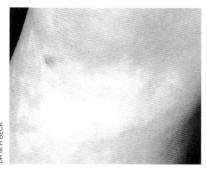

DR M H BECK

Vitiligo or leucoderma

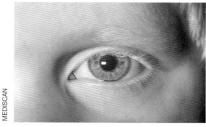

MEDISCAN

Albinism

Treatment: A barrier cream or a total sun-block will reduce the risk of the chloasmata increasing in size or number and thereby becoming more apparent.

Dermatosis papulosa nigra
Often called flesh moles, these are characterized by multiple benign, small brown to black hyperpigmented papules, common among dark-skinned people.

Infectious? No.

Appearance: Raised pigmented markings resembling moles.

Site: Usually seen on the cheeks and forehead, although they may appear on the neck, upper chest and back.

Treatment: Medical by medication or surgery.

Vitiligo or leucoderma
Patches of completely white skin which have lost their pigment, or which were never pigmented.

Infectious? No.

Appearance: Well-defined patches of white skin, lacking pigment.

Site: The face, the neck, the hands, the lower abdomen and the thighs. If vitiligo occurs over the eyebrows, the hairs in the area will also lose their pigment.

Treatment: Camouflage cosmetic concealer can be applied to give even skin colour; or skin-staining preparations can be used in the de-pigmented areas. Care must be taken when the skin is exposed to ultra-violet light, as the skin will not have the same protection in the areas lacking pigment.

Albinism
The skin is unable to produce the melanin pigment and the skin, hair and eyes lack colour.

Infectious? No.

Appearance: The skin is usually very pale pink and the hair is white. The eyes also are pink and extremely sensitive to light.

Site: The entire skin.

Treatment: There is no effective treatment. Maximum skin protection is necessary when the client is exposed to ultra-violet light and sunglasses should be worn to protect the eyes.

Vascular naevi
There are two types of naevus of concern to beauty therapists: vascular and cellular. **Vascular naevi** are skin conditions in which small or large areas of skin pigmentation are caused by the permanent dilation of blood capillaries.

Erythema
An area of skin in which blood capillaries have dilated, due either to injury or inflammation.

Infectious? No.

Appearance: The skin appears red.

Site: Erythema may affect one area (locally) or all of the skin (generally).

Treatment: The cause of the inflammation should be identified. In the case of a **skin allergy**, the client must not be brought into contact with the irritant again. If the cause is unknown, refer the client to their GP.

Dilated capillaries Capillaries near the surface of the skin that are permanently dilated.

Infectious? No.

Appearance: Small red visible blood capillaries.

Site: Areas where the skin is neglected, dry or fine, such as the cheek area.

Treatment: Dilated capillaries can be concealed using a green corrective camouflage cosmetic, or removed by qualified electrologist using diathermy.

Spider naevi or stellate haemangiomas Dilated blood vessels, with smaller dilated capillaries radiating from them.

Infectious? No.

Appearance: Small red capillaries, radiating like a spider's legs from a central point.

Site: Commonly the cheek area, but may occur on the upper body, the arms and the neck. Spider naevi are usually caused by an injury to the skin.

Treatment: Spider naevi can be concealed using a camouflage cosmetic, or treated by a qualified electrologist with diathermy.

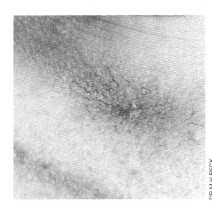

Spider naevus or stellate haemangiomas

Naevi vasculosis or strawberry marks Red or purplish raised marks which appear on the skin at birth.

Infectious? No.

Appearance: Red or purplish lobed mark, of any size.

Site: Any area of the skin.

Treatment: About 60 per cent disappear by the age of six years. Treatment is not usually necessary; concealing cosmetics can be applied if desired.

Capillary naevi or port-wine stains Large areas of dilated capillaries that contrast noticeably with the surrounding areas.

Infectious? No.

Appearance: The naevus has a smooth flat surface.

Site: Some 75 per cent occur on the head; they are probably formed at the foetal stage. Naevi may also be found on the neck and face.

Treatment: Camouflage cosmetic creams can be applied to disguise the area.

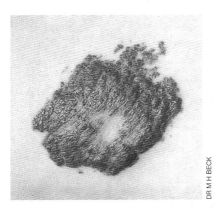

Naevi vasculosis or strawberry marks

Cellular naevi or moles **Cellular naevi** are skin conditions in which changes in the cells of the skin result in skin malformations.

Malignant melanomas or malignant moles Rapidly-growing skin cancers, usually occurring in adults.

Infectious? No.

Appearance: Each melanoma commences as a bluish-black mole, which enlarges rapidly, darkening in colour and developing a halo of pigmentation around it. It later becomes raised, bleeds and ulcerates. Secondary growths will develop in internal organs if the melanoma is not treated.

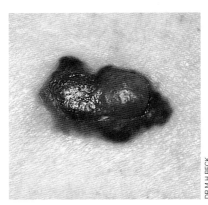

Malignant melanoma

HEALTH & SAFETY

Moles

If moles change in shape or size, if they bleed or form crusts, seek medical attention.

HEALTH & SAFETY

Malignant melanoma risk

The risk of melanoma increases as the number of naevi increases. Therefore clients with lots of naevi or moles are at highest risk.

Normal Mole	Melanoma	Sign	Characteristic
		Asymmetry	When half of the mole does not match the other half.
		Border	When the border (edges) of the mole are ragged or irregular.
		Colour	When the colour of the mole varies throughout.
		Diameter	If the mole's diameter is larger than a pencil's eraser.

PERMISSION OF THE NATIONAL CANCER INSTITUTE

Guidance images for moles

Site: Usually the lower abdomen, legs or feet.

Treatment: Medical – always recommend that a client has a mole checked if it is changing in size, structure or colour, or if it becomes itchy or bleeds.

Junction naevi Localized collections of naevoid cells that arise from the mass production locally of pigment-forming cells (melanocytes).

Infectious? No.

Appearance: In childhood junction naevi appear as smooth or slightly raised pigmented marks. They vary in colour from brown to black.

Site: Any area.

Treatment: None.

Dermal naevi Localized collections of naevoid cells.

Infectious? No.

Appearance: About 1cm wide, dermal naevi appear smooth and dome-shaped. Their colour ranges from skin tone to dark brown. Frequently one or more hairs may grow from the naevus.

Site: Usually the face.

Treatment: None.

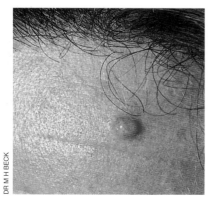

DR M H BECK

Benign naevus

Hairy naevi Moles exhibiting coarse hairs from their surface.

Infectious? No.

Appearance: Slightly raised moles, varying in size from 3cm to much larger. Colour ranges from fawn to dark brown.

Site: Anywhere on the skin.

Treatment: Hairy naevi may be surgically removed where possible and this is often done for cosmetic reasons. Hair growing from a mole should be cut, not plucked: if plucked, the hair will become coarser and the growth of further hairs may be stimulated.

Skin disorders involving abnormal growth

Psoriasis Patches of itchy, red, flaky skin, the cause of which is unknown.

Infectious? No. Secondary infection with bacteria can occur if the skin becomes broken and dirt enters the skin.

Appearance: Red patches of skin appear, covered in waxy, silvery scales. Bleeding will occur if the area is scratched and scales are removed.

Site: The elbows, the knees, the lower back and the scalp.

Treatment: There is no known treatment. Medication including steroid creams can bring relief to the symptoms.

Seborrhoeic or senile warts: Raised, pigmented, benign tumours occurring in middle age.

Infectious? No.

Appearance: Slightly raised, brown or black, rough patches of skin. Such warts can be confused with pigmented moles.

Site: The trunk, the scalp and the temples.

Treatment: Medical – the warts can be cauterized by a GP.

Verrucae filliformis or skin tags These verrucae appear as threads projecting from the skin.

Infectious? No.

Appearance: Skin-coloured threads of skin 3–6mm long.

Site: Mainly seen on the neck and the eyelids, but may occur in other areas such as under the arms.

Treatment: Medical – cauterization with diathermy, either by a GP or by a qualified electrologist.

Xanthomas Small yellow growths appearing upon the surface of the skin made up of cholesterol deposits.

Infectious? No.

Appearance: A yellow flat or raised area of skin with distinct edges.

TOP TIP

Naevi numbers and skin colour
Caucasian skin normally has up to four times as many naevi than black skin.

HEALTH & SAFETY

Skin tags
Skin tags often occur under the arms. In case they are present, take care when carrying out a wax depilation service in this area: do not apply wax over tags.

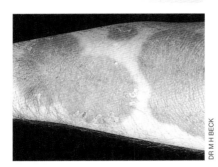

Psoriasis

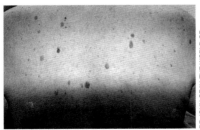

Seborrhoeic or senile warts

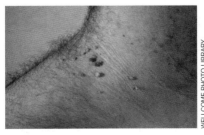

Verrucae filliformis or skin tags

Site: Common on the eyelids, but can appear anywhere on the body.

Treatment: Medical – the growth is thought to be connected with certain medical diseases, such as diabetes or high or low blood pressure. Sometimes a low-fat diet can correct the condition.

Keloids Keloids occur following skin injury and are overgrown abnormal scar tissue which spreads, characterized by excess deposits of collagen. To avoid skin discoloration the keloid must be protected from UV exposure.

Infectious? No.

Appearance: The skin tends to be red, raised, shiny and ridged.

Site: Located over the site of a wound or other lesion.

Treatment: Medical by drug therapy, such as cortisone injection, or surgery.

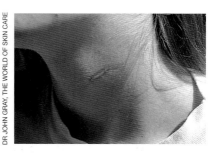

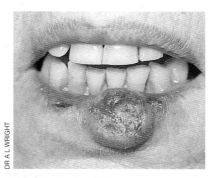

DR JOHN GRAY, THE WORLD OF SKIN CARE

Keloids

Malignant tumours

Squamous cell carcinomas or prickle-cell cancers
Malignant growths originating in the epidermis.

Infectious? No.

Appearance: When fully formed, the carcinoma appears as a raised area of skin.

Site: Anywhere on the skin.

Treatment: Includes surgical removal also radiotherapy (treatment with x-ray) or treatment with drugs as necessary.

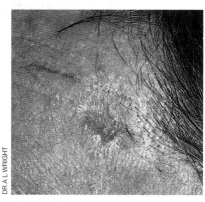

DR A L WRIGHT

Squamous cell carcinoma

Basal cell carcinomas or rodent ulcers
Slow-growing malignant tumours, occurring in middle age.

Infectious? No.

Appearance: A small, shiny, waxy nodule with a depressed centre. The disease extends, with more nodules appearing on the border of the original ulcer.

Site: Usually on the face.

Treatment: Includes surgical removal also radiotherapy (treatment with x-ray) or treatment with drugs as necessary.

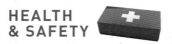

DR A L WRIGHT

Basal cell carcinomas

Skin allergies

The skin can protect itself to some degree from damage or invasion. **Mast cells** detect damage to the skin; if damage occurs, the mast cells burst, releasing the chemical **histamine** into the tissues. Histamine causes the blood capillaries to dilate, giving the reddening we call 'erythema'. The increased blood flow transports materials in blood which tend to limit the damage and begin repair.

If the skin is sensitive to and becomes inflamed on contact with a particular substance, this substance is called an **allergen**. Allergens may be animal, chemical or vegetable substances, and they can be inhaled, eaten or absorbed following contact with the skin. An **allergic skin reaction** appears as irritation, itching and discomfort, with reddening and swelling (as with nettle rash). If the allergen is removed, the allergic reaction subsides.

HEALTH & SAFETY

Record any known allergies
When completing the client record card, always ask whether your client has any known allergies.

Each individual has different tolerances to the various substances we encounter in daily life. What causes an allergic reaction in one individual may be perfectly harmless to another.

Here are just a few examples of allergens known to cause allergic skin reactions in some people:

- metal objects containing nickel
- sticking plaster
- rubber
- lipstick containing eosin dye
- nail polish containing formaldehyde resin
- hair and eyelash dyes
- lanolin, the skin moisturising agent
- detergents that dry the skin
- foods – well-known examples are peanuts, cow's milk, lobster, shellfish and strawberries
- plants such as tulips and chrysanthemums

Dermatitis An inflammatory skin disorder in which the skin become red, itchy and swollen. There are two types of dermatitis. In *primary dermatitis* the skin is irritated by the action of a substance on the skin, and this leads to skin inflammation. In *allergic contact dermatitis*, the problem is caused by intolerance of the skin to a particular substance or groups of substances. On exposure to the substance the skin quickly becomes irritated and an allergic reaction occurs.

Infectious? No.

Appearance: Reddening and swelling of the skin, with the possible appearance of blisters.

Site: If the skin reacts to a skin irritant outside the body, the reaction is localized. Repeated contact with the allergen will lead to a general hypersensitivity. If the irritant gains entry to the body it will be transported in the bloodstream and may cause a general allergic skin reaction.

Treatment: Moisturising cream can be used to help prevent drying of the skin. Personal protective equipment should be worn in the case of occupational hazards, i.e. gloves should be worn by a hairdresser to avoid developing contact dermatitis due to the hazards in the nature of the work, like contact with water for long periods. When an allergic dermatitis reaction occurs, the only 'cure' is the absolute avoidance of the substance. Steroid creams such as hydrocortisone are usually prescribed, to soothe the damaged skin and reduce the irritation.

Eczema Inflammation of the skin caused by contact, internally or externally, with an irritant.

Infectious? No.

Appearance: Reddening of the skin, with swelling and blisters. The blisters leak tissue fluid which later hardens, forming scabs.

Site: The face, the neck and the skin, particularly at the inner creases of the elbows and behind the knees.

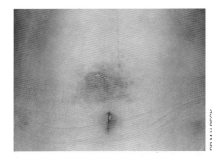

Allergic reaction to a nickel button

DR M H BECK

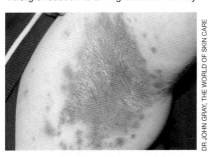

Allergic reaction to an ingredient in hair dye

DR JOHN GRAY, THE WORLD OF SKIN CARE

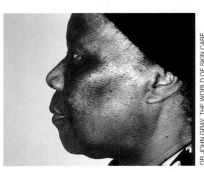

Allergic reaction to an antiperspirant

DR JOHN GRAY, THE WORLD OF SKIN CARE

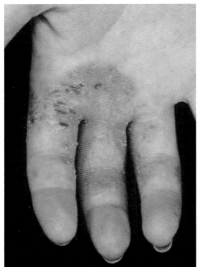

Contact dermatitis

HSE

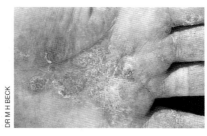

DR M H BECK

Eczema

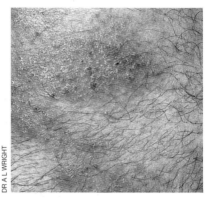

DR A L WRIGHT

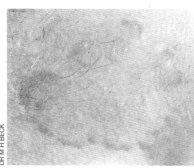

DR M H BECK

Urticaria (nettle rash) or hives

Treatment: Refer the client to their GP. Eczema may disappear if the source of irritation is identified and removed. Steroid cream may be prescribed by the GP and special diets may help.

Urticaria (nettle rash) or hives A minor skin disorder caused by contact with an allergen, either internally (food or drugs) or externally (insect bites).

Infectious? No.

Appearance: Erythema with raised round whitish skin wheals. In some cases the lesions can cause intense burning or itching, a condition known as pruritis. Pruritis is a symptom of a disease (such as diabetes), not a disease itself.

Site: At the point of contact.

Treatment: Antihistamines may be prescribed to reduce the itching. The visible skin reaction usually disappears quickly leaving no trace. Complete avoidance of the allergen 'cures' the problem.

HEALTH & SAFETY

Hypoallergenic products
The use of hypoallergenic products minimizes the risk of skin contact with likely irritants.

Allergies
You may suddenly become allergic to a substance that has previously been perfectly harmless. Equally, you may over time cease to be allergic to something.

Infection following allergy
Following an allergic skin reaction in which the skin's surface has become itchy and broken, scratching may cause the skin to become infected with bacteria.

ALWAYS REMEMBER

To avoid potential hazards and risks in the workplace you should:

- be aware of the workplace health and safety policy and your responsibility in its implementation

- ensure your personal presentation and conduct at work meets health and safety and legislative requirements in accordance with workplace policies

- follow the most recent workplace policies for your job role and manufacturers' instructions for the safe use of resources

- follow the latest health and safety legislation related to your work

- know who is responsible for health and safety in your workplace. Pass on any suggestions for reducing health and safety risks within your job role

- report or deal immediately with any risk which could be a hazard, complying with workplace policies and legal requirements

- be aware of first aid arrangements in the event of an accident or illness

- know the workplace fire evacuation advice and procedure

- ensure your working practice minimizes the possible spread of infection or disease.

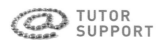

TUTOR SUPPORT

Activity 7: H&S multiple choice questions

GLOSSARY OF KEY WORDS

Accident book a written record of any accident in the workplace. Incidents in the accident book should be reviewed to see where improvements to safe working practice could be made.

Accident form a detailed report form to be completed following any accident in the workplace.

Antiseptic a chemical agent that prevents the multiplication of microorganisms. It has limited action and does not kill all microorganisms.

Aseptic The methods used to eliminate bacteria when performing treatment procedures from British standards. Glossary of terms relating to disinfectants.

Autoclave an effective method of sterilization, suitable for small metal objects and beauty therapy tools. Water is boiled under increased pressure and reaches temperatures of 121–134°C.

Bacteria minute, single-celled organisms of various shapes. Large numbers live on the skin's surface and are not harmful (they are non-pathogenic); others, however, are harmful (pathogenic) and can cause disease.

Client groups this term is used in a number of the units and it refers to client diversity. The CRE (Commission for Racial Equality) ethnic group classification is used in the range for these units. These cover white, mixed, Asian, black and Chinese.

Contra-indication a problematic symptom that indicates the service may not proceed.

Control of Risk the means by which risks identified are removed or reduced to acceptable levels.

Control of Substances Hazardous to Health (COSHH) (2002) these regulations require employers to identify hazardous substances used in the workplace and state how they should be correctly stored and handled.

Controlled Waste Regulations (1992) categorizes waste types. The Local Authority provides advice on how to dispose of waste types in compliance with the law.

Cosmetic Products (Safety) Regulations (2008) part of consumer protection legislation that requires that cosmetics and toiletries are safe in their formulation and are safe for use for their intended purpose as a cosmetic and comply with labelling requirements.

Cross-infection the transfer of contagious microorganisms.

Disinfectant a chemical agent that destroys most microorganisms.

Electricity at Work Regulations (1989) these regulations state that electrical equipment in the workplace should be tested every 12 months, by a qualified electrician. The employer must keep records of the equipment tested and the date it was checked.

Employers' Liability (Compulsory Insurance) Act (1969) this provides financial compensation to an employee should they be injured as a result of an accident in the workplace. A certificate indicating that a policy of insurance has been purchased should be displayed.

Environmental conditions this includes heating, lighting, ventilation and general comfort requirements for the workplace or service.

Fire Precautions Act (1971) legislation that states that all staff must be familiar with, and trained in fire, and emergency evacuation procedures for their workplace.

Fungi microscopic plants. Fungal diseases of the skin feed off the waste products of the skin. They are found on the skin's surface or they can attack deeper tissues.

Hazard a hazard is something with potential to cause harm.

Health and Safety at Work Act (1974) legislation that lays down the minimum standards of health safety and welfare requirements in all workplaces.

Health and Safety (Display Screen Equipment) Regulations (1992) these regulations cover the use of visual display units (VDUs) and computer screens. They specify acceptable levels of radiation emissions from the screen and identify correct posture, seating position, permitted working heights and rest periods.

Health and Safety (First Aid) Regulations (1981) legislation that states that workplaces must have appropriate and adequate first aid provision.

Health and Safety policy each employer of more than five employees must have a written health and safety policy issued to their employees outlining their health and safety responsibilities.

Hygiene requirements the expected standards as required by law, industry codes of practice or written procedures specified by the workplace.

Infestation a condition where animal parasites live off and invade a host.

Legislation laws affecting the beauty therapy business relating to products and services, the business premises and environmental conditions, working practices and those employed.

Local Government (Miscellaneous Provisions) Act (1982) legislation that requires that salons offering any form of skin piercing be registered with the local health authority. This registration includes both the operators who will be carrying out the service and the salon premises where the service will be carried out.

Management of Health and Safety at Work Regulations (1999) this legislation provides the employer with an approved code of practice for maintaining a safe, secure working environment.

Manual Handling Operations Regulations (1992) legislation that requires the employer to carry out a risk assessment of all activities undertaken which involve manual handling (lifting and moving objects).

Personal Protective Equipment (PPE) at Work Regulations (1992) this legislation requires employers to identify through risk assessment those activities that require special protective equipment to be worn.

Posture the position of the body, which varies from person to person. Good posture is when the body is in alignment. Correct posture enables you to work longer without becoming tired; it prevents muscle fatigue and stiff joints.

Provision and Use of Work Equipment Regulations (PUWER) (1998) this regulation lays down important health and safety controls on the provision and use of equipment.

Public Liability Insurance protects employers and employees against the consequences of death or injury to a third party while on the premises.

Reporting of Injuries, Diseases and Dangerous Occurrences Regulations (RIDDOR) (1995) these regulations require the employer to notify the local enforcement officer in writing, in cases where employees or trainees suffer personal injury at work.

Regulatory Reform (Fire Safety) Order (2005) this legislation requires that the employer or designated 'responsible person' must carry out a risk assessment for the premises in relation to fire evacuation practice and procedures.

Responsible persons This term is used in the Health and Safety unit to mean the person or persons at work to whom you should report any issues, problems or hazards. This could be a supervisor, line manager or your employer.

Risk the likelihood of a hazard's potential being recognized.

Secondary infection bacterial penetration into the skin causing infection.

Skin allergy if the skin is sensitive to a particular substance, an allergic skin reaction will occur. This is recognized by irritation, swelling and inflammation.

Sterilization the total destruction of all microorganisms in metal tools and equipment.

Viruses the smallest living bodies, too small to see under an ordinary microscope. Viruses invade healthy body cells and multiply within the cell. Eventually the cell walls break down and the virus particles are freed to attack further cells.

Workplace (Health Safety and Welfare) Regulations (1992) these regulations provide the employer with an approved code of practice for maintaining a safe, secure working environment.

Workplace policies This covers the documentation prepared by your employer on the procedures to be followed in your workplace. Examples are your employer's safety policy statement, or general health and safety statements and written safety procedures covering aspects of the workplace that should be drawn to the employees' (and "other persons'") attention, pricing policies and customer service policies.

Workplace practices any activities, procedures, use of materials or equipment and working techniques used in carrying out your job. Lifting techniques and maintaining good posture whilst working are also included.

ASSESSMENT OF KNOWLEDGE AND UNDERSTANDING

Having covered the learning objectives for **Make sure your own actions reduce risks to health and safety**, test what you need to know and understand by answering the following short questions below.

Actions to avoid health and safety risks

1   What are your main legal responsibilities under the Health and Safety at Work Act (1974)?

2   Name four different pieces of legislation relating to health and safety in the workplace.

3   What is the purpose of a salon health and safety policy? What sort of information does it include?

4   What is the importance of personal presentation in respect of your salon workplace policy?

5   Why is your personal conduct important to maintain the health and safety of yourself, colleagues and clients?

6   Why must regular health and safety checks be carried out in the workplace?

7   When completing a client's record card, you recognize that service is contra-indicated because the client has impetigo, an infectious skin disorder. What action do you take and why?

8   Effective sterilization and disinfection methods prevent cross-infection and secondary infection. What do you understand by the following terms:
   - sterilization?
   - disinfection?

- cross-infection?
- secondary infection?

9 How should a large box be lifted from the floor level to be placed on the work surface?

Dealing with significant risks in your workplace

1 What hazards may exist in the beauty therapy workplace?

2 Why must you always be aware of potential hazards?

3 In your role in the salon, describe four potential hazards and what precautions you would take to prevent them becoming a risk?

4 While cleaning a wax heater you notice that the wires in the lead are exposed. What action should you take?

5 If you were unable to deal with a risk because it was outside of your responsibility, what action would you take?

6 What does the abbreviation COSHH stand for? Why is it important to follow suppliers' and manufacturers' instructions for the safe use of materials and products?

7 When preparing a trolley for an eyelash tint, you drop and break a glass bottle of hydrogen peroxide. How would you deal with this spillage? How would you dispose of the broken glass?

Taking the right action in the event of a danger

1 What is the procedure for dealing with an accident in the workplace?

2 What is a fire drill? What is the fire evacuation procedure in your salon? How often should this be carried out?

3 In the event of a real fire, after having safely evacuated the building, how would you contact the appropriate emergency service?

4 In a beauty room, you discover a smoking bin in which a fire has been caused by a match used to light a fragranced candle. What action should you take and how should this fire be extinguished?

5 What actions can be taken to follow environmentally-friendly working practices?

6 The air conditioning system in the salon has broken. Who should be contacted to deal with this? What is the potential risk of inadequate ventilation?

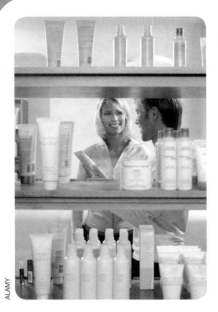

4 Selling Skills (G18)

G18 Unit Learning Objectives

This chapter covers **Unit G18 Promote additional products or services to clients**. By offering new or improved services and products, your salon benefits by sustaining client interest and increasing client satisfaction. Businesses must continuously launch new or improved products and services to be able to survive in a competitive world. However, it is equally important for a business without local competitors to encourage their clients to try new services or products to maximize service benefits.

This unit is all about your need to keep pace with new developments and to educate your clients about them. Clients expect more and more services or products to be offered to meet their needs. Their awareness of what is available will give them greater choice.

There are **three** learning outcomes for Unit G18 which you must achieve competently:

1 Identify additional services or products that are available

2 Inform clients about additional services or products

3 Gain client commitment to using additional services or products

Your assessor will observe you promoting additional products or services to different clients on different occasions over a period of time to ensure competence.

You are required to collect evidence in relation to the additional services or products offered.

(continued on the next page)

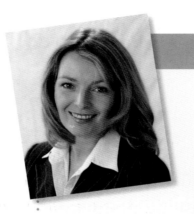

ROLE MODEL

Ruth Langley

Salon owner and beauty therapist
Pink Orchid Hair and Beauty Salon

" Ruth began her beauty therapy career in 1985 by renting a tiny room inside a hair salon. After five years she opened Pink Orchid which now employs 18 hair and beauty therapists. The salon has won many regional and national awards.

Her main responsibilities are ensuring the continual growth and success of the salon, training the teams and ensuring each client receives the very best service and customer care.

Ruth works as a sales consultant for Habia and wrote their Selling Skills course. She is the author of the book *Beautiful Selling* which was written to help and encourage therapists everywhere to sell. Ruth says that she is very proud of the book and the wonderful feedback which she has received.

(continued)

Communication with clients may be face-to-face, in writing, by telephone, text message, email, internet, intranet or other system used within your workplace for this purpose.

> **TOP TIP**
>
> **Seeking selling opportunities**
> The client's skincare preparations need to alter throughout the different seasons. As such, the client should be advised on products that are most suitable to maintain skin health and appearance. This gives you the opportunity to promote additional products and maintain client interest.

> **TOP TIP**
>
> **Client refreshments**
> Healthy light refreshments may be promoted as an additional retail opportunity.

The importance of product or services promotion

When clients select a beauty therapy service or product they do so for one or a number of reasons. This may be:

- to improve their appearance, e.g. an eyelash tint or manicure
- for a special occasion, e.g. make-up application
- for therapeutic reasons, to receive a quality professional service in tranquil surroundings, e.g. a de-stress facial massage
- for aspirational reasons, to imitate the appeal of an advertising campaign for example
- to seek professional guidance on what would best suit their needs, e.g. skincare advice
- for performance, the product or service has guaranteed results
- to maintain the benefits of a particular service they have received before, e.g. repeat booking for leg waxing service
- for social reasons, they enjoy visiting the salon as much as receiving the service
- to give a friend a service or product as a gift, e.g. a **gift voucher**

Whatever the reason, you want the client to feel satisfied with their choice, enjoy their experience and tell others – thus promoting the business.

Retail sales are of considerable importance to the beauty salon: they are a simple way of greatly increasing the income without too much extra time and effort. Beauty therapy services are time-consuming and labour-intensive; selling a product in addition to providing the service will greatly increase the profitability.

Clients need to be regularly informed about what products and services the business is promoting. This will maintain their motivation and their experience of the salon. In Chapter 3 we looked at the importance of creating an initial positive impression to the client. Staff knowledge of products and services is vital to ensure personal effectiveness and helps in gaining client loyalty

If you have got it right the client will maintain their loyalty to you and this enables the business to grow. For example, a facial service might take one hour and cost the client £40. You might then sell the client a moisturiser costing £40, of which £10 might be clear profit.

ACTIVITY

Express services
Increasingly clients are requiring a fast service often received in their lunch break. Examples include express artificial lashes for that unexpected special occasion. Find out what other services may be offered as an express service.

HEALTH & SAFETY

Contra-indications
If the client has a contra-indication to a service they wish to receive, recommend they seek their GP's approval first. You may require written evidence of this.

> **Give good advice**
> You have a duty to provide your clients with good home-care advice and help them to buy. Do your best to make the buying process easy and enjoyable for the client.
>
> **Ruth Langley**

Supposing that you sold eight products each day each yielding £10 profit. That would be a profit of £80 per day or £400 per week, or £1600 each month and thus, £19 200 profit over the whole year: a significant sum.

Outcome 1: Identify additional services or products that are available

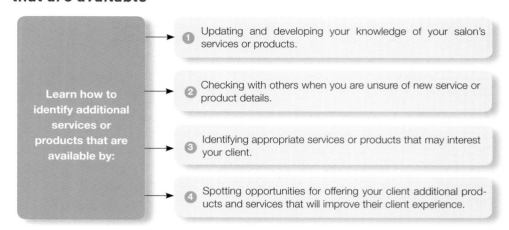

Learn how to identify additional services or products that are available by:

1. Updating and developing your knowledge of your salon's services or products.

2. Checking with others when you are unsure of new service or product details.

3. Identifying appropriate services or products that may interest your client.

4. Spotting opportunities for offering your client additional products and services that will improve their client experience.

BEST PRACTICE

Testers for products

Encourage your client to try the testers. Make-up can look very different on the face compared with its appearance on the palette. You can also take the opportunity to apply the product to show it at its best effect to suit the client.

When promoting products or services, find out first about the client's needs and expectations. This will help you identify appropriate services or products. Consider the following.

● What is the client's main priority? What would they like to achieve? This information will guide you on selecting and advising them of the most suitable product or service.

● Is a skin sensitivity test necessary before the service? Ensure there will be sufficient time to carry out any necessary tests when promoting a service.

● Is the client allergic to any particular substance, contact with which should be avoided?

● Does the client have a skin disorder or nail disease which might contra-indicate use of a particular product? Contra-indications to products must always be noted and the action to take explained to the client.

● Is the client planning to use the product over a skin disorder, i.e. cuts and abrasions? If so, is this safe?

● Find out what services the client has received before. Were they satisfied or disappointed in any way with them? If so, find out why.

● How much is the client used to spending on products? Ask about what they are presently using: this will give you an idea of the types of product they have experience with using, and the sort of prices they are used to paying.

Bearing in mind the client's needs, you can now guide them to the most suitable service or product. This is where your expertise and knowledge are so important: you can describe fully and accurately the features and benefits of the services and products you can offer.

Features and benefits

This can be repeated later to help the client make a purchase decision when there are several items to consider.

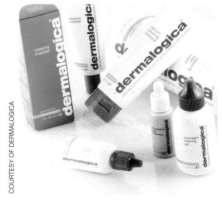

Skincare retail products

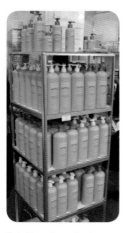

Retail product display

A **feature** is the uniqueness or individuality of a product or service, e.g. new technology in the ingredient formulation of a product or the design technology of a piece of equipment.

A **benefit** is the gain to be made by the client from using the product or service.

Selling products

The products themselves must be presented to the client in such a way that they seem both attractive and desirable: the presentation should encourage the client to purchase them. The packaging and the product should be clean and in good condition, and **testers** should be available wherever possible so that the client can try the product before purchasing it.

The final choice of product is with the client, of course, but often the client will ask for a recommendation, for example if they cannot decide between two possibilities. It is in these circumstances that your ability to answer technical questions fully, from a complete knowledge of the product, will help in closing the sale. Speaking with confidence and authority on the one product that will particularly suit the client's requirements may well persuade them to buy it.

Product suitability

If the client has not used the product or received the service before there is always a possibility of an allergic reaction.

If the client does not know what an **allergic reaction** is – or how to recognize an allergy – it is important that you describe it to them (red, itchy, flaking and even swollen skin). If they experience this sort of contra-action they should contact you immediately or in the case of product intolerance stop applying the product the client suspects is producing it.

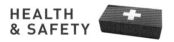

HEALTH & SAFETY

Skin sensitivity tests
If the client has not tried a product before, or if there is doubt as to how their skin will react, a skin patch test must be carried out.

1   Select either the inner elbow or the area behind the ear. The skin here is thinner and more sensitive.

2   Make sure the skin is clean.

3   Apply a little of the product, using a clean applicator.

4   Leave the area alone for 24 hours.

5   If there is no reaction after 24 hours, the client is not allergic to the product: they can go ahead and use it. If there has been any itching, soreness, erythema, or swelling in the area where the product has been applied, the client is allergic to it and should not use it.

Techniques in selling

The first rule of selling is: *know your products*. This applies to all retail products and to all salon services.

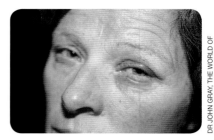

Allergic reaction to a cosmetic product that has affected the eyes

TOP TIP

Features and benefits
A *feature* is the product's specialist ingredients and the effects they can achieve.

A *benefit* is what the client can expect from buying the product.

ACTIVITY

Increasing product knowledge
With colleagues, discuss and note down the features, functions and benefits of a range of cosmetic products sold in your training establishment.

Know your clients
The products that you recommend must be the right choice for your clients and deliver the results they require.

Ruth Langley

ACTIVITY

Updating your knowledge
Professionally it is recommended that you update your skills and knowledge annually, referred to as **continuous professional development (CPD)**. This allows you to be aware of current skills and trends. Keep a record or log of the different training activities you have been on.

ALWAYS REMEMBER

Consumer protection legislation
Legally you are required to comply with legislation including the **Prices Act (1974)** and the **Trade Descriptions Acts (1968 and 1972)**. These Acts prohibit false descriptions and prices of goods and services by the business. You must ensure accuracy of all media information provided in relation to products and services.

TOP TIP

Promotional launch events
Promotions are an ideal opportunity to establish your new product line with special offers.
Clients may have the opportunity to:
- purchase products at a special discounted rate
- purchase products with complimintary gifts
- receive complimentary samples

Clearly signpost these offers at different areas of the salon, i.e. reception and service rooms, using professional marketing materials. Provide the opportunity for the client to try the products.

Staff training

It is important that everybody is knowledgeable and able to answer the client's questions – this includes the receptionist who is often the first and last person the client comes into contact within a salon. In conversation, especially during quieter periods, they have opportunities to discuss products and services informally.

Often product companies provide training either at the business or at another venue. This is a great opportunity to update your knowledge and skills, which you will be able to share enthusiastically with your clientele. Often certificates to prove training are issued and these should be professionally displayed in the salon.

If not all staff can participate it is important that new information is passed on to them to make them effective in their jobs. Team meetings are a good opportunity to discuss salon policy and new products and promotions.

Information on products and services must be supplied for clients to read, and **displays** should be set up to gain attention. Be aware of your **competitors** and their current advertising displays and campaigns.

If your business has a website ensure this is kept updated. It is a great resource for sharing any product or service promotions. If you have the software facility, clients may be able to purchase products or services online also.

Methods of promoting products and services

When promoting products and services it is good to raise client interest and awareness by considering the following.

- Eye-catching promotional material (usually provided by the product supplier): displays in the window will encourage new clients! This should be changed regularly to maintain interest.

- Updated salon literature discussing benefits and costs of products and services may be provided.

- A promotional launch event, where clients can enjoy a social event and perhaps book services or buy products at discounted prices, may be held.

- Promotional packages may be presented at reduced cost or limited edition products can be purchased.

- Sample products may be given following a service for the client to try at home.

- Products to enhance the service may be promoted, e.g. specially formulated mascara to wear with individual false lashes.

- If you have a website you may wish to promote products and services on your homepage. Special offers may be featured and you may have the facility for clients to book online.

- Special events or occasions: e.g. if the client is going on holiday, recommend travel-size products.

Know your products **Product usage** must be discussed with clients, as necessary, and advice given on which product will best suit each of them. The only way to be able to do this is to memorize the complete range: all your products, including for example which skin types or service conditions each is for, what the active ingredients are, when and how each should be used, and its cost. Any questions asked must be answered with authority and confidence. Clients expect the staff in the beauty salon to be professionals, able to provide expert advice.

● Speak with confidence and enthusiasm.

● Avoid confusing technical words.

● Explain the benefits and personalize these, matching them to the needs of each client.

If the client requests advice on products or services that are outside of your responsibility refer them to the relevant colleague who has the expertise. You may have information literature you are able to provide to your client that will prevent possible loss of a sale, so pass it on.

Information to read The **information** available to clients can start from the window display. Use the **window adverts** if supplied with product ranges, and include information that advertizes the salon's services. Few salons use windows for product displays, but you could consider doing so.

Posters are supplied with good-quality product ranges, and most suppliers provide **information leaflets** for clients. Use the posters and **display cards** in the reception area; clients can then help themselves, and read about the products and their benefits. This will generate questions – and sales.

Product and retail displays Two types of display can be used in the beauty salon. In the first, the display is there simply to be looked at, and seen as part of the decor. It should be attractive and artistically arranged, and can use dummy containers. It is not meant to be touched or sold from, so it can be behind glass or in a window display.

On the other hand, in the second, products are there to be sold. In this case products must be attractive but also accessible. The display should include testers so that clients can freely smell and touch. Each product must be clearly priced, and small signs placed beside the products or on the edge of the shelves to describe the selling points of each product.

This sort of active display must always be in the part of the salon where most people will see and walk past it -– the area of 'highest traffic'. A large proportion of cosmetic and perfume sales are **impulse buys**. It is no accident that perfumery departments are beside the main entrances to department stores, or right beside access points such as escalators.

Product displays must always feature in the beauty service area. As the beauty therapist uses the products, she can discuss and recommend them for the client. If displays are there to see and to take from, the sale can be closed even before the client returns to reception. Although in theory clients can of course change their minds between the service area and actually paying, in practice once they have the product in their hands they will go on to buy it.

Most small salons will design and create their own displays using the counter **display packs** provided by the product companies. Some will have a professional **window dresser** to regularly change the window displays for the best effect.

Displays should always be well stocked, with smart undamaged packaging. Eye-level displays are best and ideally should be accessible. Change the display regularly according to the promotion, for example UV skin protection products in summer.

TOP TIP

Product knowledge
Use the products yourself. It is always good to be able to speak from experience and shows your confidence in them. You will also be able to give tips on how best to use them.

Be a great salesperson
Believe in yourself. You have the potential to become a great salesperson. Most sales are lost because they were never asked for.

Ruth Langley

ACTIVITY

Learning the product range
Learn about and memorize the product range sold in the training establishment you attend. Once you have learnt about the range, memorize the cost of the products.

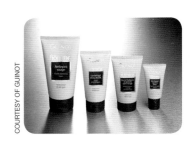

A range of men's skincare products

HEALTH & SAFETY

Maintaining hygiene and preventing cross-infection
Spatulas must be used so customers do not put their fingers into the pots either when testing or during home use. (You may also like to sell spatulas for clients to use at home.)

ACTIVITY

Collecting information
Collect information leaflets from local salons and beauty product or perfume counters in department stores. Is this literature attractive? Will the presentation encourage sales?

Write to wholesalers and product companies for information about the display packs they supply with their products.

Look at websites also. What are the features of a good business website?

ACTIVITY

Evaluating displays
Whenever you can, look at displays and make a note of neatness, cleanliness, availability, pricing and information. Compare the best with the worst.

Displays must be checked and cleaned regularly – in busy salons this will usually mean daily. A window display will need to be dusted, straightened, and looked at from outside to make sure that it looks its best. The display from which products are being sold will also need to be dusted, perhaps wiped over (if testers have dripped), and straightened up. Testers need to be checked to make sure they are not sticky and spilt, and that no one has left dirty fingerprints on them.

The range of products

It is not enough to stock just a few items and expect clients to fit in with the range you carry: different ranges must be available for each skin type, and a number of specialist products – such as eye gel, skin serums or creams – that will suit all skin types. Make-up and nail polish should be attractive to all ages and types of customer. Sales must not be lost because of a lack of product range.

Information provided to the client should be accurate and not false or misleading. Legal action could follow in the case of non-compliance with consumer protection legislation.

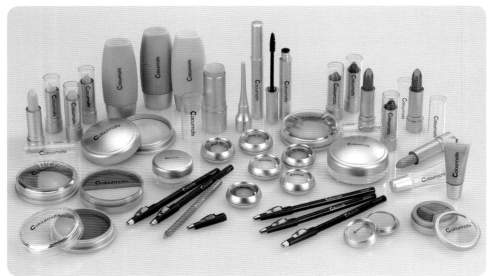

A product range

Consumer protection legislation

The salon has a legal obligation to implement and/or abide by the following legislation, designed to protect the rights of clients.

Consumer Protection Act (1987)

The Consumer Protection Act (1987) follows European Union (EU) directives to protect the customer from unsafe, defective services and products that do not reach safety standards. It is important, therefore, to only use reputable products, purchased from a reliable source and that adequate information is provided to the client on their correct use. All staff should be trained in using products and maintaining them so they are in consistently good condition. It also covers misleading price indications about goods or services available from a business. Up-to-date prices for products and services must be available. Local authorities are responsible for protecting consumers. Trading Standards or Consumer Protection Departments check that trading standards and laws are adhered to and investigate any complaint. If proven at fault and an offence has occurred the business may face legal action. For more information visit htttp://www.ico.gov.uk.

Consumer Safety Act (1978)

The Consumer Safety Act (1978) aims to reduce risk to consumers from potentially dangerous products. It outlines the minimum safety standards to be met.

Prices Act (1974)

The Prices Act (1974) states that the price of products or services has to be displayed in order to prevent the buyer being misguided.

Trade Descriptions Acts (1968 and 1972)

The Trade Descriptions Acts (1968 and 1972) prohibit the use of false descriptions of goods and services provided by a business. Products must be clearly labelled. When retailing, the information supplied both in written and verbal form must always be accurate. The supplier must not:

- supply misleading information
- describe products falsely
- make false statements

In addition they must not:

- make false comparisons between past and present services
- offer products at what is said to be a 'reduced' price, unless they have previously been on sale at the full price quoted for a 28-day minimum
- make misleading price comparisons

The Acts also require accurate information to be included in advertisements.

Resale Prices Acts (1964 and 1976)

Under the provisions of the Resale Prices Acts (1964 and 1976) the manufacturer can supply a recommended retail price (MRRP), but the seller is not obliged to sell at the recommended price.

Sale and Supply of Goods Act (1994)

This Act amended the previous Sale of Goods Act (1979) but the customers' rights as outlined in 1979 remain unchanged. The Sale and Supply of Goods Act (1994) provides that goods must be as described, of satisfactory quality including fit for their intended purpose, in appearance and finish, free from minor defects and safe and durable. The Act also covers the conditions under which customers can return goods. It is the responsibility of the retailer to correct a problem where the goods are not as described. This may be by refund, credit note, repair or replacement.

Cosmetic Products (Safety) Regulations (2004)

The Cosmetic Products (Safety) Regulations (2004) consolidates earlier regulations and incorporates current European Union directives. Part of consumer protection

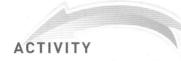

ACTIVITY

Siting of displays
In your nearest large town, go into the big department stores and note where the cosmetic and perfumery department displays are situated.

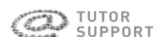

TUTOR SUPPORT

Activity 2: Product and retail display project

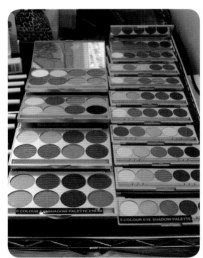

A range of eye cosmetics for make-up services

legislation, it requires that cosmetics and toiletries are safe in their formulation and are safe for use for their intended purpose as a cosmetic and comply with labelling requirements.

Data Protection Act (DPA) (1998)

The Data Protection Act (1998) applies to any business that uses computers or paper-based systems to store information about its clients and staff.

Through communication with your client it is necessary to ask clients a series of questions before the service plan can be finalized. Client details are recorded on the client record card. This information is confidential and should be stored in a secure area. The client should understand the reason behind the questions asked of them and how it will be used. Confidential information on staff or clients should only be made available to persons to whom consent has been given.

Clients who have given information need to know how it will be used; otherwise they have a right to withhold it. Information stored must be accurate and up to date. It is necessary to register with the Data Protection Registrar who will place the business on a public register of data users. A code of practice is provided which must be complied with. For more information visit htttp://www.ico.gov.uk.

Consumer Protection (Distance Selling) Regulations (2000)

These regulations, as amended by the Consumer Protection (Distance Selling) (Amendment) Regulations (2005) are derived from a European Union directive and cover the supply of goods/services made between suppliers, acting in a commercial capacity, and consumers. They are concerned with purchases made where there is no face-to-face contact, that is, by telephone, fax, internet, digital television or mail order, including catalogue shopping.

Consumers must receive clear information on goods or services, including delivery arrangements and payment, suppliers' details and consumers' cancellation rights, which should be made available in writing. The consumer also has a seven working day cool-off period where they may cancel their purchase. The point at which the right to cancel services is reached is detailed in the 2005 amendment to the 2000 Regulations.

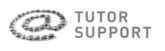

TUTOR SUPPORT

Activity 1: Customer rights task

The Disability Discrimination Act (DDA) (1996)

Under the Disability Discrimination Act (1996), as a provider of goods, facilities and services your workplace has the duty to ensure that clients are not discriminated against on the grounds of disability. It is unlawful to use disability as a reason or justification to:

- refuse to provide a service
- provide a service to a lesser standard
- provide a service on worse terms
- fail to make reasonable adjustments to the way services are provided

From 2004 this includes failure to make reasonable adjustments to the physical features of service premises to overcome physical barriers to access. Service can be denied to a disabled person if justified and if any other client would be treated in the same way. Your employer has a responsibility under the DDA to ensure that you receive adequate training to prevent discrimination in practice, and as such is responsible for your actions. Also they must make reasonable adjustments to the premises to facilitate access for disabled persons.

Equal opportunities policy

The Equal Opportunities Commission (EOC) states it is best practice for the workplace to have a written **equal opportunities policy**. This will include a statement of the commitment to equal opportunities by the employer and the details of structure for implementing the policy.

All employees should know this policy and it should be monitored regularly to review effectiveness.

Professional codes of practice

There is a code of behaviour and expected standards for the professional beauty therapist to follow, which will uphold the reputation of the industry and ensure best working practice for the safety of the industry and members of the public.

Beauty therapy professional bodies produce codes of practice for their members. Although not a legal requirement, this code may be used in criminal proceedings as evidence of improper practice. A business may have its own code of practice in relation to product and service promotion.

Insurance

Product and service liability insurance is usually included within public liability insurance, but should be checked with the insurance company. Product liability insurance covers risk, which might occur as a result of the products you are selling.

Informing clients about additional products or services

Outcome 2: Inform clients about additional services or products

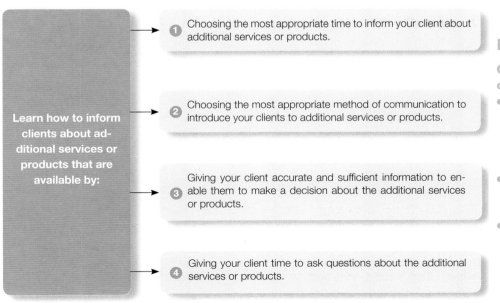

Learn how to inform clients about additional services or products that are available by:

1. Choosing the most appropriate time to inform your client about additional services or products.

2. Choosing the most appropriate method of communication to introduce your clients to additional services or products.

3. Giving your client accurate and sufficient information to enable them to make a decision about the additional services or products.

4. Giving your client time to ask questions about the additional services or products.

BEST PRACTICE

Create your own selling opportunity

- If the client is having a manicure and has weak nails, you could recommend a course of nail services and an appropriate nail strengthener.
- If the client is going away on holiday tell them about the special 'holiday package promotion'.
- If the client is having an eyelash tint, tell them how quick and simple an eyebrow wax is and the difference it can make!

ACTIVITY

Product and service promotion
Think of different services or products that your workplace offers that are not as popular as they once were. Consider a promotion you could offer to gain client interest. How would this promotion be presented?

> **Use initiative**
> Be a leader, not a follower. Put forward your ideas, but be prepared to listen to other people's ideas. Think big and take control of your career. Remember that great success starts from small ideas. Believe in yourself, but show modesty in all things. Never forget what Walt Disney said when referring to his immense success: 'I only hope that we never lose sight of one thing – that it was all started by a mouse!'.
>
> **Ruth Langley**

TOP TIP
Always pay careful attention to your client and their responses. Remember: question, listen, answer:
- *Question* your client as to their needs.
- *Listen* to the answer.
- *Answer* with the relevant information.

Knowing when to promote the product or service

Choose the most appropriate time to inform the client about additional products and services. Present information on the product or service at a pace relevant to the client's knowledge and experience. If the information is new this may be slower and detailed. If the client is receiving a service this may be at the consultation, when discussing the service objectives, during service delivery when you have the opportunity to recommend and share advice, or when discussing aftercare. Here you will be able to reinforce the importance of further products and services to enhance the service benefits gained. This may be further use of products or services that the client has used before or of those that are new to the client.

Use good communication techniques

Communication with clients, both verbal and non-verbal, is important. Establish a rapport with your client and give your attention fully to the client above any other tasks. Use your client's name: this increases their sense of self-importance and value.

- At all times remain polite, friendly and respect the client's individual opinions and preference. Never be critical this may lose a sale.

- A client may be already considering purchasing a product or service and the type of questions they ask will signal this. The most common question is 'How much is it?'

- Make eye contact, observe the client's body language: are they interested in what you are telling them? If the client is interested, they will agree with you and their body language will be relaxed yet attentive. There are many customer types: those that are decisive, indecisive, chatty, quiet, opinionated, awkward and disbelieving. This should be considered in your approach: it is important that the client gains confidence in you and ultimately your products or service. This will be secured through your appearance, communication, style and manner.

- **Questions** must be accurate and detailed. You are the expert: show your knowledge. Do not ask the client what sort of skin they have – they are not the expert, and will probably give the wrong answer. Instead, ask more detailed questions, such as 'Does your skin feel tight?' (which may indicate dryness), or 'Do you have spots in a particular area?' (which may indicate an oily patch). Use open questions. These are questions that may not be answered with yes or no. Open questions usually start with 'why,' 'how,' 'when,' 'what' and 'which'.

- **Listening** is a skill. Listen to your client; this will help you to identify their service requirements and personality. Always listen carefully to the answers your customer gives: do not talk over their answer or interrupt. Only when they have finished should you give a considered, informed reply. You may need to ask another question, or you may be able straightaway to direct them to the best product or service for their needs.

- Ensure that the client receives adequate attention in providing them with the products that they have agreed to purchase. Present the products to them and explain any specific requirements in their use in order to gain maximum benefit from their use.

- Allow time for the client to think about the purchase.

- In the case of a service, make an appointment and provide the client with an appointment card and relevant literature relating to the service. If the client has made a decision to receive a service or purchase a product, you may find there is a delay in its availability. Ensure any delay is minimal. Do not be tempted to offer unsuitable alternatives, which are not as suited to the client's needs or service requirements. Inform the client honestly and realistically of their availability. In the case of a product you may be able to give the client a sample to use until the product is available.

- Record all sales on the client's record card. This is a useful reference point for the therapist and client to refer back to.

- Ensure that the client has sufficient information to make a confident selection in their service or product choice.

- Give the client opportunity to ask questions and answer these confidently.

- Questions may lead to the opportunity to increase the sale of more products or services.

- Ensure the environment is conducive to the client feeling comfortable to ask questions.

- If a sale is achieved, be positive – smile, this will help to make the client feel they have made a good decision.

- Ask the client if there is anything else they need when closing the sale on the product. Confirm the size of product the client wishes to purchase, explaining any financial benefit to their selection.

- Be appreciative, thank the client when they are about to leave even if an enquiry has not resulted in a purchase.

TOP TIP

Competitions and free gifts are a popular incentive for clients to purchase products. Make your client aware of any promotions.

BEST PRACTICE

Gift bags and a wrapping provide a thoughtful customer care service. If packaging carries the salon name and contact details this may generate future business.

Promotion

Promotions are another way of informing your clients about products or services that are available. They are also a great way of gaining interest in a product or service from a wider audience.

General benefits of a promotion

- Clients may take the opportunity of using a product or service because it is on offer at a reduced cost. If they do not like, it is less of a costly mistake.

- A service or product on promotion may cost less and therefore be accessible to a wider client base.

- Limited editions or offers are a way of gaining client interest as the product or service may not be available or on offer at a later date.

- The enthusiasm of some clients will motivate others to purchase.

BEST PRACTICE

Effective stock control
It is important that you endeavour to always have retail stock available. It is disappointing for the client if they are unable to purchase a retail item and could potentially result in the loss of a sale – especially if they source an alternative.

Demonstration

Demonstrating to an audience needs particularly careful planning if the demonstration is to achieve the maximum benefit. Everything required must be available, and all the relevant literature to be given out to the audience or clients.

Consider all possibilities in your planning. What type of demonstration is required? Will you be working on one client, to demonstrate and sell a product, or demonstrating to a group? Is a range of products or services to be demonstrated, or just one item?

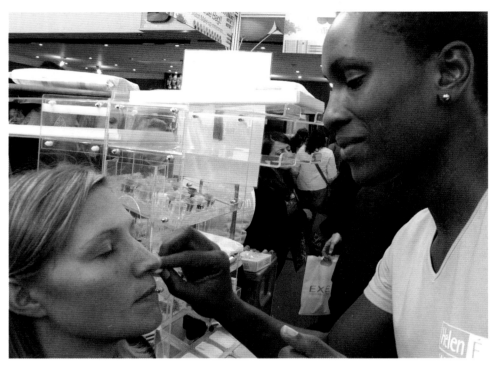

Trade demonstration

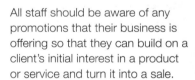

BEST PRACTICE

All staff should be aware of any promotions that their business is offering so that they can build on a client's initial interest in a product or service and turn it into a sale.

Team working

It takes all kinds of personalities to make a successful team. Learning to accept each other's differences is essential. A good team is one of the reason a salon becomes successful.

Ruth Langley

Outcome 3: Gain client commitment to using additional services or products

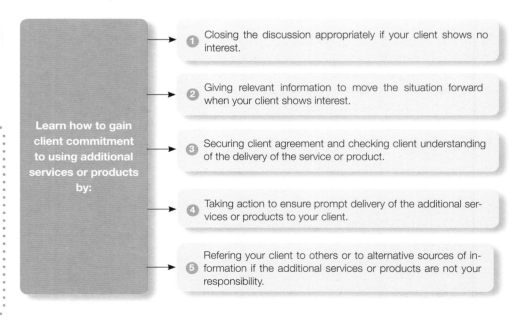

Learn how to gain client commitment to using additional services or products by:

1. Closing the discussion appropriately if your client shows no interest.
2. Giving relevant information to move the situation forward when your client shows interest.
3. Securing client agreement and checking client understanding of the delivery of the service or product.
4. Taking action to ensure prompt delivery of the additional services or products to your client.
5. Refering your client to others or to alternative sources of information if the additional services or products are not your responsibility.

Client suitability

If the client is not interested they will probably not engage with you, and will appear disinterested in what you are saying. If this occurs go back to the beginning and suggest alternatives to attempt to regain their interest, but avoid pressuring the client. Following discussion about a product or service, you may feel that the client is unsuitable. Tactfully explain to the client why this is. If it is for medical reasons, ask them to seek permission from their GP before the product or service is provided. The expectations of some clients may be unrealistic. If this is the case, patiently and diplomatically explain why and aim to agree to a realistic service programme. Remember your legal duty under the **Health and Safety at Work Act (1974)** to take reasonable care to avoid harm to yourself and others.

Single client When demonstrating on a client, have a mirror in front of them so that you can explain as you go along and the client can watch. They can then see the benefit of the product and learn how to use it at the same time. This is a simple but effective way to sell products. Demonstrations may be used to discuss facial skincare or make-up application and removal techniques.

A group The presentation should include an introduction to the demonstrator and the product, the demonstration itself, and a conclusion with thanks to the audience and model. Written **promotional material** can be placed on the seats before the audience arrives, or handed out at an appropriate point during the demonstration; **samples** can be handed around the audience to try while being discussed.

The demonstration itself must be clear, simple and not too long. The audience *must* be able to see what is being done and hear the commentary. Maximize the impact of the demonstration by giving the audience the opportunity to buy the product immediately.

If this is not possible – because the demonstration is in another room, away from the products or at another venue, not the salon business premises – ensure that members of the audience leave with a **voucher** to exchange for the product. This should offer some incentive, such as a **discount**, to encourage potential buyers to make the effort to come to the salon and buy. Never sell the features and benefits to potential customers, creating the desire for the product, without also giving them the chance to buy it.

Targets

The setting of financial targets for the business and for individuals is important to enable analysis of overall performance. The salon owner must have an overall idea of productivity against the targets set. Targets may vary for different employees depending upon experience, length of service and workload.

Productivity

Levels of performance will take into account expected services and retail product sales. Services are normally costed on the products used, including consumables such as cotton wool and tissues, and should include other hidden costs such as laundering of towels. Productivity can be increased through:

- incentives
- promotions
- personal targets

TOP TIP

Demonstrations
An effective demonstration will always create sales. Have the product ready to sell, or give out vouchers to encourage clients to purchase the product or service at a discounted rate.

TOP TIP

Visual promotional resources
You may wish to have the demonstration professionally recorded. This may then be used as a video on your website (if available) or in reception to capture client's interest and generate questions from those who did not attend.

Employability skills
Showing a willingness to learn and improve is paramount. Having a warm, friendly personality is an essential characteristic. You should aspire to be a good team player and show that you have the essential beauty therapy skills. Demonstrate that you have a passion for the industry and most importantly, remember to smile.

Ruth Langley

Poor levels of performance and productivity may indicate a need for additional training. Some companies provide rewards for employees who develop ideas for increased productivity and commission is one method of rewarding individuals who achieve and exceed targets.

Always evaluate any activity to increase productivity, reviewing sales reports and feedback from clients.

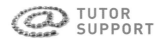

TUTOR SUPPORT

Activity 3: Designing a client questionnaire

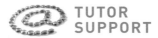

TUTOR SUPPORT

Activity 4: Multiple choice questions

Gaining client feedback

In the service industry feedback from clients is important when measuring levels of service and satisfaction. It enables you to evaluate marketing methods, salon image and service.

Client feedback can be gathered in a variety of ways, both formally and informally.

- Client questionnaires can be used at random to evaluate performance, for example following a promotion. The results should be analyzed and appropriate action taken to improve areas of weakness, build on strengths and investigate potential areas of development.

- Simply asking the client if they have enjoyed or been satisfied with the service received is another method of service evaluation.

GLOSSARY OF KEY WORDS

Additional products and services products and services offered by your salon that a client may receive or purchase to enhance their service benefits.

Body language communication involving the body.

Client groups this term is used in a number of the units and it refers to client diversity. The CRE (Commission for Racial Equality) ethnic group classification is used in the range for these units. These cover white, mixed, Asian, black and Chinese.

Code of practice the expected standards and behaviour for the professional beauty therapist to follow, which will uphold the reputation of the industry and ensure best working practice for the industry and protect members of the public. Beauty therapy professional bodies produce codes of practice for their members. A business may have its own code of practice.

Communication the exchange of information and the establishment of understanding between people.

Consumer Protection Act (1987) this act follows European Union directives to protect the customer from unsafe, defective services and products that do not reach safety standards.

Consumer Protection (Distance Selling) Regulations (2000) these Regulations, (as amended by the Consumer Protection (Distance Selling) (Amendment) Regulations (2005), are derived from a European Union directive and cover the supply of goods/services made between suppliers acting in a commercial capacity and consumers. They are concerned with purchases made by telephone, fax, internet, digital television and mail order.

Consumer Safety Act (1978) this act aims to reduce risks to consumers from potentially dangerous products.

Cosmetic Products (Safety) Regulations (2004) part of consumer protection legislation that requires cosmetics and toiletries be safe in their formulation and safe for use for their intended purpose as a cosmetic and comply with labelling requirements.

Data Protection Act (1998) legislation designed to protect client privacy and confidentiality.

Disability Discrimination Act (1996) implemented to prevent disabled persons being discriminated against. Employers have a responsibility to remove physical barriers and to adjust working conditions to prevent discrimination on the basis of having a disability.

Gift voucher a pre-payment method for beauty therapy services or retail sales.

Legislation laws affecting the workplace in relation to services, systems and procedures, the premises, employers and employees.

Prices Act (1974) this act states that the price of products has to be displayed in order to prevent the buyer being misguided.

Promotion ways of communicating products or services to clients to increase sales.

Resale Prices Acts (1964 and 1976) this act states that the manufacturer can supply a recommended price (MRRP), but the seller is not obliged to sell at the recommended price.

Sale and Supply of Goods Act (1994) goods must be as described, of merchantable quality and fit for their intended purpose.

Targets goals or objectives to achieve, usually set within a timescale.

Trade Descriptions Acts (1968 and 1972) legislation that states that information when selling products both in written and verbal form should be accurate.

ASSESSMENT OF KNOWLEDGE AND UNDERSTANDING

Having covered the learning objectives for **Promote additional products and services to clients**, test what you need to know and understand answering the following short questions below. The information covers:

- salon systems and procedures for promoting additional products and services
- benefits of effective service an product promotion

Salon systems and procedures for promoting additional products or services

1 Why are retail sales important to the beauty salon?

2 Why is it important that you have a good knowledge about the products and services available in your salon?

3 How can you keep up to date with the beauty products and service you have on offer? Why is this important?

4 What are the opportunities that occur where you can promote a product or service? Think of examples from your experience.

5 Communication is important when selling. Why is it important to observe the client's body language?

6 As well as direct advice, what other ways can you make clients aware of the products and services available in your salon?

7 If the client required advice about a product or service on which you were not qualified to advise, what action would you take?

8 How must displays of retail stock be kept? Why is this important?

9 Clients have 'consumer rights'. Why is it important to give accurate information about products or services?

10 Name three pieces of legislation/regulations relating to the way products or services are delivered to clients which protect their legal rights.

Benefits of effective service and product promotion

1 Why must the client's needs be confirmed before selling them products or services?

2 What are the benefits to the client of using additional products, as advised by the therapist?

3 Why is it important to stock a range of products?

4 How do you think speaking with confidence and authority on a product will influence the client?

5 Staff training is important to ensure that everybody is knowledgeable and able to advise clients on their questions. What other benefit does this have to the clients, employees and salon?

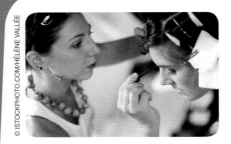

5 Effectiveness at Work (G8)

G8 Unit Learning Objectives

This chapter covers **Unit G8 Develop and maintain your effectiveness at work**.

This unit is all about taking personal responsibility to improve your performance at work. This also includes ensuring positive, professional relationships are established with colleagues, the team of people you work with, to contribute to the effectiveness and ultimately the success of the business.

There are **two** learning outcomes for Unit G8 which you must achieve competently:

1   Improve your personal performance at work

2   Work effectively as part of a team

Your assessor will observe your contributions to effective teamwork on **at least one occasion** which will be recorded.

From the **range** statement, you must show that you:

● have participated in all the listed **opportunities** to learn

● have agreed and reviewed your progress towards both productivity and personal development **targets**

● have offered **assistance** to both an individual colleague and in a group of your colleagues

You will need to collect evidence to show how you have met the standard for developing and maintaining your effectiveness at work.

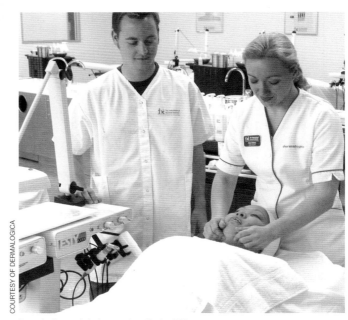

Beauty therapists improving their skills

Improve your personal performance at work

Outcome 1: Improve your personal performance at work

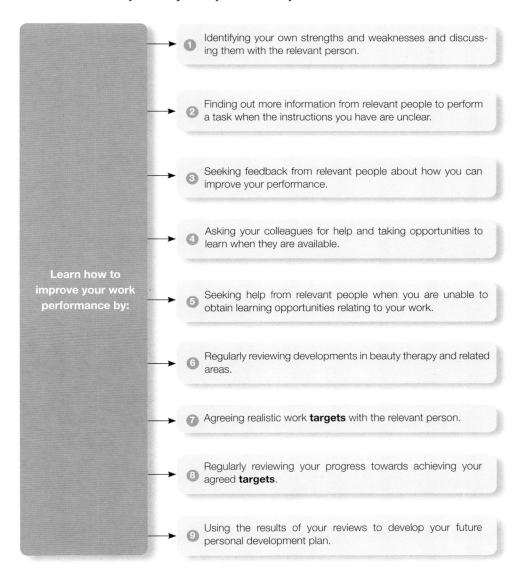

Learn how to improve your work performance by:

1. Identifying your own strengths and weaknesses and discussing them with the relevant person.

2. Finding out more information from relevant people to perform a task when the instructions you have are unclear.

3. Seeking feedback from relevant people about how you can improve your performance.

4. Asking your colleagues for help and taking opportunities to learn when they are available.

5. Seeking help from relevant people when you are unable to obtain learning opportunities relating to your work.

6. Regularly reviewing developments in beauty therapy and related areas.

7. Agreeing realistic work **targets** with the relevant person.

8. Regularly reviewing your progress towards achieving your agreed **targets**.

9. Using the results of your reviews to develop your future personal development plan.

For any beauty therapy business, to be a success requires the commitment of each employed individual to ensure quality at all levels and in all services.

For this to occur it is important both that you are effective in your job role and that you develop and maintain positive working relationships with your colleagues and clients which will create the right work environment.

Good working relationships in the workplace are essential. Each employee, whatever their job role, is valuable as part of the team in ensuring the success of the business. All staff at **induction** should be told of the goals of the business, and their role in achieving them. The induction should take place as soon as you start work, or progress into a new job role. Its aim is to provide you with general and essential information such as a description of the work environment facilities, health and safety, security, the

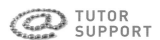

TUTOR SUPPORT

Activity 1: Code of conduct poster

TOP TIP

Image

A professional image creates confidence in clients, who learn to trust that they will be treated in a certain way – professionally and with respect.

TOP TIP

Team meetings

The team should meet at least every two weeks to ensure that it remains focused on targets to be achieved and that communication within the team is effective.

ACTIVITY

Roles and responsibilities

List the different roles and responsibilities of personnel in your workplace. Clients and business callers may require this information.

staffing structure, roles and responsibilities of colleagues in the organization and how they relate to your welfare. For example who to report to if you require advice in area outside of your responsibility or you have a concern. The induction should leave you more confident about the expectations required from you and how you will be supported. Relevant responsibilities should be clearly defined in a job description.

Your workplace will have certain salon service standards with regard to the expected standard of behaviour and appearance to perform successfully in the job role. These are often referred to as codes of conduct.

General beauty therapy codes of conduct

- Have a smart, professional appearance at all times and follow the expected dress code – it creates an impression of the quality standard that can be expected.
- Always have high standards of personal hygiene.
- Never eat, drink or chew gum in front of the client.
- Ensure that you follow your health and safety responsibilities, never putting yourself or anybody else at risk through your actions.
- Communicate clearly and positively, both verbally and non-verbally.
- Be polite and courteous at all times to both clients and colleagues.
- Never lose your temper, or swear in front of a client.
- Avoid controversial and personal topics of conversation.
- If you are unable to give the client information they need, quickly find somebody suitably qualified to assist.
- If there are any personal issues among staff or towards a client, do not let these show in front of the client. Settle the grievances (reasons for complaint) as soon as possible, to avoid job satisfaction and productivity being affected.

Job roles and responsibilities

Each team member should have a job description. This details:

- the job title
- the specific job role
- the duties and responsibilities
- the work location
- any extra special circumstances affecting duties, such as attending salon promotional events

The job description enables each employee to know what is expected of them and to whom and for what they are responsible. A job description may also be used when appraising your performance in your job role.

For reasons of safety and effectiveness it is important that you know what jobs and roles you are qualified to undertake. At all times work only within your job role, providing the skills that you are qualified to undertake. Performing additional responsibilities outside your job description may mean you are not meeting the requirements of the Beauty Therapy

Job description

Job description – Beauty Therapist

Location:	Based at salon as advised.
Main purpose of job:	To ensure customer care is provided at all times.
	To maintain a good standard of technical and client care, ensuring that up-to-date methods and techniques are used following the salon training practices and procedures.
Responsible to:	Salon manager.
Requirements:	To maintain the company's standards in respect of beauty therapy services.
	To ensure that all clients receive service of the best possible quality.
	To advise clients on services.
	To advise clients on products and aftercare.
	To achieve designated performance targets.
	To participate in self-development or to assist with the development of others.
	To maintain company policy in respect of:

- personal standards of health/hygiene
- personal standards of appearance/conduct
- operating safely while at work
- public promotion
- corporate image

as laid out in employee handbook.

To carry out client consultation in accordance with company policy.

To maintain company security practices and procedures.

To assist your manager in the provision of salon resources.

To undertake additional tasks and duties required by your manager from time to time.

National Occupational Standards (NOS). These standards state the skills required to be completed competently as well as the things you must know and understand. The result could cause harm to yourself and others and you could be liable for any misdemeanour.

A contract of employment should also be provided, this is made as soon as you accept a job offer. It is an agreement between an employer and employee stating your employment rights, responsibilities and duties. A written contract of employment should be given to an employee within two months of being employed. This contains details of the job description and employment including hours of work, holiday entitlement and length of notice requirements. It also identifies disciplinary rules and what disciplinary action will be applied when set rules or working conditions are broken. Ultimately this could lead to dismissal. Instant dismissal occurs where there is sufficient reason, for example, in cases such as theft or breach of health and safety practice that endangers others, termed as **gross misconduct**. Where an employee feels that they have been treated unfairly in their dismissal they may take this to an employment tribunal.

The contract is legally binding until circumstances change such as giving notice to terminate employment or terms of the contract are changed.

Therefore, to be aware of the standards expected, your job responsibilities and limits of your own authority you should receive an induction, job description and contract of employment.

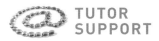 **TUTOR SUPPORT**

Activity 5: Job description project

ACTIVITY

Client care

Find out whether your organization has a customer care statement. If so, how well do you do in providing that Level of customer care? Monitor yourself against the statement, and ask colleagues for feedback.

ACTIVITY

Telephone calls

A telephone call is often the first contact the client has with the salon and is an important method of communication.

- How should the phone be answered?
- What should you confirm if the client requires an eyelash tint?
- What action would you take if there was not sufficient time for the appointment at the time requested?
- How would you handle a complaint about a service?

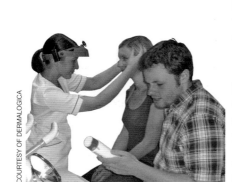

COURTESY OF DERMALOGICA

Client consultation

Customer care

Many organizations have a customer care statement, which outlines the standards of service customers can expect.

Clients want to enjoy their visits to the beauty salon and they are paying for a service. It is important that during each visit they are made to feel relaxed and comfortable and their needs are met.

Client care

Remember that each client has a different personality and different service needs, requiring an individual service approach.

A client can be made to feel intimidated, uncomfortable or ignored – and this can happen without your saying anything! Even without speaking you communicate with your eyes, your face and your body, transmitting some of your feelings. This is called **non-verbal communication**. How you look and how you behave in front of your clients is important.

Positive relationships with clients

On meeting a client, always smile, make eye contact and greet her cheerfully – however bad your own day is! As you communicate you can:

- promote yourself, and gain the client's confidence in your professionalism and technical expertise
- develop a professional relationship with the client
- establish the client's needs
- promote services

Verbal communication occurs when you talk directly to another person, either face to face or over the telephone. Always speak clearly and precisely, and avoid slang. It is important to be a good listener: this will help you identify the client's service requirements and understand their personality. You can then guide the conversation appropriately.

Conversing with a client

Having developed a professional relationship with your client, centre the conversation on them, so that they feel special. Avoid interrupting the client while they are speaking, listen carefully and be patient.

Listening skills When you listen, give the person all your attention, the other person then knows you are listening. You must ensure that you *hear* what the other person is saying and you *understand* what they are saying. Then you will be able to *respond* appropriately to what they have said or asked. Do not be afraid of silence, allow the other person to think and consider when listening.

A nervous client may need to be reassured. Gain their confidence by being pleasant and cheerful without chattering constantly. When asking questions, don't interrogate your client. Never talk down to them, and avoid technical jargon – instead, use commonly understood words.

Questioning skills Asking questions allows you to find out information you need to know and learn more to make a decision. Ask open questions; those that encourage the other person to talk and cannot be answered with *yes* or *no* (these are called closed questions). Open questions start with 'how,' 'why,' 'what,' 'when,' and 'which.' Probing questions can used and are necessary when you need to gain further detail or information. These may ask for precise detail e.g. 'How long exactly do you want to wear your false lashes for?'.

Certain technical information may not appear complicated, but if for example a client has bought several skincare products it is important that they know how to use them safely and efficiently. Always check tactfully with the client to ensure that they have fully understood the information provided.

Avoid all controversial topics, such as sex, religion and politics! When a relationship has been established, value it but be discreet – clients will often share confidences with you. Never pass judgement, and ensure that you deserve clients' trust by maintaining confidentiality.

Responding appropriately

It may be that the client requests information that you are unable to help with or which lies outside your responsibility. If this occurs politely inform them that you are not able or qualified to deal with their request but will get somebody else to assist. Always indicate how long this will take if it will not be immediately.

Keeping your client informed is reassuring and important to avoid dissatisfaction with the service provided.

Non-verbal communication

Non-verbal communication is also referred to as **body language**. Interpreting body language is an important skill: learn to notice how the client is behaving, including their voice, their eyes, their body and their arm and hand movements. An instinctive 'feel' for customers' behaviour can be developed with experience.

Noticing client behaviour will help you to recognize the client's different needs and expectations. You must be able to adapt to these.

When approaching potential customers in a situation, such as a client who shows an interest in a product on a retail display, be aware that conflicting signals may be given. For example, a person may smile and nod as if interested but may, in fact, not be. On the other hand, if the customer makes the first approach then they obviously have an active interest already

Initially the customer may be formal and may even have a stiff body posture and a reserved manner. As they become more interested, however, their posture will relax: they may begin to lean forward. It will become obvious at this stage that they are interested, and they then will go on to nod and agree, and to listen actively.

You must use your own body language to good effect. You must be relaxed but attentive, and listen actively – nodding and shaking your head, and smiling in agreement. Use relaxed, gentle hand movements: do not twitch or turn away from the customer.

TOP TIP

Client care
Make notes on the client's record card of topics that interest them. You can introduce these topics in conversation next time the client receives a service, and they will be pleased that you have taken the trouble to remember.

TOP TIP

Client confusion
If a client is confused about the information you have given them, identify which part is confusing.

Repeat the information clearly and logically to clarify your instructions, checking for understanding.

Always allow time for clients to consider your response and provide further explanation as necessary.

Confirm the client's understanding with them and ensure that they are now clear and satisfied.

TOP TIP

Using the correct title
It is important that a client is greeted appropriately according to their expectations.

Never use a client's first name unless invited to do so.

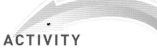

ACTIVITY

Evaluating customer care
Visit a local salon. Beforehand, think of questions you would like to ask in relation to services offered. Then evaluate the customer care and services you received. Were the staff:

- friendly?
- dressed smartly?
- knowledgeable?
- efficient and eager to assist you?
- helpful?

If you answered 'no' to any of these questions, discuss your reasons with your colleagues. What have you learnt from this experience?

ACTIVITY

Handling customer complaints
List five complaints that might be made by a client. How would you handle each situation to ensure a positive outcome?

BEST PRACTICE

Handling and monitoring complaints

A complaint from a dissatisfied client gives us the opportunity to put things right and turn a negative into a positive!

Complaints received should be logged however minor, and reviewed at team meetings. There may be patterns to the complaints which if not fixed could affect long-term customer satisfaction.

If the customer is not agreeing with you, or is not interested, they may look bored, tap their fingers, fiddle with their shopping, look away, or even look at their watch. If these signs are evident, go back to the beginning and try to find out why they are not interested. This is important when selling. Perhaps they do not want the product you have recommended? Or perhaps it is too expensive? Suggest alternatives and see whether you can get their interest again.

When the customer has decided to buy, smile – help them to feel that they have made an excellent decision. They should leave feeling proud to have purchased the product.

Avoiding client dissatisfaction

Some dissatisfied clients will voice their dissatisfaction; others will remain silent and simply not return to the salon. This situation can often be prevented through good customer care and effective communication.

- Always ensure that the client has a thorough consultation before any new service. This should be carried out by a colleague with the appropriate technical expertise.

- Regularly check the client's satisfaction. If there is any concern, make the supervisor aware of this immediately.

- Inform the client of any disruption to service – do not leave them wondering what the problem may be. Politely inform them of the situation, for example 'I'm sorry but we are running ten minutes late – are you able to wait?' If your salon has the facilities, you may offer them a drink.

- Inconvenience caused by disruption to service can usually be compensated in some way. It is important to resolve problems and keep clients satisfied.

Customer care is vital: clients provide the salon's income and your wages. The success of the business depends upon satisfied clients.

Complaints procedure

Unfortunately problems do sometimes arise in which the client cannot be appeased. Many complaints are easily resolved but require a procedure to deal with them. A complaints procedure is a formal, standardized approach adopted by the organization to handle any complaints. It should also be used to handle complaints of discrimination.

Whatever the procedure for handling a complaint, all employees should be familiar with it.

Clients should be advised of the standard complaint procedure and if not able to be dealt with immediately, they should be left with confidence knowing how it is to be dealt with, and how and when they will be contacted with an update or outcome.

Dealing with client dissatisfaction or complaint

If a client is dissatisfied they may appear angry and complain or they may say nothing. However they react, remember that a dissatisfied client is bad for business.

You may be required to deal with a dissatisfied client.

- Stay calm and listen to the client's complaint.

- If you are unable to handle it refer it as quickly as possible to somebody who can. Inform the client of your actions at all times. (It is important that you know the limits of your authority when handling a complaint.)

- Establish the facts and take appropriate action as laid down in your client complaints procedure.

- Always aim to repair the relationship, although at times this may not be possible.

- Not all clients are always genuine in their complaint – establish the facts and tactfully advise the client of the outcome.

- Always remain courteous, professional and create a positive impression.

Legal requirements

The salon has a legal obligation to implement legislation designed to protect client's rights.

Health and safety Following the consultation you may feel that the client is unsuitable for service. Explain tactfully why this is and ask them to seek permission from their GP before the service is given. Some clients may have unrealistic expectations. If this is the case, tactfully explain why and aim to agree to a realistic service programme.

Remember your legal duty under the **Health and Safety at Work Act (1974)** to take reasonable care to avoid harm to yourself and others. Never use equipment for which you do not have the professional expertise. As well as the obvious potential hazards, you would not have the expertise to adapt the service to suit the client's service needs, and you would not be able to provide the relevant service advice in order to obtain the optimum service results.

Data Protection Act (1998) Before treating your client it is necessary to ask them a series of questions so that a service plan can be finalized.

Client details are recorded on the client record card. This information is confidential and should be stored in a secure area. The client should understand the reason behind the questions asked of them.

Confidential information on staff or clients should only be made available to persons to whom consent has been given.

Equal opportunities The United Kingdom has specific legislation on equal opportunity that outlaws discrimination, protecting employees. This legislation also covers the provision of goods and services.

The **Race Relations Act (1976 and 2000)** makes it unlawful to discriminate on the grounds of colour, race, nationality, ethnic or national origin. The **Commission for Racial Equality** has produced a code of conduct to eradicate racial discrimination.

The **Disability Discrimination Act (DDA) (1995 and 2005)** makes it unlawful to discriminate on the grounds of disability.

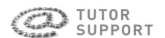

TUTOR SUPPORT

Activity 3: Communicating to clients

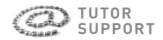

TUTOR SUPPORT

Activity 2: Evaluating client care project

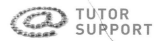

TUTOR SUPPORT

Activity 4: Which Act? handout

The **Sex Discrimination Act (1975 and 1985)**, and the **Equal Pay Act (1970) Amendment Regulations (2003)**, prevent discrimination or less favourable service of men or women on the basis of gender. This covers pay and conditions as well as promotion.

Improving your performance

In order to develop personally and to improve your skills professionally, it is important to set yourself targets against which you can measure your achievement.

To an employer it is important that you are *consistent*. You must always perform your skills to the highest standard, and present and promote a positive image of the industry and the organization in which you are employed and which you represent.

Performance review or appraisal

Appraisal is a process whereby a designated colleague performs the role of appraiser and identifies and discusses with individuals their strengths and weaknesses, and areas within their job role that require further training and development. The job description is used as a key document during appraisal.

Appraisals should focus on current performance in the job role including achievement of targets' set. They should be carried out regularly and work best when the appraisee, yourself, welcomes feedback both positive and negative and seeks guidance on where and how personal performance can be improved.

In preparing for an appraisal you should appraise your personal performance to date, a self-appraisal.

- What are your strengths, your personal attributes, accomplishments, the achievements you are proud of?
- What are your weaknesses, the things that you are not as good at and need to improve on?
- Have you achieved all targets set, and if not why?

At the appraisal you should:

- Seek feedback on how you can improve your performance. Ask for specific examples where comments on your performance are made. Feedback is essential to learning.
- Accept comments where valid – avoid being defensive.
- Respond to ideas suggested – avoid resisting them.

This may seem daunting, but it is an important and useful process. You can also use it to your advantage to:

- identify opportunities for further or specialist training
- identify obstructions that are affecting progression
- identify and amend any changes to your role
- identify and focus on your achievements to date against targets set
- make an action plan which will help you achieve your targets

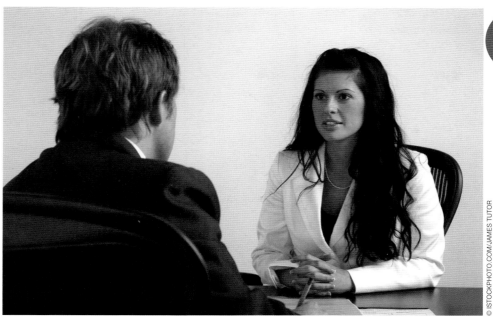

A performance appraisal

TOP TIP

Internal verification

When you are being assessed, all assessment is checked for validity using a process called *internal verification*. An appointed person titled *internal verifier* will investigate an appeal if it is thought by the candidate that the assessment decision outcome by the assessor was incorrect.

A date should be set to review your performance against the targets set.

At the next appraisal date the agreed objectives and targets set for the previous period are reviewed and the results measured. Additional accomplishments and contributions should also be looked at. Keep your personal development action plan up to date. A revised action plan will then be set for review at the next performance review or appraisal. A sample performance appraisal is shown on the next page. The agreed actions produce your **personal development plan**.

Targets

In order to develop personally and to improve your skills professionally, it is important to have personal targets against which you can measure your achievement.

If these are confidential, salon policy regarding confidentiality should be observed.

Targets should be **SMART**

- **Specific** – clearly defined
- **Measurable** – quantifiable in some way
- **Agreed** – between both parties
- **Realistic** – achievable
- **Timed** – for the duration of the fixed period

Targets to be achieved may be set by the employer or appraiser either for individuals or for the team as a whole. These may review quality, efficiency and results. Computer systems are often able to provide relevant data about the salon's performance, including sales performance against target for individuals and the team.

Targets set must be realistic and agreed between yourself and the appraiser.

ACTIVITY

Peer observation

In preparing for an appraisal you could ask a colleague to review your performance in your job role and give you feedback. This will make you more aware of what are your strengths and weaknesses. It will also improve your motivation and confidence if others recognize and appreciate what you are good at.

Where you have weaknesses you need to plan on how these can be improved.

TOP TIP

Feedback

Enable us to get information about ourselves.

Without feedback we do not know how we are doing or how our actions affect others.

Performance Appraisal

Name:	Jeanette Manners
Job title:	Trainee junior beauty therapist
Date of appraisal:	19 February 2010
Objectives:	To obtain competence within: improving and maintaining facial skin condition across the range.
Notes on achievement:	Competence has been achieved for most facial skin condition range requirements.
Training requirements:	Further training and practice is *needed* within the area of facial massage.
Any other comments on performance by appraiser:	Jeanette has achieved most of the objectives set out during the last appraisal.
Any comments on the appraisal by the staff member appraised:	I feel that this has been a fair appraisal of my progress although I did not achieve all of my performance targets. *J Manners*
Action plan: Targets to be achieved.	• To achieve occupational competence across the range for facial skin condition. • To undergo training and practice in hair removal techniques. • To take assessment for hair removal.
Date of next appraisal:	20 October 2010

TOP TIP

Productivity targets

Productivity targets can be achieved by:

- being aware of retail opportunities. For example, if a client receives a leg wax you could sell her a body lotion that slows hair re-growth
- informing your client of any special offers
- keeping up to date with current trends, encouraging your client to receive new products and services which will help to ensure client motivation and loyalty

You should set your *own* targets, however, to monitor your effectiveness and performance. In training situations your personal targets will include:

- what training activities will take place and when
- what tasks need to be performed
- what standards are expected to be reached
- when assessment should be expected
- productivity targets, e.g. with regard to technical and retail sales
- when a review of progress towards the agreed targets is to take place

In the same way, you can set targets for yourself and appraise your effectiveness at achieving them.

Sometimes achievement of productivity targets will be rewarded with additional financial payment called commission or complimentary products or training.

Personal effectiveness against targets set

Your ability to meet the expected standards is referred to as personal effectiveness.

Standards that you are assessed against include:

- The National Occupational Standards for Beauty Therapy.

- Organizational Codes of Conduct.

- Personal targets and their achievement, identified in appraisal and short- and long-term reviews.

- Your productivity targets, e.g. with regard to technical and retail sales.

If you meet the standards before the due target date, your appraiser should be informed to review new targets for completion. This will ensure that you remain motivated in your work role and it will enable you to progress more quickly.

If personal targets are not being met it is important to identify the problem with the relevant person and constructive performance targets should be put in place to resolve this and prevent unsatisfactory performance.

Your future personal objectives and targets should be agreed with a date set for completion. At the next appraisal the agreed objectives and targets set for the previous period will be reviewed.

Being positive about negative feedback

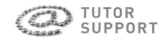

TUTOR SUPPORT

Activity 6: Effectiveness at work wordsearch

TOP TIP

National Occupational Standards for Beauty Therapy

The NVQ/SVQ Level 2 Beauty Therapy qualification is used to plan your training needs and assessment requirements.

The National Occupational Standards for Beauty Therapy are identified in the examination-awarding body's candidate logbook. They can also be obtained from the Hairdressing and Beauty Therapy Industry Authority (Habia) www.habia.org.

An *individual learning plan*, negotiated with your assessor, sets short-term targets for completion and records valuable feedback on assessment completion and where there is a need for further training to meet the expected standards. This may be used when reviewing your personal performance.

TOP TIP

Job promotion

Internal promotion may require an employee to put in extra work, take on more responsibility or come up with new ideas.

TOP TIP

Continuous professional development (CPD)

Those involved in the training and assessment of candidates formally record activities undertaken to further develop their technical skills for continuous professional development (CPD) and provide evidence of current, professional experience in the beauty therapy industry.

Your appraisal may not always be a positive experience. It is important to be positive about recommendations to improve your performance and work towards achieving these. Not meeting targets may ultimately result in disciplinary procedure which may lead to dismissal. Your achievements of the productivity targets set lead to the financial effectiveness of the business.

If you are unhappy about your appraisal there should be a process of grievance or appeal where an independent, impartial review can take place to assess if your appeal is valid or not.

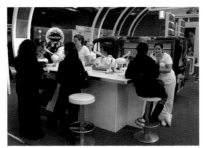

Trade fair

Developing within the job role

There will be many opportunities to develop your skills and experience, and your understanding of your work:

● By attending trade seminars: this will maintain your awareness of emerging trends and industry developments.

● By subscribing to professional trade magazines.

● By active participation in training and development activities.

● By watching and talking to colleagues who have more advanced qualifications or experience.

● By developing your portfolio to include evidence and examples of experience gained.

● By using time effectively, and by practising – all tasks take time to master: the more you practise, the more skilled and efficient you will become.

Outcome 2: Work effectively as part of a team

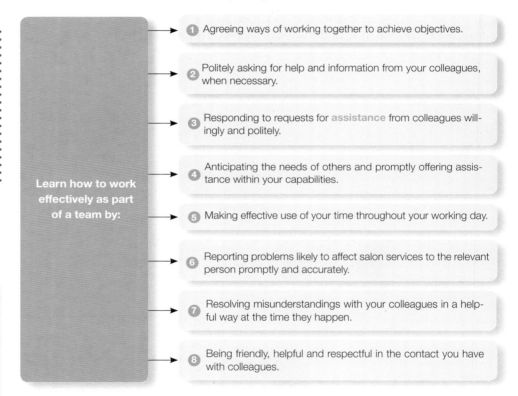

Learn how to work effectively as part of a team by:

1 Agreeing ways of working together to achieve objectives.

2 Politely asking for help and information from your colleagues, when necessary.

3 Responding to requests for assistance from colleagues willingly and politely.

4 Anticipating the needs of others and promptly offering assistance within your capabilities.

5 Making effective use of your time throughout your working day.

6 Reporting problems likely to affect salon services to the relevant person promptly and accurately.

7 Resolving misunderstandings with your colleagues in a helpful way at the time they happen.

8 Being friendly, helpful and respectful in the contact you have with colleagues.

Positive relationships with colleagues

There can be no place in a customer care industry for poor working relationships. A great portion of your time is spent in the workplace alongside your colleagues, and if the environment becomes stressful this will affect your effectiveness. It will also be apparent to clients, and relationships between staff members should not trouble them. Disputes must be resolved immediately.

When handling a dispute:

● Your behaviour can affect others for the worse or the better, remember 'behaviour breeds behaviour'. Stay calm and the other person will become calm, become angry and so will the other person.

ACTIVITY

In your organization do you know:

● who to report an accident to?

● who to report a client complaint to?

● who carries out your performance review or appraisal?

● who you would report a staff sickness to?

● who you would report a stock shortage to?

● who you report a grievance to?

● who you would discuss any concern you had with achieving your targets?

- Do not be defensive, this is a negative behaviour.

- Behave appropriately for the workplace, remembering your salon 'codes of conduct': there may be clients in the work environment.

- Explain your case clearly and what your issues are. Avoid repeating yourself.

- Listen to the other person's case without interrupting.

- Suggest ideas to resolve the dispute. What outcomes do you need?

- Agree a solution, negotiate, including the other person's ideas also.

- Agree mutually to move forward.

If the dispute cannot be resolved report this to a senior colleague who has the responsibility to deal such personnel issues.

Personnel problems may occur if there are ineffective communication systems. Time should be made to hold regular staff meetings where any concerns can be shared. A staff meeting can also be an exciting opportunity to share ideas to improve the efficiency of the job role and to look together at ways of improving the business.

It is important that you understand the salon's **staffing structure**. You need to know who is responsible for what, and who you should approach in various circumstances.

Each person will have a job description which states their roles and responsibilities.

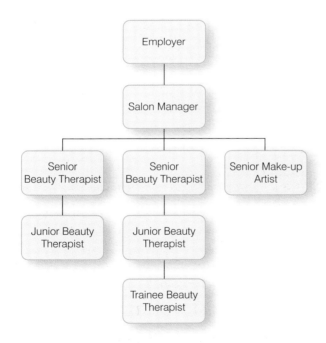

A salon staffing structure

Grievances

If you felt that you were being treated unfairly. Any grievance should be reported to a supervisor. You should familiarize yourself with the **grievance and appeals procedure**.

This includes what action to take if you:

- have a disagreement with a colleague that you cannot resolve

- feel you are being treated unfairly

- are being discriminated against

To do	By when	Done ✓

Task pad

TOP TIP

Electronic communication
Check emails regularly if this is a form of communication within your business.

• are unhappy with feedback on your personal performance

• are working outside the limitations of your job role

The grievance and appeals procedure should ensure that the issue is fully investigated and appropriate action is taken or implemented. In some cases this will mean that disciplinary action against an individual is taken. For a team to work effectively, problems should be addressed as soon as they arise and it is important that harmonious relationships are rebuilt.

Support and guidance should be requested, but only when needed. It is important to use your initiative whenever possible while operating within your job role. When seeking support or guidance, any request should be courteously asked for at an appropriate time from the appropriate person, this may be the senior therapist, trainer or supervisor.

If you are unclear how to perform any task you should request further support.

Any request for support or guidance should be responded to clearly and courteously.

Use your time effectively. Make a list of tasks you need to complete (listing each task, when it needs to be done by and ticking it off when it is done) and prioritize them in importance. If you are not busy, offer to help your colleagues.

Service times allowed for the completion of beauty therapy services within a 'commercially viable time' should be adhered to, to ensure clients receive their service on time, customer satisfaction is maintained and potential profits are achieved.

Don't ignore problems – always report these to the relevant person.

Maximum service times for Level 2 beauty therapy services

Service	*Maximum service time allowed (minutes)	Service	*Maximum service time allowed (minutes)
Eyebrow shape	15 mins	Half leg, bikini and underarm wax	60 mins
Eyelash tint	20 mins	Full leg, bikini and underarm wax	75 mins
Facial	60 mins	Threading	10 mins
Make-up	45 mins	Facial including lash tint and eyebrow shape	80 mins
Manicure	45 mins	Eyebrow shape and eyelash tint	30 mins
Pedicure	45 mins	Eyebrow tint	10 mins
Eyebrow wax	15 mins	Eyebrow tint, shape and lash tint	30 mins
Underarm wax	15 mins	Ear piercing	15 mins
Half leg wax	30 mins	Facial and make-up	90 mins
Bikini line wax	15 mins	Nail art	5–10 mins (per nail)
Arm wax	30 mins	False lashes	20 mins
Full leg	50 mins		

*Specialist services may require longer following manufacturers' instructions.

Punctuality

It is important to the efficient working of the salon that you are punctual for work. This ensures that you are composed, that clients are not kept waiting and that you are able to support other members of the team. You thereby minimize stress for yourself and for your colleagues. While being punctual, you should also have the necessary smart appearance to commence your working day,

Working under pressure

Sometimes you will be extremely busy and you may be feeling tired and weary. This is not the client's problem however! Remain cheerful, courteous and helpful. You should also use your initiative in helping others, for example by preparing a colleague's work area when you are free and they are busy.

You must be able to cope with the unexpected such as:

- clients arriving late for appointments
- clients' services overrunning the allocated service times
- double bookings, with two clients requiring service at the same time
- the arrival of unscheduled clients
- changes to the bookings

With effective teamwork such situations can usually be overcome.

Absence from work

If a member of staff is absent from work, other staff will need to review the daily work schedule to minimize disruption. In the case of holiday cover this can be planned for, but if a staff member is absent unexpectedly, teamwork will be needed to get the work done.

When you learn that someone is to be absent, find out, if you can, for approximately how long. Then do the following:

- Check the work schedule of the person who is absent.
- With authority to do so, reschedule clients, but without affecting the quality of the salon's service.
- Determine whether any clients' appointments can or must be cancelled, especially if there are double bookings or if the client must be treated specifically by the person who is away. Contact clients as soon as possible, so that they can reschedule their own time.

If you yourself are ill, to minimize disruption you must report your sickness as early as possible to the relevant person. You may be required to complete sickness forms.

Effective teamwork

An effective team member:

- knows who to report to for guidance
- is supported in their job role by their supervisor and other colleagues
- communicates freely

ACTIVITY

Dealing with the unexpected
How would you deal with the unexpected situations listed opposite? With colleagues, discuss your experiences and record your ideas.

ACTIVITY

How good are we?
A questionnaire may be useful in monitoring client satisfaction. Questionnaires can be anonymous, and collected at a central point.

Ask questions that are important to the team and the business. Collate the findings and use them to evaluate effectiveness and identify areas requiring development. Simple changes can make all the difference!

ACTIVITY

Teamwork
What personal characteristics do you need to work effectively in a team? From your own experience, discuss times when you have worked in a team. What was your role?

Ask a colleague: are you seen by others as a team player? If not, how can you develop the necessary skills?

- has targets to work towards that are regularly reviewed
- is flexible and willing to change to meet organizational needs
- operates in a supportive, friendly atmosphere
- feels valued

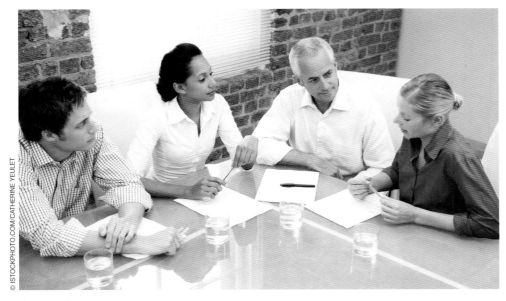

© ISTOCKPHOTO.COM/CATHERINE YEULET

Team meeting

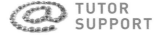

TUTOR SUPPORT

Activity 7: Multiple choice quiz

GLOSSARY OF KEY WORDS

Appraisal a process whereby a supervisor, referred to as an appraiser, identifies and discusses with an individual their performance and achievements in their job role, against previously set targets.

Assistance providing help or support.

Body language communication involving the body.

Client groups this term is used in a number of the units and it refers to client diversity. The CRE (Commission for Racial Equality) ethnic group classification is used in the range for these units. These cover white, mixed, Asian, black and Chinese.

Code of conduct workplace service standards with regard to appearance and behaviour while in the working environment.

Complaints procedure a formal, standardized approach adopted by the organization to handle any complaints.

Continuous Professional Development (CPD) activities undertaken to develop technical skill and expertise to ensure current, professional experience in the beauty industry is maintained.

Customer care statement defined customer service standards that are expected.

Equal opportunity non-discrimination on the basis of sex, race, disability, age, etc.

Grievance a cause for concern or complaint.

Induction an introductory activity delivered when you start or progress into a new job role. Its aim is to provide you with general and essential information related to the work environment, welfare and your job roles and responsibilities.

Job description written details of a person's specific work role, duties and responsibilities.

Limits of own authority the extent of your responsibility as determined by your own job description and workplace policies.

National Occupational Standards for Beauty Therapy standards that set the relevant performance objectives, range statements and knowledge specifications to support performance. These can be obtained from the Hairdressing and Beauty Industry Authority (Habia) website: www.habia.org.uk.

Punctual arriving at the correct time.

Responsible persons this term is used in the Health and Safety unit to mean the person or persons at work to whom you should report any issues, problems or hazards. This could be a supervisor, line manager or your employer.

Target a goal or objective to achieve, usually set within a timescale.

Teamwork supportive work by a team.

Verbal communication occurs when you talk directly to another person either face to face or over the telephone.

Workplace policies this covers the documentation prepared by your employer on the procedures to be followed in your workplace. Examples are your employer's safety policy statement, or general health and safety statements and written safety procedures covering aspects of the workplace that should be drawn to the employees' (and "other persons'") attention, pricing policies and customer service policies.

ASSESSMENT OF KNOWLEDGE AND UNDERSTANDING

Having covered the learning objectives for **Develop and maintain your effectiveness at work**, test what you need to know and understand answering the following short questions below. The information covers:

- salon roles, procedures and targets
- improving your performance
- working with others

Salon roles, procedures and targets

1 What is a job description? How does the job description guide you in your work role?

2 List five important service standards expected of you while in the salon environment. Consider professional appearance and behaviour.

3 Where would you be able to find out more information about other people's areas of responsibility?

4 If a client requested information that was outside your responsibility how would you respond to ensure that dissatisfaction was avoided?

5 A client requests a service that you are not qualified to offer. They insist that they receive the service. You have seen other therapists carrying out the service before. What action should you take and why?

6 If a beauty therapist had an unprofessional attitude, how would this affect the reputation of the salon?

7 What is a salons code of conduct? Why is it important to follow these at all times?

8 What is an appeals and grievance procedure used for in the workplace?

9 What is the purpose of setting staff personal targets and productivity targets?

10 How will achievement of your training targets improve your personal performance?

11 Why is it important to have an awareness of and allocate the appropriate amount of time when booking and performing different beauty therapy services?

Improving your performance

1 Why is it important to know what are your personal strengths and weaknesses in your job role?

2 When and who can you discuss your ongoing training and developments needs with?

3 What are the National Occupational Standards (NOS) and where can you find them?

4 How can they help you identify your training and development needs?

5 What is continuous professional development (CPD) and how will it affect you in your job role?

6 Why is it important to regularly refer to and ongoing update your personal development plan?

7 A client arrives for a service to find that there has been a mistake with the booking and an appointment has not been made for them. What action should be taken?

8 Why is it important to keep up to date with current trends, products and services in beauty therapy?

Working with others

1 Why are positive working relationships with your colleagues important?

2 Action points for your personal development are identified at a performance review appraisal. Why is it important to respond positively to reviews and feedback on performance?

3 If you have a dispute with a colleague, why is it important that it is quickly resolved? What actions would you take?

4 All colleagues should be treated equally. The Equal Opportunities Commission (EOC) states that it is best practice to have a written Equal Opportunities Policy. What should this include?

5 Why is it important to cooperate with and willingly assist colleagues in the workplace? Think of three examples where you have acted using your initiative to help others or resolve a problem during the working day.

6 Give four examples of how can you make best use of your time to be an effective team member in the work place.

7 Sometimes disputes are not immediately resolved leading to poor working relationships which can create a stressful working environment. If you were experiencing relationship difficulties when and who would you report this to?

8 Why are good listening and questioning skills important when you are trying to gain more information and help your understanding about something.

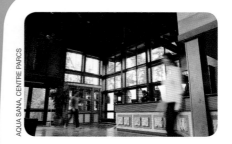

AQUA SANA, CENTRE PARCS

6 Salon Reception (G4)

G4 Unit Learning Objectives

This chapter covers **Unit G4 Fulfil salon reception duties**. It explains how to carry out the important reception skills of welcoming and receiving people entering the beauty therapy work area, handling enquiries, making appointments, dealing with client payments and generally maintaining the appearance of the reception area. Dealing with people in a polite, efficient manner while questioning them to find out what they require forms an important part of this unit.

There are **four** learning outcomes for Unit G4 which you must achieve competently:

1 Maintain the reception area

2 Attend to clients and enquiries

3 Make appointments for salon services

4 Handle payments from clients

Your assessor will observe your performance on at least three occasions. These observations must cover all four main outcomes of this unit.

From the range statement, you must show that you have:

* handled three of the four types of **people**
* handled two of the three types of **enquiries**
* handled both types of **appointment**
* obtained all of the **appointment details**
* handled all the **methods of payment**
* dealt with all types of **discrepancy**

However, you must prove that you have the necessary knowledge, understanding and skills to be able to perform competently for all items in the range.

When providing reception service it is important to use the skills you have learnt in the following units.

* Unit G20 Make sure your own actions reduce risks to health and safety.
* Unit G8 Develope and maintain your effectiveness at work.

(continued on the next page)

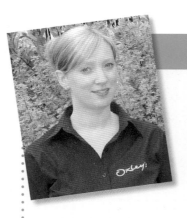

ROLE MODEL

Sally-Anne Braithwaite

Sally-Anne Braithwaite
Front of House Manager
Oxley's at Ambleside
Blue Fish Spa

" My current job role as front of house manager includes all sorts of responsibilities such as running reception, meeting and greeting customers, product sales and helping with marketing and accounts.

When I first started the job in October 2006 I was new to the beauty industry and had to learn all aspects of the job as I went along. I was trained up to have a good knowledge of all the treatments we have to offer, which I feel is a very important part of my role. Now I am part of a great team and have a very rewarding and enjoyable job.

(continued)
- **Unit G18 Promote additional products or services to clients.**

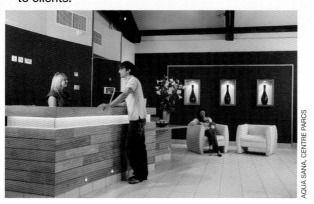

AQUA SANA, CENTRE PARCS

Spa reception

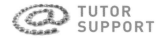

TUTOR SUPPORT

Activity 1: Requirements of the reception area task

Reception introduction

Reception is a client's first and also final impression of the business, whether this is on the telephone or in person when they visit. Clients observe the quality of service, making judgements through every contact they have with the business. It is important that the attitude of the receptionist and their response to any query is knowledgeable and extremely helpful. First impressions count, so ensure that the client gets the *right* impression!

Clients need to feel valued. **Interpersonal skills** are essential in a receptionist. Interpersonal skills are behaviours – everything you say and do. Clients will reach conclusions based upon your behaviour. Always:

- act positively and confidently
- speak clearly
- be friendly, and smile
- look at the client and maintain eye contact
- use good listening skills
- be interested in everything that is going on around the reception area
- give each client individual attention and respect

Outcome 1: Maintain the reception area

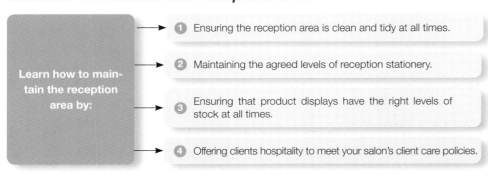

Learn how to maintain the reception area by:

1. Ensuring the reception area is clean and tidy at all times.

2. Maintaining the agreed levels of reception stationery.

3. Ensuring that product displays have the right levels of stock at all times.

4. Offering clients hospitality to meet your salon's client care policies.

> **Selling skills**
> A good knowledge of the products and treatments is essential for good sales. Having confidence and passion for what you are selling helps a great deal.
>
> **Sally-Anne Braithwaite**

TOP TIP

Cleanliness
An attractive heavy-duty foot mat at the entrance to reception will protect the main floor covering from becoming marked. Keep the entrance clean and smart at all times and reduce accidents from slipping.

ACTIVITY

Magazines
What magazines do you think would be appropriate for the beauty salon? Consider your clientele.

TOP TIP

DVD promotion presentation

Facilities in reception may be used to promote salon services. Many suitable DVDs are available from beauty manufacturers and suppliers.

HEALTH & SAFETY

Disability Discrimination Act (DDA) (2005) – wheelchair access.

The Disability Discrimination Act (2005) is a piece of legislation that promotes civil rights for disabled people and protects disabled people from discrimination. Your business provides an everyday service that those with disabilities have a right to get access to. It is important every effort is made to comply with this legislation and the appointment of reception and access design should take this into account.

HEALTH & SAFETY

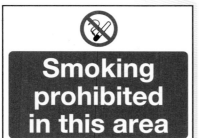

No smoking sign

HEALTH & SAFETY

Ventilation

Ensure that the air is fresh and the room adequately ventilated to remove any smells created from services such as nail services performed in the reception area.

Reception area

Location Reception is usually situated at the front of a beauty salon; in a large department store, reception may be a cosmetic counter. It should be clean, tidy and inviting.

With a salon, the advantage of having reception at the front is that the window can be used to attract and capture the attention and interest of potential clients. Clients who are waiting in reception, however, may seek privacy, so the window should be attractively curtained and the seating should be situated away from the view of the main window if possible.

Size The entrance to reception should be large enough for wheelchair access. There should be adequate seating, and an area in which to hang clients' coats and wet umbrellas. If the entrance floor becomes wet for any reason, all necessary action should be taken immediately to avoid slippage.

It may be that small services, such as manicures, are carried out at reception. These services can then be seen by others, and may attract further clients.

Hospitality is important and shows the salon's commitment to client care. If the client arrives early or their service is likely to be delayed, offer magazines or refreshments such as coffee or water. Clients may also like refreshments following their service for example while waiting for their nail polish to dry or while waiting between different services. It is also a pleasant gesture to have boiled sweets on reception for the client to take.

Magazines should be stored in an area of the reception. They should be collected as necessary and returned to this area. Magazines should be renewed regularly and if in poor condition, disposed of.

Smoking It is illegal to smoke on enclosed or partially enclosed business premises and you are required by law to display a mandatory sign stating this. Out of courtesy if you have an area where clients are able to smoke outside you may inform them of this.

Decoration The reception area should be decorated tastefully in keeping with the décor in the rest of the salon. Attractive posters promoting proprietary cosmetic ranges/services may be displayed on the walls. Framed certificates of the staff's professional qualifications can be displayed, as well as health-legislation registration certificates.

Decorative plants or fresh flowers displayed on reception are attractive. Avoid heavily fragranced flowers which could cause irritation to some people.

Reception resources The reception area should be uncluttered. The main equipment and furnishings required for an efficient reception include the following:

- **A reception desk** The size of the desk will depend on the size of the salon; some salons may have several receptionists. The desk should include shelves and drawers; some have an in-built lockable cash or security drawer. The desk should be at a convenient height for the client to write a cheque, note down the appointment time etc. It should also be large enough to house the appointment book or computer (or both).

- **A comfortable chair** The receptionist's chair should provide adequate back support.

- **A *computer*** Computers are becoming more and more popular in the salon as they can perform many functions. They can be used to store data about clients, to book appointment schedules, to carry out automatic stock control, and to record business details such as accounts and marketing information. They can also be programmed to recommend specific services on the basis of personal data about the client! Space should be provided for a printer if required.

- **A *calculator*** This is used for simple financial calculations, especially if the salon does not have a computer.

- ***Stationery*** This should include price lists, gift vouchers, appointment cards and a receipt pad. Keep a supply available in line with your salon policy.

- **A *notepad*** This is for taking notes and recording messages.

- ***Address and telephone contact details*** All frequently used telephone numbers should be available in an electronic or non-electronic format.

- ***Sales-related equipment*** Items such as till rolls, credit card equipment and a cash book if used.

- **A *telephone and an answering machine*** The answering machine allows clients to notify you, even when the salon is closed, of an appointment request, or an unavoidable change or cancellation. You can then re-schedule appointments as quickly as possible. If you are working on your own, the answering machine avoids interruptions during a service, yet without losing custom.

- **A *fax machine*** This may be available at reception. The fax is capable of transmitting text and image via a telephone line to another fax machine. This is useful when information needs to be passed on quickly.

- ***Record cards*** Record cards are confidential cards that record the personal details of each client registered at the salon. They should be kept in alphabetical order in a filing cabinet or a card-index box, and should be ready for collection by the therapist when treating new or existing clients. See the general beauty therapy units of this book for complete unit-specific examples of record cards. Each card records:

  - the client's name, address and telephone number
  - any medical details
  - any contra-indications (such as allergies and contra-actions)
  - service aims and outcomes
  - a base on which to plan future services
  - services received, products used and merchandise purchased

  These records may be updated by the receptionist at a later stage following the client's service if a central electronic database is used for this purpose.

- **Pens, pencils and a rubber** Make sure these stay at the desk!

- **A display cabinet** This may be used to store proprietary skincare and cosmetic products, and any other merchandise sold by the salon.

- **Waste bin** A covered, lined waste bin may be provided at the reception area. Ensure this is emptied regularly following salon policy.

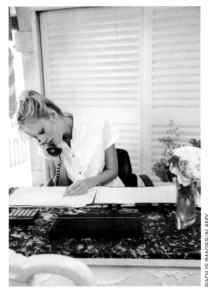

A receptionist booking an appointment

Employability skills Someone who is well presented, willing to learn, adaptable and a confident communicator makes a good impression.

Sally-Anne Braithwaite

 HEALTH & SAFETY

Eating and drinking
The receptionist and other employees should not eat or drink at reception.

 ALWAYS REMEMBER

Data Protection Act (1998) Client records
The record card records confidential information about your client. Ensure that how client information is stored and used complies with the Data Protection Act (1998).

A sample client record card

BEAUTY WORKS		
Date	Beauty therapist name	
Client name		Date of birth
Address		Postcode
Evening phone number	Daytime phone number	
Name of doctor	Doctor's address and phone number	
Related medical history (Conditions that may restrict or prohibit service application.)		
Are you taking any medication (especially antibiotics, steroids, the pill etc.)?		

CONTRA-INDICATIONS REQUIRING MEDICAL REFERRAL

(Preventing facial service application.)

☐	bacterial infection (e.g. impetigo)
☐	fungal infection (e.g. tinea corporis)
☐	viral infection (e.g. herpes simplex)
☐	eye infections (e.g. conjunctivitis)

CONTRA-INDICATIONS WHICH RESTRICT SERVICE

(Service may require adaption.)

☐	cuts and abrasions
☐	recent scar tissue
☐	skin allergies
☐	styes
☐	bruising and swelling
☐	eczema
☐	vitiligo
☐	hyper keratosis

Data Protection Act (DPA) (1998)

The Data Protection Act (1998) was passed by Parliament to control the way information is handled and to give legal rights to people who have information stored about them. With more and more organizations using computers to store and process personal data, access to confidential information has become increasingly possible.

This legislation is designed to protect the client's privacy and confidentiality. It is necessary to ask the client questions before the service plan can be finalized. The relevant information gathered on the client is confidential and should be stored in a safe and secure area following client service, whether on a computer or organized paper filing system. Inform the client that their personal details are being stored and will only be accessed by those individuals who are authorized to do so. Remember also, do not provide confidential information over the telephone or in email correspondence.

The receptionist duties

Outcome 2: Attend to clients and enquiries

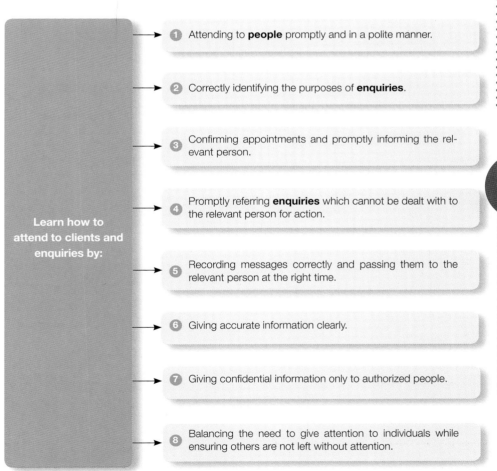

Learn how to attend to clients and enquiries by:

1. Attending to **people** promptly and in a polite manner.

2. Correctly identifying the purposes of **enquiries**.

3. Confirming appointments and promptly informing the relevant person.

4. Promptly referring **enquiries** which cannot be dealt with to the relevant person for action.

5. Recording messages correctly and passing them to the relevant person at the right time.

6. Giving accurate information clearly.

7. Giving confidential information only to authorized people.

8. Balancing the need to give attention to individuals while ensuring others are not left without attention.

TOP TIP

Client attention at reception

It is important to give the right amount of attention to all clients according to their specific requirements, to ensure client satisfaction. This must always be considered in a busy situation where a client may be kept waiting. Always acknowledge their arrival.

TOP TIP

Price lists

Some salons' price lists are in booklet form, detailing the services offered and explaining their benefits. Ensure adequate supply is available at the reception area. Your prices should be kept updated if shown on a website.

TOP TIP

Business cards

Visitors to the salon may leave a business card, stating the name of the company, and the representative's name, address and telephone number. These cards should be filed by the receptionist for future reference. At a convenient time, store these electronically for ease of reference in the future.

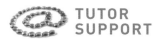

Receptionists should have a smart appearance and be able to communicate effectively and professionally, creating the right impression.

The receptionist's duties include:

- maintaining the reception and product displays
- looking after clients and visitors on arrival and departure
- answering telephone calls
- dealing with enquiries face-to-face, by telephone, fax or possibly email
- scheduling appointments
- dealing with complaints and compliments
- telling the appropriate therapist that a client or visitor has arrived
- assisting with retail sales
- operating the payment point and handling payments
- filing client records (increasingly this is performed electronically)

The receptionist should know:

- the name of each member of staff, their role and their area of responsibility
- who to refer enquiries to that cannot be dealt with
- the salon's hours of opening, and the days and times when each beauty therapist is available
- the range of services or products offered by the salon, their duration and their cost
- any booking service restrictions such as skin testing requirements
- who to refer different types of enquiries to
- the person in your salon to whom you should refer reception problems
- any current discounts and special offers that the salon is promoting
- the benefits of each service and each retail product
- the approximate time taken to complete each service
- how to schedule follow-up services

ACTIVITY

Designing record cards/salon service menu

Design a record card to be used to record the client's requirements and the service details. Alternatively, you could design a salon service menu explaining the different services available and their cost. Be creative, and include a business name you may wish to use in the future. Relate the design of each to the NVQ/SVQ Level 2 services.

Skin sensitivity (patch) tests Before clients receive certain services it may be necessary to carry out skin sensitivity tests to test skin sensitivity. The skin sensitivity test is often carried out at reception, and the receptionist or NVQ/SVQ Level 1 therapist will be able to perform the test once they have been trained. Every client should undergo a skin test before a permanent tinting service to the eyelashes or eyebrows. Further tests may be necessary, depending on the sensitivity of the client, before services such as those for artificial eyelashes, or wax depilation. Refer to the relevant chapters to familiarize yourself with the test required.

As a reception duty it may be your responsibility to check that the necessary test has been received on client arrival following the salon policy for this.

The importance of good communication

As discussed previously clients make quality judgements based on their contact with the business. Effective communication is important to the success of the business. This may be verbal communication, that is face-to-face, over the telephone or written communication – including email – and remember non-verbal communication – we speak through our bodies' gestures. Conclusions about how we see other people are based on their behaviour both spoken and unspoken.

Always remember the **diversity** or range of people you will come into contact with. Diversity includes:

- personality
- beliefs and attitudes
- age
- religion, morality
- background and culture

Diversity should be considered in communication, respond to any enquiry and allow time for the client to respond. Consider if you feel you have dealt with their enquiry adequately. It is important that a client is listened to and responded to appropriately.

Communication should always suit the situation. In all situations you should speak slowly and clearly, avoid rushing the conversation even in busy trading situations. Avoid slang words and informal phrases such as 'hang on a minute'. Your tone of voice is important; you should always sound calm, cheerful, helpful, knowledgeable and professional. Your voice and manner should inspire confidence and trust.

Adopting good posture will also positively affect your speech and professional appearance. You will sound and look more energized.

Non-verbal communication This is often referred to as body language and is how we communicate using our face, body movements and gestures.

Often we do this unconsciously and our body language may contradict what we are actually saying. It is an important skill to be able to interpret body language and the mood of clients. Observing clients' behaviour will help you to recognize their needs and expectations. Your body language should also show you to be attentive, examples include nodding your head and smiling in agreement.

Asking questions It is important to ask verbal questions to ensure, for example, that you are confident and understand what the client has asked you, do not be embarrassed to do this. It will ensure you give an appropriate answer, make the correct decision and that client satisfaction will be achieved. You may ask 'open' or 'closed' questions.

ACTIVITY

Planning a reception area
Design a reception area, to scale, appropriate to a small or large beauty salon. Discuss the choice of wall and floor coverings, furnishings and equipment, and give the reasons for their selection. Consider clients' comfort, and health and safety.

To help you plan this you may refer to a specialist equipment suppliers' brochure or online information.

HEALTH & SAFETY

Cleaning
In a large salon a cleaner may be employed to maintain the hygiene of the reception area. In a smaller salon this may be the responsibility of the receptionist, assistant therapist or a junior therapist. Reception must be maintained to a high standard at all times. Use quieter periods for this purpose and to check stock levels etc.

BEST PRACTICE

Data Protection Act (DPA) (1998)
Be aware of the full legislation requirements for the DPA visit www.hmso.gov.uk.

BEST PRACTICE

Name badges
It is a good idea for the receptionist to wear a badge indicating their name and position.

BEST PRACTICE

Client care

If you are engaged on the telephone when a client arrives, look up and acknowledge their presence. This is positive body language and an example of good interpersonal skills, which makes the client feel welcome.

HEALTH & SAFETY

Fire drill

As the receptionist you should be familiar with the emergency procedure in case of fire.

ACTIVITY

Reception

Pair up with a colleague and share your experiences of a well managed and a badly managed reception.

TOP TIP

Do's and don'ts

List *five* important do's and *five* don'ts for the receptionist. Think also of things that *should not* be discussed at reception.

TOP TIP

Clients matter most

Don't regard the phone ringing as an interruption. Always remember that clients matter – it is they ensure the success of your business!

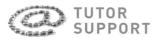

TUTOR SUPPORT

Activity 9: Telephone technique task

Always ask open questions if you need more information as these questions cannot be answered with 'yes' or 'no'. Open questions start with 'what', 'when', 'who' and 'why' etc. Closed questions are used when you need to confirm something quickly. These are answered 'yes' or 'no'.

Telephone calls: communication

A good telephone technique can gain clients; a poor technique can lose them. Here are some guidelines for good technique:

- **Answer quickly** On average, a person may be willing to wait up to nine rings: try to respond to the call within six rings.

- **Build a rapport** by introducing yourself.

- **Be prepared** Have information and writing materials ready to hand. It should not normally be necessary to leave the caller waiting while you find something.

- **Be welcoming and attentive** Speak clearly without mumbling, at the right speed. Pronounce your words clearly, and vary your tone. Sound interested, and never abrupt.

ACTIVITY

Listening to yourself

A pleasant speaking voice is an asset. Do you think you could improve your speech or manner?

Record your voice as you answer a telephone enquiry, then play it back. How did you sound? This is how others hear you!

> **Helping clients**
> Recognise the needs of each individual client and work to build a rapport with them. Show a genuine interest in them and their lifestyle, family and hobbies etc. and your customer will come to trust you and listen to your recommendations.
>
> **Sally-Anne Braithwaite**

TOP TIP

Telephone services

Telephone directories, codebooks and guides to charges provide a great deal of useful information. Read them carefully to make yourself familiar with the telephone services that are available.

Remember: the caller may be a new client ringing several salons, and their decision whether to visit your salon may depend on your attitude and the way you respond to their call.

Here are some more ideas about good telephone technique:

- **Smile** – this will help you put across a warm, friendly response to the caller.

- **Alter the pitch of your voice** as you speak, to create interest.

- **As you answer give the standard greeting for the salon** – for example: 'Good morning, Visage Beauty Salon, Susan speaking. How may I help you?'

- **Listen attentively** to the caller's questions or requests. You will be speaking to a variety of clients: you must respond appropriately and helpfully to each.

- **Evaluate the information** given by the caller, and be sure to respond to what they have said or asked.

- **Use the client's name** if you know it; this personalizes the call.

- **In your mind summarize the main requests from the call**. Ask for further information if you need it.

- **If you have an enquiry that you cannot deal with yourself** refer to the relevant person promptly for assistance. Tell the client what you are doing.

- **At the end** repeat the main points of the conversation clearly to check that you and the client have understood each other.

- **Close the call pleasantly** – for example, 'Thank you for calling, Mrs Smith. Goodbye.'

If you receive a business call, or a call from a person seeking employment, always take the caller's name and telephone number. Your supervisor can then deal with the call as soon as they are free to do so.

Transferring calls

If you transfer a telephone call to another extension, explain to the caller what you are doing and thank them for waiting. If the extension to which you have transferred the call is not answered within nine rings, apologize and explain to the caller that you will ask the person concerned to ring back as soon as possible. Take the caller's name and telephone number and offer to take a message. Always make sure the person gets the message.

Taking messages

Messages should be recorded neatly on a memorandum ('memo') pad. Each message should record:

- who the message is for

- who the message was from

- the date and the time the message was received

- accurate details of the message including the reason for the call, details of information requested or to be passed on

- the telephone number or address of the caller

- the signature of the person who took the message

ACTIVITY

Open and closed questions
Think of an open question you could ask a client to check their suitability for leg waxing, when making a waxing appointment.

Think of a closed question you may ask to confirm client satisfaction with their service that day.

ACTIVITY

Non-verbal communication
In conversation you give signals through your behaviour that tell others whether you are listening or not.

1 What do you think the following signals indicate:
   - a smile?
   - head tilted, and resting on one hand?
   - frowning?
   - eyes semi-closed?
   - head nodding?
   - fidgeting?

2 Can you think of further facial or body signals that indicate your mood?

ACTIVITY

Communicating with clients
Listen to experienced receptionists and notice how they communicate with clients.

TOP TIP

Personal calls

Check the salon's policy on personal calls. Usually they are permitted only in emergencies. This is so that staff are not distracted from clients, and to keep the telephone free for clients to make appointments.

ACTIVITY

What do you need to know?
Think of different questions that you might be asked as a receptionist. Then ask an experienced receptionist what the most common requests are.

TOP TIP

A client who has received a poor response to their telephone call may tell others about it.

TOP TIP

If the salon uses a cordless phone or a mobile phone, keep it in a central location where it can easily be found when it rings. After each call, be sure to return the phone to its normal location.

When taking a message listen actively and attentively. Repeat the details you have recorded so that the caller can check that you've got it right. Pass the message directly to the correct person as soon as possible. The message should be received in time to be acted upon.

A memo

TELEPHONE MESSAGE RECEIVED			
To	Angela	Date	10.7.10
From	Jenny Heron	Time	9.30 am
Number	273451	Taken by	Sandra

Please ring Jenny Heron regarding her appointment on Saturday

Listening skills

It is important to listen closely to what people are saying to you in your role to ensure you correctly identify the purpose of any enquiry in order to choose the correct response when dealing with it.

Listening skills include:

- being focused on the other person, paying them your full attention
- ensuring that your facial expressions show your interest
- not interrupting the other person speaking
- using positive body language to show your interest; maintain eye contact; nod your head and lean forward
- observing the other person's body language reading what it is telling you while you listen
- summarizing what the other person has said to confirm understanding
- asking further questions as necessary if unsure in order to give the right response
- asking a client to rephrase what you have said in their own words if they appear confused

How to deal with a dissatisfied client or complaint

Occasionally a client may be dissatisfied and wish to complain. The receptionist is usually the first contact with the client (either face-to-face or through telephone contact) and may have to deal with dissatisfied, angry or awkward customers. Considerable skill is needed if you are to deal constructively with a potentially damaging situation.

If your business has a procedure for handling complaints this should be followed. Procedures are useful as these can be audited to identify emerging problems that may require correction. If ignored these problems could be harmful to the business.

Never become angry or awkward yourself. Always remain courteous and diplomatic, and communicate confidently and politely.

1 Listen to the client as they describe their problems, without making judgements. Do not make excuses for yourself or for colleagues. Do not interrupt.

2 Ask questions to check that you have the full background details. Summarize the client's concerns to confirm this.

3 If possible, agree on a course of action, offering a solution if you can. Check that the client has agreed to the proposed course of action. It may be necessary to consult the salon supervisor before proposing a solution to the client: if you're not sure, always check first.

4 Log the complaint: the date, the time, the client's name, the nature of the complaint and the course of action agreed.

5 There should also be a system for handling compliments. Again it is good to see those aspects of the business that are particularly successful. This can also be rewarding and motivational for staff to hear. Such compliments can be used in marketing materials.

Appointments

Outcome 3: Make appointments for salon services

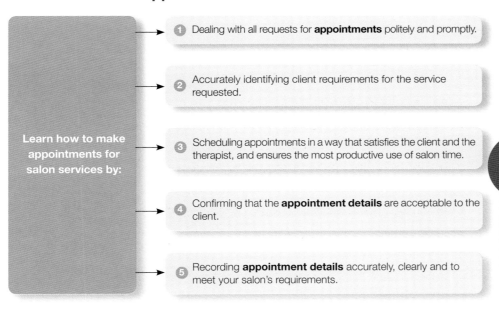

Learn how to make appointments for salon services by:

1 Dealing with all requests for **appointments** politely and promptly.

2 Accurately identifying client requirements for the service requested.

3 Scheduling appointments in a way that satisfies the client and the therapist, and ensures the most productive use of salon time.

4 Confirming that the **appointment details** are acceptable to the client.

5 Recording **appointment details** accurately, clearly and to meet your salon's requirements.

Making correct entries in the **appointment book** or salon **computer** is one of the most important duties of the receptionist. As receptionist you must familiarize yourself with the salon's appointment system, column headings, service times and any abbreviations used.

Each therapist will usually have their name at the head of a column. Entries in columns must not be reallocated without the consent of the therapist or supervisor, unless they are absent.

Bookings

When a client calls to make an appointment, record the client's name and the service they want. Allow adequate time to carry out the required service (as indicated in the

ACTIVITY

Reception role play
With colleagues, act out the following situations, which may occur when working as a receptionist. You may wish to video the role plays for review and discussion later.

1 A client arrives very late for an appointment but insists that she be treated.

2 A client questions the bill.

3 A client comes in to complain about a service given previously. (Choose a particular service.)

Alternatively you may choose to do this as a written activity with a discussion of your answers.

following chapters). Take the client's telephone number or other contact details in case the therapist falls ill or is unable to keep the appointment for some other reason. If the client requests a particular therapist, be sure to enter the client's name in the correct column.

In addition, software enabling online appointment booking and scheduling is becoming more popular. This is accessed through the business website and clients can book appointments and view the business's information (services offered, specials offers etc.) at any time. The business can make the final decision to accept or reject the appointment. As receptionist this may be your responsibility.

Finally the hours of the day are recorded along the left-hand side of the appointment page, divided into 15-minute intervals. You must know how long each service takes so that you can allow sufficient time for the therapist to carry out the service in a safe, competent, professional manner. If you don't allow sufficient time, the therapist will run late, and this will affect all later appointments. On the other hand, if you allow too much time, the therapist's time will be wasted and the salon's earnings will be less than they could be. Suggested times to be allowed for each service are given in the service chapters.

Ensure that you regularly check scheduled appointments and plan ahead where you can see any potential problem – put a strategy in place to rectify it. This may involve asking others to help you.

Confirm the name of the therapist who will be carrying out the service, the date and the time.

Finally, confirm or estimate the cost of the service to the client.

Services are usually recorded in an abbreviated form. All those who use the appointment page must be familiar with these abbreviations.

Service	Abbreviation	Service time allowed*
Cleanse and make-up	C/M/up	45 mins
Eyebrow shaping	E/B reshape or trim	15 mins
Eyebrow tint	EBT	10 mins
Eyelash tint	ELT	20 mins
Manicure	Man	45 mins
Pedicure	Ped	45 mins
Leg wax: half	½ leg wax	30 mins
three-quarter	¾ leg wax	30–40 mins
full	Full leg wax	50 mins
Bikini wax	B/wax	15 mins
Underarm wax	U/arm wax	15 mins
Arm wax	F/arm wax	30 mins
Facial wax	F/wax	10–15 mins

Service	Abbreviation	Service time allowed*
Eyebrow wax	E/B wax	15 mins
Threading	EB/Thread	10–15 mins
	F/Thread	10–15 mins
Ear pierce	E/P	15 mins
Facial	F	60 mins
Artificial eye lashes strip/individual flare	F/Lash	20 mins

*Service time does not include preparation for service and consultation.

HEALTH & SAFETY

Health and Safety (Display Screen Equipment) Regulations (1992)
These regulations cover the use of visual display units and computer screens. They specify acceptable levels of radiation emissions from the screen, and identify correct posture, seating position, permitted working heights and rest periods.

If an appointment book is used, write each entry neatly and accurately. It is preferable to write in pencil: appointments can be amended by erasing and rewriting, keeping the book clean and clear.

THERAPIST	JAYNE	SUE	LIZ
9.00	Mrs Young		
9.15	1/2 leg wax	Jenny Newley	
9.30	Carol Kreen	EL T/EBT	
9.45	Full leg wax	EB trim	
10.00	B /Wax		
10.15		Sandra Smith	Fiona Smith
10.30	Ms Lord E/B wax	C / M / up	C / M / up
10.45			Strip / lash
11.00		Mrs Jones	
11.15		W/arm wax	
11.30		F/arm wax	Carol Brown
11.45			E/P
12.00			
12.15			
12.30	Nina Farrel		
12.45	Man		
1.00	Ped		
1.15		Sue Uip E/P	
1.30	1/2 leg wax	T Scott	
1.45		3/4 leg wax	
2.00	Karen Davies	W/arm wax	
2.15	Facial		
2.30			
2.45			Pat king
3.00			C / M / up
3.15	Anna Wood		Man
3.30	Man		
3.45	E/B Reshape		
4.00			

DAY SATURDAY   DATE 15th JANUARY

DNA

> **Teamwork**
> A good team member has the ability to listen and communicate well, respect their colleagues and be able to get their point across in the appropriate manner.
>
> **Sally-Anne Braithwaite**

TOP TIP

Software business management features
The software which can be used for booking and scheduling appointments often has the benefits of stock control and ordering, managing client data, and issuing gift cards.

TOP TIP

Appointment reminder
Some software can email and text your clients an appointment reminder directly to their mobile phone.

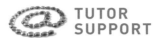

TOP TIP

Service time allowed

Dependent upon the manufacturers' guidelines and the service needs of the client including any procedure modifications required, the service times may take less or more time.

TUTOR SUPPORT

Activity 3: Treatment list task

ALWAYS REMEMBER

Appointments can usually be made up to six weeks in advance. Often clients will book their next appointment while still at the salon. How far ahead the receptionist is able to book appointments will vary from salon to salon.

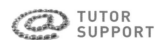

TUTOR SUPPORT

Activity 8: Reception book scheduling task

> **Using Initiative**
> If you see something that needs to be done, do it without having to be asked. If you think a procedure could be done better or more efficiently, don't be afraid to suggest it to your employer.
>
> **Sally-Anne Braithwaite**

Electronic appointment booking systems, if used, allow you to read the appointment schedule and add or edit appointments immediately.

Appointment cards may be offered to the client, to confirm the client's appointment. The card should record the service, the date, the day and the time. The therapist's name may also be recorded.

When the client arrives for their service, draw a line or checkmark through their name to indicate that they have arrived.

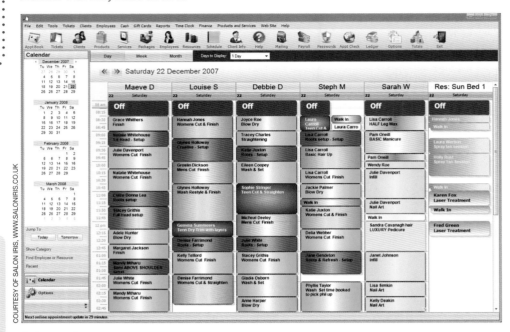

COURTESY OF SALON IRIS, WWW.SALONIRIS.CO.UK

Online appointments page

If the client cancels, indicate this on the appointment page *immediately*, usually with a large C, placed through the booking. This enables another client to take the appointment.

If a client fails to arrive, the abbreviation DNA ('did not arrive') is usually written over the booking. The client's telephone number should then be used to see if a re-booking is required.

Use the relevant recording icon if using an online appointment booking system.

Some salons will have a policy to charge for a missed appointment.

Dealing with appointment problems

You are often required to use your initiative in helping colleagues and clients and be able to cope with the unexpected such as:

- clients arriving late for appointments
- double-bookings, with two clients requiring service at the same time
- the arrival of unscheduled clients
- staff absence with a column of appointments!

Effective teamwork can usually overcome any of these situations. Inform your colleague/supervisor of the problem and, dependent upon your experience, state what action needs to be taken or ask them to support you in identifying a solution. You must always:

- aim to accommodate clients
- not disadvantage or compromise any clients in terms of quality of service

- keep the client informed of what action is being taken
- state how long any delay to service will be and if this is unsuitable offer an alternative future appointment
- use your excellent communication skills!

Outcome 4: Handle payments from clients

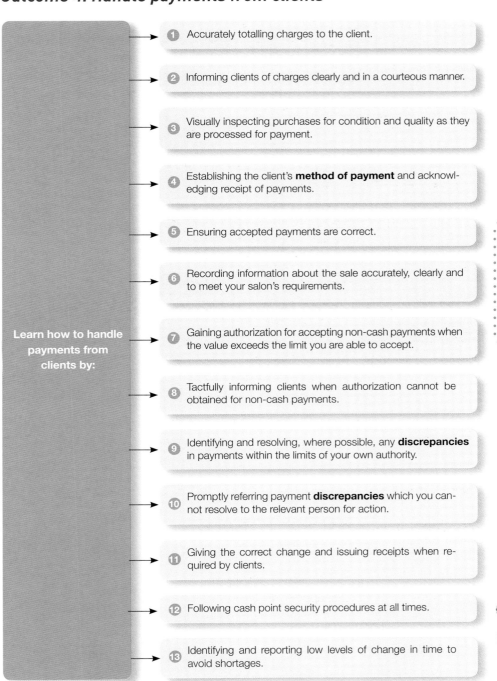

Learn how to handle payments from clients by:

1. Accurately totalling charges to the client.

2. Informing clients of charges clearly and in a courteous manner.

3. Visually inspecting purchases for condition and quality as they are processed for payment.

4. Establishing the client's **method of payment** and acknowledging receipt of payments.

5. Ensuring accepted payments are correct.

6. Recording information about the sale accurately, clearly and to meet your salon's requirements.

7. Gaining authorization for accepting non-cash payments when the value exceeds the limit you are able to accept.

8. Tactfully informing clients when authorization cannot be obtained for non-cash payments.

9. Identifying and resolving, where possible, any **discrepancies** in payments within the limits of your own authority.

10. Promptly referring payment **discrepancies** which you cannot resolve to the relevant person for action.

11. Giving the correct change and issuing receipts when required by clients.

12. Following cash point security procedures at all times.

13. Identifying and reporting low levels of change in time to avoid shortages.

ACTIVITY

How would you deal with the following reception problems:

- a client arriving late for a service?
- a double-booking?
- the arrival of an unscheduled client?

> **Customer service**
> A friendly and helpful approach is the key to good customer service.
>
> **Sally-Anne Braithwaite**

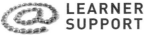

LEARNER SUPPORT

Reception mini crossword

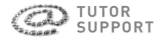

TUTOR SUPPORT

Activity 4: Handling payments handout

Every beauty therapy or cosmetic business will have a policy for handling cash and for handling the payment. Clients can choose from a wide range of payment methods. It's important that you handle each payment efficiently and correctly. Not all businesses accept every **method of payment** so this should be checked in your training.

TOP TIP

Advertisement vouchers

Sometimes the salon may publish other offers, such as a discount on producing a newspaper advertisement for the salon or a website voucher. The advertisement voucher is a form of payment, and must be collected.

ALWAYS REMEMBER

Sale and Supply of Goods Act (1994)

You have a duty to comply with the responsibilities of this Act, ensuring all products sold are of merchantable quality. They must 'conform to contract'. This means fit for purpose and of satisfactory quality.

It is important that you have received training and are confident to take payment in the client's preferred method, which may be cash or cash equivalent (i.e. gift voucher), cheque or payment card.

Before processing payment confirm what it is the client is paying for i.e. the services received and/or the products to be purchased. Confirm the price; ask how they would like to pay. Gaining client confirmation will reduce discrepancies later. Always check for any defects in products as you process a sale, i.e. breakage or leakage. If you are responsible for stock control when a product is found to be defective a replacement product is required.

The payment point

Kinds of payment points

Manual tills With **manual tills** a lockable drawer or box is used to store cash: this may form part of the reception desk. Each transaction must be recorded by hand.

At the end of the working day, record the total cash register in a book, to ensure that accurate accounts are kept. Records of petty cash, small amounts of monies used for expenditures, e.g. milk for clients' coffee, must also be kept so that the final totals will balance.

Automatic tills **Electrical automatic tills** use codes, one for each kind of service or retail sale. These are identified by keys on the till. Using these with each transaction makes it possible to analyze the salon's business each day or each week.

With each sale during the day a receipt is given to the client; the total is also recorded on the till's **audit roll**.

Automatic tills also provide **subtotals** of the amounts taken: these can be cross-checked against the amount in the till, to determine the daily takings:

- The X reading provides subtotals throughout the day, as required.
- The Z reading provides the overall figures at the end of the day.

Computerized tills **Computerized tills** provide the same facilities as automatic tills, with additional features to help with the business, record-keeping, including client service cards and stock records.

Both electronic and computerized tills help calculate the client's bill for you, including change to be given.

Equipment and materials required

- **Calculator** This is useful in totalling large amounts of money or when using a manual till.
- **Credit card equipment** If your business is authorized to accept credit cards you may use either an *imprinter* or *electronic terminal*. An imprinter is a manual system whereby the client's credit card is placed on a self-carbonating voucher within the machine and a manual sliding mechanism imprints the details of the card upon the voucher. If this system is used you require a supply of vouchers. Alternatively, where an electronic payment system is used a special till roll which provides a printout for yourself and a copy for the client is required.

- **Cash float** At the start of each day you need a small sum of money comprising coins and perhaps a few notes, to provide change: this is called the **float**. (At the end of the day there will be money surplus to the float: if no mistakes have been made, this should match the takings.)

- **Till roll** This records the sales and provides a receipt. Keep a spare to hand. If you're using a manual cash drawer, you'll need a **receipt book**.

- **Audit roll** The retailer's copy of the till roll.

- **Cash book** This is a record of income and expenditure, for a manual till.

- **Other stationery** A date stamp and a salon name stamp (for cheques), pens, pencils and an eraser, and a container to hold these.

ACTIVITY

Fraud

Find out about your salon's policy in the case of fraudulent monetary transactions, using either cash or cards. What actions should you take?

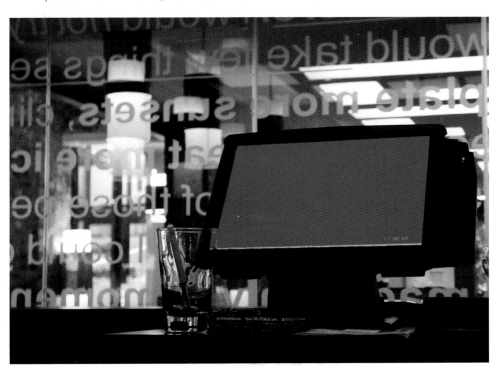

Computerized till

Security at the payment point

Having placed money in the cash drawer and collected change as required, always close the cash drawer firmly – never leave it open. Do not leave the key in the drawer, or lying about reception unattended.

Some members of staff will be appointed to authorize cheques and credit card payments; one of these should initial each cheque.

Errors may occur when handling cheques or when operating an electronic or computerized payment point. Don't panic! If you can't correct the error yourself, seek assistance – but don't leave the cash drawer unattended and open.

Be aware of stolen cards and forged notes and coins. Check at every payment transaction and follow the salon policy if presented. Remember that this must be handled sensitively as the client may not know they are in receipt of a cash forgery.

You may periodically be informed of cards that are invalid, on a credit card warning list from the service provider. If you receive a card that is on a credit card warning list, politely

LEVEL 2 BEAUTY THERAPY

TOP TIP

Forgeries

Hold notes to the light to check for forgeries. You should be able to see the watermark (picture of the Queen's head), the continuous metal strip that runs through the note and a hologram decal in the mid-left section of the note.

An ultra-violet detector machine may also be used to check for forgeries.

The police will often provide a list of forged bank note numbers to businesses to be aware of.

TOP TIP

Cheques

Most cheques may only be valid for six months from the date on the cheque – however this is at the discretion of the bank.

detain the customer, hold onto the card, and contact your supervisor, who will implement the salon's procedure. If the card is unsigned, do not allow the cardholder to sign the card unless you first get authorization from the credit card company's service provider. (The service provider's telephone number should be kept near the telephone.)

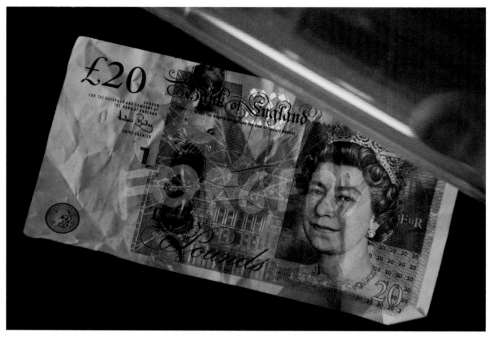

Forged note detector

Methods of payment

Cash When receiving payment by **cash**, follow this sequence:

1 Accurately total the charge for the services/products received. Inform the client of the amount to be paid.

2 Check that the money offered is **legal tender** – that is, money you will be able to pay into your bank. (Your salon will probably not accept foreign currency, for example.)

3 Place the customer's money on the till ledge until you have given change, or at least state to the customer verbally the sum of money that they have given you.

4 Aloud, count the change as you give it to the client. This will help avoid payment disputes.

5 Thank the client, and give them a receipt.

6 If a client disputes the change given as too little, ask how much money they are missing. Inform the client that when the takings are cashed at the end of the day if there is a surplus and it matches that amount they will be reimbursed. Ensure that you have the client's details so that you can inform them of the outcome the next day.

Cheques **Cheques** are an alternative form of payment, and must be accompanied by a **cheque guarantee card**. This proves identity and guarantees the spending limit, usually £100. The debit card is usually the same card as the cheque guarantee card. Your salon may be willing to accept cheques for larger amounts if the client can show some

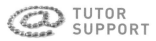

TUTOR SUPPORT

Activity 5: Cheque payment handout

other identification, such as a driving licence, but you must always check first with your supervisor.

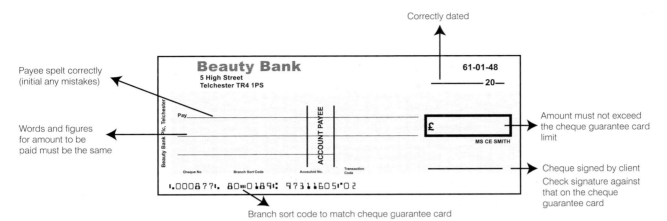

A cheque

Some businesses are no longer accepting cheques as it is becoming more costly to accept as a form of payment.

When receiving payment by cheque, follow this sequence of checks:

1   The cheque must be correctly dated.

2   The cheque must be made payable to the salon (you may have a salon stamp for this).

3   The words and figures written on the cheque must match those in the box.

4   Any errors or alterations must have been initialled by the client.

5   The signature on the back of the cheque guarantee card must match that on the cheque – compare these as the customer writes their signature on the cheque.

6   The bank's 'sort code' numbers on the cheque must match those on the cheque guarantee card.

7   The date on the cheque guarantee card must be valid.

8   The value on the cheque must not exceed the cheque guarantee card limit.

9   The cheque card number must be recorded on the back of the cheque.

10   The cheque must be signed by the client.

Debit cards Debit cards include Switch/Maestro and Solo. The card authorizes immediate debit of the cash amount from the client's account and is an alternative to writing a cheque. (This card may also be a cheque guarantee card.) You cannot perform this kind of transaction unless your salon has an electronic terminal. This processes payment automatically through a telephone connection (chip and PIN). The card processing company applies a fixed fee for each transaction made. Duplicated receipts are produced following authorization; one copy is given to the client, the other kept by the salon. If there is a connection problem a manual imprinter is used as an alternative, details of the sale are written on the voucher which is signed by the client. The client is then given one copy of the sales voucher; a copy is sent to the debit card company; the third copy is kept by the salon.

TOP TIP

Security

When paying for goods with a debit or credit card the client will need to enter their PIN (personal identity number). This is usually entered into an electronic handheld device, but in some cases they may have to sign.

Debit and credit cards can also be used to make payments by phone or over the internet. In this case the client will need to provide certain details that are printed on their card.

TOP TIP

Card non-authorization

If a card is declined when processing, it may be requested that the card is retained. Refer this to the designated responsible person without causing embarrassment to the client following salon policy.

TOP TIP

Cards

If cards are accepted as a method of payment, those that are accepted by the business will usually be displayed at the payment point.

Types of credit and debit card

embossed account number should be valid – not on a credit card company's warning list

card logo

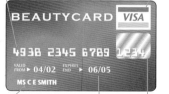

sex and name should fit your client

hologram: clear sharp image

valid to (expiry) date

Credit card checks

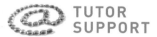

TUTOR SUPPORT

Activity 6: Credit and debit card payment handout

Credit cards Credit cards can be used only if your business has an arrangement with the relevant credit card company. In this case the company will give the salon a credit limit (a **ceiling**), the maximum amount that may be accepted with the card. Any amount greater than this must be individually authorized by the credit card company. (This is done by telephone at the time of transaction.)

Credit cards allow the client to 'buy goods now and pay later' with interest paid each month on the outstanding balance if not paid off in full.

Electronic payment systems An electronic computerized terminal may be used for payment by both credit and debit cards.

1 Check that the terminal display is in 'SALE' mode.

2 Confirm that a sale is to be made by pressing the YES button.

3 The terminal will request that you swipe the card. Do this, ensuring that the magnetic strip passes over the reader head and that you retain the card in your hand. In some cases the magnetic strip cannot be read by the swipe card reader: in this situation you will have to key the complete card number into the terminal manually. This does not necessarily mean that there is any reason for suspicion, but do look carefully at it for any signs that the card has been tampered with.

4 When prompted, use the 'AMOUNT' button on the keypad to input the purchases and total them. (If you make a mistake, you can clear the figures using the CLEAR button.)

5 Press ENTER, which will automatically connect the terminal to the credit card company. A message will indicate first 'DIALLING', and then 'CONNECTION MADE'.

6 Customer details are accessed automatically. After a few moments you should receive one of two messages. If the payment is authorized you will see 'AUTH CODE', and a code number will be printed on the receipt with the other purchase details. If the transaction is declined, you will see 'CARD NOT ACCEPTED'.

7 While holding the card, check the details and tear off the two-part receipt and ask the cardholder to sign in ballpoint pen, in the space provided. Alternatively the 'chip and PIN' system may be used, where the client enters their personal identity number instead of signing their name. The transaction will be declined if the PIN is incorrect.

8 Where a signature is used, check the signature matches the signature on the card, and give the customer the top, signed copy, with the card.

9 Place the copies in the till. One copy is for the debit/credit card company, the other for your records.

When receiving payment by debit or credit card, check these points:

1 The card logo for a credit card is at the upper right-hand corner on the front of the card. For a debit card, it should be at the lower right-hand corner of the card.

2 The hologram should have a clear, sharp image and be in the centre right of the card.

3   The date on the card must be valid: if it is out of date ask for another form of payment.

4   The sex (Ms, Miss, Mrs, Mr) and the name of the customer must fit your client.

5   The cardholder's signature on the reverse of the card must match the name on the front of the card.

6   The cardholder's card number should be embossed and across the width on the front of the card.

7   The cardholder's card number must not be one of those on the credit card company's warning list.

Travellers' cheques   **Travellers' cheques** are pre-printed fixed-amount cheques. They may be acceptable, provided they are in particular currencies (usually sterling). Such cheques must be compared with the client's passport for validity. Also available are travellers' cheque cards.

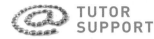

Activity 7: Reception area Wordsearch

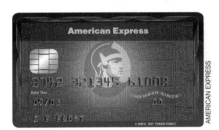

A charge card

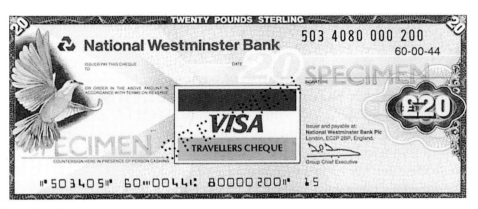

A travellers' cheque

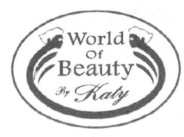

Charge cards   Some businesses accept **charge cards** such as American Express. These differ from credit cards in that the account holder must repay to the card company the complete amount spent each month. They are considered a more convenient alternative to cash.

Gift vouchers   Gift vouchers are purchased from the salon as pre-payments for beauty therapy services or retail sales. Check the following:

● There is usually a specific time period in which gift vouchers must be used. Check to see if this is the case and if they are still valid.

● Check the value of the voucher, and remember to request another form of payment if the cost of the service is higher than the voucher.

It is important that all financial transactions are handled competently. However busy you are always follow the guidelines for handling each method of payment.

If you are ever unsure when handling a financial transaction or make a mistake, inform your supervisor immediately. It may be that you have to be discreet when doing this, for example if a client has handed you a forged bank note!

A gift voucher

GLOSSARY OF KEY WORDS

Appointment arrangement made for a client to receive a service on a particular date and time.

Body language communication involving the body.

Charge card an alternative form of payment where the complete amount of credit spent must be repaid by the card-holder each month to the card company.

Cheque an alternative form of payment to that of using cash. A cheque must be accompanied by a cheque guarantee card.

Client groups this term is used in a number of the units and it refers to client diversity. The CRE (Commission for Racial Equality) ethnic group classification is used in the range for these units. These cover white, mixed, Asian, black and Chinese.

Communication the exchange of information and the establishment of understanding between people.

Credit card an alternative form of payment to that of using cash. These cards are held by those who have a credit account, where there is a pre-arranged borrowing limit. These can only be used if your business has an arrangement to deal with the relevant credit card company.

Data Protection Act (1998) legislation designed to protect client privacy and confidentiality.

Debit card alternative method of payment where the card authorizes immediate debit of the cash amount from the client's account.

Discrepancy a disagreement over amounts of money etc. This is referred to in instances where a client disagrees with what they are being asked to pay or the amount of change received.

Enquiries questions presented by clients or business contacts to find out more information.

Gift voucher a pre-payment method for beauty therapy services or retail sales.

Health and Safety (Display Screen Equipment) Regulations (1992) these regulations cover the use of visual display units (VDUs) and computer screens. They specify acceptable levels of radiation emissions from the screen and identify correct working posture, seating position, permitted working heights and rest periods.

Hospitality this covers welcoming the client, being helpful and offering refreshments and magazines, and ensuring the client is comfortable while at reception.

Messages communication of information to another person in written, electronic or verbal form.

Method of payment different forms of payment that may be accepted to pay for a product or service including cash, cash equivalents, cheque and payment cards.

Non-verbal communication communicating using body language, i.e. using your eyes, face and body to transmit your feelings.

Reception the area where clients are received.

Receptionist person responsible for maintaining the reception area, scheduling appointments and handling payments.

Record cards confidential cards recording the personal details of each client registered at the business. This information may be stored electronically on the salon's computer.

Sale and Supply of Goods Act (1994) goods must be as described, of merchantable, satisfactory quality and fit for their intended purpose.

Salon services covers all the services offered in your workplace.

Skin sensitivity test method used to assess skin tolerance/sensitivity to a particular substance or service.

Travellers' cheques alternative form of payment used when travelling abroad and must be compared with the client's passport.

Verbal communication occurs when you talk directly to another person, either face to face or over the telephone.

ASSESSMENT OF KNOWLEDGE AND UNDERSTANDING

Having covered the learning objectives for **Fulfil salon reception duties**, test what you need to know and understand answering the following short questions below. The information covers:

- salon and legal requirements
- communication
- salon services, products and pricing
- calculating and taking payments
- making appointments

Maintain the reception area

1 What are the main duties of the salon receptionist?

2 Hospitality is important to show the salon's commitment to customer care. What examples of hospitality may be offered to clients at reception?

3 What equipment and materials do you need at the reception desk?

4 How should the reception be maintained?

5 What is a float? When must this be checked, and why?

6 Client records are often stored at reception. How should this information be used and stored to comply with the Data Protection Act (1998)?

Attend to clients and enquiries

1 What interpersonal skills are essential in a receptionist?

2 How should clients be greeted on arrival?

3 What information should be sought by the receptionist from a visitor to the reception desk?

4 What are the important details to record when taking a message?

5 If as receptionist you were unable to give appropriate information to a client, what action should you take?

6 For what different reasons may people telephone the salon?

7 A client rings up to check the time of an appointment. What information do you need from them?

8 A client complains at reception about a leg wax service they have received. What questions should you ask? What action should you take?

Make appointments for salon services

1 A client telephones the salon, how should you:
- answer the telephone and introduce yourself?
- speak on the telephone?
- seek information from the client?
- finish the telephone conversation?

2 What are the common systems used in salons to make appointments?

3 Why is it necessary to confirm an appointment with a client verbally before they leave the salon?

4 A client wishes to make an appointment for an eyelash tint. What information is required from the client before making the appointment?

5 How long should you allow when making an appointment for the following services:
- full leg wax?
- ear piercing?
- eyelash extensions?
- pedicure including a foot conditioning service?
- full facial and eyelash tint?

Handle payment from clients

1 If you make an error when operating the till, why must you report this?

2 When taking cash from a client, what is the correct procedure to follow?

3 Why is it important to inspect the quality and condition of goods before payment is processed?

4 If you made a mistake in giving the client their change, how would you deal with this?

5 What would you check when receiving payment by cheque?

6 What is the procedure for receiving payment by credit card?

7 If a client has presented an invalid cheque card, what should you say to them?

8 If your salon accepts vouchers in exchange for salon services, how are these handled?

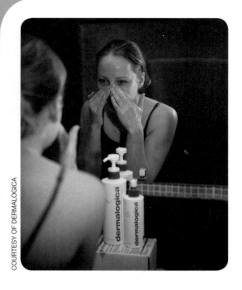

COURTESY OF DERMALOGICA

7 Facial Skincare (B4)

B4 Unit Learning Objectives

This chapter covers **Unit B4 Provide facial skincare treatments**.

This unit is all about improving and maintaining your client's facial skin condition. A facial includes the application of facial products, use of associated equipment and facial massage techniques adapted to suit your client's skin type and condition.

There are **four** learning outcomes for Unit B4 which you must achieve competently:

1. **Maintain safe and effective methods of working when improving and maintaining facial skin condition**

2. **Consult, plan and prepare for facials with clients**

3. **Improve and maintain facial skin condition**

4. **Provide aftercare advice**

Your assessor will observe your performance on **at least three occasions**, each involving a different client.

From the **range** statement, you must show that you have:

- used all **equipment**
- used all **consultation techniques**
- treated all **skin types**
- treated two out of three **skin conditions**
- taken the necessary action where a contra-action, contra-indication or service modification occurs

(continued on the next page)

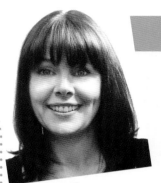

Sally Penford

Education Manager, UK and Ireland
The International Dermal Institute

"

As Education Manager for the International Dermal Institute, I am responsible for training and development of a highly specialized team of lecturers, along with overall operations of eight training centres across UK and Ireland.

I studied at the London College of Fashion and achieved a Higher National Diploma in Beauty Therapy. From this I gained extensive experience in spas and industry consultancy and went on to run my own skin centre. It was 15 years ago that I joined the International Dermal Institute, the world's largest and most influential postgraduate education centre for professional skin therapists.

I share my knowledge in various ways such as traditional lecturing and more recently, through contemporary media methods, such as Twitter. As skincare services evolve, it is important to keep up with new advances.

(continued)

- applied all **facial products**
- applied both types of **massage medium**
- applied all classification of **massage techniques**
- applied a setting and non-setting **mask service**
- provided relevant service **advice**
- You must prove that you have the necessary knowledge, understanding and skills to be able to perform competently for all skin conditions.

When providing facial service it is important to use the skills you have learnt in the following units:

Unit G20 Make sure your own actions reduce risks to health and safety

Unit G18 Promote additional products or services to clients

Unit G8 Develop and maintain your effectiveness at work

Essential anatomy and physiology knowledge for this unit, **B4**, is identified on the checklist in Chapter 2, page 16.

LEARNER SUPPORT

Health multiple choice quiz

TUTOR SUPPORT

Activity 4: Healthy living task

Basics of skincare

Healthy eating

If the skin is to function efficiently the skin must be cared for both internally and externally.

Internally, a nutritionally balanced diet is vital to the health and appearance of the skin. A number of skin allergies and disorders are in part the result of poor nutrition, caused by a poorly balanced diet, including highly processed food, alcohol and lack of essential nutrients.

Foods contain the chemical substances we need for health and growth, the **nutrients**: a healthy diet contains all the essential nutrients. The nutrients are carried to the skin in the blood, where they nourish the cells in the processes of growth and repair.

A balanced diet prevents malnutrition (undernourishment) and vitamin/mineral deficiencies. The following food triangle diagram illustrates the different food groups. The daily recommended amounts to be consumed are:

Fats/oils	1 serving*
Fruit	2–4 servings
Milk and yoghurt	2–3 servings
Proteins	2–3 servings
Starch	6–11 servings
Sugar	1 serving*
Vegetables	3–5 servings

*use scarcely

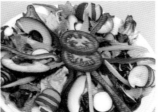

TOP TIP

Five a day rule
Eat at least the recommended five servings of fruit and fresh vegetables every day. These foods provide vital vitamins and minerals that keep the skin healthy. A serving is:

- 1 small glass of pure fruit juice
- 3 heaped tablespoons of fruit salad
- 4 heaped tablespoons of vegetables
- 1 medium fruit (an orange); 2 small fruits (plums)
- 1 dessert bowl of salad

LOW Fat

 LOW Saturates

HIGH Sugar

MED Salt

Traffic light system food label

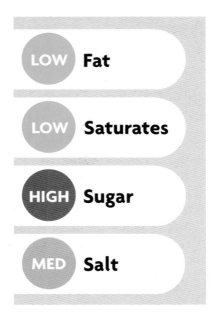

HEALTH & SAFETY

Vegan diets

Proteins are composed of many smaller units called *amino acids*. Animal protein sources contain all the amino acids essential to health. A *vegetarian* consuming dairy food will likewise obtain all the essential amino acids. A *vegan*, however, must be careful to eat an adequate quantity and variety of vegetables and other foods, in order to be sure that they receive all the amino acids they need.

Vegans must take vitamin B$_{12}$ as a vitamin supplement as this vitamin occurs naturally only in animal-derived foods.

HEALTH & SAFETY

Special diets

Warn your clients about the danger of very low-fat, low-carbohydrate or low-protein diets: these can deprive the body of the nutrients it needs for growth, repair and energy.

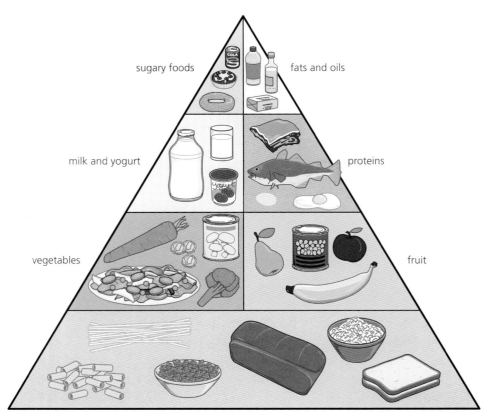

sugary foods

fats and oils

milk and yogurt

proteins

vegetables

fruit

starches

Chart for a balanced diet

A traffic light system of food package labelling shows information on the nutritional content of foods to inform healthy food choice.

There are six principal groups of nutrients:

Carbohydrates Carbohydrates provide energy quickly. They are either simple sugars or starches that the body can turn into simple sugars.

Food sources: Carbohydrates are found in fruit, vegetables, milk, grains and honey.

Fats Fats provide a concentrated source of energy, and are also used in carrying certain vitamins (see below) around the body. Fat is stored in the body around organs and muscles and under the skin. However, if too much fat is deposited under the skin, the elastic fibres there may be damaged by the expansion of the adipose tissue. Fat is also used in the formation of sebum, the skin's natural lubricant.

Food sources: Although this is not always evident, fats are present in almost all foods, from plants and from animals.

Proteins Proteins provide material for the growth and repair of body tissue, and are also a source of energy. Severe protein deficiency in children gives the skin a yellowish appearance, known as **jaundice**.

Food sources: Proteins are found in meat, fish, eggs, dairy products, grains and nuts.

Minerals Minerals provide materials for growth and repair and for regulation of the body processes. The major minerals are calcium, iron, phosphorus, sulphur, sodium, potassium, chlorine and magnesium. Of these, the most important to the skin is iron. A pale, dry skin may indicate **anaemia**, caused by a shortage of iron.

Food sources: Fruit and vegetables; iron is found in liver, egg yolks and green vegetables.

Vitamins
Vitamins regulate the body's processes and contribute to its resistance to disease. Vitamins are divided into two groups, according to whether they are soluble in water or in fat:

- the fat-soluble vitamins are A, D, E and K
- the water-soluble vitamins are B and C

The vitamins most important to the condition of the skin are vitamins A, B_2, B_3, C and E.

Vitamin A Essential for the growth and renewal of skin cells. Insufficient vitamin A in the diet leads to **hyperkeratinization** (production of too much keratin). This causes blockages in the skin tissue. The skin becomes rough and dry, and eye disorders such as styes may occur.

Food sources: Vitamin A is found in red, yellow and green vegetables, and in egg yolk, butter and cheese.

Vitamin B_2 Vitamin B_2 (also called **riboflavin**) helps to break down other foodstuffs, releasing energy needed by cells to desquamate and function efficiently. A deficiency of vitamin B_2 causes the skin at the corners of the mouth to crack.

Food sources: Vitamin B_2 is found in brewer's yeast, milk products, leafy vegetables, liver and whole grains.

Vitamin B_3 Vitamin B_3 (also called **niacin**) has the same function as vitamin B_2, but is also vital in the maintenance of the tissues of the skin.

Food sources: Vitamin B_3 is found in meat, brewer's yeast, nuts and seeds.

Vitamin C Vitamin C (also called **ascorbic acid**) maintains healthy skin and is important for the production of collagen, providing tone and elasticity. A lack of vitamin C causes the capillaries to become fragile, and haemorrhages of the skin, such as bruising, may occur. Severe deficiency results in **scurvy**.

Food sources: Vitamin C is found in fruit and vegetables.

Vitamin E Vitamin E is found in most foods. It is an antioxidant and helps prevent premature skin ageing. It helps to rehydrate the skin, calms inflammation, helps healing and maintains healthy skin.

Food sources: Vitamin E is found in most foods. The richest sources are vegetable oils, cereal products, eggs and meat.

Water
Water forms about two-thirds of the body's weight, and is an important component both inside and outside the body cells. Water is essential for the body's growth and maintenance. It helps remove waste from the body through urine and sweat and regulates temperature. Water must be regularly replaced through the diet. At least one and a half litres of water should be drunk every day, to avoid dehydration of the body and the skin. Aim to drink 6–8 medium glasses daily.

Food sources: Water is also a constituent of many foods, including fruits and vegetables.

TOP TIP

Antioxidant foods

As we know, antioxidants are essential to maintain the health of the skin, fighting the damaging effects of free radicals in your body. Vitamins A, C and E and the mineral selenium all have good antioxidant properties. These can be found in significant amounts in the following foods: blueberries, kale, strawberries, spinach, avocado and broccoli.

ACTIVITY

How do each of the following vitamins benefit the skins appearance and its function: A, B, C and E?

HEALTH & SAFETY

Weight loss

If you lose weight too quickly, your skin will sag and wrinkle. A healthy weight loss plan should be followed, drinking the recommended amount of water to stay hydrated.

HEALTH & SAFETY

Effects of dehydration

Adequate water consumption means that we avoid being dehydrated which can lead to symptoms such as headaches, tiredness and loss of concentration.

In hot weather or following active physical exercise more water must be consumed.

HEALTH & SAFETY

Alcohol intake

Alcohol intake is measured in units — one unit is one centilitre of pure alcohol and is equivalent to:

- 1 single measure of spirits
- 1/2 pint lager, beer or cider
- 1 small glass of wine

A maximum of three units a day are recommended for men and a maximum of two units for women. It is increasingly recommended to have two alcohol-free days per week.

TOP TIP

Caffeine

Advise your clients to replace tea with herbal infusions and to drink decaffeinated coffee (in moderation) rather than regular coffee.

Caffeine is a diuretic causing increased urination and loss of water leading to dehydration.

HEALTH & SAFETY

Smoking

Smoking depletes the body of vital nutrients, preventing their absorption.

ACTIVITY

Causes of stress

1 Can you think of everyday situations that may trigger stress?
2 How do you react physically when put in a stressful situation?
3 How can you create a relaxing environment in the salon?

Fibre Fibre is not broken down into nutrients, but it is very important for effective digestion.

Food sources: Fibre is found in fruit, vegetables and cereals.

Threats to the skin

Internal

Alcohol Alcohol deprives the body of its vitamin reserves, especially vitamins B and C, which are necessary for a healthy skin. Alcohol also tends to dehydrate the body, including the skin. Skin conditions such as acne rosacea, eczema and psoriasis are often aggravated by the consumption of alcohol.

Caffeine Coffee, tea, cocoa and soft fizzy drinks contain a mild stimulant drug called **caffeine**. In moderate doses, such as two or three cups of coffee per day, caffeine is safe. If you drink too much, however, caffeine can cause nervousness, interfere with digestion, block the absorption of vitamins and minerals, dehydrate and spoil the appearance of the skin, stimulating skin ageing.

Drugs Drugs are chemical substances that affect the way our body performs. When they enter the body they are transported throughout the body in the blood. Recreational drugs are taken because they cause a particular effect or sensation which may feel good initially. Long term, they are harmful and addictive. Most affect the blood pressure and heart rate. Stimulants, for example, can cause sweating, shaking and headaches. Heroin, in the class of painkillers called *narcotics*, ravages the skin, causing chronic dryness and premature ageing.

Smoking Smoking interferes with cell respiration and slows down the circulation. This makes it harder for nutrients and oxygen to reach the skin cells and for waste products to be eliminated. Cigarette smoking also releases a chemical that destroys vitamin C. This interferes with the production of collagen, and thereby contributes to premature wrinkling. Nicotine is a **toxic** substance – a poison!

Medication Certain medicines taken by mouth can cause skin dehydration, oedema – swelling of the tissues – (this may for example be caused by steroids) or irregular skin pigmentation (sometimes caused by the contraceptive pill). During the initial consultation with the client, find out whether they are taking any medication – and take this into account in your diagnosis and service plan.

Stress Stress is shown in the face as tension lines where the facial muscles are tight. Because blood and lymph cannot circulate properly, this causes a sluggish skin condition and poor facial nutrition. A person suffering from stress usually experiences disturbed sleep or sleeplessness (**insomnia**). Lack of sleep causes the skin to become dull and puffy, especially the tissue beneath the eyes, where dark circles also appear. Too *much* sleep can also cause the facial tissue to become puffy – because the circulation is less active, body fluids collect in the tissues.

If someone is suffering from stress, they may drink more tea, coffee or alcohol, or smoke more cigarettes: this too damages the skin.

Stress and anxiety are often the underlying cause of certain skin disorders. Some skin conditions, such as boils and styes, appear at times of stress; others, such as psoriasis and eczema, may become much worse. At the consultation, try to determine whether the client is suffering from stress: if they are, make sure that the salon services promote relaxation.

External

As well as looking after the skin from the *inside*, by diet, it needs care from the *outside* – it must be kept clean, and it must be nourished.

With normal physiological functioning, the skin becomes oily, and sweat is deposited on its surface. The skin's natural oil (**sebum**) can easily build up and block the natural openings, the hair **follicles** and **pores**: this may lead to infection. Facial cosmetics too affect the health of the skin; if not regularly removed, they may cause congestion. Skincare services help to maintain and improve the functioning of the skin.

Ultra-violet light

Although recently ultra-violet (UV) has been identified as a hazard to skin, it also has some *positive* effects. One of these is its ability to stimulate the production of **vitamin D**, which is absorbed into the bloodstream and nourishes and helps to maintain bone tissue. Second, UV light activates the **pigment** **melanin** in the skin, and thereby creates a **tan**. Many people feel better when they have a tan, as it gives a healthy appearance.

Ultra-violet light is divided into different bands. The most important to skin tanning are UVA and UVB. **UVA** stimulates the melanin in the skin to produce a rapid tan, which does not last very long. UVA penetrates deep into the dermis where it can cause premature ageing of the skin. **Free radicals** – highly reactive molecules which cause skin cells to degenerate – are also formed. These molecules disrupt production of collagen and elastin, the fibres that give skin its strength and elasticity. Reduced elasticity leads to wrinkling.

UVB stimulates the production of vitamin D. Melanin activation by UVB produces a longer-lasting tan than that produced by UVA. UVB is partially absorbed by the atmosphere – it has a shorter wavelength than UVA – and only 10 per cent reaches the dermis. UVB causes thickening of the stratum corneum layer, which reflects ultra-violet away from the skin's surface. UVB causes **sunburn**: the skin becomes red as the cells are damaged, and the skin may blister. UVB is also implicated in skin cancers, especially malignant melanoma.

The relaxing, warming effect of the sun is caused by the **infra-red (IR)** light. This penetrates the skin to the subcutaneous layer and is thought to speed skin ageing and possibly to cause a cancer called squamous cell carcinoma. The tan is actually a sign of skin damage, therefore, and both UV and IR probably contribute to photo-ageing – the premature ageing of the skin by light.

Although black skin has a high melanin content, which absorbs more ultraviolet and allows less to reach the dermis, it is not fully protected against the UV and still requires additional protection.

Chemical skin protection, or sunscreens, are designed to absorb ultra-violet light (UVA and UVB), reducing the rate of skin ageing in all skin types. Various sunscreens are available, classified by number according to their sun-protection factor (SPF). This is the amount of protection that the sunscreen gives you from the sun. A SPF of at least 15 is recommended in winter and 30 in summer. The application of the sunscreen extends your natural skin protection, allowing you to stay in the sun for longer without burning. For example, if normally you can be in the sun for ten minutes before the skin begins to go red, a sunscreen with an SPF of 10 will allow you 10×10 minutes' (i.e. 100 minutes') safe exposure in the sun. Always check the expiry date of sunscreens, they only have a shelf life of 2–3 years.

Artificial UV light produced by sun beds, used for cosmetic skin tanning, also causes premature ageing. Most sun beds use concentrated UVA, which causes dermal tissue damage resulting in lines and wrinkles.

It may take years to see the effects of the dermal damage caused by unprotected UV exposure, but once they have occurred the effects are irreversible. UVA rays are present

HEALTH & SAFETY

Sunbathing

Never wear perfume, cosmetic products or deodorants when sunbathing, either in natural sunlight or in artificially produced (sun-canopy) ultra-violet. The chemicals in these products can sensitize the skin, causing an allergic skin reaction.

Ultra-violet can penetrate water to a depth of one metre, so even when swimming you need to wear a sunscreen. Special waterproof products are designed for this purpose.

BEST PRACTICE

To acquire a tan without the damaging effects of the sun or sun beds, your client can use a *fake tanning* preparation. This service is becoming popular in the beauty therapist's salon.

ALWAYS REMEMBER

At the consultation, ask the client their occupation: this will guide you as to their likely skincare requirements. The client who works outdoors, for example, will have different service needs from the one who works indoors.

ACTIVITY

Geographical variations

Consider the effects of climate on the skin. Name four different geographical locations, and state the humidity level and climate you would expect at each location.

Think of the probable effects on the skin. What services by a beauty therapist might be needed in each country?

all year round, so to prevent premature ageing, cosmetic preparations containing sun-screens should be worn at all times.

Climate Sebum, the skin's natural grease, provides an oily protective film over the surface of the skin that reduces evaporation. Despite this, unprotected exposure of the skin to the environment allows evaporation from the epidermis which results in a dry, de-hydrated skin condition.

The climate has several effects on the skin:

- **Sebum production** When the skin is exposed to the cold, less sebum is produced. The skin has reduced protection, allowing moisture to evaporate.

- **Perspiration** In very hot weather more moisture is lost as **perspiration**: perspiration increases to cool the skin and regulate the body's temperature.

- **Humidity** Moisture loss from the skin is also affected by the **humidity** (water content) of the surrounding air. In hot, dry weather humidity will be low, so water loss will be high. In temperate, damp conditions humidity will be high, so water loss will be low.

- **Extremes of temperature** Alternating heat and cold often leads to the formation of **broken capillaries**. These appear as fine red lines on Caucasian skin, and as discolouration on black skin.

- **Stratum corneum** The cells of the stratum corneum multiply with repeated unprotected exposure to the climate, as the body's natural defence.

The damaging effects caused by the climate can be reduced by using protective skincare preparations such as moisturisers. These spread a layer of oil over the skin's surface, reducing evaporation.

HEALTH & SAFETY

Ashiness

A black skin can sometimes appear ashen, with patches of skin becoming grey and flaky. This is caused by sudden changes in temperature combined with low humidity, which can cause the skin to lose moisture. Moisturisers help in alleviating this problem.

Environmental stress and pollution Further causes of moisture loss include harsh alkaline chemicals such as detergents and soaps – which remove sebum from the skin's surface – and air conditioning and central heating.

Environmental **pollutants** such as lead, mercury, cadmium and aluminium can accumulate in the body. One result is the formation of dangerous chemicals that attack proteins in the cells. Such pollutants find their way into food through polluted waters, rain and dust. To protect the body, always wash vegetables thoroughly, and eat a diet rich in vitamins C and E.

Air pollution, involving carbon from smoke, chemical discharges from factories, and fumes from car exhausts, should be removed from the skin by effective cleansing. Absorption of these pollutants is reduced by the application of moisturiser: this forms a barrier over the skin's surface.

Skincare services

The beauty therapist has the professional expertise to help each client improve the appearance and condition of their skin by the application of appropriate skincare services and products. The facial skin services the beauty therapist offers include:

- consultation and skin analysis
- skin cleansing
- specialized skincare services
- manual massage of the face, neck and shoulders
- the application of face masks
- facial make-up

The beauty therapist cannot change the underlying skin type, which is genetically determined, but they can keep the physiological characteristics of each skin type in check.

Skin types

The basic structure of the skin does not vary from person to person, but the physiological functioning of its different features does; it is this that gives us skin types, recognized by specific visible characteristics.

The first and most important part of a facial service is the correct diagnosis of the skin type. This is carried out at the beginning of each facial service. The beauty therapist must choose the correct skincare products and facial services for the client's skin type. This assessment is called a skin analysis.

Basic types

There are four main skin types:

- normal
- dry
- oily
- combination

Normal skin Normal skin is often referred to as **balanced**, the water and oil content is constant, it is neither too oily nor too dry. Because when young, this skin type seldom has any problems, such as blemishes, it is often neglected. Neglect causes the skin to become dry, especially around the eyes, cheeks and neck, where the skin is thinner.

HEALTH & SAFETY

Air pollution

There are many components to air pollution. Car exhaust fumes, for example, release nitrogen oxide and volatile organic compounds. These react with sunlight to form ozone, a highly reactive form of oxygen. This can penetrate deep inside the skin and damage the cells' DNA (their main component), which can lead to skin cancer. Also, accelerated skin ageing is caused by free radical damage caused by unstable molecules, which affect the skin's elasticity. Moisturisers containing antioxidants are essential and should be recommended to neutralize free radicals or repel them from the skin before skin damage is caused.

TOP TIP

Dry skin in winter

Central heating creates an environment with humidity similar to that of the desert. Unless you use a moisturiser, the loss of moisture from the skin will cause a dry, dehydrated skin condition.

HEALTH & SAFETY

Effects of water loss

Water loss can sometimes be sufficient to disrupt living cells in the skin to the extent that some actually die. This results in skin irritation and reddening.

ACTIVITY

Environmental factors

It is important that you are aware of all the factors that can affect the health of a client's skin: this knowledge allows you to assess each client's service needs. Summarize the different factors you have learnt about.

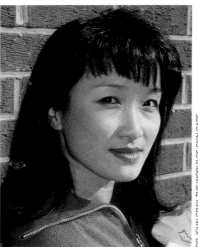

DR JOHN GRAY, THE WORLD OF SKIN CARE

Normal skin

ACTIVITY

Recognizing skin types and conditions

Refer to the illustration below. What skin characteristics conditions would you expect to see in each of the numbered areas if performing a skin analysis on a:

- dry skin type?
- oily skin type?
- combination skin type?

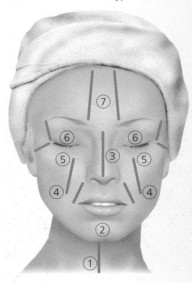

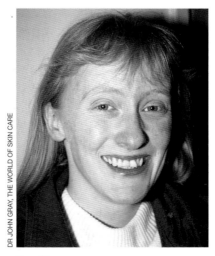

Dry skin

DR JOHN GRAY, THE WORLD OF SKIN CARE

A normal skin type in adults is very rare. It has these characteristics:

- the pore size is small or medium
- the moisture content is good
- the skin texture is smooth and even, neither too thick nor too thin
- the colour is healthy (because of good blood circulation)
- the skin elasticity is good, when young
- the skin feels firm to the touch
- the skin pigmentation is even-coloured
- the skin is usually free from blemishes

Dry skin Dry skin is lacking in either sebum or moisture, or both. Because sebum limits moisture loss by evaporation from the skin, skin with insufficient sebum rapidly loses moisture. The resulting dry skin is often described as **dehydrated**.

Dry skin has these characteristics:

- the pores are small and tight
- the moisture content is poor
- the skin texture is coarse and thin, with patches of visibly flaking skin
- there is a tendency towards sensitivity (broken capillaries often accompany this skin type)
- premature ageing is common, resulting in the appearance of fine lines leading to deeper wrinkles, seen especially around the eyes, mouth and neck
- skin pigmentation may be uneven, and disorders such as ephelides (freckles) usually accompany this skin type
- milia are often found around the cheek and eye area

Oily skin In oily skin the sebaceous glands become very active at puberty, when stimulated by the male hormone **androgen**. An increase in sebum production often causes the appearance of skin blemishes. Sebaceous gland activity begins to decrease when the person is in their twenties.

Oily skin has these characteristics:

- the pores are enlarged
- the moisture content is high
- the skin is coarse and thick
- the skin is sallow in colour, as a result of the excess sebum production, dead skin cells become embedded in the sebum, and the skin has sluggish blood and lymph circulation
- the **skin tone** is good, due to the protective effect of the sebum
- the skin is prone to shininess, due to excess sebum production
- there may be uneven pigmentation
- certain skin disorders may be apparent – comedones, pustules, papules, milia or sebaceous cysts

Acne vulgaris and **seborrhoea** are skin disorders that occur when the skin becomes excessively oily due to the influence of hormones. Treatment of these skin disorders should be carried out to control and reduce sebum flow.

Combination skin   Combination skin is partly oily and partly dry. The oily parts are generally the chin, nose and forehead, known as the **T-zone**. The upper cheeks may show signs of oiliness, but the rest of the face and neck area is usually dry.

Combination skin is the most common skin type. It has these characteristics:

- the pores in the T-zone are enlarged, while in the cheek area they are small to medium
- the moisture content is high in the oily areas, but poor in the dry areas
- the skin is coarse and thick in the oily areas, but thin in the dry areas
- the skin is sallow in the oily areas, but shows sensitivity and high colour in the dry areas
- the skin tone is good in the oily areas, but poor in the dry areas
- there is uneven pigmentation, usually seen as ephelides and lentigines
- there may be blemishes such as pustules and comedones on the oily skin at the T-zone
- milia and broken capillaries may appear in the dry areas, commonly on the cheeks and near the eyes

Additional skin conditions

While looking closely at the skin, further **skin characteristics** may become obvious. The skin may be:

- sensitive
- dehydrated
- moist
- oedematous (puffy)

Sensitive skin   Sensitive skin usually accompanies a dry skin type, but not always. The characteristics of sensitive skin are these:

- the skin may show high colouring as it is easily irritated
- there are usually broken capillaries in the cheek area
- the skin feels warm to the touch
- there is superficial flaking of the skin
- the skin may show high colouring and tightness after skin cleansing, if it is sensitive to pressure

In black skin, instead of the redness shown by Caucasian skin, irritation shows up as a darker patch.

Allergic skin   Allergic skin is irritated by external **allergens**, including chemicals in some cosmetics. The allergens inflame the skin and may damage its protective function. At the consultation, always try to discover whether the client has any allergies, and if so, to what.

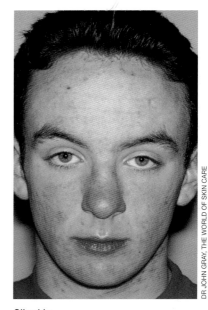

Oily skin

DR JOHN GRAY, THE WORLD OF SKIN CARE

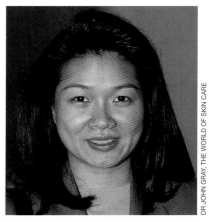

Combination skin

DR JOHN GRAY, THE WORLD OF SKIN CARE

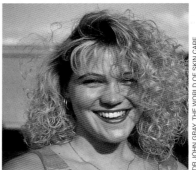

Sensitive skin

DR JOHN GRAY, THE WORLD OF SKIN CARE

BEST PRACTICE

Dehydrated skin

Encourage clients especially with dehydrated skin to drink six to eight glasses of water a day to replenish the moisture in the body.

DR JOHN GRAY, THE WORLD OF SKIN CARE

DR JOHN GRAY, THE WORLD OF SKIN CARE

BEST PRACTICE

Oedematous skin

While completing the record card you may be able to recognize aspects of your client's lifestyle that probably contribute to the oedematous skin. If so, you can advise the client accordingly.

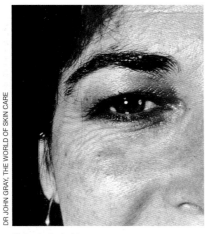

Dehydrated skin

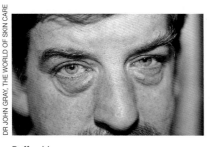

Puffy skin

ALWAYS REMEMBER

Sensitive skin

Use hypoallergenic products – these do not contain any of the known common skin sensitizers such as perfume that can cause skin irritation.

Skin that is sensitive may also be allergic to certain substances such as adhesives that may be used in false lash application.

Recommend avoiding lifestyle factors that can make sensitive skin worse. These include alcohol, smoking, poor diet and stress.

The allergies of most concern to the beauty therapist are those caused by substances applied to the skin. The therapist must be aware of such substances and avoid their use. Contact with an allergen, especially if repeated, may cause skin disorders such as eczema or dermatitis (see Chapter 3, pages 91–104, where skin diseases and disorders are dealt with in more detail).

Dehydrated skin Dehydrated skin is skin that has lost water from the skin tissues. The condition can affect any skin type, but most commonly accompanies dry or combination skin types. The problem may be related to the client's general health. If they have recently been ill with a fever, for example, the skin will have lost fluid through sweating. If they are taking medication, this too may cause dehydration, as may drastic dieting. In many cases the dehydration is caused by working in an environment with a low humidity, or in one that is air-conditioned. You must try to discover the cause, and provide both corrective service and advice.

The characteristics of dehydrated skin are as follows:

- the skin has a fine orange-peel effect, caused by its lack of moisture
- there is superficial flaking
- fine, superficial lines are evident on the skin
- broken capillaries are common

Moist skin Moist skin appears moist and feels damp: this is due to the over-secretion of sweat. The beauty therapist cannot correct this skin condition, which is often caused by some internal physiological disturbance such as a hormonal or metabolic imbalance.

Advise the client to use lightweight cleansing preparations. The client should avoid skin-toning preparations with a high alcohol content; these would stimulate the skin, causing yet further perspiration and skin sensitivity. They should avoid highly spiced food, and be aware that alcoholic or hot drinks will cause dilation of the skin capillaries, thereby increasing the skin's temperature.

Oedematous (puffy) skin Oedematous skin is, and appears, swollen and puffy: this is because the tissues are retaining excess water. The condition may be caused by a medical disorder, or may be a side-effect of medication. Hot weather can cause temporary swelling of the tissues, as can local injury to the tissues. Poor blood circulation and lymphatic flow may cause puffy skin, too; this is often seen around the eyes. In this case the condition may benefit from gentle massage around the eye area. Tissue-fluid retention in the facial skin may be caused by an incorrect diet, such as one that includes too much salt or the drinking of too much alcohol, tea or coffee and insufficient water.

Unless you are quite sure about the cause of the oedema, always seek permission from your client's doctor before treating the skin.

The sex of the client

Men have a more acidic skin surface than females and the stratum corneum is thicker on males than females. However, males have coarse facial hair and shaving daily removes cells of the stratum corneum before they are ready to desquamate naturally. This can sensitize and dry the skin, especially if aftershave lotions with a high alcohol content are directly applied. A moisturiser should be applied to protect the skin.

The collagen content of the skin is different in men and women. Collagen and sebum production falls in menopausal women causing skin ageing. Skin does not appear to age as quickly in males as females because collagen, elastin and sebum production remain constant. The skin of males typically feels firmer.

The main reason males choose to have a facial is for relaxation, to improve the appearance of the skin, and increasingly for the anti-ageing benefits.

The age of the skin

Having identified the skin type, the beauty therapist must classify the age of the skin. This can vary between people of different race because of evolution which may delay the visible signs of ageing due to differences in sebaceous gland and melanin activity in skin.

Often the age of a client will relate to skin problems that are evident. A young client, for example, may have skin blemishes such as comedones, pustules and papules. These disorders are caused by over-activity of the sebaceous gland at puberty, when the body is developing its secondary sexual characteristics. It is at this time that acne vulgaris is most likely to occur, due to the hormonal imbalance. The skin of clients aged over 25 years, however, is generally termed **mature skin**.

The beauty therapist should also consider the client's skin tone and muscle tone in relation to their age. A young skin will probably have good skin tone, and the skin will be supple and elastic. This is because the collagen and elastin fibres in the skin are strong. Poor skin tone, on the other hand, is recognized by the appearance of facial lines and wrinkles.

A healthy young skin will also have good muscle tone, and the facial contours will appear firm. With poor muscle tone, the muscles becomes slack and loose.

Poor lifestyle choices and general health will also affect how quickly our skin shows visible signs of aging.

Mature skin The change in appearance of women's skin during ageing is closely related to the altered production of the hormones oestrogen, progesterone and androgen at the menopause.

Mature skin has the following characteristics:

- The skin becomes dry, as the sebaceous and sudoriferous glands become less active.
- The skin loses its elasticity as the elastin fibres harden, and wrinkles appear due to the cross-linking and hardening of collagen fibres.
- The epidermis grows more slowly and the skin appears thinner, becoming almost transparent in some areas such as around the eyes, where small veins and capillaries show through the skin.
- Broken capillaries appear, especially on the cheek area and around the nose.
- The facial contours become slack as muscle tone is reduced.
- The underlying bone structure becomes more obvious, as the fatty layer and the supportive tissue beneath the skin grow thinner.
- Blood circulation becomes poor, which interferes with skin nutrition, and the skin may appear sallow.
- Due to the decrease in metabolic rate, waste products are not removed so quickly, and this leads to puffiness of the skin.
- Patches of irregular pigmentation appear on the surface of the skin, such as lentigines and chloasmata.

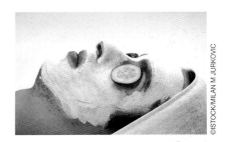

©ISTOCK/MILAN M JURKOVIC

Male facial

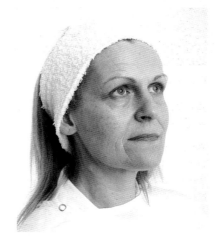

Mature skin

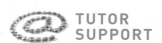

TUTOR SUPPORT

Activity 1: Consultation sheet task

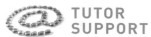

TUTOR SUPPORT

Activity 2: Skin analysis handout

HEALTH & SAFETY

UV light and ageing
The ageing process is accelerated when the skin is regularly exposed to ultra-violet light.

TOP TIP

Skin appearance
As the surface of the skin reflects light and shows the skin colour, the therapist's aim is for the skin surface to be smooth and healthy. This is achieved by the removal of dead skin cells and ensuring it is adequately moisturised.

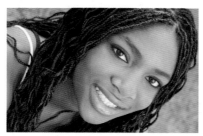

African-Caribbean skin

The skin may also exhibit the following skin conditions, although these are not truly *characteristic* of an ageing skin:

- Dermal naevi may be enlarged.
- Seborrhoeic warts may appear on the epidermal layer of the skin.
- Verruca filliformis warts may increase in number.
- Hair growth on the upper lip or chin, or both, may become darker or coarser, due to hormonal imbalance in the body.
- Dark circles and puffiness may occur under the eyes.

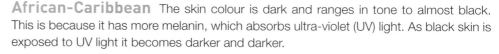

ACTIVITY

The ageing process
Cut out photographs from magazines or newspapers showing men and women of different cultures and various ages.

1 Can you identify the visible characteristics of ageing?
2 Does ageing occur at the same rate in men and women and in different cultures?
3 Discuss your findings with your colleagues and tutor.

Differences in skin

Although there is no difference between skin functions such as sweat and sebaceous gland activity in white and black skin, the amount of pigment, called *melanin*, varies, resulting in different skin and hair colour.

There are two forms of the melanin pigment: *eumelanin*, produced in black and brown skin colours, and *phaeomelanin*, found in lighter skins. Both forms of pigment can be present together but the amount of each can vary.

People who originate from hot countries and are nearer the equator have more melanin and a darker skin pigment. This is because the UV is very intense and the skin requires more protection. Those who originate from cooler countries have less melanin and a lighter skin pigment. The pigmentation of the skin is the result of millions of years of evolution.

African-Caribbean The skin colour is dark and ranges in tone to almost black. This is because it has more melanin, which absorbs ultra-violet (UV) light. As black skin is exposed to UV light it becomes darker and darker.

Care must be taken when dealing with blemishes on darker skins as scars may occur as the skin heals. The scars may become keloids, scarring that becomes enlarged and projects above the skin's surface. Even minor scratches may result in keloid formation.

Hyperpigmentation (uneven patches of skin tone which are darker than the surrounding skin) may also occur with exposure to UV light. It is more common in darker skinned people due to increased melanin. Hyperpigmentation most commonly occurs following skin inflammation, such as acne vulgaris. Keloids may become hyperpigmented if exposed to the sun in the early stages of their formation.

DR JOHN GRAY, THE WORLD OF SKIN CARE

ALWAYS REMEMBER

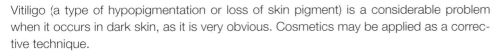

Hyperpigmentation and **hypopigmentation** can affect the skin of any race.

Chloasma or 'liver spots' are an example of hyperpigmentation and are commonly seen as dark brown marks on the backs of the hands. These occur as a result of skin damage caused by sun damage, skin trauma or hormonal imbalance.

Freckles or ephelides are another example of hyperpigmentation. These become darker when the skin is exposed to the sun.

Prescription creams containing hydroquinone bleach and laser treatment may be used to lighten the skin. However, care must be taken using hydroquinone bleach on black and Asian skin as hypopigmentation and skin allergy can occur.

Increasing in popularity are botanical brighteners which include the professional application of an exfoliant to remove the pigmented surface cells and serum.

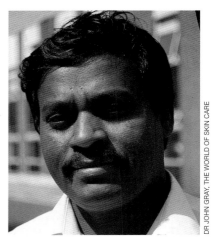

Asian skin

Vitiligo (a type of hypopigmentation or loss of skin pigment) is a considerable problem when it occurs in dark skin, as it is very obvious. Cosmetics may be applied as a corrective technique.

Male African-Caribbean clients may have a tendency towards *pseudo folliculitis*, an inflammatory skin disorder. This occurs as the hair is coarse and curly and has a tendency as it grows out of the skin to curl back and re-enter it, becoming ingrown. This foreign object in the skin becomes irritated and inflamed. Hyperpigmentation may also accompany this condition.

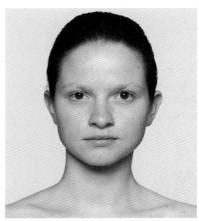

Caucasian skin

Dermatosis papulosis nigra, also called flesh moles, can occur. These are brown or black hyperpigmented markings, resembling moles, usually seen on the cheeks. Their cause is unknown but they are sometimes found to be hereditary. They also occur more frequently in women than men.

Hair colour is dark brown to black.

Asian The skin colour has a light to dark tone due to increased melanin, with yellow undertones. There is a tendency towards hyperpigmentation, appearing as dark patches of skin, and scarring can appear following skin inflammation. Dermatosis papulosis nigra can occur. In women there is a normal tendency towards superfluous facial hair.

Hair colour is dark brown to black.

Caucasian The skin colour is pink. This skin has less melanin and so less defence in the presence of UV light; sun damage results in skin burning and premature ageing. Caucasian skin has a tendency to show freckles (ephelides), as a result of uneven melanin distribution in the skin.

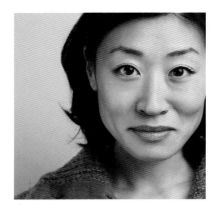

Oriental skin

Hair colour is usually fair, red or brown.

Oriental The skin colour has more melanin present and has a yellowish tone. Oriental skin is usually oily and prone to hyperpigmentation. Blemishes should be treated with caution as hyperpigmentation and scarring could result due to increased levels of melanin. Female skin generally appears smooth and has little facial hair.

Hair colour is usually mid-brown to black.

ALWAYS REMEMBER

Skin and UV light defence
Very dark skin offers up to 30 times more protection against the sun than lighter skin.

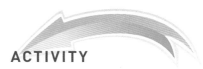

ACTIVITY

Which countries do the skin types listed below originate from:

- Caucasian?
- Oriental?
- Asian?
- African-Caribbean?

HEALTH & SAFETY

Habia Health and Safety

Hygiene for Hairdressers and Beauty Therapists booklet is available as a download from habia.org providing practical advice on how to avoid infection in the workplace.

Outcome 1: Maintain safe and effective methods of working when improving and maintaining facial skin condition

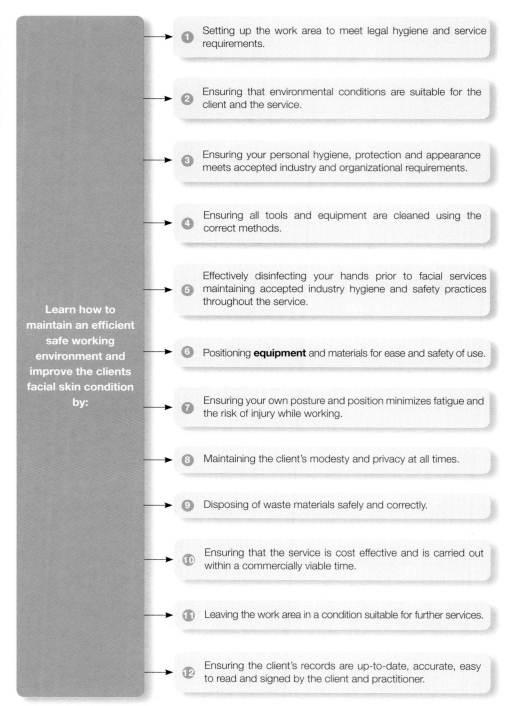

Learn how to maintain an efficient safe working environment and improve the clients facial skin condition by:

1. Setting up the work area to meet legal hygiene and service requirements.

2. Ensuring that environmental conditions are suitable for the client and the service.

3. Ensuring your personal hygiene, protection and appearance meets accepted industry and organizational requirements.

4. Ensuring all tools and equipment are cleaned using the correct methods.

5. Effectively disinfecting your hands prior to facial services maintaining accepted industry hygiene and safety practices throughout the service.

6. Positioning **equipment** and materials for ease and safety of use.

7. Ensuring your own posture and position minimizes fatigue and the risk of injury while working.

8. Maintaining the client's modesty and privacy at all times.

9. Disposing of waste materials safely and correctly.

10. Ensuring that the service is cost effective and is carried out within a commercially viable time.

11. Leaving the work area in a condition suitable for further services.

12. Ensuring the client's records are up-to-date, accurate, easy to read and signed by the client and practitioner.

Beauty salons differ in how much floor space is available and how much of that is allocated to each beauty service. There may be one or several facial-service work areas. In the case of a salon having only one such work area, it is important that the range of facial services offered can all be delivered safely and hygienically.

Chapter 3, **Health and safety** covers general legal hygiene and safety practice which you are legally obliged to implement. You will learn about further specific health and safety legislation service requirements in **Outcome 3, Improve and maintain facial skin condition**.

Remember to always:

- Give due consideration to general health and safety legislation throughout the service.

- Implement any hygiene, health and safety requirements as identified in the National Occupational Standard.

- Follow industry hygiene, health and safety practices throughout the service application. Refer to the Habia website to keep up to date with current health and safety practice.

- Dispose of any service waste materials safely and correctly.

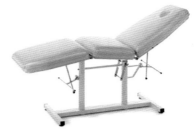

Service couch

Setting up the work area

Basic equipment

Consideration should be given to the positioning of equipment for ease and safety of use.

Each facial work area should have the following basic equipment a **service couch or beauty chair** The couch or chair should be covered with easy-to-clean upholstery: it must withstand daily cleaning with warm water and detergent. It must have an adjustable **back rest**, for the comfort of both the client and the therapist. If possible, purchase a couch that also has an adjustable **leg rest**, as this allows services such as pedicure to be carried out.

Hydraulic couches are useful as they can be adjusted in height to enable the client to position herself on the couch with ease.

If you are a freelance beauty therapist you will require a lightweight, durable beauty couch for facial services. These beds are also useful to have when carrying out demonstrations at a different location.

- **Equipment trolley** The equipment trolley should be large enough to accommodate all the necessary equipment and products; trolleys are usually of a two- or three-shelf design. Like the chair or couch, the trolley should be made of a material that will withstand regular cleaning. Some models have restraining bars to prevent objects sliding off the trolley. Drawers are useful in storing tools and small consumables. The trolley should have securely fixed easy-glide castors. Some salons may use a large surface work area to display and store equipment and products.

- **Beauty stool** The stool should be covered in a fabric similar to that covering the service couch. It may or may not have a back rest; in some designs the back rest is removable. For the comfort of the therapist, it should be adjustable in height; to allow mobility, it should be mounted on castors.

- **Step-up stool** To assist clients as necessary to position themselves on the couch, have available a step-up stool.

- **Magnifying lamp** The magnifying lamp is available in three models: floor-standing, wall-mounted and trolley-mounted.

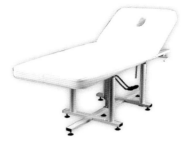

Hydraulic service couch

> **Be thorough**
> Creating a unique, personalized experience is essential. Think about how you can go the extra mile, and what extra special touches you can add to make it an out-of-this world treatment every time. Your client will see excellent results, and you'll never get bored!
>
> **Sally Penford**

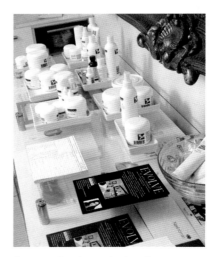

A prepared and organised work area

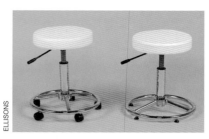

ELLISONS

Beauty stools

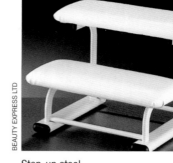

BEAUTY EXPRESS LTD

Step-up stool

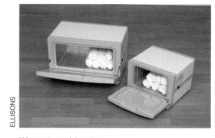

ELLISONS

Warm towel heater

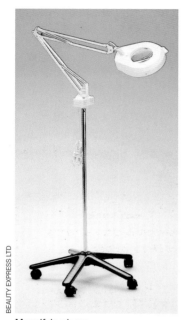

BEAUTY EXPRESS LTD

Magnifying lamp

HEALTH & SAFETY

The couch and chair

The couch should be wiped over with a disinfectant solution after each client, and should be cleaned thoroughly with hot water and detergent at the end of each day. If protected with a towelling couch cover this must be protected with a covering that is replaced after each client, i.e. large towel or disposable paper.

- **Warm towel heater** The warm towel heater is used to prepare hot steam towels used to soften and warm the skin and remove excess facial skincare products from the skin's surface.

- **Covered waste bin** A covered waste bin should be placed unobtrusively within easy each. It should be lined with a disposable bin-liner. You should also have a 'sharps' box for the disposal of contaminated equipment.

Arrangements for the collection and disposal of contaminated waste should be made with your local environmental health office.

Preparing the work area

The following equipment guidelines describe the basic preparation of the **facial service work area**. Further equipment and materials relevant to other beauty services are discussed within the appropriate chapters.

EQUIPMENT AND MATERIALS LIST

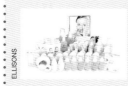

ELLISONS

Headband
A clean headband should be provided for each client. Use either a material headband or disposable. Disposable are useful as they can be discarded after the service

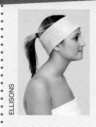

ELLISONS

Skin-cleansing preparations
The trolley should carry a display of facial skin-cleansing preparations to suit all skin types

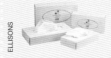

ELLISONS

Cotton wool
There should be a plentiful supply of both damp and dry cotton wool, sufficient for the service to be carried out. Dry cotton wool should be stored in a covered container; damp cotton wool is usually placed in a clean bowl

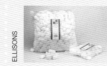

ELLISONS

Tissues
Facial tissues should be large and of a high quality. They should be stored in a covered container

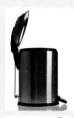

ELLISONS

Waste bin
A covered container for waste may be placed on the bottom shelf of the trolley or it can be put into the waste bin at once

Spatulas
Several clean spatulas (preferably disposable) should be provided for each client. One should be used in tucking any stray hair beneath the headband. Others will be used in removing products from their containers

YOU WILL ALSO NEED:

Towel drapes There should be a large towel to cover the client's body, and a small hand towel to drape across the client's chest and shoulders

Trolley The surface of each shelf can be protected with a sheet of 500mm disposable bedroll

Towel A clean towel should be placed on the trolley for the therapist to wipe their hands on as necessary

Gown A clean gown should be provided for each client as necessary

Facial sponges, facial mitts or towels Are used to remove facial products from the skin during service. They are particularly useful when working on a male client where cotton wool would collect on coarse facial hair

Mirror A clean hand mirror should be available for use in consulting with the client before during and after their service

Container for jewellery A container may be provided in which the client can place their jewellery if they need to remove it prior to service – follow your salon procedures in respect of client possessions

TOP TIP

It is bad practice to leave the client in order to fetch more cotton wool. It is also bad practice to prepare too much and be wasteful!

Pre-shaped cotton wool discs are ideal for facial services. Alternatively, cut high-quality cotton wool into squares (6cm × 6cm).

TOP TIP

Towel racks
Wall-mounted towel racks save storage space.

HEALTH & SAFETY

Containers
Bottles and other containers should be clean and clearly labelled.

On arrival

When the client arrives for the service, generally the **record card** is completed. Record the client's personal details, such as their name and address. Check that there are no contra-indications to facial service.

If a client is a minor, under the age of 16 years of age, it is necessary to obtain signed written consent before service is carried out. It is also necessary that the parent or guardian is present when the service is given.

The beauty therapist will add further information to the record card at the consultation and during service.

Clients should not be kept waiting on arrival for their appointment. It is important that the work area is ready to proceed. The work area should always be maintained in a condition suitable for further services.

TOP TIP

Disposable paper roll may be placed over the surface of the treatment couch if desired. This should be changed for each client.

HEALTH & SAFETY

Poor health
If the client is in poor health, or is taking medication that affects their skin condition, it may not be possible to treat them until the medical condition has been treated by their general practitioner.

Reception

When a new client telephones to make an appointment for a service, always allocate extra time for the consultation beforehand. Explain to the client how long they should allow for the appointment. For example, if a client is seeking a basic skin cleansing and mask service, allow 30 minutes; if they are a new client allow 45 minutes so that there is time for the consultation and filling in the record card. If it is necessary to remove facial blockages and to carry out other specialized services, allow 45 minutes to one hour. For a full facial service, allow one hour.

ALWAYS REMEMBER

Compliance with the Data Protection Act (1998)

Ensure all client records are stored securely, with only those staff who have the client's permission having access to them.

ALWAYS REMEMBER

Service timing

Full facial service: service time allow one hour.

HEALTH & SAFETY

Consultation check

Check if a client has received any specialist electrical facials such as micro-dermabrasion or chemical peels. These treatments involve removing the surface epidermal cells from the skin, which may cause it to be sensitive. Ensure that you check at the consultation if the client has been receiving any specialised treatments for the facial skin, and if so what and when. Seek guidance as necessary from a senior therapist as to client suitability.

Outcome 2: Consult, plan and prepare for facials with clients

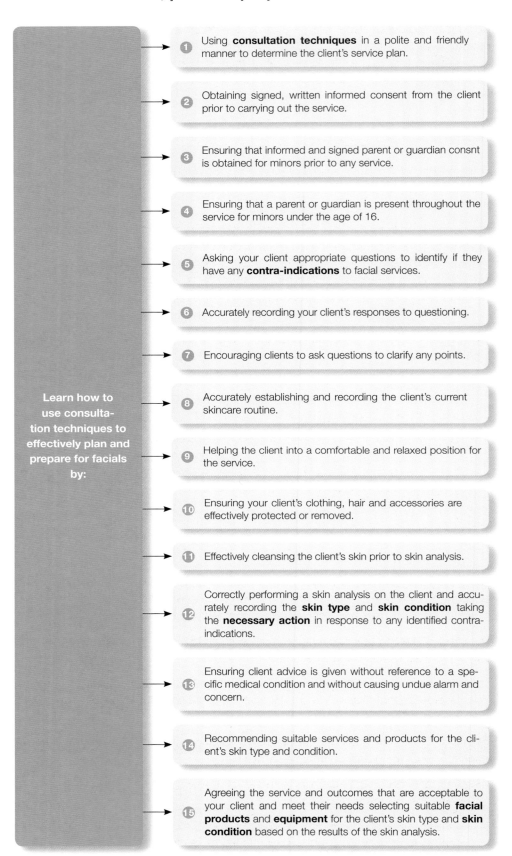

Learn how to use consultation techniques to effectively plan and prepare for facials by:

1. Using **consultation techniques** in a polite and friendly manner to determine the client's service plan.

2. Obtaining signed, written informed consent from the client prior to carrying out the service.

3. Ensuring that informed and signed parent or guardian consnt is obtained for minors prior to any service.

4. Ensuring that a parent or guardian is present throughout the service for minors under the age of 16.

5. Asking your client appropriate questions to identify if they have any **contra-indications** to facial services.

6. Accurately recording your client's responses to questioning.

7. Encouraging clients to ask questions to clarify any points.

8. Accurately establishing and recording the client's current skincare routine.

9. Helping the client into a comfortable and relaxed position for the service.

10. Ensuring your client's clothing, hair and accessories are effectively protected or removed.

11. Effectively cleansing the client's skin prior to skin analysis.

12. Correctly performing a skin analysis on the client and accurately recording the **skin type** and **skin condition** taking the **necessary action** in response to any identified contra-indications.

13. Ensuring client advice is given without reference to a specific medical condition and without causing undue alarm and concern.

14. Recommending suitable services and products for the client's skin type and condition.

15. Agreeing the service and outcomes that are acceptable to your client and meet their needs selecting suitable **facial products** and **equipment** for the client's skin type and **skin condition** based on the results of the skin analysis.

Depending on the facial service to be carried out, the client may need to remove some clothing. Offer them a **gown** to wear for modesty. Privacy must be maintained at all times.

Before carrying out *any* facial services, the beauty therapist must consult with the client to determine their service needs and to discuss the services that are available. **Consultation** is a service that should be offered separately: there should be no pressure on the client to book a service following the consultation. Excellent communication skills should be used at consultation to ensure your judgements on the needs of the client are correct.

The consultation

In the privacy of the facial treatment work area, carry out the consultation. This takes place when the client first meets the therapist and again whenever a new treatment is to be carried out.

The consultation is the time when the beauty therapist can assess whether the client is actually suited to treatment. The therapist must look for contra-indications, and must give no treatment if there are any – this is to safeguard the therapist, the client and, in the case of a client with a contagious skin disorder, other clients who would be at risk of cross-infection. Remember you are not qualified to diagnose a contra-indication. Refer the client to their GP without causing unnecessary cause for concern.

Ask the client specific questions about their present skincare routine and their general health. Listen carefully to their responses to guide you in your assessment.

> **Be empathetic**
>
> Being able to 'connect' with your client is invaluable as a therapist. Try to see the world through the other person's eyes, think about how they might feel and adapt your communication as necessary. For instance, if it is their first ever skin treatment, are they shy or embarrassed? How can you help them to feel more at ease?
>
> **Sally Penford**

The beauty therapist's knowledge of facial treatments and advice on skincare will instil confidence in the client. Explain what is involved with each service, how long it takes and the aftercare that is required. This will demonstrate your professional expertise.

The client is likely to ask which is the most suitable treatment for them, and you must advise them as to which would best meet their needs.

Make the client aware of the cost of the individual treatment – or treatment programme, if necessary – so that they can decide whether or not to undertake the financial commitment involved.

Invite the client to ask questions during the consultation. By the end, they should understand fully what the proposed treatment involves.

The client may receive the treatment immediately, following the consultation, or go away to consider the proposals.

During the consultation, details are noted on the client's record card. You can fill this in as you speak to them, without diverting your attention away from them.

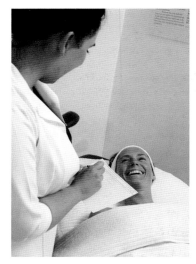

Confirming details following the consultation

ALWAYS REMEMBER

Treatment modification
Examples of facial treatment modification include:

- altering the pressure or choice of manipulations during massage to suit the client's skin and muscle tone
- altering the distance and application of steam heat to take into account skin sensitivity

ALWAYS REMEMBER

Never make assumptions about what the client can afford. Usually the client will indicate to you what they are prepared to spend.

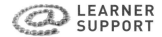

LEARNER SUPPORT

Facial skincare: match the statements

A sample client record card

Date		Beauty therapist	
Client name		Date of birth (identifying client age group.)	
Home address		Postcode	
Email address	Landline		Mobile phone number
Name of doctor	Doctor's address and phone number		

Related medical history (Conditions that may restrict or prohibit service application.)

Are you taking any medication? (This may affect the appearance of the skin or skin sensitivity.)

CONTRA-INDICATIONS REQUIRING MEDICAL REFERRAL
(Preventing facial service application.)

- ☐ bacterial infection (e.g. impetigo)
- ☐ viral infection (e.g. herpes simplex)
- ☐ fungal infection (e.g. tinea corporis)
- ☐ parasitic infection (e.g. pediculosis and scabies)
- ☐ eye infections (e.g. conjunctivitis)
- ☐ watery eyes
- ☐ systemic medical condition
- ☐ severe skin condition

SKIN GROUP

- ☐ oily
- ☐ young
- ☐ dry
- ☐ combination
- ☐ mature

FACIAL PRODUCTS

- ☐ cleanser
- ☐ mask – non-setting
- ☐ toner
- ☐ massage medium
- ☐ eye cleanser
- ☐ moisturiser
- ☐ exfoliant
- ☐ specialist skin services (e.g. eye cream)
- ☐ mask – setting
- ☐ facial service
- ☐ skincare instruction

MASSAGE MEDIUMS

- ☐ oil
- ☐ cream

CONTRA-INDICATIONS WHICH RESTRICT SERVICE
(Service may require adaptation.)

- ☐ cuts and abrasions
- ☐ bruising and swelling
- ☐ recent scar tissue
- ☐ eczema
- ☐ skin allergies
- ☐ vitiligo
- ☐ styes
- ☐ hyper keratosis
- ☐ watery eyes

SKIN CONDITION CHARACTERISTICS

- ☐ sensitive
- ☐ mature
- ☐ dehydrated
- ☐ milia
- ☐ broken capillaries
- ☐ comedones
- ☐ pustules
- ☐ papules
- ☐ open pores
- ☐ hyperpigmentation
- ☐ hypopigmentation
- ☐ dermatitis papulosa nigra
- ☐ keloids
- ☐ ingrowing hairs
- ☐ pseudo folliculitis
- ☐ hyperikeratosis

Following skin analysis identify on the illustration below skin condition characteristics found and in which numbered area they appear.

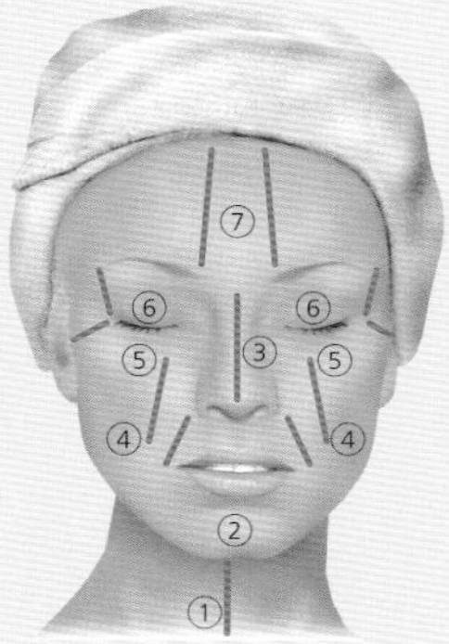

EQUIPMENT AND MATERIALS

- ☐ magnifying light
- ☐ skin warming devices
- ☐ consumables

MASSAGE TECHNIQUES

- ☐ effleurage
- ☐ petrissage
- ☐ tapotement

Beauty therapist signature (for reference)

Client signature (confirmation of details)

A sample client record card (continued)

SERVICE ADVICE

Full facial service – this service will take 60 minutes (1 hour).

SERVICE PLAN

Record relevant details of your service and advice provided for future reference.

Ensure the client's records are up-to-date, accurate and fully completed following service. Non-compliance may invalidate insurance.

DURING

Find out:

- what products the client is currently using to cleanse and care for the skin of the face and neck
- how regularly the products are used
- satisfaction with their current skincare routine

Explain:

- how the products used should be applied and removed

Note:

- any adverse reaction, if any occur

AFTER

Record:

- specific areas treated
- any modification to service application that has occurred
- what products have been used in the facial service
- the effectiveness of service
- any samples provided (review their success at the next appointment)

Advise on:

- product application and removal in order to gain maximum benefit from product use
- use of make-up following facial service
- recommended time intervals between services
- the importance of a course of service to improve the skin condition

RETAIL OPPORTUNITIES

Advise on:

- progression of the service plan for future appointments
- products that would be suitable for the client to use at home to care for their skin
- recommendations for further facial services
- further products or services that you have recommended that the client may or may not have received before

Note:

- any purchase made by the client

EVALUATION

Record:

- comments on the client's satisfaction with the service
- how you will progress the service to maintain and advance the service results in the future

HEALTH AND SAFETY

Advise on:

- avoidance of activities or product application that may cause a contra-action
- appropriate action necessary to be taken in the event of an unwanted skin reaction

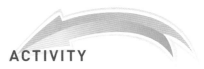

ACTIVITY

Recognizing contra-indications

Think of six skin disorders and six skin diseases. List them in a chart.

Briefly describe how you would recognize each skin condition. Why would it be inappropriate to treat each?

HEALTH & SAFETY

Herpes simplex (cold sore)
A small skin lesion due to herpes simplex may initially appear to be simply a pustule with a scab. At the consultation, always check whether the client knows if they suffer from any skin disease or disorder.

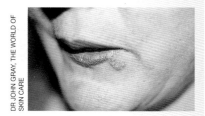

DR JOHN GRAY, THE WORLD OF SKIN CARE

Herpes simplex

> **Be attentive**
> When talking with your client give them your undivided attention. Even if you have only ten minutes to give. By being truly present when engaging in interpersonal communication, such as product sampling, you will add value and worth over and above your competitors.

Sally Penford

Contra-indications

The consultation and skin analysis will draw your attention to any contra-indications or aspects that require special care and attention.

Remember that not all contra-indications are visible. Refer to the checklist of contra-indications on the client's record card.

The following contra-indications are relevant to *all* facial services:

- **skin disorder**, such as acne vulgaris (unless medical approval has been sought and given)
- **skin disease**, such as impetigo
- **bruising** in the area
- **haemorrhage**, if recent – wait until the condition has healed
- **operation** in the area, if recent – wait for six months
- **fracture**, if recent – wait for six months
- **furuncle** (boil)
- **inflammation or swelling** of the skin
- **scar tissue,** if recent – wait for six months
- **sebaceous cyst**
- **eye disorder**, such as conjunctivitis

Certain contra-indications restrict service; that is, the service may have to be adapted or delayed until the contra-indication has gone. For example, if eczema is present but the skin is not broken, the service can proceed but the area should be avoided as much as possible.

If the client has an allergy to an ingredient in the cosmetic preparations used, service cannot proceed until an alternative, non-allergenic product suited to the client is obtained. If the client has a stye, service cannot proceed. However, when the eye disorder has gone service may be carried out.

These are referred to in Chapter 3, pages 91–104, where skin diseases and disorders are illustrated and discussed.

Following the consultation, the client's answers will indicate to the therapist what is required, and what is achievable, from a skincare programme.

When finalizing the most suitable service plan:

- explain what is involved in each service, how long it takes, and what aftercare and home care are required (if relevant)
- assess how much the client is willing to spend, and design a service programme within their budget

This allows the client to:

- discover what the beauty therapist can offer to meet their needs
- ask questions, and receive honest professional advice concerning the most appropriate choice of skincare service
- decide how much they are willing to spend

The beauty therapist should ensure that the client fully understands and is realistic about what the proposed service involves and what can be achieved.

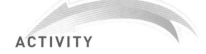

ACTIVITY

Answering questions

You should be able to answer honestly, competently and tactfully any questions related to the beauty services you offer. Below are examples of the questions you may be asked at consultation.

- 'I have always used soap and water upon my face. Is this a satisfactory way to cleanse my face?'
- 'Why do I need to use a separate night cream as well as a day moisturiser?'
- 'How often should I have a facial?'
- 'I have extremely oily skin. Why do I need to wear a moisturiser?'
- 'What can I do to treat these fine lines around my eyes?'

What answers would you give? Think of further questions you might be asked with regard to skincare. A senior beauty therapist will be able to advise you.

> ❝ **Be a receptive communicator**
>
> Employers often ask for a range of skills, however often two skills come from the opposite end of the spectrum. Which do you have your strength in? For example, communication in writing versus communicating face-to-face, or following rules versus thinking creatively. One skill will be your natural preference but by developing the opposite skill you will be more appealing to potential employers.
>
> **Sally Penford**

When the service plan has been agreed, prepare and position the client for service.

1. Position the client on the couch according to the service to be given. Ensure the client is comfortable and relaxed. Cover the client with the clean, large bath towel. If necessary, drape a small hand towel across her shoulders. Some salons offer a quilt cover to keep the client warm and relaxed.

2. If facial, neck and shoulder massage is to be given, ask the client politely to remove her arms from her bra straps in preparation: this avoids disturbance later.

3. Fasten a clean headband around the client's hairline. Position the headband so that it does not cover the skin of the face. If using an electronic vapour unit, cover the hair to stop it getting damp.

4. After preparing the client, wash your hands: this demonstrates to the client your concern to work hygienically.

The skin should than be cleansed prior to completing the skin analysis where you can correctly diagnose the skin type and condition.

Choice of products selected will be decided upon from the information you have gained so far.

All **facial products** and equipment should be used with due regard to health and safety following manufacturers' instructions.

BEST PRACTICE

Client care

Always give clear instructions to your client. This will help to ensure that they are not embarrassed or uncomfortable at any time.

Headbands

Check that the headband is comfortable. A tight headband will cause tension and eventually a headache.

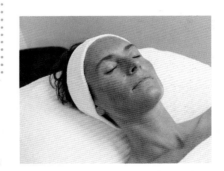

Client prepared and positioned for service

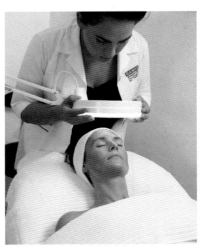

Skin analysis

Outcome 3: Improve and maintain facial skin condition

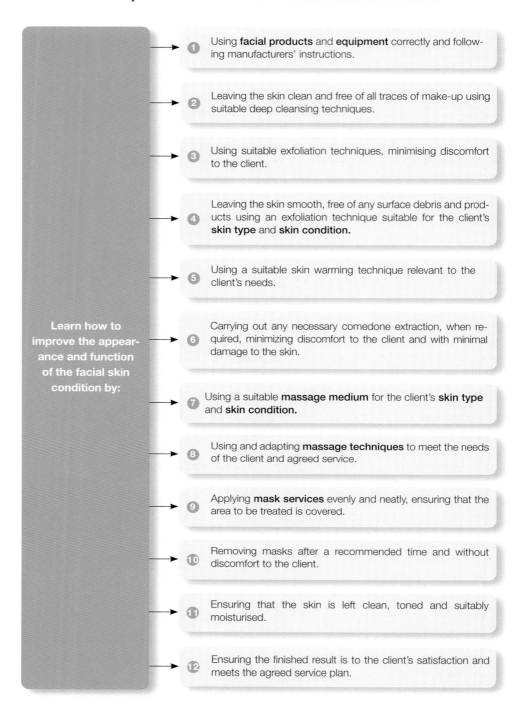

Learn how to improve the appearance and function of the facial skin condition by:

1. Using **facial products** and **equipment** correctly and following manufacturers' instructions.

2. Leaving the skin clean and free of all traces of make-up using suitable deep cleansing techniques.

3. Using suitable exfoliation techniques, minimising discomfort to the client.

4. Leaving the skin smooth, free of any surface debris and products using an exfoliation technique suitable for the client's **skin type** and **skin condition.**

5. Using a suitable skin warming technique relevant to the client's needs.

6. Carrying out any necessary comedone extraction, when required, minimizing discomfort to the client and with minimal damage to the skin.

7. Using a suitable **massage medium** for the client's **skin type** and **skin condition.**

8. Using and adapting **massage techniques** to meet the needs of the client and agreed service.

9. Applying **mask services** evenly and neatly, ensuring that the area to be treated is covered.

10. Removing masks after a recommended time and without discomfort to the client.

11. Ensuring that the skin is left clean, toned and suitably moisturised.

12. Ensuring the finished result is to the client's satisfaction and meets the agreed service plan.

Cleansing

Skin cleansing is essential in promoting and maintaining a healthy skin. There are various cleansing preparations to choose from; basically their action is the same in each case:

- to gently exfoliate dead skin cells from the stratum corneum, exposing younger cells and improving the skin's appearance

- to remove make-up, dirt and pollutants from the skin's surface, reducing the possibility of blemishes and skin irritation

ALWAYS REMEMBER

Seasonal changes

Seasonal changes affect the skin. You may need to alter the client's basic skincare routine through the year.

- to remove excess sweat and sebum from the skin's surface, reducing congestion of the skin and the subsequent formation of comedones and pustules

- to prepare the skin for further services

> ## Be positive
> Having a positive attitude will not only help you to continually improve yourself, it will also rub off on your fellow team members. Show your initiative with suggestions and ideas that make moves towards the goals of your skin centre. Don't be scared to get creative and think outside of the box with new ideas for treatments, promotions or events.
>
> **Sally Penford**

Cleansing preparations

A **cleanser** is required that will remove both oil-soluble and water-soluble substances without drying the skin. Oil is capable of dissolving grease; water will dissolve other substances. Usually, therefore, a cleanser is a combination of both oil and water.

Oil and water do not combine: if you simply mix the two together they separate again, with the oil floating on the top of the water. If the two substances are shaken together vigorously, however, one substance will break up and become suspended in the other. The result is known as an **emulsion**.

Emulsions are used in many cosmetic preparations. They are either:

- **oil-in-water** (O/W) – minute droplets of oil, surrounded by water

- **water-in-oil** (W/O) – minute droplets of water, surrounded by oil

To give the emulsion stability, and to stop it separating out again, an **emulsifier** is added.

Various cleansing preparations are available to the beauty therapist, with formulations designed to suit the different skin types. They include:

- cleansing milks

- cleansing creams

- cleansing balms

- cleansing lotions

- facial gel or foaming cleansers

- cleansing bars

- eye make-up removers

Whichever cleanser is chosen, it should have the following qualities:

- it should cleanse the skin effectively, without causing irritation

- it should remove all traces of make-up and grease

- it should feel pleasant to use

- it should be easy to remove from the skin

- ideally, it should be pH-balanced

HEALTH & SAFETY

Sensitive skin

When treating a sensitive skin, choose a cleansing product that does not contain common known allergens such as mineral oil, alcohol or lanolin. Such products are usually referred to as *hypoallergenic* or *dermatologically* tested.

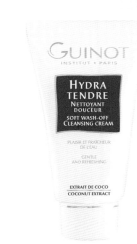

COURTESY OF GUINOT

Cleansing preparation cream

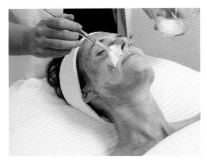

Facial foaming cleanser being applied

TUTOR SUPPORT

Activity 3: Facial products handout

ACTIVITY

Acidic or alkaline?

To discover whether a liquid product is acidic or alkaline, carry out a simple test using litmus paper. Litmus changes colour according to the pH:

- litmus paper turns *blue* if an *alkali* is present

- litmus paper turns *red* if an *acid* is present

Test the pH of various cleansing preparations.

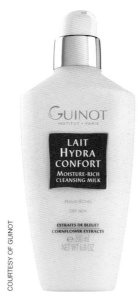

Cleansing milk

Be different

What makes you stand out from the crowd? As well as a good all-round basic knowledge, try to offer something that no other skin therapist in your area offers. There are plenty of postgraduate training facilities to help you progress, so step outside of the treatment room and learn something new!

Sally Penford

TOP TIP

Dry skin

If a client has very dry skin, advise them to avoid them use of tap water on the face – tap water contains salts and chlorine, which can dry the skin.

Male skin

Cleansing rinse-off formulations are very popular with male clients.

The use of a soft nylon bristle face brush is beneficial to use with a facial foaming cleanser or bar to prevent ingrowing hairs forming.

The pH scale
The **pH scale** is used to measure the **acidity** or **alkalinity** of a substance. Using a numbered scale of 1–14, acids have a pH less than 7; alkalis have a pH greater than 7. Substances with a pH of 7 are **neutral**.

The skin is naturally slightly acidic: it has an acid mantle. Alkalis strip the skin of its protective film of sebum, making it feel dry and taut. To avoid skin irritation it is preferable to use a product that matches the acid mantle, a product whose pH is 5.5–5.6.

Cleansing milks
Cleansing milks are usually oil-in-water emulsions, with a relatively high proportion of water to oil, making the milk quite fluid and light in its consistency.

Cleansing milks have these specific treatment uses:

- treating normal to dry skin that is prone to sensitivity
- treating sensitive skin

Cleansing creams
Cleansing creams have a relatively high proportion of oil to water, making the emulsion thicker and richer in its consistency than cleansing milks. The high oil content allows the product to be massaged over the skin surface without dragging the tissues. The cream is also more effective in removing grease and oil-based make-up from the skin.

Cleansing creams have these specific service uses:

- removing facial cosmetics
- treating by deep cleansing massage
- treating very dry skin

Cleansing balms
Cleansing balms are usually light weight cleansers which quickly transform from a solid balm to a fluid. They moisturise and improve the texture of the skin while cleansing.

Cleansing balms have these specific service uses:

- moisturising, non-drying effect
- improvement of skin texture
- suitable for all skin types except oily

Cleansing lotions
Cleansing lotions are solutions of detergents in water. They do not usually contain oil, and are therefore unsuitable for the removal of facial cosmetics.

Cleansing lotions have these specific service uses:

- cleansing a normal to combination skin type
- treating oily skin (where a high oil content could aggravate the skin, causing yet further sebum production)

Medicated ingredients may be included in a cleansing formulation: these are only suitable for oily, congested, pustular skin types.

If the client has a mature, normal or combination skin, a cleansing lotion may not be effective because of the reduced oil content. A mature skin benefits from oil content to compensate for reduced sebum production.

Facial gel or foaming cleansers **Facial gel or foaming cleansers** usually contain a mild detergent which foams when mixed with water. Additional ingredients are selected for the treatment of different skin types. These cleansers are quick to use and afford a suitable alternative for the client who likes to cleanse their face with soap and water. If the client wears an oil-based make-up, advise them to use a cleansing cream first to remove make-up thoroughly before using this cleanser.

Facial foaming cleansers have a general application:

- treating most skin types except very dry or sensitive skin

- particularly suitable for oily and combination skin due to their formulation which effectively removes sebum without drying the skin

Cleansing bars Although it is efficient as a cleanser, **soap** is usually considered unsuitable for use on the skin. It has an alkaline pH, which disturbs the skin's natural acidic pH balance. Soap strips the skin of its protective acid mantle, leaving insoluble salts on the skin's surface. The skin may be left feeling itchy, taut and sensitive.

Cleansing bars are a milder alternative to soap, and are specially formulated to match the skin's acidic pH of 5.5–5.6. They are less likely to dry out the skin.

Cleansing bars have this specific application:

- treating oily to normal skin that is not sensitive

Eye make-up remover Eye tissue is a lot finer than the skin on the rest of the face. It readily puffs if aggravated by oil-based cleansing preparations, and becomes very dry if harsh cleansing preparations are used.

To remove make-up from this area, use an **eye make-up remover.** This product cleanses the eyelid and lashes, gently emulsifying the make-up. It also conditions the delicate skin. Formulated as a lotion or a gel, it is designed to remove either water-based or oil-based products (or both) from the eye area.

Oily eye make-up removers have these specific service uses:

- treating clients who wear waterproof mascara

- removing wax or oil-based eye shadow

Non-oily eye make-up removers have these applications:

- treating clients with sensitive skin around the eyes

- treating clients who wear contact lenses

- treating clients who wear individual false eyelashes

Cleansing service

There are two manual processes involved in the cleansing routine: *the superficial cleanse* and the *deep cleanse*.

The superficial cleanse uses lightweight cleansing preparations to emulsify surface make-up, dirt and grease. This is followed by the more thorough deep cleanse, in which a heavier cleansing cream is applied to the face. The high percentage of oil contained in the cream formulation allows the cream to be massaged over the skin's surface without evaporation of the product.

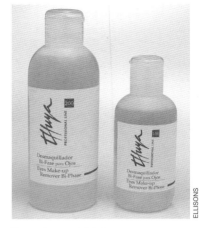

ELLISONS

Eye make-up remover

TOP TIP

Eye treatments

Many eye make-up removers are also eye treatments. If your workplace uses a commercial product in this way apply it to the dampened eye pads used during mask treatment. This may also assist your retail sales, as the client may wish to buy some for home use.

HEALTH & SAFETY

Eye care

Never apply pressure over the eyeball when cleansing the eye area.

The ring finger is always used in the eye area when applying products as it provides the least pressure.

HEALTH & SAFETY

Hygiene

Never use the reverse side of the cotton wool pad – this is unhygienic.

Never use the same piece of cotton wool to cleanse both eyes, use a separate piece for each eye to avoid cross-infection.

ALWAYS REMEMBER

Unlike the muscles of the body, which attach to bones, most of the facial muscles are attached to the facial skin itself. You should therefore avoid stretching the skin unnecessarily – if you do, you may also stretch the facial muscles and contribute to premature ageing.

Step-by-step: Superficial cleansing

Each part of the face requires a special technique in the application and removal of the cleansing product. The face is cleansed in the following order:

- the eye tissue and lashes
- the lips
- the neck, chin, cheeks and forehead

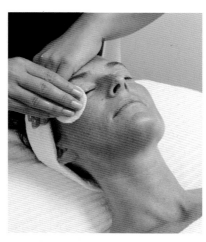

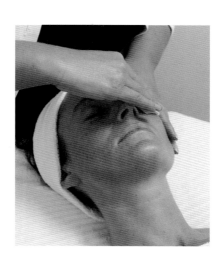

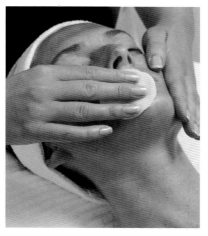

1 Wash your hands.

   Ensure that contact lenses are removed if worn.

2 Cleanse the eye area, using a suitable eye make-up remover. Each eye is cleansed separately. Your non-working hand lifts and supports the eye tissue while the working hand applies the eye make-up remover.

   If a water-based eye make-up remover is used, this is applied directly to a clean piece of cotton wool. Stroke down the length of the eyelashes, from base to points. Next, cleanse the eye tissue in a sweeping circle, outwards across the upper eyelid, circling beneath the lower lashes towards the nose. Repeat, regularly changing the cotton wool until the eye area and the cotton wool show clean.

   Sometimes a cleansing milk is used to remove eye make-up. In this case, apply a little of the product to the back of one hand. The ring finger is then used to apply the cleansing milk to the lashes.

   Use damp cotton wool to remove the emulsified product.

   Repeat the cleansing process until the eye area is clean.

3 Cleanse the lips, preferably with a cleansing milk or lotion (as this readily emulsifies the oils or waxes contained in lipstick if worn).

   Apply a little of the product to the back of your non-working hand. Support the left side of the client's mouth with this hand. With the working hand, apply the product in small circular movements across the upper lip, from left to right; and then across the lower lip, from right to left.

   Remove the cleanser from the lips. Support the corner of the mouth; using a clean damp piece of cotton wool wipe across the lips.

   Repeat the cleansing process as necessary, until the lips and the cotton wool show clean.

4   Select a cleansing product to suit your client's skin type.

Place the product into one hand – sufficient to cover the face and neck, and to massage gently over the surface of the skin. Massage the surface of the hands together when using a milk, cream or balm: this warms the product (so that it isn't cold on the client's skin) and distributes it over your hands.

Clasp the fingers together at the base of the neck, and unlink them as you move up the neck.

Clasp the fingers together again at the chin, drawing the fingers outwards to the angle of the jawbone.

Stroke up the face, towards the forehead, with your fingertips pointing downwards and your palms in contact with the skin.

Using a series of light circular movements with your fingertips, gently massage the product into the skin, beginning at the base of the neck and finishing at the forehead.

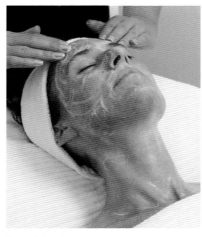

Superficial cleanse

HEALTH & SAFETY

Safe pressure
Reduce pressure when working over the *hyoid bone* at the throat and bony prominences such as the *zygomatic bone* (the cheekbone) and the *frontal bone* (the forehead).

Pressure must always be *upwards* and *outwards*, to avoid stretching the tissues.

HEALTH & SAFETY

Client comfort
When cleansing around the nose, avoid restricting the client's nostrils.

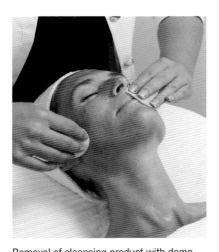

Removal of cleansing product with damp cotton wool

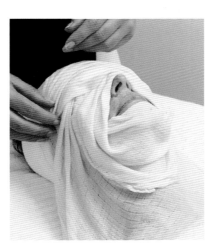

Removal of products with hot towels

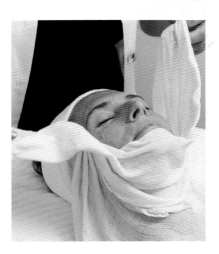

5   Remove the cleanser thoroughly with clean damp cotton wool, facial sponges, facial mitts or hot towels, simultaneously stroking over the skin surface, upwards and outwards. Repeat this process as necessary, using clean cotton wool, if used. each time. Facial sponges and mitts will require regular rinsing with clean, warm water. The facial towel is unwrapped and its surface stroked over the skin to remove facial cleanser.

TOP TIP

If there is any make-up left at the base of the lower lashes after eye cleansing, this may be removed with a cotton bud or a thin piece of damp, clean cotton wool. Ask the client to look upwards, support the eye tissue with the other hand and gently draw the cotton wool along the base of the lower lashes, towards the nose.

If the client is wearing facial make-up, it is usual to perform the superficial cleanse twice to ensure all cosmetics are effectively removed.

HEALTH & SAFETY

When cleansing, be careful that cleanser does not enter the eyes or mouth.

Step-by-step: Deep cleansing

The deep cleanse involves a series of massage manipulations which reinforce the cleansing achieved with the cleansing product. Blood circulation is increased to the area; this has a warming effect on the skin, which relaxes the skin's natural openings, the hair follicles and pores. This aids the absorption of cleanser into the hair follicles and pores, where it can dissolve make-up if worn, sebum and skin debris.

There are various deep-cleansing sequences; all are acceptable if carried out in a safe, hygienic manner, and all can achieve the desired outcomes. Here is one sequence for deep cleansing.

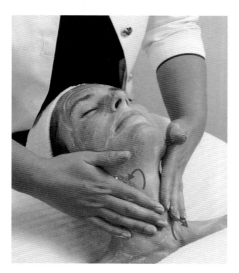
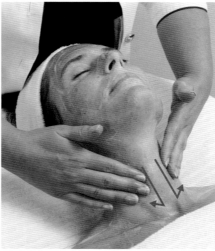
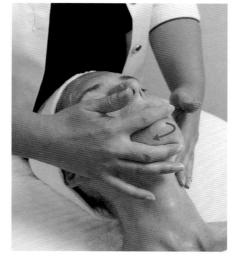

1 Select a cleansing medium to suit your client's skin type. The procedure for application is the same as that for the superficial cleanse.

2 Stroke up either side of the neck, using your fingertips. At the chin, draw the fingers outwards to the angle of the jaw, and lightly stroke back down the neck to the starting position.

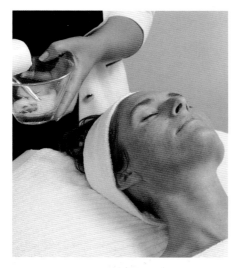
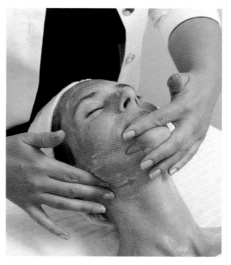

3 Apply small circular manipulations over the skin of the neck.

4 Draw the fingertips outwards to the angle of the jaw. Rest each index finger against the jawbone (you will be able to feel the lower teeth in the jaw). Place the middle finger beneath the jawbone. Move the right hand towards the chin where the index finger glides over the chin; return the fingers beneath the jawbone, to the starting position. Repeat with the left hand.
Repeat step 4 a further 5 times.

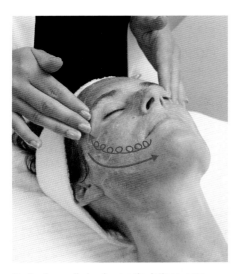

5 Apply small circular manipulations, commencing at the chin working up towards the nose, and finishing at the temples. Slide the fingers from the temples back to the chin.

*Repeat step **5** a further 5 times.*

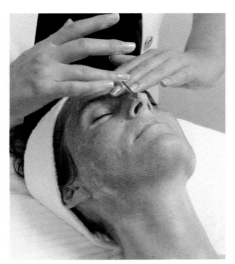

6 Position the ring finger of the right hand at the bridge of the nose. Perform a running movement, sliding the ring, middle and index fingers off the end of the nose. Repeat immediately with the left hand.

*Repeat step **6** a further 5 times with each hand.*

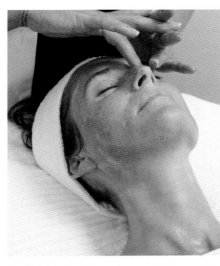

7 With the ring fingers, trace a circle around the eye orbits. Begin at the inner corner of the upper brow bone; slide to the outer corners of the brow bone, around and under the eyes, and return to the starting position.

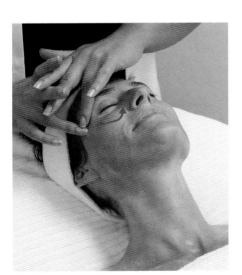

*Repeat step **7** a further 5 times.*

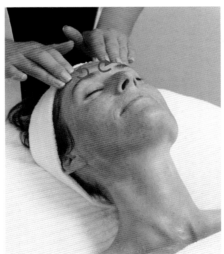

8 Using both hands, apply small circular manipulations across the forehead. *Repeat step **8** a further 5 times.*

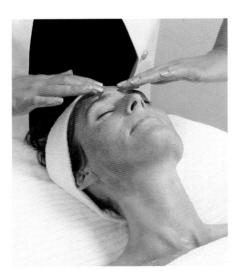

9 Open the index and middle fingers of each hand and perform a cross-cross stroking movement over the forehead.

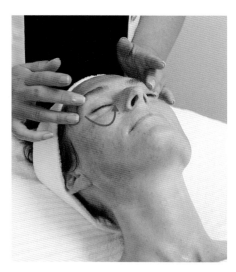

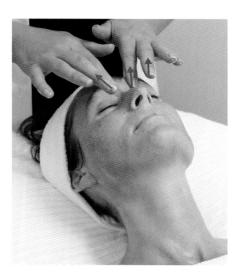

10 Slide the index finger upwards slightly, lifting the inner eyebrow. Lift the centre of the eyebrow with the middle finger. Finally, lift the outer corner of the eyebrow with the ring finger. Slide the ring fingers around the outer corner and beneath the eye orbit. *Repeat step **10** a further 5 times.*

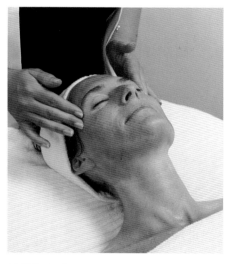

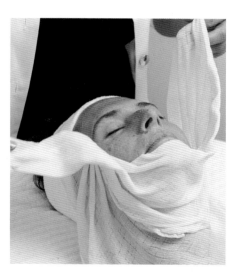

TOP TIP

Check that the brow hair and the skin beneath the chin are free of grease: it is easy to overlook some cleansing product in these areas.

11 With the finger pads of each hand, apply slight pressure at the temples. This indicates to the client that the cleansing sequence is complete.

12 Remove the cleansing cream from the skin, using damp cotton wool, facial sponges, facial mitts or towels.

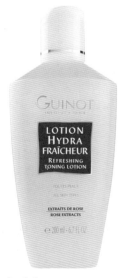

COURTESY OF GUINOT

Toning lotion

Toning

After the skin has been cleansed it is then toned with an appropriate lotion.

Toning preparations

Toning lotions remove from the skin all traces of cleanser, grease and skincare preparations. The toning lotion's main action is as follows:

● It produces a cooling effect on the skin when the water or alcohol in the toner evaporates from the skin's surface. (When a liquid evaporates it changes to a gas, which takes energy. In the case of toner, the energy is taken from the skin, which therefore feels cooler.)

● It creates a tightening effect on the skin, because of a chemical within the toner called an astringent. This causes the pores to close, thereby reducing the flow of sebum and sweat onto the skin's surface.

● It helps to restore the acidic pH balance of the skin. Milder skin toners have a pH 4.5–4.6; stronger astringents disturb the pH more severely, and may cause skin irritation and sensitivity.

There are three main types of toning lotions, the main difference being the amounts of alcohol they contain. They include:

● bracers and fresheners

● tonics

● astringents

Skin bracers and fresheners

Skin bracers and **skin fresheners** are the mildest toning lotions: they contain little or no alcohol. They consist mainly of purified water, with floral extracts such as **rose water** for a mild toning effect.

Skin bracers and fresheners are recommended for:

● dry, delicate skin

● sensitive skin

● mature skin

Skin tonics

Skin tonics are slightly stronger toning lotions. Many contain a little of some astringent agent such as orange flower water.

Skin toners are recommended for:

● normal skin

Astringents

Astringents are the strongest toning lotions; they have a high proportion of alcohol which can be very drying. They may contain antiseptic ingredients such as witch hazel or tea tree oil; these are for use on blemished skin, to reduce the growth of bacteria and promote skin healing. Strong astringents can cause the skin to become dry and irritated if there is any skin sensitivity – so care must be taken.

Astringents are recommended for:

● oily skin with no skin sensitivity

● mild acne in young skin

Toning lotions which are suitable for oily skin are becoming increasingly available and rely upon their botanical formulations to control sebum flow and promote skin healing.

Application

Toning lotion may be applied in several ways. Whichever method you choose, it should leave the skin thoroughly clean and free of grease.

The most popular method of application is to apply the toner directly to two pieces of clean damp cotton wool, which are wiped gently upwards and outwards over the neck and face.

TOP TIP

Toning lotions
All toning lotions have some astringent effect on the skin, but those that contain a relatively high alcohol content are actually marketed as astringents.

Do not use toning lotions that contain more than 20 per cent alcohol on dry skin – they may cause skin irritation.

Avoid the excessive use of astringent on oily skin – the astringent will make the skin dry, and it will then produce more sebum.

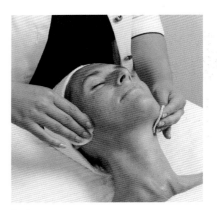

Toning

TOP TIP

Combination skin
When applying toning lotion to a combination skin, you may need to apply different toning lotions to treat separate skin conditions.

For home use, advise the client to apply toning lotion using dampened cotton wool: this is more economical.

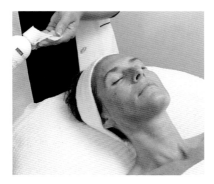

Application of toning lotion

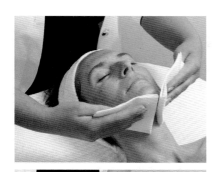

Blotting the skin

Alternatively, the toner may be applied under pressure as a fine spray, using a vaporizer. This produces a fine mist of the toning lotion over the skin. If using this method, always protect the eye tissue with cotton wool pads and hold the vaporizer about 30cm from the skin, directing the spray across the skin in a sweeping movement. This is preferable when treating a male client, where the cotton wool application technique would be unsuitable.

To produce a stimulating effect, the toning lotion can be applied to dampened cotton wool: hold this firmly at one corner, and gently tap it over the skin.

Blotting the skin

After applying toning lotion, immediately blot the skin dry with a soft facial tissue to prevent the toner evaporating from the skin's surface (which would stimulate the skin). Alternatively you can make a small tear in the centre of a large facial tissue for the client's nose. Place the tissue over their face and neck, and mould it into position to absorb excess moisture. Alternatively, blot over the face with large facial tissues as shown.

When skin is thoroughly cleansed and toned a thorough skin analysis can occur using a magnifying lamp. If the client is sensitive to light protect the client's eyes with damp cotton wool pads. The skin's surface will be magnified enabling you to comment further and note any characteristics of skin type and skin conditions requiring attention. Record these on a record card.

Moisturising

The skin depends on water to keep it soft, supple and resilient. Two thirds of our body is composed of water and the skin is an important reservoir, containing about 20 per cent of the body's total water content. Most of the fluid is in the lower layers of the dermis, but it circulates to the top layer of the epidermis, where it evaporates.

The skin protects its water content in these ways:

- sebum keeps the skin lubricated, and reduces water loss from skin
- the skin cells have **natural moisturising factors** (**NMFs**), a complex mix of substances which are able to fix moisture inside the cells
- a cement of fats (lipids) between the skin cells forms a watertight barrier

The natural moisture level is constantly being disturbed. The application of a cosmetic **moisturiser** helps to maintain the natural oil and moisture balance by locking moisture into the tissues, offering protection and hydration.

The basic formulation of a moisturiser is oil and water to make an oil-in-water emulsion. The water content helps to return lost moisture to the surface layers; the oil content prevents moisture loss from the surface of the skin. Often a **humectant**, such as **glycerine** or **sorbitol**, is included: this attracts moisture to the skin from the surrounding air and stops the moisturiser from drying out. If a humectant is included, less oil is used in the formulation: this results in a lighter cream.

Moisturiser also has the following benefits:

- it protects the skin from external damage caused by the environment
- it softens the skin and relieves skin tautness and sensitivity

- it plumps the skin tissue with moisture, which minimizes the appearance of fine lines
- it provides a barrier between the skin and make-up cosmetics
- it may contain additional ingredients which improve the condition of the skin (such as vitamin E, which has a humectant action and is an excellent skin conditioner)
- it may contain ultra-violet filters, which protect the skin against the age-accelerating sunlight

Moisturisers are available for wear during the day or the night. These are available in different formulations, to treat all skin types and conditions.

Moisturisers are applied at the final stage of the facial when the skin is clean and toned, providing a protective barrier.

ALWAYS REMEMBER

Oily skin

Even oily skin requires a moisturiser. This skin can become dehydrated by the over-use of harsh cleansers and astringents.

HEALTH & SAFETY

UV light

Even on an overcast day, as much as 80 per cent of the sun's age-accelerating UVA can penetrate the skin.

TOP TIP

Tinted moisturisers

If your client likes a natural look for the day, they may wish to wear a moisturiser that is tinted; this gives the skin a healthy appearance.

Antioxidant moisturisers

Antioxidant moisturisers protect against free-radical damage from UV exposure, cigarette smoke, pollution and stress.

Moisturisers for daytime use

Moisturising lotions Moisturising lotions contain up to 85–90 per cent water and 10–15 per cent oil. They have a light, liquid formulation, and are ideal for use under make-up.

Moisturising lotions have these specific applications:

- oily skin
- young combination skin
- dehydrated skin
- normal skin

TOP TIP

Moisturising creams

Some clients dislike heavier cream, feeling that it is too heavy for their skin. Offer them a suitable moisturising lotion alternative.

Moisturising creams Moisturising creams contain up to 70–85 per cent water and 15–30 per cent oil. They have a thicker consistency, and cannot be poured.

Moisturising creams have these specific applications:

- mature skin
- dry skin

HEALTH & SAFETY

Allergies

Hypoallergenic moisturisers are available for clients with sensitive skin. These are screened from all common sensitizing ingredients, such as lanolin and perfume, and they also have soothing properties.

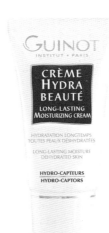

Moisturising lotion

Step-by-step: How to apply moisturiser

Moisturiser is applied after the final application of toning lotion. If the moisturiser is being applied before make-up, use a light formulation so that it does not interfere with the adherence of the foundation.

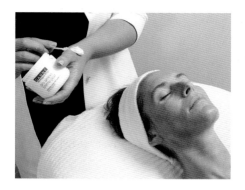

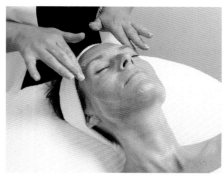

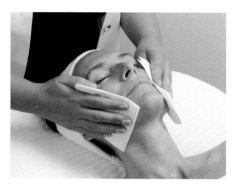

1. Remove some moisturiser from the jar, using a disposable spatula or disinfected plastic spatula. Place it on the back of the non-working hand, then take it on the fingertips of your working hand.

2. Apply the moisturiser in small dots to the neck, chin, cheeks, nose and forehead. Quickly and evenly spread it in a fine film over the face, using light upward and outward stroking movements.

3. Blot excess moisturiser from the skin using a facial tissue.

BEST PRACTICE

If the moisturiser is very fluid, apply it directly to the fingertips of the non-working hand – it would run if applied to the back of the hand.

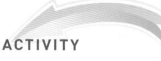

ACTIVITY

Moisturisers
Collect information on different moisturisers from various skin-care suppliers. You could visit local beauty salons, retail stores or beauty wholesale suppliers, or write to professional skincare companies.

BEST PRACTICE

Weight loss
Advise the client against losing weight quickly, especially when older – the neck tissue can look loose and very wrinkled as the underlying fat is lost.

Moisturisers for night-time use

Moisturisers are applied to the skin in the evening, after the skin has been cleansed, toned and blotted dry.

An emulsion **night cream** with a higher proportion of oil is the most effective for application in the evening: by this time the surrounding air is dry and warm, which encourages water loss from the skin; the oil seals the surface of the skin, preventing this water loss.

A small amount of **wax** (such as beeswax) may be included in the formulation: this improves the *slip* of the product, making it easier to apply and helping its skin-conditioning effect.

Specialist skin service products

In addition to basic skincare products, specialist skincare treatment products are available to target improvement for specific facial areas.

Throat creams The neck can become dry as it is exposed to the weather, often without the protection of a moisturiser. As a client ages, the collagen molecules in the dermis become increasingly cross-linked; they are then unable to retain the same volume of water, and the skin loses its plump appearance.

The formulation for a **throat cream** is similar to that for a night cream; it also contains various skin conditioning supplements, such as collagen or vitamin E, which help maintain moisture in the stratum corneum.

Encourage your client to include the neck in their cleansing routine, applying facial moisturiser to the neck during the day and either a night cream or specially formulated throat cream in the evening. Recommend that they always apply the throat cream gently in an upward and outward direction, using their fingertips.

To improve the appearance of the neck, good posture is important. If the client is round-shouldered the head often drops forwards, putting strain on the muscles of the neck. This causes tension in the muscles, which become tight and painful. Correct the client's posture, and advise them to massage the neck when applying the throat cream to relieve tension.

Eye creams The eye tissue is very thin and readily becomes very dry, emphasizing fine lines and wrinkles (**crow's feet**). Special care must be taken when applying products near this area: it contains a large number of **mast cells**, the cells that respond to contact with an irritant by causing an allergic reaction.

Eye cream is a fine cream formulated specifically for application to the eye area. A small quantity of the product is applied to the eye tissue using the ring finger of one hand, gently stroking around the eye, inwards and towards the nose. Support the eye tissue with the other hand. Do not apply the product too near to the inner eyelid or you will cause irritation to the eye.

Eye gel **Eye gel** is usually applied in the morning: it has a cooling, soothing, slightly astringent effect. (This is caused partly by the evaporation of the water in the gel, and partly by the inclusion of plant extracts such as **cornflower** or **camomile**.)

Eye gel is recommended for all clients, but especially for those suffering with slightly puffy eye tissue. It may also be applied following a facial service, to normalize the pH of the skin.

Eye gel may be applied with a light tapping motion, using the pads of the fingers. This will mildly stimulate the lymphatic circulation in the area and help to reduce any slight swelling.

Ampoule service **Serums** are chemicals used to revitalize the skin. They are supplied in **ampoules**, sealed glass or plastic phials which prevent the content from evaporating and losing their effectiveness. Serums are usually applied for 7–28 days as a skin tonic course for the service of different skin types and conditions.

Blemished skincare preparations Professional products are available for the client to apply specifically to blemishes such as pustules and papules. Benzoyl peroxide is an example of a product ingredient that dries and promotes healing of skin blemishes. The skincare aims to purify the skin while keeping it hydrated.

After cleansing the skin thoroughly the skin is exfoliated.

Exfoliation

The natural physical process of losing dead skin cells from the stratum corneum layer of the epidermis is called **desquamation**. **Exfoliation** is a salon technique used to accelerate this process. It is normally carried out after the skin has been cleansed and toned, and before further facial services.

Exfoliation has the following benefits:

- dead skin cells, grease and debris are removed from the surface of the skin
- fresh new cells are exposed, improving the appearance of the skin
- skin preparations such as moisturising lotions are more easily absorbed

TOP TIP

Specialist eye and lip products
Products designed to firm the skin around the eyes resulting in visible lines is becoming popular to treat the lip area also. The result aims to smooth and firm the lip line reducing the appearance of visible lines caused by lifestyle factors such as smoking and stress.

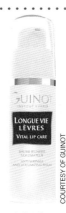

COURTESY OF GUINOT

Specialist lip product

ACTIVITY

Eye conditions
Think of different *non-medical eye* conditions for which a client might seek your advice. Discuss with colleagues the possible cause of these conditions, and what you could recommend to improve the appearance in each case.

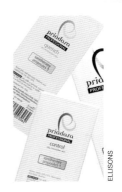

ELLISONS

Ampoule products

ACTIVITY

Exfoliants

Apply an exfoliant to the back of your own – or a colleague's – hand or arm. Compare the appearance and the feeling of the skin before and after application.

This technique produces a particularly marked effect on black skin, as it reduces the greyish appearance of the skin. (This is due to the skin having a thicker stratum corneum.)

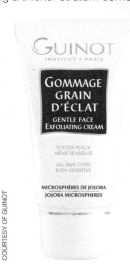

COURTESY OF GUINOT

Exfoliator product

TOP TIP

Steaming

Steaming before exfoliation softens the outer skin cells, making them easier to remove. This is particularly beneficial when treating a male client.

HEALTH & SAFETY

Exfoliants

Avoid exfoliating products that contain sharp grains of nut shells: these can scrape, split and damage the epidermis. Before purchasing, test the exfoliating product on the back of your own hand to feel its action.

- the blood circulation in the area is mildly stimulated, bringing more oxygen and nutrients to the skin cells and improving the skin colour
- hyperpigmentation is improved in appearance by the removal of the pigmented surface skin cells

TOP TIP

Male skin

A man who shaves, exfoliates every day, as shaving removes the top layer of skin. You can recommend that he also uses a cosmetic exfoliating product on areas such as the nose and forehead. If a male client suffers from pseudo folliculitis, recommend an electric shave rather than a wet shave, which tends to make this disorder worse.

Contra-indications

Exfoliation is beneficial for most skin types; however, avoid application if the client has the following:

- highly sensitive skin
- a vascular skin disorder such as telangiectases or damaged broken veins in the area of service application
- pustular, blemished skin

Exfoliants Various exfoliants are available; they may be of chemical or vegetable origin. Alternatively, mechanical exfoliation may be used.

Biochemical skin peel **Natural acids** (alpha-hydroxy acids – AHAs), derived from fruits, sugar cane and milk, are applied to the skin as a face mask. The natural acids dissolve dead surface cells and stimulate circulation in the underlying skin. These masks are available to suit all skin types.

AHAs may be combined with enzymes derived from fruits such as papaya (papain) to help remove surface dead skin to achieve maximum effect.

When you apply this type of face mask, warn the client that there will be a stinging sensation and then a tightening effect as the mask sets.

Pore grains **Pore grains** are the most popular exfoliants: a base of cream or liquid containing tiny spheres of polished plastic or crushed nuts is gently massaged over the skin's surface.

Clay exfoliants Gentler **clay exfoliants** have a clay base which is applied like a face mask. As it dries, the clay absorbs dead skin cells and sebum. The mask is then gently stroked away, using the pads of the fingers. A mask style exfoliant is more suitable for a blemished skin accompanying an oily skin type.

Mechanical exfoliation **Mechanical exfoliation**, or 'facial brushing', softens and cleanses the skin. Dead skin cells and excess sebum are removed as the soft hair bristles rotate over the skin's surface. The rotary action also increases the cleansing action of exfoliation.

If steam is applied before mechanical exfoliation, this will soften the dead skin cells, and **skin peeling cream** may be applied: together these will maximize the result of exfoliation.

Be careful to avoid over-stimulation, and over-exfoliation resulting in sensitizing the skin's surface, or disturbing the skin's natural protective qualities. Permanent sensitization could result from incorrect exfoliation techniques or over-exfoliation.

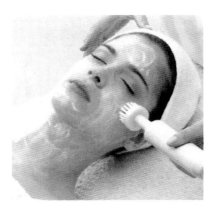
Mechanical exfoliation

TOP TIP

Exfoliation

Exfoliation should be strongly recommended for the mature client. The removal of the surface dead cells has a rejuvenating effect on the skin's appearance.

Teenagers regenerate external skin cells every 14 days. This increases to 30–40 days as a client reaches their forties.

Step-by-step: Exfoliation service

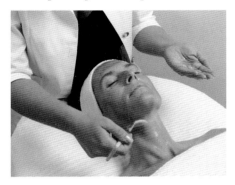

Exfoliant lotion is applied to a dry, sensitive skin type.

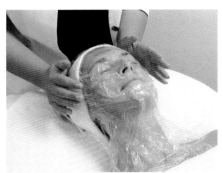

Plastic film is placed over the exfoliant to speed up the action of the exfoliant lotion.

1 Facial cream exfoliant is applied manually to the skin following cleansing and steaming to warm and soften the skin. The exfoliant containing hydroxy acids is applied, which removes dead skin cells and stimulates skin renewal. Warn the client a mild stinging sensation may be experienced, but will disappear quickly upon removal.

2 A soft facial brush may be used in a rotary action to further enhance the effectiveness of the exfoliant to remove areas of dead skin and sebum. A client may purchase the brush to use as part of their home care programme.

ALWAYS REMEMBER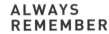

Body exfoliants

Point out to clients that exfoliants designed for use on the *body* are unsuitable for use on the *face* – their action is not as gentle.

Advice on home use

The client can be advised to use exfoliants at home as a specialized cleansing service after normal cleansing and toning. Exfoliants should be applied once a week for all skin types except oily, for which it may be applied twice a week.

Advise the client to massage the product gently over the skin using their fingertips. Application should always be upwards and outwards. The application and removal technique will differ according to the exfoliant product type.

After application, any product residue should be thoroughly rinsed from the face using clean, tepid water. The client may then apply a face mask or tone the skin and apply a nourishing skin moisturiser.

A UV sun block should be used to protect the skin to avoid skin damage.

TOP TIP

Retail opportunity

To encourage sales of this skin-care product, demonstrate the product on the back of one of the client's hands. They will be amazed when they compare the appearance of their hands.

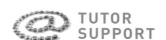

TUTOR SUPPORT

Activity 5: Comparing exfoliant treatments task

Following the exfoliation technique applied to suit your client's skin type a suitable skin warming technique is used relevant to the client's needs.

HEALTH & SAFETY

Exfoliants

- Tell the client how the skin should look after exfoliation service. The skin's colour should be *slightly* heightened; but too vigorous a massage application may cause the formation of broken capillaries.
- Tell the client to avoid contact with the delicate eye tissue.
- A client with a pustular skin should not use exfoliant products – they would probably cause discomfort, and any lesions present might burst.

Warming the skin

A **steam service** is the ideal means of producing the required warming effect on the skin to achieve both cleansing and stimulation. Skin warming is often incorporated into a facial service after the manual cleansing, so as to stimulate the skin and make it more receptive to subsequent services.

The effects are these:

- the pores are opened
- locally the blood circulation and the lymphatic circulation are stimulated
- the surface cells of the epidermis are softened, which helps desquamation
- sebaceous gland activity is improved, which benefits a dry mature skin type
- skin colour is improved

Steam is provided by an electric **vapour unit**. In this, distilled water is heated electrically until it boils to create steam.

The resulting steam is applied as a fine mist over the facial area. As the steam settles upon the skin it is absorbed by the surface epidermal cells. These cells are softened and can be gently loosened with an exfoliation service.

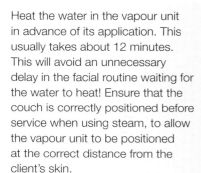

BEST PRACTICE

Heat the water in the vapour unit in advance of its application. This usually takes about 12 minutes. This will avoid an unnecessary delay in the facial routine waiting for the water to heat! Ensure that the couch is correctly positioned before service when using steam, to allow the vapour unit to be positioned at the correct distance from the client's skin.

HEALTH & SAFETY

Vapour application
Keep the vapour directed away from the client's face until a visible jet of steam can be seen. To avoid skin sensitization, consider carefully where to position the steam so as to ensure even heat distribution.

HEALTH & SAFETY

Safe use and care of the vapour unit

- Always follow manufacturer's instructions on correct usage. Have the unit tested annually by a qualified electrician to ensure its safety in compliance with the Electricity at Work Regulations (1989).
- Always use distilled water to avoid lime scale build-up in the heating element.
- Never fill the water vessel past the recommended level or 'spitting' could occur, where hot droplets of water are ejected and could burn the client's skin.
- Never use the equipment if the water vessel is below the recommended level or the heating element could be damaged. Most units have a cut-out feature so that the machine switches off if this occurs.
- Never leave the lead trailing across an area where somebody could trip and fall.

Contra-indications Although the service is suitable for most clients, do not use steam if you discover that the client has any of the following:

- **Respiratory problems**, such as asthma or a cold.

- **Vascular skin disorders** – these would be aggravated by the heating action and increased blood circulation.

- **Claustrophobia** – fear of enclosure or confined space.

- **Excessively dilated capillaries**.

- **Skin with reduced sensitivity**.

- **Diabetes**, unless the client's GP has given permission.

- **Rosacea –** a vascular skin disorder, where excess sebum production combined with a chronic inflammatory condition is caused by dilation of the blood capillaries. The skin becomes coarse, the pores enlarge, and the cheek and nose become inflamed.

- **Dilated capillaries**, where capillaries near the surface of the skin are permanently dilated.

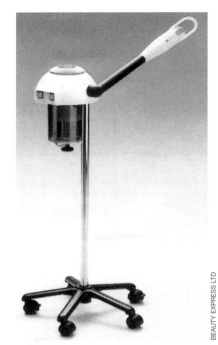

BEAUTY EXPRESS LTD

A vapour unit

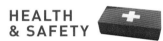

HEALTH & SAFETY

Steam application

Oily skin will tolerate a shorter application distance and a longer application time. For sensitive skin, increase the application distance and reduce the time. What are the manufacturer's guidelines for your equipment? Remember that these are only *guidelines* – observe the skin's reaction and check that the client is comfortable.

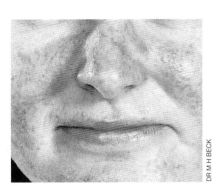

DR M H BECK

Rosacea

Explain to the client:

- how long the service is to be applied for

- the sensations that will be experienced

- the physical effect on the skin

The duration of the application and the distance differ according to the skin type.

The client should be positioned in a semi-reclined position for facial application.

Before applying steam, protect the client's eyes with damp cotton wool. Areas of delicate skin should be protected with damp cotton wool and if necessary a barrier cream.

The distance between the vapour outlet and the client's skin to be treated should be approximately 30–35cm. The application time will depend on the service effect and the type of skin that is being treated. Generally allow:

- 10 minutes for the face

- 15 minutes for the body

Ensure that an even flow of steam covers all the area being treated; reposition as necessary.

If you are using ozone, this is applied following the steam application for the final few minutes, as directed by the manufacturer. The steam will change in appearance to a bluish-white cloud.

After applying steam vapour, blot the skin dry with a soft facial tissue and proceed to remove any blockages.

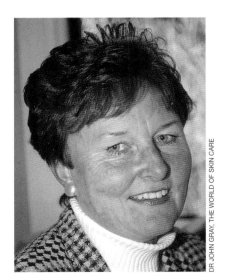

DR JOHN GRAY, THE WORLD OF SKIN CARE

Dilated capillaries

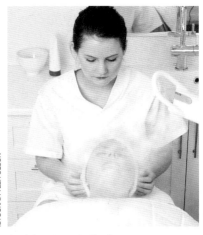

ISTOCK©TYLER OLSON

Applying steam to the face

HEALTH & SAFETY

Ozone

Most vapour units produce ozone when the oxygen in the steam is passed over a high-intensity quartz mercury arc tube. Ozone is thought to be beneficial in the treatment of blemished skin, as it kills many bacteria, but it may also be carcinogenic (liable to cause cancer) if inhaled. Use a vapour unit only in a well-ventilated room, and only for short periods of time.

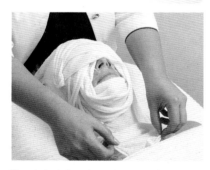

Towel steaming

TOP TIP

Aromatic oils

Provided that you have received instruction in the use of aromatic oils, and provided that the client has no contra-indications to them, you may add oils to the water.

At the end of the service, turn off the machine and unplug it. Check that you have tidied away the trailing lead so that there is no risk of it causing an accident.

ACTIVITY

Vapour units

Collect literature on different vapour units. Compare their efficiencies and features. Which would be the best buy? Consider:

- Is the unit transportable, for marketing demonstrations?
- Is it height-adjustable, to suit the height of the treatment couch?
- Is it easy to clean?
- If floor-standing, does it move easily?
- Does it allow the addition of aromatic oils?
- Does it havesafety features to prevent overheating or the vessel running dry?

Contra-actions Contra-actions to steaming include the following:

- *over-stimulation of the skin*, caused by incorrect application distance and duration of the steam
- *scalding*, caused by spitting from a faulty steam jet or by the vessel being over-filled
- *discomfort*, caused by the steam being too near the skin, leading to breathing difficulties, or by the treatment being applied for too long

Towel steaming Towel steaming is an alternative to steaming which can be used if an electrical vapour unit is not available to achieve the same beneficial effects. Several clean small towels are required: these are heated in a bowl of clean hot water, or specialized unit, and are then applied to the face. The towels must not be too hot to handle or you could burn the client's skin.

Application Seat the client in a semi-reclined position. Neatly fold a small clean towel and immerse it in very warm water. Wring it out quickly and, standing behind the client, transfer it to her face – with the towel folded in half, place it over the lower half of the face, directly under the client's lower lip; then unfold it to cover the upper face, leaving the mouth and nostrils uncovered.

Press the towel gently against the face for two minutes; during this time the towel will begin to cool. Remove the towel and replace it with another heated towel. Continue in this way, heating and replacing the towels, for approximately ten minutes.

After towel steaming, blot the skin dry with a soft facial tissue and proceed to remove any blockages.

HEALTH & SAFETY

Service programme

If the client suffers from severe congestion, do not attempt to carry out all the removals in one session. This would sensitize the skin, making it appear very red, and would be most uncomfortable for the client. Instead they should visit the salon weekly for you to clear the skin gradually as part of an overall service programme.

Removing skin blockages

After the skin has been cleansed, you may wish to remove minor skin blemishes such as comedones (blackheads) and milia (whiteheads). It is preferable to warm the tissues first: this softens the skin and relaxes the openings of the skin that are blocked.

Equipment and materials

You will need the following equipment and materials:

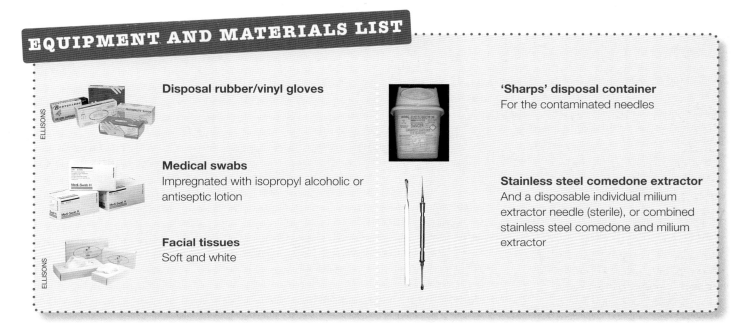

EQUIPMENT AND MATERIALS LIST

Disposal rubber/vinyl gloves

Medical swabs
Impregnated with isopropyl alcoholic or antiseptic lotion

Facial tissues
Soft and white

'Sharps' disposal container
For the contaminated needles

Stainless steel comedone extractor
And a disposable individual milium extractor needle (sterile), or combined stainless steel comedone and milium extractor

Sterilization and disinfection

You must put the disposable milium extractor in a 'sharps' container. All waste material from this service (such as facial tissues and gloves) should be disposed of in an identified waste container, as directed by your local health authority.

After use the stainless steel comedone extractor should be cleaned with an alcohol preparation and then sterilized in an autoclave.

Wear disposable gloves while carrying out the service.

Service

Comedone removal For comedone removal the loop end of the extractor tool, apply gentle pressure around the comedone. The comedone should leave the skin, apparent as a plug. You may need to apply gentle pressure with your fingers at the sides of the comedone to ensure that it is effectively removed; when doing this, wrap a tissue around the pads of the index fingers.

Contra-actions:

● Skin bruising could occur if too much pressure is applied.

● Capillary damage could result if too much force is used when squeezing the comedone. The surrounding blood capillaries can rupture, causing permanent skin damage.

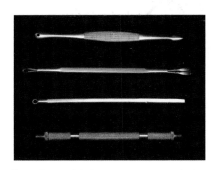

Comedone extractors

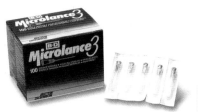

Microlance milia extractors

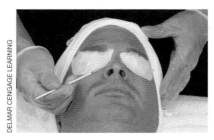

DELMAR CENGAGE LEARNING

Milium extraction

Milium extraction When supplying a milium extraction hold the point of the extractor tool parallel with the skin's surface, and *superficially* pierce the epidermis. This makes an opening through which the sebaceous matter can pass to the skin's surface. Using either the comedone extractor or tissue wrapped around the index fingers, apply gentle pressure. A mild antiseptic soothing lotion applied after extraction will help the skin to heal.

Mask service

The **face mask** is a skin-cleansing preparation which may contain a variety of different ingredients selected to have a deep cleansing, toning, nourishing or refreshing effect on the skin. The mask achieves this through the following actions. If it contains:

- *absorbent* materials, dead skin cells, sebum and debris will adhere to it when it is removed
- *astringent* ingredients, the pores and the skin will tighten
- *emollient* ingredients, the skin will be softened and nourished
- *soothing* ingredients, the skin can be desensitized to reduce skin irritation

There are basically two types of mask: setting and non-setting.

Setting masks

Setting masks are applied in a thin layer over the skin and then allowed to dry. The mask need not necessarily set solid – a solid mask can become uncomfortable, and be difficult to remove.

Setting masks come in these varieties:

- clay packs
- peel-off masks – gel, polyvinyl acetate (PVA) or paraffin wax
- thermal masks

Clay masks The **clay mask** absorbs sebum and debris from the skin surface, leaving it cleansed. It can also stimulate or soothe the skin, according to the ingredients chosen. Various clay powders are available – select from these according to the physiological effects you require:

- *Calamine* A light pink powder which soothes surface blood capillaries. For sensitive or delicate skin.
- *Magnesium carbonate* A very light, white powder which creates a temporary astringent and toning effect. For open pores on dry and normal skins.
- *Kaolin* A cream-coloured powder which has a very stimulating effect on the skin's surface capillaries, thereby helping the skin to remove impurities and waste products. For congested, oily skin.
- *Fuller's earth* A green, heavy clay powder. It has a very stimulating effect, such that the skin will show slight reddening. It also produces a whitening, brightening effect. For oily skin with a sluggish circulation. Due to its strong effect, it is not suitable for a client with sensitive skin.
- *Flowers of sulphur* A light, yellow clay powder, which has a drying action on pustules and papules. Applied only to specific blemishes (pustules).

HEALTH & SAFETY

Client comfort

- Never obstruct the client's nostrils when removing a comedone from the nose area.
- Never apply pressure on the soft cartilage of the nose.

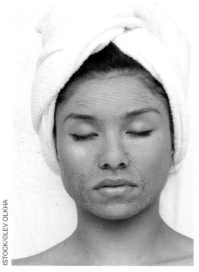

ISTOCK/©LEV OLKHA

A setting face mask

HEALTH & SAFETY

Avoiding infection

Clay mask ingredients must always be made from sterilized materials, because of the danger from tetanus spores.

Ensure that *all* contents of the skin blockage are removed, or infection may occur.

To activate these masks it is necessary to add a liquid – an **active lotion** – which turns the powder to a liquid paste. Active lotions are selected according to the skin type of the client and the mask to be used; they reinforce the action of the mask. Examples are:

- *Rose water and orange-flower water* These are very popular; they have a very mild stimulating and toning effect.

- *Witch-hazel* This has a soothing effect on blemished skin; it is also an astringent and is suitable for use on oily skin.

- *Distilled water* This is used on highly sensitive skins.

- *Almond oil* This is mildly stimulating. Because it is an oil, it does not allow the mask to dry: it is therefore recommended for highly sensitive skin or dehydrated skin.

- *Glycerol* A humectant, which prevents the mask drying and is suitable for dry mature skin.

Clay masks have the disadvantage when treating a black skin in that they tend on removal to leave streaks of white residue. Choose a mask that does not have this effect.

The mask should be kept in place for about 10–15 minutes.

Peel-off masks

Peel-off masks may be made from gel, latex or paraffin wax. Because perspiration cannot escape from the skin's surface, moisture is forced into the stratum corneum. The mask also insulates the skin, causing an increase in temperature.

The **gel mask** is either a suspension of biological ingredients, such as starches, gums or gelatine, or a mixture of synthetic non-biological resin ingredients. The mask is applied over the skin; on contact with the skin it begins to dry. When dry it is peeled off the face in one piece. Depending on the biological ingredients added, the gel mask can be used to treat all skin types. (If the client has excessive facial hair, such as at the sides of the face, this mask may cause discomfort on removal. To avoid this place a lubricant under the mask, or use a different sort of mask.)

The **latex mask** is an emulsion of latex and water: when applied to the skin, the water evaporates to leave a rubber film over the face. This produces a rise in temperature, thereby stimulating the skin. In alternative peel-off masks, latex is replaced by a synthetic resin emulsion such as **polyvinyl acetate** (PVA) resin. Latex masks tighten the skin temporarily, and are suitable for mature skin; they can also be used with dry skin. Algae may be used as an ingredient which causes rapid setting.

The **paraffin-wax mask** is stimulating in its action. The paraffin wax is blended with petroleum jelly or acetyl alcohol which improve its spreading properties. The wax is heated to approximately 37°C and is then applied to the skin as a liquid. It sets on contact, so speed is essential if the mask is to be effective. The wax mask is loosened at the sides and removed in one piece after 15–20 minutes. The paraffin-wax mask is suitable for dry skin. Because of its stimulating action, it is unsuitable for oily skin or highly sensitive skin.

Thermal masks

The **thermal mask** contains various minerals. The ingredients are mixed and applied to the face and neck, avoiding the mouth and eye tissue. The mask warms on contact with the skin: this causes the pores to enlarge, thereby cleansing the skin. As the mask cools it sets, and the pores constrict slightly. The mask is removed from the face in one piece. Thermal masks have a stimulating, cleansing action, suitable for a normal skin or for a congested, oily skin with open pores.

ALWAYS REMEMBER

Face packs
The term *face pack* is sometimes used instead of face mask: a face pack does not set, but remains soft; a face mask sets and becomes firm.

ACTIVITY

Choosing face masks
Which clay powder and which active lotion would you mix for clients with the following skin types:
1 A mature, sensitive skin type.
2 A young, normal skin type.
3 A combination skin type: cheeks, neck area dry; forehead, nose and chin area oily.

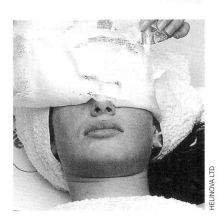

HELINOVA LTD

Removal of paraffin-wax mask

HEALTH & SAFETY

Contra-indications
Do not use thermal masks on a client with a circulatory disorder or one who has lost tactile sensation.

HEALTH & SAFETY

Client comfort
If a client is particularly nervous, choose an effective non-setting mask. Some clients feel claustrophobic when wearing a setting mask.

HEALTH & SAFETY

Client comfort

Before applying the wax to the client's skin always test the temperature of the wax on your own inner wrist.

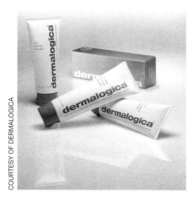

COURTESY OF DERMALOGICA

Selection of face masks

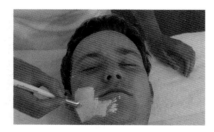

Applying a cream face mask

BEST PRACTICE

Gauze masks

Ensure that you position the gauze correctly so that the nose and eye holes are properly placed.

HEALTH & SAFETY

Allergies

When using biological masks, always check first whether the client has any food allergies.

Non-setting masks

Some **non-setting masks** stay soft on application; others become firm, but they do not tighten like a setting mask. For this reason they do not tone the skin as effectively as setting masks. Non-setting masks include:

- warm oil
- natural masks – fruit, plant and herbal
- cream

Warm-oil masks A plant oil, typically **olive oil** or **almond oil**, is warmed and then applied to the skin. It softens the skin and helps to restore the skin's natural moisture balance. Warm-oil masks are recommended for mature skin and dry or dehydrated skin.

Gauze masks A **gauze mask** is cut to cover the face and neck, with holes for the eyes, nostrils and lips. This is then soaked in warm oil. A dampened cotton wool eye pad is placed over each eye. The gauze is then placed over the face and neck. It is usually left in place for 10–20 minutes.

Natural masks **Natural masks** are made from natural ingredients rich in vitamins and minerals. Fresh **fruit** and **vegetables** have a mildly astringent and stimulating effect. Usually the fruit is crushed to a pulp and placed between layers of gauze, which are laid over the face.

Honey is used for its toning, tightening, antiseptic and hydrating effect. **Egg white** has a tightening effect and is said to clear impurities from the skin. **Avocados** have a nourishing effect; **bananas** soften the skin, and are used for sensitive skins.

Cream masks **Cream masks** are pre-prepared for you. They have a softening and moisturising effect on the skin. Each mask contains various biological extracts or chemical substances to treat different skin types or conditions. Instructions will be provided with the mask, stating how the product is to be used professionally.

These masks are popular in the beauty salon: they often complement a particular facial treatment range used by the salon, and they are available for retail sale to clients.

Contra-indications

The contra-indications to general skincare apply also to face mask application. In addition, observe the following:

- **Allergies** Check whether your client knows if they have allergies. If so, avoid all contact with known allergens.
- **Claustrophobia** Do not use a setting mask on a particularly nervous client. Some clients feel claustrophobic under its tightening effect.
- **Sensitive skins** Do not use stimulating masks on clients with highly sensitive skin.

HEALTH & SAFETY

Natural masks

Because natural masks are prepared from natural foods, they must be prepared *immediately* before use – they very quickly deteriorate.

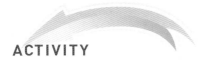

ACTIVITY

Creating natural masks

Create some masks, listing the ingredients to suit each of the following skin types:

- dry
- oily
- mature, with superficial wrinkling
- sensitive

If possible, arrange to carry out one of the masks on a suitable client in the workplace. Evaluate the natural face mask. Consider: cost, preparation, application, removal and effectiveness. Remember to ask your client for *their* opinion!

HEALTH & SAFETY

Acidic fruit

Lemon and grapefruit are generally considered too acidic for use on the face.

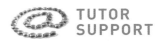

TUTOR SUPPORT

Activity 6: Face masks handout

EQUIPMENT AND MATERIALS LIST

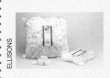

Clean, dampened and clean, dry cotton wool

With sit-up and lie-down positions and an easy-to-clean surface

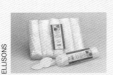

Cotton wool eye pads

(2) Pre-shaped, round and dampened

Scissors

To cut cotton wool eye pads (if cotton wool discs are not used)

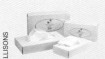

Facial tissues (white)

To blot the skin dry after applying toner following mask removal

Protective headband (clean)

Clean spatulas (several)

To mix individual masks (if required) and remove products from containers

Face-mask ingredients

Gauze

Used in applying certain masks

Waste bin (covered and lined)

For waste consumables

YOU WILL ALSO NEED:

Disposable tissue roll Such as bedroll

Towels (2) Freshly laundered for each client

Flat mask brushes (3) Disinfected

Trolley To display all facial treatment products to be used in the facial service

Client's record card To record all the details relevant to the client's service

Facial toning lotions (a selection) To suit various types of skin

Sterilized mask-removal sponges (2) or facial mitts/ towels For use when removing the mask using clean warm water

Large bowl To hold warm water during removal of the mask

Lukewarm water If required for mask removal

Moisturisers (a range) To suit different skin types for use after mask removal

Hand mirror (clean) To show the client their skin following the facial service

Equipment and materials

When applying masks you will need the following equipment and materials:

Sterilization and disinfection After applying the mask, clean the mask brush thoroughly in warm water and detergent. Next, place it in a chemical disinfecting agent; rinse it in clean water; allow it to dry; and then store it in the ultra-violet cabinet.

When you use a paraffin-wax mask, remove as much mask residue as possible from the brush, then place the brush in boiling water to remove excess wax. Disinfect the brush as usual before use.

If you use sponges to remove the mask, place them in warm water and detergent. After rinsing them in clean water, place them ready for disinfection in an autoclave. (With re-peated disinfection, sponges will begin to break up.)

Thermal mitts and towels should be washed at a temperature of 60°C.

A large high-quality cotton wool disc may be purchased to use in mask removal.

Preparing the work area Check that you have all the materials you need to carry out the service. You may like to place a paper roll at the head of the couch, under-neath the client's head, to collect any mask residue on mask removal.

The head of the couch should be flat or slightly elevated. Don't have it in a semi-reclined position during the mask application, as some masks are liquid in consistency and may run into the client's eyes and behind their neck.

Service

Preparing the client For maximum effect, the mask must be applied on a clean, grease-free surface. If the mask application follows a facial massage, ensure that the massage medium has been thoroughly removed.

Select the appropriate mask ingredients to treat the skin type and the facial conditions that require attention.

How to apply and remove the mask The mask is usually applied as the *final* facial service, because of its cleansing, refining and soothing effects upon the skin. The methods of preparation, application and removal are different for the various face mask types, so the guidelines below are a general outline of effective service technique.

1 Having determined the client's service requirements, select the appropriate mask ingredients. If you use a commercial mask, always read the manufacturer's in-structions first.

2 Discuss the service procedure with the client, explain:

- what the mask will feel like on application

- what sensation, if any, they will experience

- how long the mask will be left on the skin

Generally the mask will be left in place for 10–20 minutes, but the exact time depends on the client's skin type, the type of mask and effect required.

3 Prepare the mask ingredients for application.

4 Using the sterilized mask brush or spatula, begin to apply the mask. The usual sequence of mask application is neck, chin, cheeks, nose and forehead.

If you are using more than one mask to treat different skin conditions, apply first the one that will need to be on longest.

Apply the mask quickly and evenly so that it has maximum effect on the whole face. Don't apply it too thickly; as well as making mask removal difficult, this is wasteful as only the part that is in contact with the skin has any effect.

Keep the mask clear of the nostrils, the lips, the eyebrows and the hairline.

5 To relax the client, apply cotton wool eye pads dampened with clean water.

6 Leave the mask for the recommended time or according to the effect required. Take account also of the sensitivity of the skin and your client's comfort.

7 Wash your hands.

8 When the mask is ready for removal, remove the eye pads.

Explain to the client that you are going to remove the mask. Briefly describe the process, according to whether this is a setting or a non-setting mask.

Remove the mask using an appropriate technique, i.e. make-up sponges or warm towel method. Mask sponges, if used, should be damp, not wet, so that water doesn't run into the client's eyes, nose or mouth.

9 When the mask has been completely removed, apply the appropriate toning lotion using dampened cotton wool. Blot the skin dry with a facial tissue.

10 Apply an appropriate moisturiser to the skin.

11 Remove the headband, and tidy the client's hair.

12 With a mirror, show the client their skin. Evaluate the service.

13 Record the results on their record card.

Contra-actions Before you apply the mask, explain to the client what the action of the mask will feel like on the skin. This will enable them to identify any undesirable skin reaction, evident to them as skin irritation – a burning sensation.

Ask the client initially whether they are comfortable: this will give them the opportunity to tell you if they are experiencing any discomfort. Should there be a contra-action to the mask, remove the mask immediately and apply a soothing skincare product.

If on removal of the mask you can see that there has been an unwanted skin reaction (that is, if you see inflammation), apply a soothing skincare product. In either case, note the skin reaction on the record card, and choose a different mask next time.

Advice on home use The client may be given a sample of the face mask for use at home. Explain to them the procedure for application and removal, so that they achieve maximum benefit from the mask. Encourage them to aply a mask once or twice a week, depending on their skin type, to dislodge dead skin cells and to cleanse and stimulate the skin.

ALWAYS REMEMBER

Paraffin wax
If you are using paraffin wax, remember to heat it in advance.

HEALTH & SAFETY

Allergies
When using a commercial mask, try to find out *exactly* what it contains, so that you don't apply a sensitizing ingredient to an allergic skin type.

Setting masks
When using a setting mask, ensure that the mask is evenly applied or it will dry unevenly.

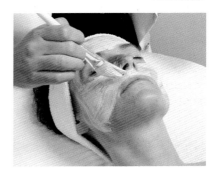

Applying the mask around the lips

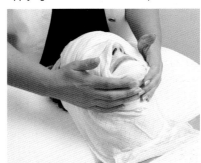

Applying warm towel to the mask

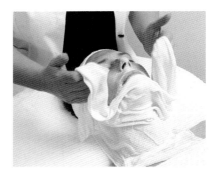

Removing the mask with a warm towel

ALWAYS REMEMBER

Mask removal

When using water to remove a mask you may need to renew the water as you work.

BEST PRACTICE

While the mask is on the face you can tidy the working area and collect together the materials required for mask removal. Do not disturb the client, who will be relaxing at this time. A hand massage may also be offered.

HEALTH & SAFETY

Peel-off masks

When using a peel-off mask, make sure that the border of the mask is thick enough – if it isn't, it will be difficult to remove and the client may experience discomfort.

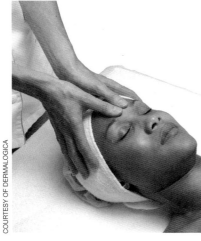

COURTESY OF DERMALOGICA

Facial massage

Advise the client not to apply the mask directly before a special occasion, in case it causes blemishes, as sometimes happens.

The skin should be toned and moisturised after removing the mask.

Facial massage

Manual massage is the external manipulation, using the hands, of the soft tissues of the face, neck and upper chest. Massage can improve the appearance of the skin and promote a sensation of stimulation or relaxation.

Each massage performed is adapted to the client's physiological and psychological needs. The skin's physiological needs are observed during the skin analysis; the client's psychological needs are usually discovered during the consultation.

The benefits of the facial massage include the following:

- Dead epidermal cells are loosened and shed. This improves the appearance of the skin, exposing fresh, younger cells.

- The muscles receive an improved supply of oxygenated blood, essential for cell growth. The tone and strength of the muscles are improved, firming the facial contour.

- The increased blood circulation in the area warms the tissues. This induces a feeling of relaxation, which is particularly beneficial when treating tense muscles.

- As the blood capillaries dilate and bring blood to the skin's surface, the skin colour improves.

- The lymphatic circulation and the venous blood circulation increase. These changes speed up the removal of waste products and toxins, and tend therefore to purify the skin. The removal of excess lymph improves the appearance of a puffy oedematous skin (provided that this does not require medical treatment).

- The increased temperature of the skin relaxes the pores and follicles. This aids the absorption of the massage product, which in turn softens the skin.

- Sensory nerves can be soothed or stimulated, depending on the massage manipulations selected.

- Massage stimulates the sebaceous and sudoriferous glands and increases the production of sebum and sweat. This increase helps to maintain the skin's natural oil and moisture balance.

Reception

Facial massage is carried out as required, usually once every four to six weeks. Before the facial massage is given, the skin is cleansed; afterwards it is usual to apply a cleansing face mask, which absorbs any excess grease from the skin.

When booking a client for this service, allow one hour. The facial massage itself should take approximately 20 minutes, but this may vary according to the client's skin type.

Warn the client that the skin may appear slightly red and blotchy after the service, due to the increase in blood circulation to the area: this reaction will normally subside after four to six hours.

Because of the stimulating effect on the skin recommend to the client that they receive this service when they do not have to apply any cosmetic products directly afterwards.

Sometimes the skin develops small blemishes after facial massage; this is due to its cleansing action. If the client is preparing for a special occasion, therefore, such as a wedding, make the appointment for at least five days in advance.

Massage manipulations

The facial massage is based on a series of classic massage movements, each with different effects. There are four basic groups of massage movements:

- effleurage
- petrissage
- percussion (also known as tapotement)
- vibrations

The therapist can adapt the way each of these movements is applied, according to the needs of the client. Either the *speed of application* or the *depth of pressure* can be altered.

Effleurage Effleurage is a stroking movement, used to begin the massage, as a link manipulation, and to complete the massage sequence. This manipulation is light, has an even pressure, and is applied in a rhythmical, continuous manner to induce relaxation.

The pressure of application varies according to the underlying structures and the tissue type, but it must *never* be unduly heavy.

Effleurage has these effects:

- desquamation is increased
- arterial blood circulation is increased, bringing fresh nutrients to the area
- venous circulation is improved, aiding the removal of congestion from the veins
- lymphatic circulation is increased, improving the absorption of waste products
- the underlying muscle fibres are relaxed

Uses in treatment: to relax tight, contracted muscles

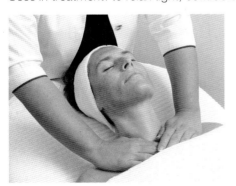
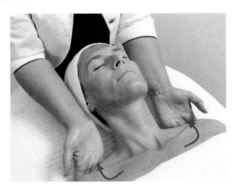

Effleurage

Petrissage Petrissage involves a series of movements in which the tissues are lifted away from the underlying structures and compressed. Pressure is intermittent, and should be light yet firm.

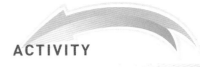

ACTIVITY

Planning a massage
How will observations from the skin analysis and the client consultation influence the facial massage service?

ALWAYS REMEMBER

Client care
The headband can spoil the hair, and the massage medium may enter the hairline. Recommend that the client does not style their hair directly before the facial service.

BEST PRACTICE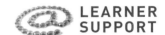

Neck and shoulders
Pressure may be increased when working on larger muscles in the neck or shoulders, especially if the client has tension in this area.

LEARNER SUPPORT

Facial skincare: mini crossword

Petrissage has these effects:

- improvement of muscle tone, through the compression and relaxation of muscle fibres

- improvement in blood and lymph circulation, as the application of pressure causes the vessels to empty and fill

- increased activity of the sebaceous gland, due to the stimulation

Movements include picking up, kneading, knuckling, pinching, rolling, frictions, and scissoring.

Uses in treatment: to stimulate a sluggish circulation; to increase sebaceous gland and sudoriferous gland activity when treating a dry skin condition.

BEST PRACTICE

Stimulation
When a stimulating massage is required, incorporate more petrissage and tapotement into the massage sequence.

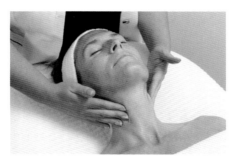
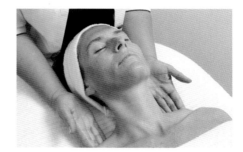

Petrissage

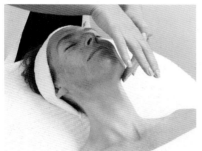

Percussion

Percussion Percussion, also known as **tapotement**, is performed in a brisk, stimulating manner. Rhythm is important as the fingers are continually breaking contact with the skin; irritation could occur if the movement were performed incorrectly

Percussion has these effects:

- a fast vascular reaction because of the skin's nervous response to the stimulus – this reaction, **erythema**, has a stimulating effect

- increased blood supply, which nourishes the tissues

- improvement in muscle and skin tone in the area

Movements include clapping and tapping. In facial massage, only light tapping should be used.

Uses in treatment: to tone areas of loose, crepey skin around the jaw or eyes.

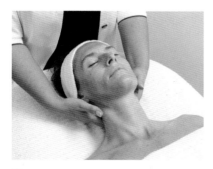

Vibrations

Vibrations **Vibrations** are applied on the nerve centre. They are produced by a rapid contraction and relaxation of the muscles of the therapist's arm, resulting in a fine trembling movement.

Vibration has these effects:

- stimulation of the nerves, inducing a feeling of wellbeing

- gentle stimulation of the skin

Movements include *static* vibrations, in which the pads of the fingers are placed on the nerve, and the vibratory effect created by the therapist's arms and hands is applied in one position; and *running* vibrations, in which the vibratory effect is applied along a nerve path.

Uses in treatment: to stimulate a sensitive skin in order to improve the skin's functioning without irritating the surface blood capillaries.

HEALTH & SAFETY

Contra-indications
Do not apply percussion over highly sensitive or vascular skin conditions to avoid excessively increasing blood circulation in the area and over-stimulating the skin.

Equipment and materials

The massage is carried out using a **massage medium** which acts as a lubricant. A massage cream or oil may be used; these are slightly penetrating, and soften the skin. Choose a product that contains ingredients to suit the client's skin type and the age of the skin.

Whichever product you choose, it should provide sufficient slip while allowing you to control the massage movements.

ACTIVITY

Choosing a massage medium
Compare two professional skincare ranges. Look at:
- the choice of facial-massage preparations
- the ingredients used in their formulation, and the effects claimed

Step-by-step: Massage service

There are many different massage sequences, but each uses one or all of the massage manipulations discussed above. What follows is a basic sequence for facial massage.

TOP TIP

It is important to maintain good posture during facial massage. If you slouch, you will experience muscle fatigue and long-term postural problems!

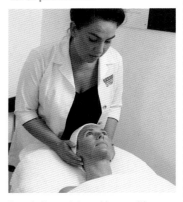

Beauty therapist working position

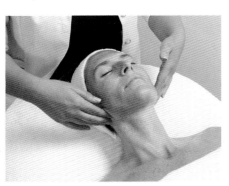
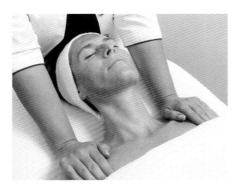
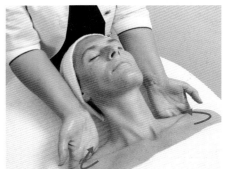

1 Effleurage to the neck and shoulders Slide the hands down the neck, across the pectoral muscles around the deltoid muscle, and across the trapezius muscle. Slide the hands up the back of the neck to the base of the skull.

Repeat step 1 a further 5 times.

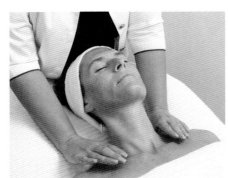
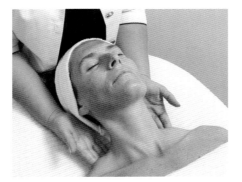
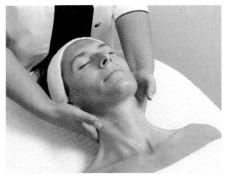

2 Thumb kneading to the shoulders Using the pad of both thumbs, make small circles (frictions) along the trapezius muscle, working towards the spinal vertebrae.

Apply each movement 3 times; then repeat the sequence (step 2) a further 2 times.

3 Finger kneading to the shoulders Position the fingers of each hand behind the deltoid, and make large rotary movements along the trapezius.

Apply each rotary movement 3 times; repeat the sequence (step 3) a further 2 times.

4 Vibrations Place the hands, cupped, at the base of the neck: perform running vibrations up the neck to the occipital bone.

Repeat step 4 a further 6 times.

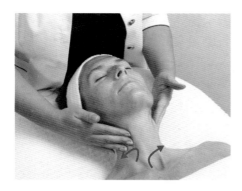

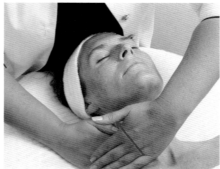

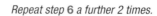

5 Circular massage to the neck Perform small circular movements over the platysma and the sternomastoid muscle at the neck.

6 Hands cupped to the neck Cup your hands together. Place the hands at the left side of the neck, above the clavicle. Slide the hands up the side of the neck, across the jaw line, and down the right side of the neck; then reverse.

Repeat step 6 a further 2 times.

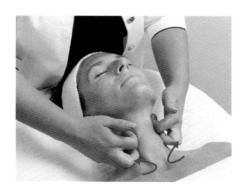

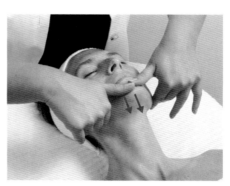

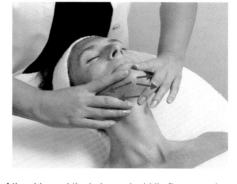

7 Knuckling to the neck Make a loose fist: rotate the knuckles up and down the neck area.

Repeat step 7 to cover, a further 2 times.

8 Up and under Place the thumbs on the centre of the chin, and the index and middle fingers under the mandible. Slide the thumbs firmly over the chin. Bring the index finger onto the chin, and place the middle finger under the mandible forming a V shape. Slide along the jaw line to the ear. Replace the index finger with the thumb, and return along the jaw to the chin.

Repeat step 8 a further 5 times.

HEALTH & SAFETY

The trachea
Never apply pressure when working on the neck over the trachea which could cause discomfort.

HEALTH & SAFETY

Sensitive skin
Do not use knuckling on sensitive skin to avoid over-stimulation.

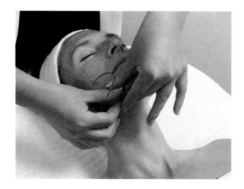

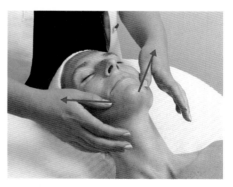

9 Circling to the mandible Place the thumbs one above the other on the chin, and proceed with circular kneading along the jaw line towards the ear. Reverse and repeat.

Repeat step 9 a further 2 times.

10 Flick-ups Place the thumbs at the corners of the mouth. Lift the orbicularis oris muscle, with a flicking action of the thumbs.

Repeat step 10 a further 5 times.

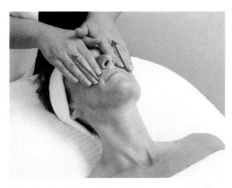

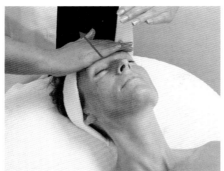

11 Half face brace Clasp the fingers under the chin; turn the hands so that the fingers point towards the sternum. Unclasp, and slide the hands up the face towards the forehead.

Repeat step **11** *a further 2 times.*

12 Lifting the eyebrows Place the right hand on the forehead at the left temple, and stroke upwards from the eyebrow to the hairline. Repeat the movement with the left hand. Alternate each hand; repeat the movement across the forehead.

Repeat step **12** *a further 2 times.*

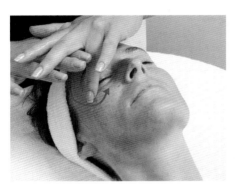

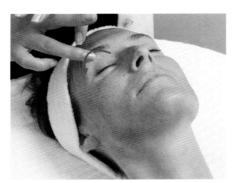

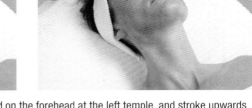

HEALTH & SAFETY

Massage manipulation 'flick-ups': the lips

Do not flick the lips. Position the thumbs 5mm from the corner of the mouth to avoid this.

13 Inner and outer eye circles Using the ring finger, *gently* draw 3 outer circles and 3 inner circles on each eye, following the fibre direction of the orbicularis oculi muscle.

Repeat step **13** *a further 2 times.*

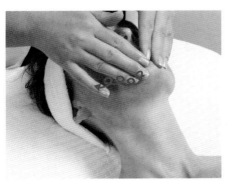

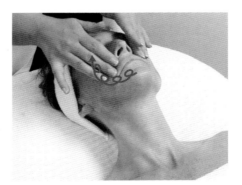

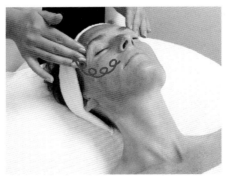

15 Circling to the chin, the nose and the temples Apply circular kneading to the chin, the nose and the temples. Return to the starting position.

Repeat step **15** *a further 2 times.*

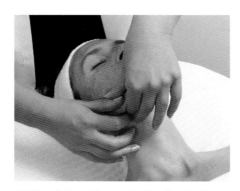

16 Thumb kneading under the cheeks Place the thumbs under the zygomatic bones. Carry out a circular kneading over the muscles in the cheek area.

Repeat step 16 a further 5 times.

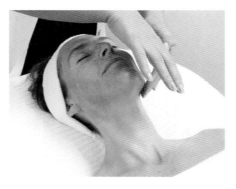

17 Tapping under the mandible Tap the tissue under the mandible, using the fingers of both hands. Work from the left side of the jaw to the right; then reverse.

Repeat step 17 a further 5 times.

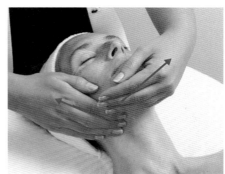

18 Lifting the masseter Cup the hands. Using the hands alternately, lift the masseter muscle.

Repeat step 18 a further 5 times.

HEALTH & SAFETY

Sensitive skin
Avoid the use of tapotement over areas of sensitivity.

ALWAYS REMEMBER

Massage medium
If the skin appears to drag during massage, stop and apply more massage medium. If you keep going you may cause skin irritation or discomfort.

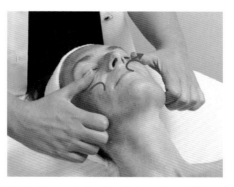 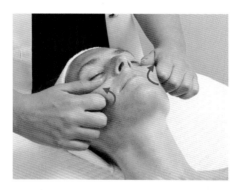

19 Rolling and pinching Using a deep rolling movement, draw the muscles of the cheek area towards the thumb in a rolling and pinching movement.

Repeat step 19 a further 5 times.

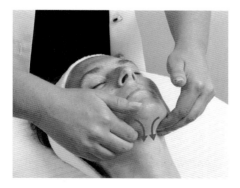 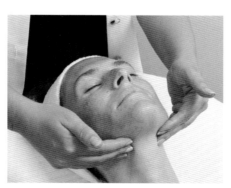

20 Lifting the mandible Place the pads of the fingers underneath the mandible and pivot diagonally. Lifting the tissues work towards the ear.

Repeat step 20 a further 2 times.

21 Knuckling along the jaw line Knuckle along the jaw line and over the cheek area.

Repeat step 21 a further 2 times.

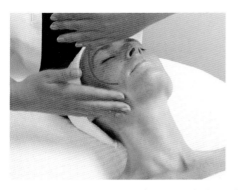

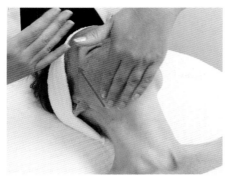

22 Upwards tapping on the face Using both hands, gently slap along the jaw line from ear to ear, lifting the muscles.

Repeat step 22 a further 5 times.

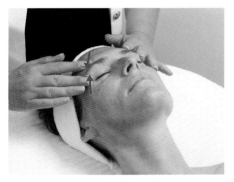

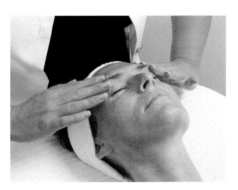

24 Scissor movement to the forehead Open the index and middle fingers to make a V shape at the outer corner of each eyebrow. Open and close the fingers in a scissor action towards the inner eyebrow.

Repeat step 24 a further 2 times.

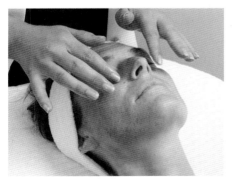

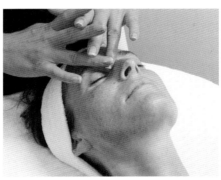

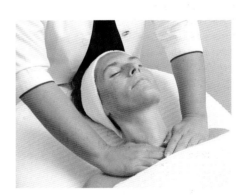

25 Tapotement movement around the eyes
Using the pads of the fingers, tap gently around the eye area.

Repeat step 25 a further 2 times.

26 Eye circling Repeat step 13, 3 times.

TOP TIP

Practise
When learning the facial massage you need to practise. Practise the movements on a Styrofoam® head block with facial features, or mannequin head as used in hairdressing, to perfect the manipulations. If these are unavailable, practise each manipulation on your knee – this will increase the agility and strength of your fingers and wrists.

BEST PRACTICE

Massage medium can easily be overlooked in the following areas: the eyebrows; the base of the nostrils; under the chin; in the creases of the neck; behind the ear and on the shoulders. Ensure all massage medium is thoroughly removed.

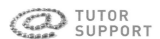 TUTOR SUPPORT

Activity 7: Facial treatment wordsearch

After the massage

After the facial massage, remove the massage medium thoroughly using clean, damp cotton wool, facial mitts or towels. Check thoroughly that all product has been removed.

Apply toner to remove traces of oil, leaving the skin grease-free. Finally, blot the skin dry.

You may then proceed with further skin services, such as a face mask, or simply apply an appropriate moisturiser to conclude the service.

Advice on home care

Encourage your client to use massage movements when applying emollient skincare products. Show them how to perform such movements correctly.

Facial exercises may be given to the client to practise at home. These should be carried out at least four times per week.

Specialist facial service

Specialist services should be offered to your client when there is a specific need or if they feel they would like to benefit from such a service. Specialist training in these advanced techniques is usually offered by the main product companies.

Step-by-step: Specialist facial

The model for this specialist facial service is a mature client with dry dehydrated skin with areas of sensitivity. One hour and 15 minutes was allowed for this facial.

The following facial service will:

- stimulate the blood circulation
- aid with the removal of toxins and waste products
- have a skin cleansing action
- remove dead skin cells (desquamation)
- improve the moisture content of the skin
- firm skin tone

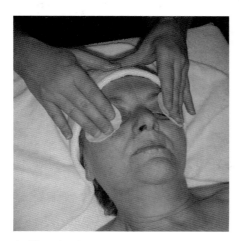

1 Cleansing the eye area

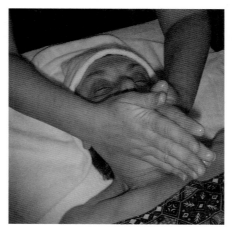

2 Application of facial cleanser.

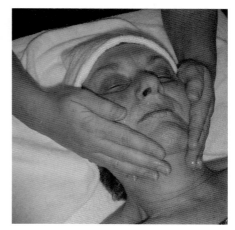

3 The cleanser is selected to rehydrate the skin.

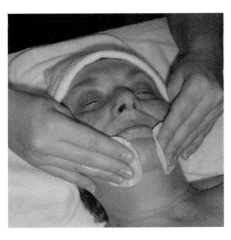

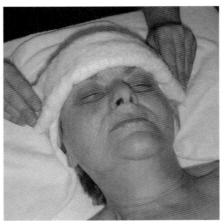

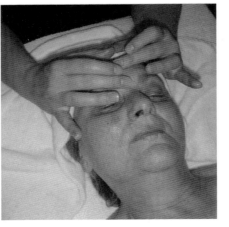

4   Removal of facial cleanser using dampened cotton wool in an upwards and outwards direction.

5   Application of a hot towel, infused with lavender oil, to the face. This will have a skin-cleansing action causing the pores to open. It also has therapeutic relaxation properties, as the client inhales the lavender oil.

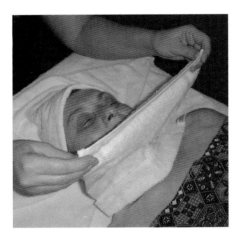

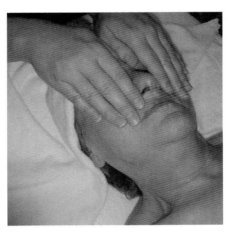

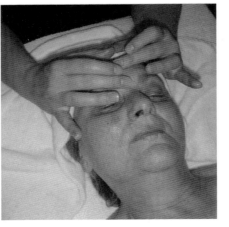

6   Removal of the hot towel.

7   Facial massage movements are applied to the shoulders and face. Eastern massage techniques are included to rebalance the mind and body.

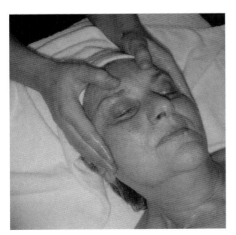

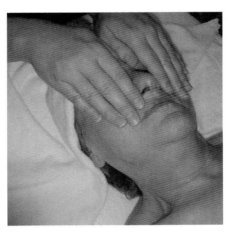

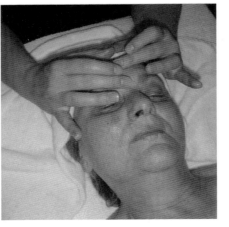

8   Pressure is applied to different points on the meridians or energy pathways based upon shiatsu massage – an ancient Eastern massage technique.

9   Application of a non-setting exfoliant cream mask.

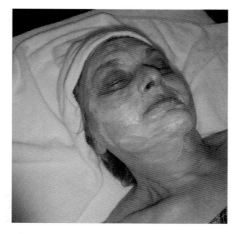

10 This mask will gently remove dead skin cells.

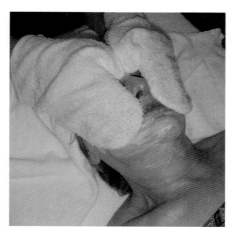

11 Exfoliant removal using warm, damp towelling mitts.

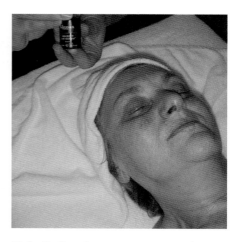

12 Application of an eye serum eye-mask to relax and strengthen the delicate skin tissue around the eye.

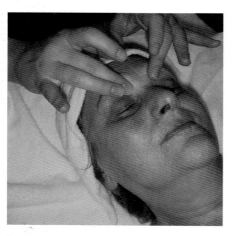

13 A specialized lifting massage is applied to increase cellular renewal around the eyes.

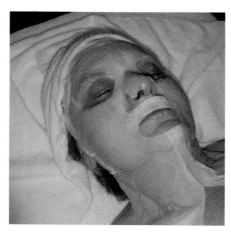

14 A Japanese silk cream mask is contoured to the face and neck, feeling like a second skin.

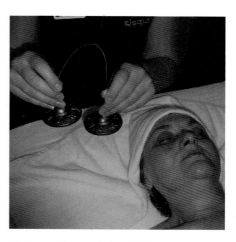

15 The service concludes with the skin being toned and moisturised and the client being gently awakened with Japanese chimes. The service will give both psychological and physiological benefits.

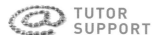

TUTOR SUPPORT

Activity 8: Revision and evaluation Re-cap task

Outcome 4 : Provide aftercare advice

> **You should learn to provide aftercare which supports the needs of your client by:**

1 Giving **advice** and recommendations accurately and constructively.

2 Giving your clients suitable **advice** specific to their individual needs.

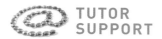

TUTOR SUPPORT

Activity 9: Multiple choice quiz

Aftercare and advice is discussed throughout the chapter in relation to each of the facial service procedures.

At the conclusion of your facial service ensure that you have covered the following in your **aftercare advice**:

- explained what products have been used in the facial service and why

- advised what products would be suitable for the client to use at home, a basic home care routine, to gain maximum benefit from the service

- advised on product application and removal, again in order to gain maximum benefit from their use

- provided contra-action advice, action to be taken in the event of an unwanted skin reaction

- discussed the use of make-up following service (only eye and lip make-up should be worn directly after a facial service; allow up to eight hours before make-up application to avoid congestion of the stimulated, cleansed skin)

- explained the recommended time intervals between services

- provided guidance on what further services you would recommend to maintain or improve further the facial skin condition

- discussed if product samples are to be provided, when and how they are to be used

- provided the opportunity for the client to ask any further questions

Update and record all details on the client record card, including products purchased. You can discuss their effectiveness at the next facial service.

Take the client to the reception to book their next appointment if required.

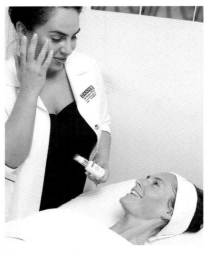

Home care routine

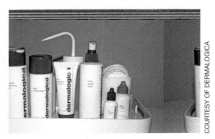

Product samples

COURTESY OF DERMALOGICA

GLOSSARY OF KEY WORDS

Acid mantle the combination of sweat and sebum on the skin's surface, creating an acid film. The acid mantle is protective and discourages the growth of bacteria and fungi. The pH scale is used to measure the acidity or alkalinity of a substance using a numbered scale. The skin's pH is acid at 5.5-5.6.

Aftercare advice recommended advice given to the client following service to continue and enhance the benefits of the service.

Antioxidant properties of some foods that maintain the health of the skin, fighting the damaging effects of free radicals (unstable molecules which can cause skin cells to degenerate) in the body. Antioxidant ingredients are increasingly being included in skincare preparations to neutralize free radicals or repel them from the skin.

Cleanser a skincare preparation that removes dead skin cells, excess sweat and sebum, make-up and dirt from the skin's surface to maintain a healthy skin complexion. These are formulated to treat the different skin types, skin characteristics and facial areas.

Client groups this term is used in a number of the units and it refers to client diversity. The CRE (Commission for Racial Equality) ethnic group classification is used in the range for these units. These cover white, mixed, Asian, black and Chinese.

Comedone removal facial techniques used to extract comedones (blackheads) from the skin. A small tool called a comedone extractor is used for this purpose.

Consultation assessment of client's needs using different assessment techniques, including questioning and natural observation.

Contra-action an unwanted reaction occurring during or after service application.

Contra-indication a problematic symptom which indicates that the service may not proceed or may restrict service application. Contra-indications identified for facial services are discussed in more detail in Chapter 3.

Effleurage a stroking massage manipulation used to begin the massage, as a link manipulation, and to complete the massage sequence. Applied in a rhythmic, continuous manner, it induces relaxation.

Equipment tools used within a facial to enhance the effects and application of facial products and procedures e.g. magnifying light and skin warming devices.

Erythema reddening of the skin caused by increased blood circulation to the area.

Exfoliant a service used to remove excess dead skin cells from the surface of the skin, which has a skin cleansing, cell rejuvenating action. This process can be achieved using a specialized cosmetic, or mechanically by using facial equipment where a brush is rotated over the skin's surface.

Facial a service to improve the appearance, condition and functioning of the skin and underlying structures.

Facial products skincare used with a facial service which have specific benefits to care for and improve the function and appearance of the skin.

Hyperpigmentation increased pigment production.

Hypopigmentation loss of pigmentation.

Mask a skin-cleansing service preparation applied to the skin, which may contain different ingredients. It can have a deep cleansing, toning, nourishing or refreshing effect. It may be applied to the face, hands and feet.

Massage manipulation of the soft tissues of the body, producing heat and stimulating the muscular, circulatory and nervous systems.

Massage manipulations movements which are selected and applied according to the desired effect, and which may be stimulating, relaxing or toning. Massage manipulations include effleurage, petrissage, percussion (also known as tapotement) and vibrations.

Massage medium a skincare product which acts as a lubricant to allow sufficient slip over the skin's, surface while performing facial massage.

Milium extraction skincare technique used to extract milia (whiteheads) from the skin. A small tool called a milia extractor is used for this purpose, which superficially pierces the epidermis, allowing effective removal of the milia.

Minor a person classed as a child who requires by law to have a guardian or parent present.

Moisturiser a skincare preparation whose formulation of oil and water helps maintain the skin's natural moisture by locking moisture into the skin, offering protection and hydration. The formulation is selected to suit the skin type, facial characteristics and facial area.

Muscle tone the normal degree of tension in healthy muscle.

Necessary action the action taken to deal safely with a contra-action or contra-indication.

Nutrition the nourishment derived from food, required for the body's growth, energy, repair and production.

Oedema extra fluid in an area, causing swelling.

Petrissage a massage manipulation in which the tissues are lifted away from the underlying structures and compressed. Petrissage improves muscle tone by the compression and relaxation of the muscle fibres.

Pigment the skin's and hair's colour, called melanin. The amount of pigment varies for each client, resulting in different skin/hair colour.

Service plan after the consultation, suitable service objectives are established to treat the client's conditions and needs.

Skin analysis assessment of the client's skin type and condition.

Skin characteristics while looking at the skin type, the skin's additional characteristics may be seen. These include skin that may be sensitive, dehydrated, moist or oedematous (puffy).

Skin condition while looking at the skin type, additional characteristics may be seen that indicate its condition. These include skin that may be sensitive, dehydrated or mature.

Skin tone the strength and elasticity of the skin.

Skin type the different physiological functioning of each person's skin dictates their skin type. There are four main skin types normal (balanced), dry (lacking in oil), oily (excessive oil) and combination (a mixture of two skin types, e.g., dry and oily).

Specialist skincare service products additional skincare preparations available to target improvement. These products include eye gels, throat creams and ampoule services.

Steam service a warming effect created by boiling water, which is then vaporized and used on the skin to achieve both cleansing and stimulation.

Tapotement also known as percussion. A massage manipulation that is used for its general toning and stimulating effect.

Toning lotion a skincare preparation formulated to treat the different skin types and facial characteristics. It is applied to remove all traces of cleanser from the skin. It produces a cooling effect on the skin and has a skin-tightening effect.

Towel steaming an alternative to facial steaming using an electrical vapour unit. Small, clean facial towels are heated in a bowl of warm water or specialized heater before application to the face to warm, cleanse and stimulate the skin.

Vapour unit an electrical appliance that heats water to produce steam which is applied to the skin of the face and neck, to warm, cleanse and stimulate the skin.

Vibrations massage manipulations applied on the nerve centre. They stimulate the nerves to induce a feeling of well-being and to provide gentle stimulation of the skin.

ASSESSMENT OF KNOWLEDGE AND UNDERSTANDING

Having covered the learning objectives for **Provide facial skincare treatments**, test what you need to know and understand by answering the following short questions below.

The information covers:

- organizational and legal requirements
- how to work safely and effectively when performing facial services
- consultation service planning and preparation
- contra-indications
- facial services
- aftercare advice for clients

Anatomy and physiology questions required for this unit are found in Chapter 2.

Organizational and legal requirements

1   What are your responsibilities under the relevant health and safety legislation?

2   What actions must be taken before a client under 16 years of age receives facial?

3   How can you ensure you comply with the legislation of the Disability Discrimination Act?

4   Why must a client's signature be obtained before commencing facial service?

5   Taking into account health and safety hygiene requirements, how would you prepare yourself for service?

6   How should all client records be stored to comply with the Data Protection Act (1998)?

7   How long would you allow to complete a facial service?

8   Why is it important for staff to be familiar with the facial pricing structures?

9   What details should be recorded on the client's record card and why is it important to keep accurate records which are maintained?

How to work safely and effectively when performing facial services

1   What environmental conditions should be considered when setting up for a facial service? Why are these important?

2   What do you understand by the terms disinfection and sterilization? State two methods used in a facial service and when?

3   How can you ensure that skincare products and equipment are used hygienically?

4   How can you ensure that you and the client are correctly positioned for the facial service to avoid discomfort?

5   It may be necessary when preparing for the facial service to dispense products for use in the service. Why should these be dispensed only in the amounts according to your needs?

6   When should electrical equipment, such as the facial steamer be checked for good repair?

7   Give five examples of how the work area should be prepared ready for the next client following a facial service. Why is this important?

Consultation, service planning and preparation

1   Why is the client consultation important before service is provided?

2   Describe the different communication skills that you would need to use when performing a client consultation.

3   At the consultation you notice that the client has herpes simplex. What action do you take?

4   At the consultation a client asks your advice about a small lump on her skin that occasionally bleeds. What advice do your give her?

5   What is the legal relevance of client-questioning and recording the client's responses?

6   How can you ensure that the client will be relaxed and confident during the facial service?

7   How do you identify a client's skin type and their service requirements?

8   How can the client's current skincare routine relate to its appearance, condition and service requirements?

Contra-indications

1 Name three contra-indications that would prevent service being provided.

2 Name three contra-indications that would restrict service being provided.

3 How would you select and apply skin products for a client with an allergic skin type?

Facial services

1 How would you adapt facial techniques for a male client?

2 Design a facial service lasting one hour for each of the different skin types; oily, dry and combination. Describe:
   - the aim of the facial service
   - the facial service products you are going to use
   - when and how you will apply them
   - the different stages of the facial and how long each stage will last
   - any specialized products you are going to use

3 Describe how you would recognize the following skin conditions: sensitive, comedone, milia, dehydrated, broken capillaries, pustules, papules, open pores, hyperpigmentation, hypopigmentation, dermatosis papulosa nigra, pseudo folliculitis, keloids and in-growing hairs.

4 How do internal and external factors affect the skin?

5 What influences the regularity of facials?

6 When and why would you use a skin warming service?

7 What is the purpose of the following skincare products:
   - cleanser?
   - toning lotion?
   - exfoliant?
   - moisturiser?
   - face masks?

8 What are names of the different massage techniques? Explain how you would adapt facial massage application for a client with mature skin.

9 What is a specialist skin product? Give an example of when you would recommend this?

10 How would you select the massage medium to perform a facial massage?

11 What is the name given excessive redness that can occur during a facial? What could be the cause of this?

12 What is a contra-action? Describe three contra-actions that could occur during or following a facial service and how you would deal with each.

Aftercare advice for clients

1 What skincare products would you recommend that a client use as part of their home care routine?

2 Why is it important to provide the client with a home care routine?

3 How would you explain the correct application and where relevant, removal of the following products for home use:
   - cleansing milk?
   - cream exfoliant?
   - toning lotion?
   - non-setting face mask?
   - eye cream?
   - night cream?

4 Why is it important to tell the client about contra-actions that may occur? What advice would you give to a client?

5 How often would you recommend a full facial service?

6 A client may visit the salon for a mini-facial. What would this consist of, and why would you recommend this additional service?

8 Eyebrows and Eyelashes Services (B5)

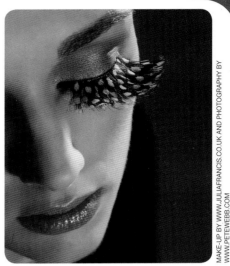

MAKE-UP BY WWW.JULIAFRANCIS.CO.UK AND PHOTOGRAPHY BY WWW.PETEWEBB.COM

B5 Unit Learning Objectives

This chapter covers **Unit B5 Enhance the appearance of eyebrows and eyelashes**.

This unit is about how to enhance and improve the appearance of the client's eyebrows and eyelashes using the practical skills of brow shaping, lash and brow tinting and application of artificial lashes. The service application will be selected and performed to meet the outcomes required.

There are **six** learning outcomes for Unit B5 which you must achieve competently:

1 Maintain safe and effective methods of working when enhancing the appearance of eyebrows and lashes

2 Consult, plan and prepare for the services with clients

3 Shape eyebrows

4 Tint eyebrows and lashes

5 Apply artificial eyelashes

6 Provide aftercare advice

Your assessor will observe you **on at least three occasions involving three different clients**. Your assessor will want to see you apply a partial set of artificial eyelashes and tinting eyebrows and eyelashes.

From the **range** statement, you must show that you have:

● used all **consultation techniques**

● taken the **necessary action** where a contra-action, contra-indication or treatment modification occurs

● provided a total **reshape** and **maintenance service** for the eyebrow

(continued on the next page)

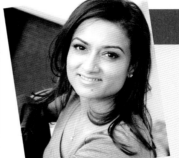

ROLE MODEL

Shavata Singh

*Brand Director
Shavata UK (encompassing
Shavata Brow Studio and
Lash Lounge by Shavata)*

" Eyebrows have always been a passion of mine. The entire process of creating the perfect arch fascinates me and I am constantly thinking of new ways to make this previously daunting beauty task simpler for my clients. This passion is one of the reasons I founded my first Brow Studio at the Urban Retreat, Harrods. This Brow Studio was my perfect solution for men and women who needed a quick, efficient, effective treatment, that takes just minutes and can transform your look. Shavata Brow Studios and Lash Lounges are now available in selected stores across the UK to help meet the demands of our clients and I have also developed my own range of fabulous products, which can help you to create the perfect brow in-between your studio appointments.

(continued)

- provided eyelash and eyebrow tinting to clients with the following hair colouring **characteristics:** fair, red, dark and white
- applied both **artificial lashes** strip and **individual flare lashes**
- applied **artificial lashes** using an **adhesive** and **solvent** to remove
- provided relevant advice

However you must prove that you have the necessary knowledge, understanding and skills to perform competently across the range.

When providing eyebrow and eyelash services it is important to use the skills you have learnt in the following units:

Unit G20 Make sure your own actions reduce risks to health and safety

Unit G18 Promote additional products or services to clients

Unit G8 Develop and maintain your effectiveness at work

Eyebrow hair removal

The eyebrows, situated above the bony eye orbits of the face, help to protect the eyes from moisture and dust, and to cushion the skin from physical injury. Misshapen bushy brows give an untidy appearance to the face; but when correctly shaped, the brows give balance to the facial features and enhance the eyes – the most expressive feature of the face.

Eyebrow shaping is offered in the salon as either an **eyebrow reshape** or **eyebrow maintenance** – the former involves removing eyebrow hair to create a new shape, the latter involves removing only a few stray hairs in order to maintain the existing shape.

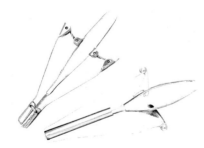

Automatic tweezers

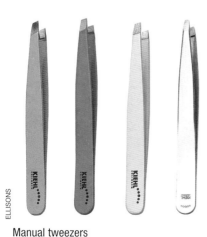

ELLISONS

Manual tweezers

Outcome 1: Maintain safe and effective methods of working when enhancing the appearance of eyebrows and eyelashes

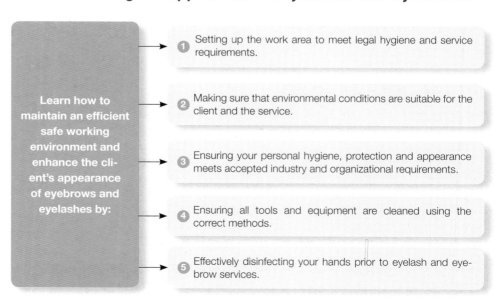

Learn how to maintain an efficient safe working environment and enhance the client's appearance of eyebrows and eyelashes by:

1. Setting up the work area to meet legal hygiene and service requirements.

2. Making sure that environmental conditions are suitable for the client and the service.

3. Ensuring your personal hygiene, protection and appearance meets accepted industry and organizational requirements.

4. Ensuring all tools and equipment are cleaned using the correct methods.

5. Effectively disinfecting your hands prior to eyelash and eyebrow services.

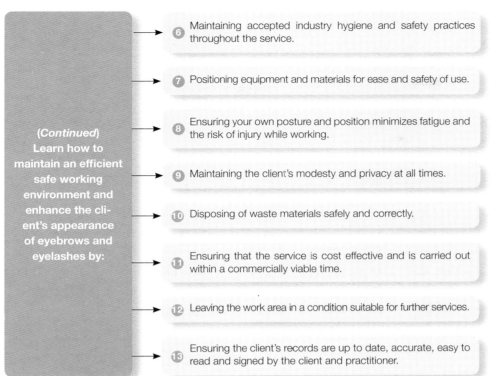

(Continued)
Learn how to maintain an efficient safe working environment and enhance the client's appearance of eyebrows and eyelashes by:

6 Maintaining accepted industry hygiene and safety practices throughout the service.

7 Positioning equipment and materials for ease and safety of use.

8 Ensuring your own posture and position minimizes fatigue and the risk of injury while working.

9 Maintaining the client's modesty and privacy at all times.

10 Disposing of waste materials safely and correctly.

11 Ensuring that the service is cost effective and is carried out within a commercially viable time.

12 Leaving the work area in a condition suitable for further services.

13 Ensuring the client's records are up to date, accurate, easy to read and signed by the client and practitioner.

HEALTH & SAFETY

Maintaining hygiene

Several pairs of tweezers must be purchased (perhaps five), due to the length of time required for sterilization. Buy good-quality stainless steel tweezers: cheaper metals rust after repeated sterilization. Disposable mascara wands are ideal for brushing the hairs during brow shaping.

Eyebrow shaping equipment

Before beginning the eyebrow shape service, check that you have the necessary equipment and materials to hand and that they meet legal hygiene and industry requirements for eye treatment services.

There are two sorts of tweezers used to shape the eyebrows. **Automatic tweezers** are designed to remove the bulk of excess hair; they have a spring-loaded action. **Manual tweezers** are used to remove stray hairs, and to accentuate the brow shape where more accurate care is required. They are available with various ends; which you use is a matter of personal preference, but slanted ends are generally considered to be the best for eyebrow shaping.

Although many beauty therapists may complete an eyebrow shaping using only one of these – automatic or manual tweezers – it is important to be skilled in the use of both these tools.

TOP TIP

Tweezers
When purchasing tweezers, make sure that the ends meet accurately so they will grasp the hair effectively.

Preparing the work area

Before the client is shown through to the work area, it should be checked to ensure that the required equipment and materials are available and the area is clean and tidy.

The plastic-covered couch should be clean, having been thoroughly washed with hot soapy water, or wiped thoroughly with a professional disinfectant cleaner. The couch or chair should be protected with a long strip of disposable paper bedroll placed to cover a freshly laundered sheet or bath towel. A small towel should be placed neatly at the head of the couch — for hygiene and protection during service. This will be draped across the client's chest. The tissue will need changing and the towels should be freshly laundered for each client.

The couch or beauty chair should be positioned flat or slightly elevated when performing the service.

Equipment materials

Before beginning the eyebrow shaping service check that you have the necessary equipment and materials to hand and that they meet the legal, hygiene and industry requirements for eye treatment services.

EQUIPMENT AND MATERIAL LIST

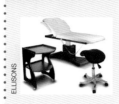

Couch or beauty chair
With sit-up and lie-down positions and an easy-to-clean surface
Trolley
On which to place everything

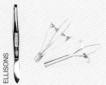

Tweezers (sterilized)
Both automatic and manual

Orange sticks
To measure the length and arch of eyebrow when planning hair removal

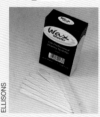

Disposable spatulas

Dry and damp cotton wool
To apply cleansing and soothing agents – and to collect hair removed during service

Scissors (stainless steel)
For trimming long hairs

Facial tissues (white)
For blotting the skin dry

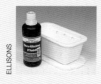

Disinfectant
For cleansing the tweezers before sterilization

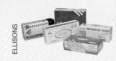

Disposable non-latex (synthetic), powder-free gloves
To be worn to prevent cross-infection

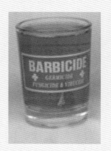

Barbicide jar
To store small stainless steel sterilized tools

YOU WILL ALSO NEED:

Disposable tissue Such as bedroll

Towels (2) (medium sized) Freshly laundered for each client

Eyebrow pencil Used to mark the skin when measuring brow length

Headband (clean) To keep hair away from the brow shaping area

Pencil sharpener (stainless steel) Suitable for use in the autoclave, used to sharpen the eyebrow pencil

Skin disinfectant To cleanse and disinfect the client's skin

Cleansing lotion Used to remove facial make-up from the eye area

Soothing lotion or gel With healing and antiseptic properties, suitable for the skin of the face

Hand mirror (clean) Used when discussing the brow shaping requirements and to show the client the finished result

Client record card To record the client's personal details, products used and details of the service

Light magnifier (cold) To magnify the area to ensure all hairs have been removed

Waste container This should be a lined metal bin with a lid

Eyebrow shaping, sterilization and disinfection

Sterilize tweezers at an appropriate time during the working day. Ensure that you always have sterile tweezers ready for use with each client. After they have been sterilized in the autoclave, the tweezers should be stored in the ultra-violet cabinet.

A fresh disinfectant solution may be used to store a spare pair of tweezers while carrying out an eyebrow service. This solution is usually dispensed into a small container stored on the trolley. (Spare tweezers are necessary in case you should accidentally drop the other tweezers during the service.) After the eyebrow shaping service, tweezers must be replaced and resterilized.

Disposable gloves may be worn for protection avoiding cross-infection during the eyebrow shaping service – the therapist may come into contact with tissue fluids from the client's skin.

As the waste from the service may contain body fluids and pose a health threat, it must be collected and disposed of carefully, in accordance with the local authority Environmental Health Department.

Permanent eyelash and eyebrow tinting

The hair of the eyelashes and eyebrows protects the eyes from moisture and dust, but the lashes and brows also give definition to the eye. Many clients, especially those with fair lashes and brows, feel that without the use of eye cosmetics their eyes lack this definition.

Further definition of the brow and lash hair can be created if a permanent dye is applied to them. Most clients will benefit from eyelash and eyebrow tinting because the tips and the bases of these hairs are usually lighter than the body of the hairs, causing the hairs to appear shorter than they actually are. Tinting the length of the lash or brow hair makes it appear longer and bolder, yet the effect created looks natural.

Because the skin around the eye area is very thin and sensitive, dyes designed for permanently tinting the hair in this area have been specially formulated to avoid any eye or tissue reactions. **The application of any other dye materials in this area is dangerous, and may even lead to blindness**.

Permanent tints are available in different forms, including jelly, liquid and cream tints. The most popular and acceptable permanent tinting product is the cream tint: this is thicker, so it does not run into the eye and it is easy to control during mixing, application and removal.

Several colours of permanent tint are available, including brown, grey, blue and black.

If the shade you want is not available, you can vary the shade of available tints by leaving the dye on the hair for different lengths of time, or by mixing different colours together. For example, to produce a navy blue colour; leave the tint to process for three to five minutes. If left to process for ten minutes, the same tint will produce a raven blue-black colour.

TOP TIP

Blue tint
When a client requests a blue eyelash tint, make clear that this will not produce an 'electric blue' fashion colour.

HEALTH & SAFETY

Permanent tinting
Always use a tint that is permitted for use under EU regulations and complies with the Cosmetic Products (Safety) Regulations 2003. If you use any other tint your insurance may be invalid.

HEALTH & SAFETY

Peroxide strength
Do not use a higher strength than 10-volume or 3% hydrogen peroxide. If you do, skin irritation or minor skin burning may occur.

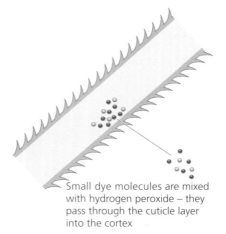

Small dye molecules are mixed with hydrogen peroxide – they pass through the cuticle layer into the cortex

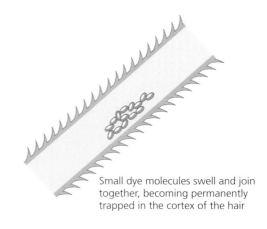

Small dye molecules swell and join together, becoming permanently trapped in the cortex of the hair

Permanent hair colouring

The development of colour

Two products are essential for the permanent tinting service:

- professional **eyelash** or **eyebrow tint**
- hydrogen peroxide (H_2O_2)

The tint contains small molecules of permanent dye called toluenediamine. These need to be 'activated' before their colouring effect becomes permanent: this is achieved by the addition of hydrogen peroxide. The peroxide is said to **develop** the colour of the tint.

Chemically, hydrogen peroxide is an **oxidant**, a chemical that contains available oxygen atoms and encourages certain chemical reactions – in this case, tinting.

The hydrogen peroxide container will state either its volume or its percentage strength. To activate the tint and for safe use around the eye area, a 3% or 10-volume strength peroxide is used.

When you add the hydrogen peroxide to the tint, the small dye molecules together form large molecules, which remain trapped in the cortex of the hair. The hair is thus permanently coloured, but in time, as it continues to grow, the new hair will show the natural colour.

Preparing the work area
Before the client is shown through to the work area, it should be checked to ensure that the required equipment and materials are available and the area is clean and tidy.

Clean and protect the couch or beauty chair as for the eyebrow-shaping service. The couch or chair should be flat or slightly elevated.

The work area should be adequately lit to ensure that service can be given, safely, but avoid bright lighting that could cause eye irritation.

Equipment and materials

Before beginning the tinting service, check that you have the necessary equipment and materials to hand and that they meet the legal hygiene and industry requirements for eye treatment services.

EQUIPMENT AND MATERIAL LIST

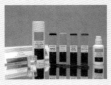

Coloured tints (a selection)

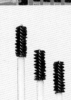

ELLISONS

Disposable brushes (2) To comb through the lash/brow hair following service

YOU WILL ALSO NEED:

Couch or beauty chair With sit-up and lie-down positions and an easy-to-clean surface

Trolley On which to place everything

Towels (2) (medium-sized) Freshly laundered for each client

Headband (clean) To protect long hair or bleached hair from the tint

Cleansing lotion Used to remove facial make-up from the eye area

Eye make-up remover (non-oily) To cleanse the eye area before service application

Hydrogen peroxide (10-volume/3%)

Petroleum jelly To protect the skin and prevent skin staining

Damp cotton wool For cleansing the eye area and for lash and brow tint removal and to soothe the area following eyelash tinting

Eye shields (commercial) To prevent skin staining during eyelash tinting

Facial tissues (white) For blotting the eye area dry

Disposable spatulas For removing the petroleum jelly from its container

Disposable non-latex (synthetic), powder-free gloves To be worn if allergic to permanent tint products

Non-metallic bowl For mixing the permanent tint (note that some metals cause immediate release of the oxygen from the hydrogen peroxide, causing ineffective processing of the tint)

Skin stain remover To remove any accidental staining

Bowl (clean) To hold dampened cotton wool

Waste container This should be a lined metal bin with a lid

Hand mirror (clean) To show the client the finished results

Client record card To record the client's personal details, products used and details of the service

Sterilization and disinfection Hygiene must be maintained in a number of ways:

- It is necessary to use disposable applicator brushes for the application of the petroleum jelly and the permanent tint because it is impossible to disinfect brushes effectively.
- Dispense products from containers, e.g. petroleum jelly.
- Maintain high standards of personal hygiene.
- Disinfect work surfaces after every client.
- All towels should be replaced with freshly laundered towels following each service.

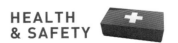

HEALTH & SAFETY

Applicator brushes

Because it is impossible to sterilize applicator brushes effectively, use disposable brushes for the application of petroleum jelly and permanent tint.

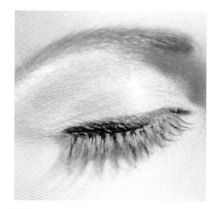

False eyelashes

Artificial eye lashes

False eyelashes are made from small threads of nylon fibre or real hair. They are attached to the client's natural lash hair imitating the natural eyelashes and making the lashes appear longer and thicker, and thereby drawing attention to the eye. There are two main types: **semi-permanent strip lashes** and **individual flare lashes**.

Artificial lashes are applied for the following reasons:

- to create shape and depth in the eye area, when completing corrective eye make-up
- simply to add definition to the eye area
- to enhance evening or fantasy make-up
- to provide thick long lashes for photographic make-up
- to provide an alternative eyelash-enhancing effect for a client who is allergic to mascara

Strip lashes Artificial **strip lashes** are designed to be worn for a short period, either for a day or an evening. They are attached to the natural eyelashes with a soft, weak adhesive. After removal the strip must be cleaned before re-application.

Individual flare lashes Artificial individual flare lashes are attached to the natural lashes with a strong adhesive. They may be worn for approximately four to six weeks, and are therefore known as **semi-permanent lashes**.

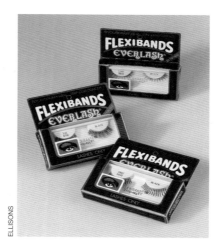

Strip lashes

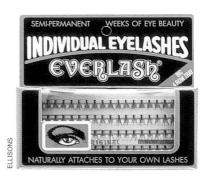

Individual flare lashes

Preparing the work area

Before the client is shown through to the work area, check it to ensure that the required equipment and materials are available and the area is clean and tidy. The plastic-covered couch should be clean, having been thoroughly washed with hot, soapy water and wiped thoroughly with a professional disinfectant cleaner. The couch or chair should be protected with a long strip of disposable tissue-paper bedroll, placed to cover a freshly laundered sheet or bath towel. A small towel should be placed neatly at the head of the couch, ready to be draped across the client's chest for protection during treatment. (The paper tissue will need changing and the towels will need to be laundered for each client.)

The couch or beauty chair should be in a slightly elevated position, to give the optimum position for the beauty therapist when applying the artificial lashes. In this position, too, the client will not be staring into the overhead light (which might cause the eyes to water).

Equipment and materials

Before beginning the artificial eyelash application, check that you have the necessary equipment and materials to hand to meet legal, hygiene and industry requirements for eye treatment services.

EQUIPMENT AND MATERIAL LIST

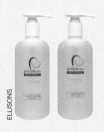

Couch or beauty chair
With sit-up and lie-down positions and an easy-to-clean surface

Trolley
On which to display everything

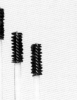

Headband (clean)
To to keep hair away from the treatment area
A large clip may be used if the hair been styled

Eye make-up remover (non-oily)
To remove make-up and general skin debris and natural oils from the area

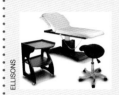

Facial tissues (white)
For blotting the eyelashes dry

Disposable mascara brush
To avoid cross-contamination

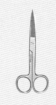

Manual tweezers (2 pairs) (sterilized)
Special tweezers are available, designed specifically to assist in attaching individual eyelashes

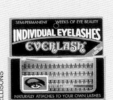

Strip eyelash lengths (a selection)
In a choice of colours

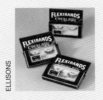

Individual eyelash lengths (a selection)
In a choice of colours

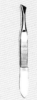

Sterilised scissors (1 pair)
Used for trimming the length of strip lashes

YOU WILL ALSO NEED:

Towels (2) (medium-sized) Freshly laundered for each client

Disposable tissue roll For example, bedroll

Cleansing lotion Used to remove facial make-up from the eye area

Damp cotton wool For removing cleansing product from the eye area

Cotton wool buds To apply solvent when removing individual flare lashes

Surgical spirit For wiping the points of the tweezers to remove adhesive

Plastic palette (disinfected) On which to place the artificial lashes prior to application

Disinfected dish (small) Lined with foil, in which to place the eyelash adhesive during lash application

Hand mirror (clean) To show the client the finished result

Client record card To record the client's personal details, products used and details of the service

Waste container Should be a lined metal bin with a lid

HEALTH & SAFETY

In order that you can effectively clean the dish containing the eyelash adhesive after the treatment, you need to line the dish with a disposable lining

Sterilisation and disinfection Hygiene must be maintained in a number of ways:

- When preparing to apply artificial *strip* lashes, clean the surface of the palette onto which you will stick the lashes once you have removed them from their packet. Use disinfectant, applied with clean cotton wool. The palette may be stored in the ultra-violet light cabinet until ready for use. *Individual* flare lashes come in a special 'contoured' package: you can hold this securely while removing individual flare lashes, so the lashes can be kept hygienically until required.

- Always have a spare pair of tweezers available during application of the individual or strip artificial lashes. Should you accidentally drop the tweezers with which you are working, you will need a clean, sterile pair available.

- Scissors, used to trim strip lashes, should be sterilized before use.

- Dispense products from containers, e.g. artificial lashes adhesive.

- Maintain high standards of personal hygiene.

- Disinfect work surfaces after every client.

- All towels should be replaced with freshly laundered towels following each service.

Outcome 2: Consult, plan and prepare for the service with clients

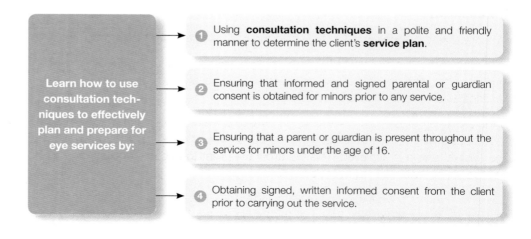

Learn how to use consultation techniques to effectively plan and prepare for eye services by:

1. Using **consultation techniques** in a polite and friendly manner to determine the client's **service plan**.

2. Ensuring that informed and signed parental or guardian consent is obtained for minors prior to any service.

3. Ensuring that a parent or guardian is present throughout the service for minors under the age of 16.

4. Obtaining signed, written informed consent from the client prior to carrying out the service.

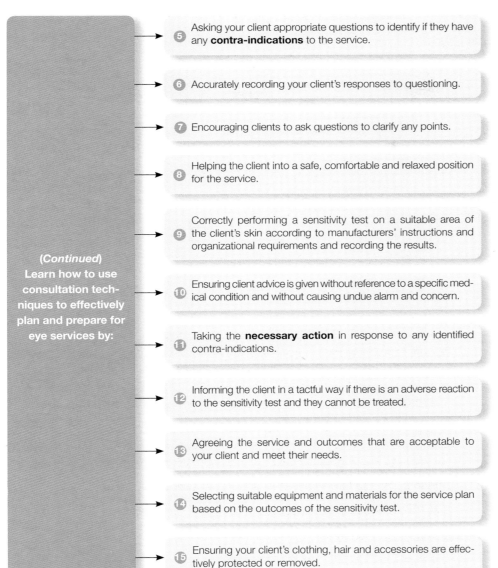

(Continued)
Learn how to use consultation techniques to effectively plan and prepare for eye services by:

5 Asking your client appropriate questions to identify if they have any **contra-indications** to the service.

6 Accurately recording your client's responses to questioning.

7 Encouraging clients to ask questions to clarify any points.

8 Helping the client into a safe, comfortable and relaxed position for the service.

9 Correctly performing a sensitivity test on a suitable area of the client's skin according to manufacturers' instructions and organizational requirements and recording the results.

10 Ensuring client advice is given without reference to a specific medical condition and without causing undue alarm and concern.

11 Taking the **necessary action** in response to any identified contra-indications.

12 Informing the client in a tactful way if there is an adverse reaction to the sensitivity test and they cannot be treated.

13 Agreeing the service and outcomes that are acceptable to your client and meet their needs.

14 Selecting suitable equipment and materials for the service plan based on the outcomes of the sensitivity test.

15 Ensuring your client's clothing, hair and accessories are effectively protected or removed.

ALWAYS REMEMBER

Permanent brow colouring
By permanently tinting brow hair before shaping you will colour any finer lighter hairs, which will then form part of the brow.

Shape eyebrows

Reception

When making an appointment it is usual to allow 15 minutes for each service.

It is wise to have a designated time between services so that there is no confusion between the two services. For example, under two weeks could be regarded as a maintenance, and over two weeks as a reshape.

If the client has thick, heavy brows, or if they do not have their brows shaped regularly, they should be encouraged to have them shaped gradually over a period of weeks, until the desired shape is achieved. This will allow the client to become accustomed to the new shape and will minimize any discomfort.

Eyebrow shaping may be carried out as an independent service, or combined with other services such as permanent tinting of the brows. In the latter case, the brows should

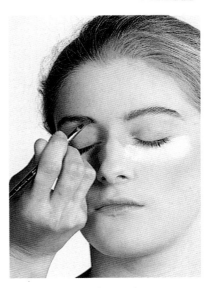

Applying temporary brow colour

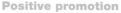

BEST PRACTICE

Positive promotion
While the client is having their eyebrows shaped, you have an ideal opportunity to discuss further possible services, such as an eyebrow tint.

Communication
At the consultation, identify any peculiarities such as bald patches or scarring in the brow area to avoid any confusion or concern later.

be tinted before shaping, to avoid the tint coming into contact with the open follicle and perhaps causing an allergic reaction.

Before brow-shaping service commences, carry out a consultation. Discuss the shape and the effect that might be achieved. Consider such factors as age, the natural shape of the brow, and fashion.

Remember for all eye services if a client is under the age of 16, it is necessary to obtain parent/guardian permission for the service. They will also have to be present when the service is received.

Contra-indications

When a client attends for an eyebrow shaping service, the therapist should always check that there are no contra-indications that might prevent the service.

If while completing the record card or on visual inspection of the skin the client is found to have any of the following in the eye area, eyebrow shaping service must not be carried out:

- **hypersensitive skin** – the skin could become excessively red and swollen
- **any eye disorder**, such as those described in the chart below
- **inflammation or swelling**– the cause may be medical
- **skin disease**
- **skin disorder**, such as psoriasis or eczema
- **bruising** – client discomfort could be caused and the condition made worse
- **cuts or abrasions** – secondary infection could occur
- **scar tissue under six months old** – the skin lacks elasticity

The following chart will help you to identify some eye disorders that contra-indicate eyebrow-shaping services and also tinting eyebrows and lashes and artificial eyelash application.

Name	Description	Name	Description
Conjunctivitis or pink eye	Infectious bacterial infection. Inflammation of the mucous membrane that covers the eye and lines the eyelid. The skin of the inner conjunctiva of the eye becomes inflamed, the eye becomes very red, itchy and sore, and pus may exude from the eye area.	Watery eye or epiphora	The eye over-secretes tears, which would normally drain into the nasal cavity.
Stye or hordeola	Infectious bacterial infection. Infection of the sebaceous glands of the eyelash hair follicles. Small lumps appear on the inner rim of the eyelid containing pus.	Blepharitis	Inflammation of the eyelid caused by infection or an allergic reaction.

Name	Description	Name	Description
Cyst	Localized pocket of sebum, which forms in the hair follicle or under the sebaceous glands in the skin. Semi-globular in shape, either raised or flat, and hard or soft. The cysts are the same colour as skin, or red if bacterial infection occurs. A cyst appearing on the upper eyelid is known as a chalazion or meibomian cyst.	Non-gloss	Benign (non-malignant) tumor. Harmless skin-coloured growths. They may appear as a 'thread' of skin on the eyelids growing between the eyelashes. Chemical services such as tinting and perming should be avoided to avoid skin irritation. Refer the client to their GP.

If you are unsure about the safety of proceeding with service – for example, if there is an undiagnosed lump in the area – ask your client to seek medical approval first. Remember you are not qualified to diagnose a contra-indication. Refer the client to their GP without causing unnecessary cause for concern.

Discuss possible contra-actions that may occur during or after the eyebrow shaping service with your client at consultation.

Contra-actions

Erythema is considered to be a **contra-action** to the service: it is recognized as a marked reddening of the skin seen over the whole area or specifically around one damaged follicle. It is usually accompanied by minor swelling of the area. If this occurs the beauty therapist must try to reduce the redness by applying a cool compress and soothing antiseptic lotion or cream to the area. In extreme cases it may be necessary to apply ice. Record details of any contra-action on the client's record card.

If the reddening reduces in response to your corrective action, you may decide in future to remove only a few stray hairs at each eyebrow-shaping service, to minimize the risk of this reaction recurring.

Planning the service: factors to be considered

Before shaping the brows you must consider the following factors.

The natural shape of the brow The natural brow follows the line of the eye socket. This varies greatly between clients, and affects what is achievable.

If the client has been shaping their own brows, it may be necessary to let them grow for a short period before shaping them professionally. If the brows are very thin or very thick, it may take several sessions before the desired shape is achieved.

If the brows have been plucked over a long period of time, they may not grow back successfully; this should be discussed with the client. In such instances, temporary eyebrow pencil or matt powder eye shadow may be used to achieve the desired effect. Temporary

HEALTH & SAFETY

Contra-action: using ice
To maintain hygiene, place the ice cube in a new small freezer food bag. Dispose of the bag hygienically after use.

Discuss possible contra-actions that may occur during or after the eyebrow shaping service with your client at consultation.

Believe in the product Believe in what you are selling, if you do not like the products it will be very hard to convince someone else that they should have them.

Be confident, when selling and use the products yourself.

Shavata Singh

TOP TIP

Temporary brow colour

A sharpened eyebrow pencil may be used to simulate brow hairs – apply feathery strokes using the pencil point. To create a natural effect, two different pencil colours may be used, for example brown and grey.

> **Practise excellent customer service**
>
> - Promote great grooming.
> - Be passionate about eyebrows.
> - A successful beauty therapist will have a natural talent with people.
> - Stay level-headed.
> - Be precise!
>
> **Shavata Singh**

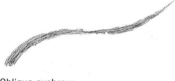

Oblique eyebrow

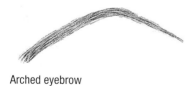

Arched eyebrow

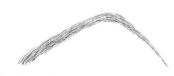

Angular eyebrow

brow colour is useful to apply when growing hairs into a new brow shape, to create a defined brow shape.

Fashion Each season sees new fashion trends, which also affect eye make-up and eyebrow shapes. This should be considered before using any form of permanent hair removal to shape the brows.

TOP TIP

Male eyebrow shaping

Men may require a result that emphasizes their natural brow shape. This generally requires removing hair as shown below:

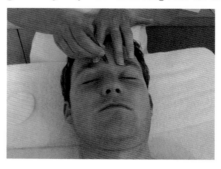

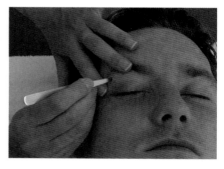

From the area between the brows where the brow hairs may meet. This brow hair if not removed can give the client a stern took.

Underneath the lower outer brow which will open up the eye area. This brow hair if not removed can create a hooded effect to the eyelid.

The age of the client The brow hair of older clients may include a few coarse, long, discoloured white or grey hairs. These may be removed provided that this does not alter the brow line or leave bald patches.

In general, thick eyebrows make the client look older, by creating a hooded appearance; and thin eyebrows will make the client look severe. Ideally the brows should therefore be shaped to a medium thickness.

The natural growth pattern The shape and effect that the client requests may be made impossible by the pattern of the natural growth of the hair, which is genetically determined. When shaping the brows of the Oriental client, for example, you will notice that the eyebrow hair grows in a downward direction. To create an arch it may be necessary to trim the hairs, using a small, sterile pair of sharp nail scissors. Alternatively, you may remove the outer eyebrow length and use a cosmetic pencil to create a new brow-line. Use your professional judgement to advise the client.

Choosing an eyebrow shape

The eyebrows should be in balance with the rest of the facial features: the right brow shape for each client will depend on the client's facial proportions and natural brow shape.

There is no single ideal brow shape; different brow shapes are shown here.

What is achievable? Obviously not all of these brow shapes are achievable for every client, but the skilful application to the eyebrows of temporary cosmetic colour can create the illusion of the desired brow shape.

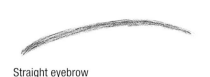

Straight eyebrow

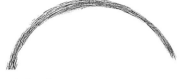

Rounded eyebrow

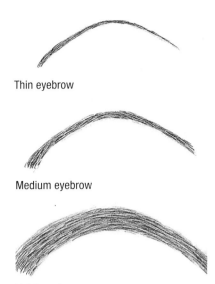

Thin eyebrow

Medium eyebrow

Thick eyebrow

The quantity of brow hair removed during shaping produces a thin, medium or thick final shape, as illustrated. Other approaches, too, may be used:

- **Semi-permanent make-up**, also referred to as micro-pigmentation, can be used to add colour permanently to the brows, for example to disguise a bald patch.

- **Hair transplants** are available for the client with sparse eyebrows.

- **False individual eyebrow hairs** are applied in the same way as individual false eyelashes.

Ideally, the distance between the two eyebrows should be the width of one eye. If this is not the case, the illusion may be created by removing hairs or by applying temporary brow colour to create this effect.

TOP TIP

Semi-permanent make-up

Suspended pigment particles in a liquid base are inserted into the outer skin using a disposable needle. Many of the popular dyes are based on plant extracts.

The effect gradually fades, lasting up to three years.

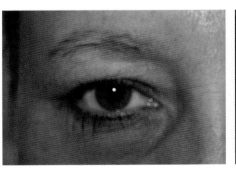

Before

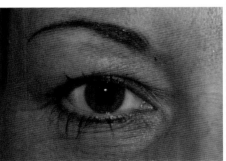

After

TOP TIP

False eyebrows

These are ideal for disguising any bald areas in the natural eyebrow hair.

Wide-set eyes can be made to appear closer together by extending the brow-line beyond the inside corner of the eye; close-set eyes can be made to look further apart by widening the distance between them.

How to measure the eyebrows to decide length

In order to determine the correct length of the client's eyebrows, there are three main guidelines:

1 Place an orange stick or spatula beside the nose and the inside corner of the eye. This is usually in line with the tear duct. Any hairs that grow between the eyes and beyond this point should be removed. If the client has a very broad nose, however, this guide is inappropriate: tweezing would commence near the middle of the brow. In this instance, use the tear duct at the inside corner of the eye as a guide (as per image).

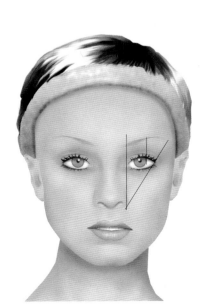

Measuring the eyebrow

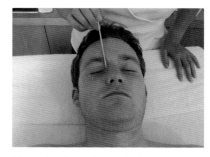

Measuring the eyebrow: the inner eye

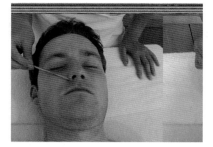

Measuring the eyebrow: the inner eye

ACTIVITY

Correcting brow shapes through brow-shaping service (2)

How would you correct the following eye shapes:

- wide-set?
- close-set?

ACTIVITY

Correcting brow shapes (3)

From magazines, collect pictures of faces showing different eyebrow shapes. Discuss which you think are correct and which incorrect for the person, explaining why.

ALWAYS REMEMBER

Accurately record your client's answers to necessary questions to be asked at the consultation.

2 Place an orange stick or spatula in a line from the base of the nose (to the side of the nostril) to the outer corner of the eye. Any hairs that grow beyond this point should be removed.

3 Place an orange stick or spatula in a vertical line from the centre of the eyelid. This is where the highest point of the arch should be.

Initially these guidelines will be needed to ensure that the correct length and brow shape are achieved, but the experienced therapist will recognize the corrective work to be carried out without the need for measuring.

ACTIVITY

Correcting brow shapes (1)

You cannot change the bone structure of the facial features without cosmetic surgery, but brow shaping can create the illusion of improved facial balance and proportion. Discuss why each of the brow shapes below would complement the accompanying face shape.

Face shape		Correct brow shape
Square	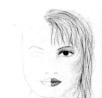	Arched
Round		Oblique
Oblong	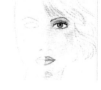	Straight
Pear (triangular)		Angular
Heart	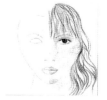	Oblique

Following the consultation, record all client details accurately on the client record card. A record card that can be used for the eye services follows.

The following record card is designed to record details of all **Eyebrow and eyelashes services**.

A sample client record card

Date	Beauty therapist name	
Client name		Date of birth (Identifying client age group.)
Home address		Postcode
Landline phone number	Mobile phone number	Email address
Name of doctor	Doctor's address and phone number	
Related medical history (Conditions that may restrict or prohibit service application.)		
Are you taking any medication? (This may affect the condition of the skin or skin sensitivity.)		

CONTRA-INDICATIONS REQUIRING MEDICAL REFERRAL
(Preventing eye service application.)
- ☐ severe skin conditions, (e.g. eczema in area)
- ☐ eye infections (e.g. conjunctivitis, styes)
- ☐ eye disease
- ☐ inflammation of the skin

EYE SERVICE
- ☐ shaping eyebrows
- ☐ tinting eyebrow hair
- ☐ tinting eyelashes
- ☐ false eyelashes
- ☐ threading

BROW SHAPE WORK TECHNIQUES
- ☐ brow shape selected following measurement of the client's natural brow and eye for brow shaping service
- ☐ opening of the pores and hair follicle to facilitate removal
- ☐ keeping the skin taut
- ☐ removal of hairs in the direction of hair growth
- ☐ protection of the eye
- ☐ hair removed to complement the shape and proportions of client's natural brow, in relation to facial features and shape and to client's satisfaction

THREADING TECHNIQUE
- ☐ mouth ☐ neck ☐ hand

TREATMENT AREA
- ☐ eyebrows
- ☐ total reshape
- ☐ maintenance of original shape

CONTRA-INDICATIONS WHICH RESTRICT SERVICE
(Service may require adaptation.)
- ☐ recent scar tissue
- ☐ eye disorders
- ☐ skin allergies
- ☐ bruising

TINTING WORK TECHNIQUES
- ☐ skin test carried out
- ☐ tint colour selection suited to client's colouring characteristics
- ☐ effectively protecting the surrounding skin
- ☐ timing, development and removal of tint adapted according to client's natural colouring characteristics
- ☐ manufacturer's instructions complied with

COLOURING CHARACTERISTIC

fair ☐   red ☐   dark ☐   white ☐

FALSE EYE LASHES
- ☐ skin test carried out
- ☐ colour and length of lash type selected to meet agreed service requirement and effect to be achieved
- ☐ individual flare lash
- ☐ strip lash
- ☐ manufacturer's instructions complied with

Beauty therapist signature (for reference)
Client signature (confirmation of details)

A sample client record card (continued)

SERVICE ADVICE

Eyebrow shape – *allow 15 minutes*
Eyebrow tint – *allow 10 minutes*
Eyelash tint* – *allow 20 minutes*
Eyebrow shape and eyelash tint* – *allow 30 minutes*

Eyebrow tint, shape and lash tint* – *allow 30 minutes*
Artificial eyelashes – *allow 20 minutes*
*Eyelash tint timing may differ according to the system used. Always follow the manufacturer's instructions.

SERVICE PLAN

Record relevant details of your service and advice provided for future reference.

Ensure the client's records are up to date, accurate and fully completed following service. Non-compliance may invalidate insurance.

DURING

Find out:
- what products the client is currently using to cleanse and care for the skin of the eye area
- satisfaction with these products

Explain:
- how the different eye products should be applied and removed

Note:
- any adverse reaction, if any occur

AFTER

Record:
- results of service
- any modification to service application that has occurred
- what products have been used in the eyelash/eyebrow service
- the effectiveness of service
- any samples provided (review their success at the next appointment)

Advise on:
- product application and removal in order to gain maximum benefit from product use
- use of aftercare products following eye service
- use of skincare/make-up products following eye service
- maintenance procedures
- recommended time intervals between services

RETAIL OPPORTUNITIES

Advise on:
- progression of the service plan for future appointments
- products that would be suitable for the client to use at home to care for the eye area
- recommendations for further services
- further products or services that the client may or may not have received before

Note:
- any purchase made by the client

EVALUATION

Record:
- comments on the client's satisfaction with the service
- if poor results are achieved, the reasons why
- how you may alter the service plan to achieve the required service results in the future, if applicable

HEALTH AND SAFETY

Advise on:
- how to care for the area following service to avoid an unwanted reaction
- avoidance of any activities or product application that may cause a contra-action
- appropriate necessary action to be taken in the event of an unwanted skin or eye irritation

ALWAYS REMEMBER

Examples of eye service modification include:

Eyebrow shape

- Avoiding removing hair that is concealing a bald area e.g. scar in the area.
- Hair removal when shaping a male client's eyebrows.

Eyelash tint

- Allowing further processing time to an area where the hair is more resistant to colour.

Artificial eyelashes

- Selecting an alternative lash length appropriate to the function of the lens, if the client wears glasses.
- If long-sighted, the lens will magnify the eye creating an unrealistic look if the artificial lash length is too long.

Tint eyebrow and lashes consultation

Reception

When making an appointment for this service, allow five minutes for a skin test, ten minutes for an eyebrow tint, and 20 minutes for an eyelash tint. When the client is booking a service, ask them:

- to visit the salon 24 hours before the appointment for a skin test
- if they wear contact lenses, to bring their lens container so that they can place the lenses in it during the tinting service

On average, a client will need their lashes tinted every six weeks, or sooner if for example they take a holiday in a climate where sun bleaches them. Eyebrow tinting, on the other hand, should be repeated when the client feels it to be necessary, perhaps every four weeks, as eyebrows seem to lose colour intensity more quickly than lash hair.

Skin sensitivity test

Some clients are sensitive to the tint, and produce an allergic reaction immediately on contact with it; others may become allergic later. For this you therefore need to carry out a **skin sensitivity test** before each lash- or brow-tinting service. (The skin sensitivity test, a hypersensitivity test, or a predisposition test – see pages 148–149.) This test should be given either on the inside of the elbow or behind the ear.

Two responses to the skin sensitivity test are possible – positive and negative:

- a **positive skin sensitivity test** result is recognized by irritation, swelling or inflammation of the skin – if this occurs, do not proceed with the service
- a **negative skin sensitivity test** result produces no skin reaction – in this case you may proceed with the service

Contra-indications

When a client attends for an eyelash or brow tinting service, the beauty therapist should always check that there are no contra-indications that might prevent service.

TOP TIP

It is acceptable for the salon receptionist – provided that they have been trained to do so – to carry out the skin test.

ACTIVITY

Eyelash and eyebrow tinting
List reasons why clients would benefit from this service. Discuss the reasons with your assessor.

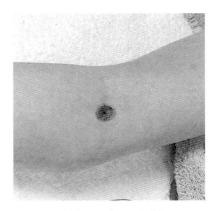

A skin sensitivity test for eyelash/brow tinting

After completing the record card and inspecting the eye area, if you have found any of the following in the eye area, do not proceed with the tinting service:

- *inflammation or swelling* – the cause may be medical
- *skin disease*
- *skin disorder*, such as psoriasis or eczema
- *cuts and abrasions* – secondary infection and irritation of the skin could occur
- *hypersensitive skin* – the skin could become excessively red and swollen
- *any eye disorders*, such as conjunctivitis, blepharitis, styes or hordeola, watery eye, or cysts
- *a positive (allergic) reaction* to the skin sensitivity test
- *contact lenses* (unless removed)

Look back at the earlier chart illustrating some contra-indications to eye services.

Remember you are not qualified to diagnose a contra-indication. Refer the client to their GP without causing unnecessary cause for concern.

A particularly nervous client would also be contra-indicated:

- it would be difficult for them to keep their eyes closed for ten minutes
- they might panic as the tint was applied, creating the possibility of tint entering the eye
- they might blink frequently, making preparation of the eye area and application of the tint both difficult and hazardous

Inform the client at consultation of any relevant contra-actions that may occur and the action to take.

Contra-actions

If the client complains of discomfort during the service, tint may have entered the eye. Take the following action:

1 Remove the tint immediately from the eye area, using clean, damp cotton wool pads in an outward sweep.

2 When you are satisfied that all excess tint has been removed (that is, when the cotton wool shows clean), carefully flush the eye with clean water. Repeat the rinsing process until discomfort has been relieved.

3 Apply a cool compress to cool and soothe the eye area.

If there is a noticeable sensitivity of the eye tissue after eyebrow or eyelash tinting it may be recommended that the client does not receive the service again. Alternatively, source an alternative tinting product to test compatibility. Record this on her record card so that the offending product may be avoided in the future.

In the event of an allergic contra-action the client should be advised to apply a cool compress and soothing agent to the skin to reduce redness and irritation. If symptoms persist they should seek medical advice.

Planning the service

For the eyelashes and eyebrows, select a colour that complements the client's hair **colouring characteristics**, fair, red, dark and white, her skin colour, her age and her usual

ACTIVITY

Allergic reactions
With colleagues, discuss the possible implications of ignoring a positive reaction to the skin test

ACTIVITY

Explaining poor results
What reasons can you think of to explain why a permanent tint applied to the eyelashes or eyebrows has not coloured the hair successfully? Discuss your answers with your tutor.

TOP TIP

Contra-action to product
Source an alternative manufacturer. The client may not be allergic to all products if the cause of the contra-action is allergy.

eye cosmetics. Always discuss the choice of colour carefully with the client to discover her preference. You may ask certain questions in order to help you in your selection:

● 'What colour mascara do you normally wear?'

● 'How dark would you like your eyelashes/eyebrows?'

● 'Do you normally wear eyebrow pencil? What colour?'

● 'Have you had your eyebrows/lashes tinted before? Were you satisfied with the result?'

Apply artificial lashes consultations

Reception

When making an appointment for false eyelash application, find out why the client wants artificial lashes and determine which type would be most appropriate.

Allow 20 minutes for the application of individual eyelashes; and again allow a further 45 minutes if applying them in conjunction with a make-up.

Although individual flare lashes can be worn for up to six weeks they look effective only for approximately three weeks. After this time, the appearance of the artificial lashes begins to deteriorate, the lash adhesive becomes brittle, and the eyelash area may become irritated.

Due to the cyclic nature of hair replacement some individual flare lashes will be lost when the natural lash falls out. These lashes may be replaced each week, as necessary; the client is usually charged a price for each individual flare lash replaced. The client must be told of this service as part of the aftercare advice.

When a client makes an appointment for an artificial lash treatment, they should be asked the following questions:

● **Have they had a similar treatment before in this salon?** If they have not, they should visit the salon beforehand for a skin test to assess any sensitivity to the adhesive (see page 447). Results should be recorded on the client record card.

● **Are they having the false eyelashes applied for any particular reason, such as a holiday or a special occasion?** In deciding which type of false eyelash would be most appropriate, take into consideration the effect required and for how long the lashes are to be worn.

If the client wears glasses, the artificial lashes must not be so long as to touch the lenses. Also, if the lens magnifies the eye, this must be taken into account. Ask the client to bring their glasses with them to the salon.

Contra-indications

If following completion of the record card or inspection of the eye area you have found any of the following, do not apply false eyelashes:

● **skin disease**

● **skin disorder in the eye area**, such as psoriasis or eczema

● **inflammation or swelling** around the eye

● **hypersensitive skin**

- **any eye disorder**, such as styes or hordeola, conjunctivitis, blepharitis, watery eye, or cysts

- **a positive (allergic) reaction** to the adhesive skin test

- **contact lenses** (unless removed)

A chart is shown pages 242–243 illustrating some contra-indications to eye treatment services.

Remember you are not qualified to diagnose a contra-indication. Refer the client to their GP without causing unnecessary cause for concern.

An unduly nervous client with a tendency to blink could also prove hard to treat in this way. Use your discretion in deciding on the suitability of a client for treatment.

Inform the client at consultation of any relevant contra-actions that may occur and the action to take.

Contra-actions

If during application of artificial lashes the eye starts to water, blot the tears with the corner of a clean tissue. The tears can cause the adhesive to take on an unsightly white crystal-lized appearance. Any possible irritation of the eyes should therefore be avoided, during both preparation of the eye area and application itself.

Never place eyelashes *underneath* the natural eyelashes – eye irritation would occur.

While practising individual eyelash application you may find at some point that you have accidentally glued a couple of the lower and upper natural lashes together. Apply adhesive **solvent** to a cotton wool-tipped orange stick, and gently roll this over the lash length to dissolve the adhesive.

If solvent or adhesive should accidentally enter the eye, remove excess product, rinse the eye thoroughly and immediately, using clean water. Repeat this until discomfort is no longer experienced.

The client should be shown through to the prepared work area after the record card has been completed.

Consult the record card and check the area for any contra-indications to service.

Remember always provide the opportunity for your client to ask any questions relating to the eye service.

The record card should be signed and dated by the client and beauty therapist following the consultation to confirm the suitability and consent with the agreed service.

It is important that accurate records are kept and stored in compliance with the Data Protection Act for future reference.

Planning the service

A variety of artificial lashes is available, including lashes intended for corrective work as well as those simply intended to enhance the natural lashes. Lash length may be short, medium or long; their texture may be fine, medium or thick, with some having a feathered effect. Strips designed for use on the lower lashes are called **partial lashes**: here small groups of hairs are placed intermittently along the length of the false-lash base.

In a commercial salon, the most popular colours are usually black and brown. For special effects, however; strip lashes are available in fantasy colours, complete with glitter and jewels!

TOP TIP

Fair lashes

If the client has fair lashes you could promote an eyelash tint service before false eyelash application to achieve a more natural, realistic effect.

TOP TIP

Individual flare lashes may be applied in a variety of lengths, short, medium and long, to create a natural look. The longest lashes are applied in the centre of the lashes.

TOP TIP

In America streaked lashes are available, to give a more subtle effect for the mature client.

Factors when choosing false eyelashes Before applying artificial lashes the beauty therapist should consider the following points, and advise the client accordingly.

The client's age Artificial lashes create a very bold, dramatic effect, which can make an older client look too hard. Remember that the skin colour and the natural hair colour change with age: the lash chosen must enhance the client's appearance.

The client's natural lashes Does the client have short or long, sparse or thick, very curly or straight lashes? Choose an artificial lash to complement the natural lash. Here are some guidelines:

- **Short and stubby lashes** These are commonly seen on older clients who have overhanging eyelids. Choose a medium lash length in a medium thickness at the outer corner of the eyelid; the lashes should become gradually shorter from the centre of the eyelid to the inner corner. Brush the artificial and natural lashes together after application to ensure that they blend.

- **Sparse lashes** Place individual short lashes along the natural lash line; or, to give a more natural appearance, you may wish to apply partial strip lashes to the upper eyelid.

- **Curly eyelashes** These are very common on African-Caribbean clients. Choose a longer, sweeping strip or individual artificial lashes, in black. The chosen lashes and colour should give emphasis and depth to the eye.

The natural eyelash colour Select artificial lashes that complement the hair and skin tone. Natural-hair false eyelashes offer the greatest choice of colour, but these are expensive and may be difficult to purchase.

Using false eyelashes for corrective purposes Here are some outlines of corrective techniques for various eye shapes.

Short and stubby lashes

Sparse lashes

Curly eyelashes

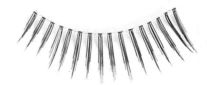

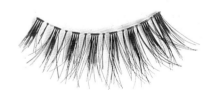

Artificial strip lashes

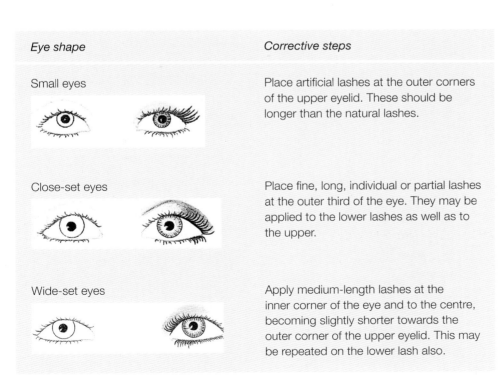

Eye shape	Corrective steps
Small eyes	Place artificial lashes at the outer corners of the upper eyelid. These should be longer than the natural lashes.
Close-set eyes	Place fine, long, individual or partial lashes at the outer third of the eye. They may be applied to the lower lashes as well as to the upper.
Wide-set eyes	Apply medium-length lashes at the inner corner of the eye and to the centre, becoming slightly shorter towards the outer corner of the upper eyelid. This may be repeated on the lower lash also.

ACTIVITY

Choosing eyelash colours
Suggest a choice of false eyelash colour for the clients below:

- a mature grey-haired client

- a young red-haired client

- a mature client with bleached hair

- a mature African-Caribbean client

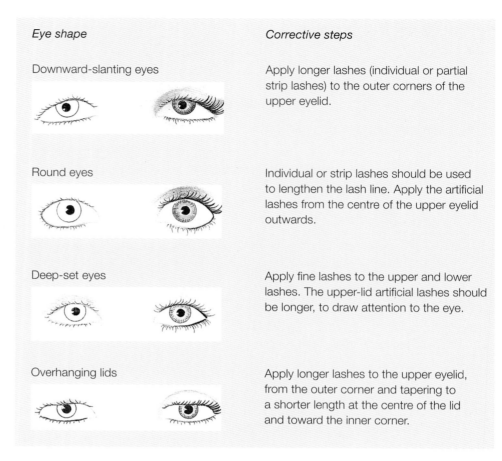

Eye shape	Corrective steps
Downward-slanting eyes	Apply longer lashes (individual or partial strip lashes) to the outer corners of the upper eyelid.
Round eyes	Individual or strip lashes should be used to lengthen the lash line. Apply the artificial lashes from the centre of the upper eyelid outwards.
Deep-set eyes	Apply fine lashes to the upper and lower lashes. The upper-lid artificial lashes should be longer, to draw attention to the eye.
Overhanging lids	Apply longer lashes to the upper eyelid, from the outer corner and tapering to a shorter length at the centre of the lid and toward the inner corner.

On completion the artificial lashes should give a balanced and well-proportioned look complementing the client's eye shape, producing the agreed desired effect.

Outcome 3: Shape eyebrows

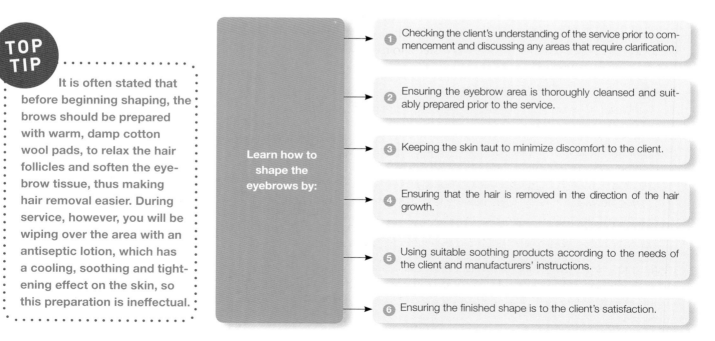

Learn how to shape the eyebrows by:

1. Checking the client's understanding of the service prior to commencement and discussing any areas that require clarification.

2. Ensuring the eyebrow area is thoroughly cleansed and suitably prepared prior to the service.

3. Keeping the skin taut to minimize discomfort to the client.

4. Ensuring that the hair is removed in the direction of the hair growth.

5. Using suitable soothing products according to the needs of the client and manufacturers' instructions.

6. Ensuring the finished shape is to the client's satisfaction.

How to shape the eyebrows

1 Position the cold-light magnifying lamp to give maximum visibility of the area.

2 Position the client on the couch.

3 Clean your hands using an approved hand cleaning technique.

4 Secure a clean headband in place, to keep client's hair away from treatment area.

5 Working from behind the client, cleanse the eyebrow area, using a lightweight cleansing lotion or eye make-up remover. Apply a mild antiseptic lotion to two damp cotton wool pads, then gently wipe each eyebrow. (This removes all grease from the area, so that the tweezers will not slip.) The brow area should then be blotted dry, using a clean, folded facial tissue.

6 Brush the brow hair with the disposable brush, first *against* the natural hair growth, then with it. This enables you to define the brow shape and to observe the natural line.

7 Measure the brows (using the guidelines on pages 245–246).

8 Place a clean piece of cotton wool in a convenient position for collecting the removed hairs, for instance at the top of the couch next to the client's head.

9 Best practice is to wear disposable gloves, as you may come into contact with body tissue fluid.

10 Begin tweezing, using a sterilized pair of automatic tweezers. These are designed to remove hairs quickly and efficiently, and are therefore used for the bulk of the hair identified for removal. It is usual to start at the bridge of the nose: the skin here is less sensitive than under the brow line.

11 Gently stretch the skin between the index and middle fingers, pressing lightly onto the skin. This will help you to avoid accidentally nipping the skin; it will also open the mouth of the hair follicle and minimize discomfort to the client.

12 Remove the hairs quickly, in the direction of growth. This prevents the hairs from breaking off at the skin's surface. Hair breakage can be seen to have occurred if a stubbly regrowth appears one or two days after shaping. Incorrect removal may also cause distortion of the hair follicle, or result in the hair becoming trapped under the skin as it starts to regrow (*ingrowing hair* – see Chapter 14, page 500).

Hairs should be removed individually, and the tweezers should be wiped regularly on the pad of clean cotton wool used to collect the removed hairs.

13 Remove the hairs from underneath the outer edge of the brow, working inwards towards the nose. It is advisable to work on each brow alternately. This ensures that the brows are evenly shaped; it also reduces prolonged discomfort in any one area during shaping. Hairs should ideally be removed only from *below* the brow, otherwise the natural line may be lost. It is sometimes necessary, however, to remove the odd stray hair growing *above* the natural line.

During shaping, show the client her brows and avoid removing too much hair.

14 At regular intervals during shaping, brush the brows to check their shape. Apply antiseptic lotion or gel to a clean, dampened cotton wool pad, and wipe this gently over the eyebrow tissue to reduce sensitivity and to sanitize the area.

HEALTH & SAFETY

Cross-infection
Use a fresh cotton wool pad for each eyebrow to avoid cross-infection.

TOP TIP

Occasionally clients start sneezing when you tweeze hairs at the bridge of the nose. If this happens, leave this area till last.

ALWAYS REMEMBER

Twenty per cent of hairs are not visible above the skin's surface at any one time. Explain this to the client so that they understand why stray hairs may appear shortly after service.

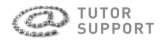

TUTOR SUPPORT

Activity 1: Methods of shaping project

HEALTH & SAFETY

Soothing lotion

Care should be taken when applying soothing lotion. If too much is applied it may run and enter the eye, causing further discomfort.

It is often best to apply a small amount of soothing lotion to a clean cotton wool pad, using a separate one for each eye to avoid cross-infection.

15 When the bulk of excess hair has been removed, manual tweezers may be used to take away any stray hairs and to define the line. Long hairs may be trimmed with scissors if necessary. Any discoloured, coarse, long, curly or wavy hairs may be removed, as long as this does not alter the line or leave a bald patch.

Brush the brows into shape and show the client the finished effect. The client may wish further hairs to be removed. Ask them to identify these. If you think this would be unsuitable explain why.

16 On completion of brow shaping, wipe the eyebrows with the antiseptic soothing lotion or gel, applied with clean, damp cotton wool. Apply a mild antiseptic cream to the area, using clean, dry cotton wool, to reduce the possibility of infection.

17 The hairs that have been removed should be disposed of hygienically.

18 Record details of the service on the client's record card.

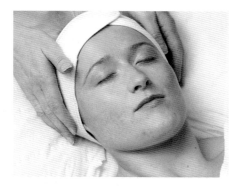

4 Protecting client's hair with headband.

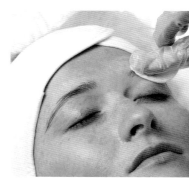

5 Cleansing the eyebrow.

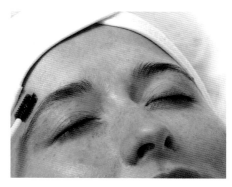

6 Brushing the eyebrow.

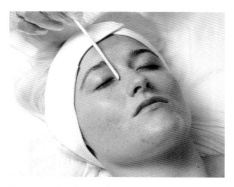

7 Measuring the eyebrow: the inner eye.

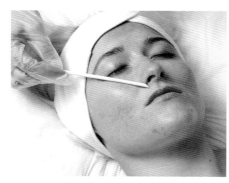

7 continued Measuring the eyebrow: the outer eye.

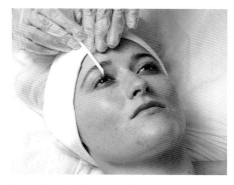

7 continued Measuring the eyebrow: the arch.

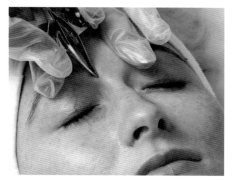

10 Tweezing at the bridge of the nose, using automatic tweezers.

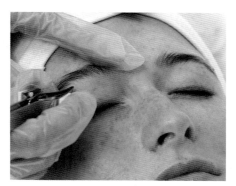

10 continued Tweezing at the outer corner of the eyebrow, using automatic tweezers.

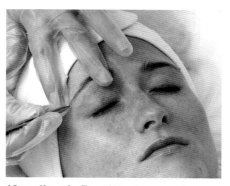

10 continued Tweezing using manual tweezers to define the finished eyebrow shape.

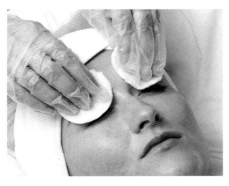
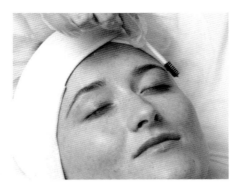
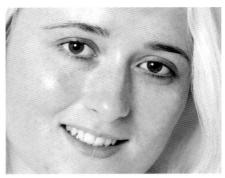

13 Applying antiseptic and soothing lotion.

14 Brushing the eyebrow into shape.

16 The completed eyebrows after shaping.

Tint the eyebrows and lashes

How to prepare the client

The client should be shown through to the cubicle after the record card has been completed.

1. Position the client comfortably, in a flat or slightly elevated position. If she is wearing contact lenses, these must be removed.

2. Drape a towel across the client's chest and shoulders, and protect her hair with a clean headband.

3. Wash your hands, which assures the client that the service is beginning in a hygienic and professional manner.

4. Consult the client's record card, then check the area for any visible contra-indications or abnormalities before proceeding.

5. Cleanse the area to be treated with a cleansing milk to dissolve facial make-up (if worn). Then use a non-oily eye make-up remover to remove eye products: apply this with clean, damp cotton wool.

6. To ensure that the area is thoroughly clean and grease-free, apply a mild toning lotion, stroked over the lash or brow hair.

7. Blot the eyelashes or eyebrows dry with a clean facial tissue. This ensures that the tint is not diluted, and also prevents the tint from being carried into the eye. Brush through the brows to separate the hair using a disposable brush. Note the fair root at the lash base.

8. Prepare the pre-shaped eye shields by applying petroleum jelly to the inner surface of each eye shield (the surface that comes into contact with the skin).

9. Ensure that the light is not shining directly into the client's eyes. If it were, the eyes might water, carrying the tint into the eye or down the face (causing skin staining).

10. Finally, check that the client is comfortable before beginning tint application.

11. Best practice is to wear disposable gloves to avoid contact with the tint that could lead to skin staining and possibly contact dermatitis. If worn, put on at this stage.

ALWAYS REMEMBER

When selecting and using permanent tint for a white-haired client, note that the hair is very often resistant to colour. The processing time may need to be increased. Note any modification on the record card for future reference.

> **Think on your feet.**
>
> For example, if a client is running late and there is a way to fit them in, then do it!
>
> Be confident with who you are and your skill set. If you give confidence, you will create it around you.
>
> Never agree to conduct a treatment that you do not feel is correct for the client. For example if the client wants to create something that you simply know will not suit her then be honest. She will appreciate it in the long run.
>
> **Shavata Singh**

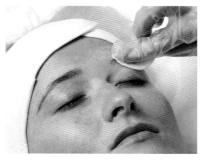

Cleansing the eye

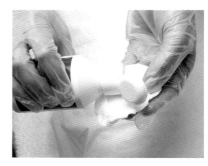

Apply a mild toning lotion

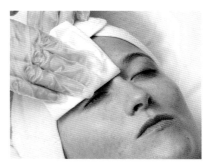

Blotting the brow hair to remove moisture

> **A great manager will...**
> - have regular updates and meetings
> - have newsletters that reward and make your team happy to be working with you
> - be a team player too
> - set high standards and lead by example
> - be a good communicator
>
> **Shavata Singh**

ALWAYS REMEMBER

The brows or lash hair to be tinted must be grease-free – the grease would be a barrier to the tint.

Outcome 4: Tint eyebrows and lashes

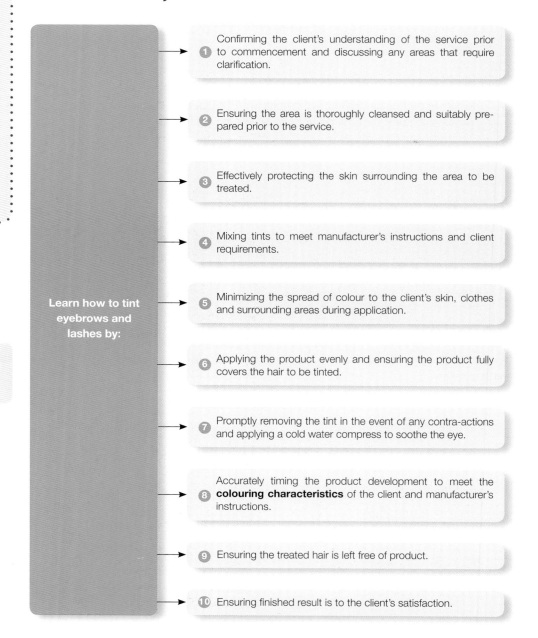

Learn how to tint eyebrows and lashes by:

1. Confirming the client's understanding of the service prior to commencement and discussing any areas that require clarification.

2. Ensuring the area is thoroughly cleansed and suitably prepared prior to the service.

3. Effectively protecting the skin surrounding the area to be treated.

4. Mixing tints to meet manufacturer's instructions and client requirements.

5. Minimizing the spread of colour to the client's skin, clothes and surrounding areas during application.

6. Applying the product evenly and ensuring the product fully covers the hair to be tinted.

7. Promptly removing the tint in the event of any contra-actions and applying a cold water compress to soothe the eye.

8. Accurately timing the product development to meet the **colouring characteristics** of the client and manufacturer's instructions.

9. Ensuring the treated hair is left free of product.

10. Ensuring finished result is to the client's satisfaction.

How to tint the eyelashes

1 Remove some petroleum jelly from its container, using a new disposable spatula.

2 Working from behind the client, ask the client to open her eyes and to look upwards towards you. Using a disposable brush, apply petroleum jelly underneath the lower lashes of one eye, ensuring that it extends at the outer corner of the eye. (This is in case the client's eyes water slightly during service, which might otherwise lead to skin staining.) The petroleum jelly must not come into contact with the lash hair, where it would create a barrier to the tint.

3 Place the prepared eye shield on the skin under the lower lashes, ensuring that it adheres to the petroleum jelly and fits 'snugly' to the base of the lower lashes.

4 Repeat the above process for the other eye.

5 Ask the client to close her eyes gently. Instruct her not to open them again until you advise her to do so, in about ten minutes' time.

6 Apply petroleum jelly to the upper eyelid, in a line on the skin at the base of the lashes.

7 Considering the length and density of the client's eyelashes, mix the required amount of tint with 10-volume (3%) hydrogen peroxide. As a guide, a 5mm length of tint from the tube, mixed with two or three drops of hydrogen peroxide, is usually sufficient. Mix the products to a smooth cream in the tinting bowl, using the disposable brush. Always recap bottles and tubes tightly after use, to avoid deterioration of materials.

ALWAYS REMEMBER

Make sure that work surfaces are protected with disposable coverings, to prevent permanent staining following spillages.

HEALTH & SAFETY

Maintaining hygiene
Do not use the same spatula in the container again, or you might contaminate the product.

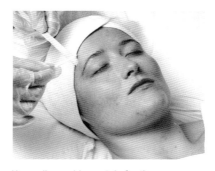

Use a disposable spatula for the petroleum jelly

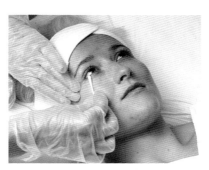

Apply petroleum jelly to prevent skin staining

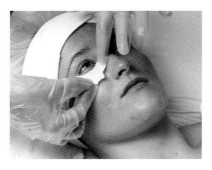

Placement of eye shield

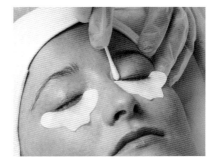

Application of petroleum jelly to upper eyelid

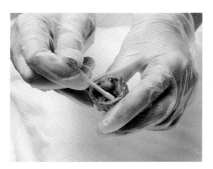

Mix the tint and hydrogen peroxide according to manufacturer's instructions

BEST PRACTICE

Client care
Speak to your clients as you apply the eyelash tint. Check that they are comfortable and understand what you are doing. Remember: the eyes are very sensitive and will water readily.

HEALTH & SAFETY

Client comfort

The client should not be left during the lash-tinting service. You must be available both to offer reassurance and to take the necessary action if the eyes water.

If the eyes do water while the eyes are closed, hold a tissue at the corner of the eye to soak up the moisture. Take further action if watering persists and the eyes begin to sting. See contra-action page 269.

8 Wipe excess tint off the brush onto the inside of the bowl. Apply the tint thinly to each hair. Work from the base of the lash to the tip, ensuring that each hair is evenly covered. Press down gently with the applicator to ensure that the lower lashes also are covered. The few inner and outer lashes should also be covered, down to the base. Remove any excess tint from the skin with a clean cotton bud.

9 Allow the tint to process, for approximately five to ten minutes from the completion of application. Discard any unused mixture as soon as the tint has been applied.

10 On completion of processing, remove the eyelash tint by applying clean, damp cotton wool pads over each eye, wiping away most of the tint and removing the protective eye shield in one movement, an outward sweep. Using fresh dampened cotton wool pads, gently stroke down the lashes from roots to tips, until all excess tint has been removed. With a sweeping action on each eye and using one cotton wool pad, wipe from the side to the middle against the lash growth, while the other hand supports the eye tissue. ***All tint must be thoroughly removed before the client opens her eyes.***

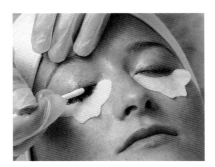

Applying the tint

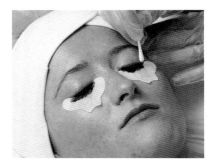

Removal of excess tint with a cotton bud

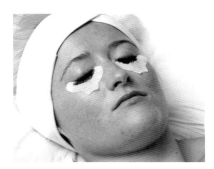

Processing the tint

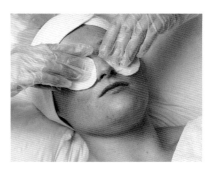

Removing the tint

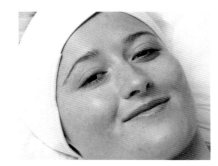

The completed eyelash tint

TOP TIP

Tint removal

Use a cotton bud to remove any excess tint from along the lash line on removal.

11 Ask the client to open her eyes. If removal has been correctly carried out, the lashes and their bases will be free from tint. (While training, if any tint remains at the base of the lashes after the eyes have been opened, ask the client to close her eyes again and finish the removal process using clean, damp cotton wool.) Check that every lash has been tinted, especially the base of each lash and the inner and outer corner lashes. Show the client the result, ensuring the colour is dark enough and that they are satisfied with the final effect.

12 Once you are satisfied that all tint has been removed, place a cool, damp cotton wool pad over each eye for two to three minutes to soothe the eye tissue.

13 Record details of the treatment on the client's record card.

HEALTH & SAFETY

Using tints

Always read the manufacturer's instructions carefully before using a permanent tint.

Step-by-step: tinting the eyebrows

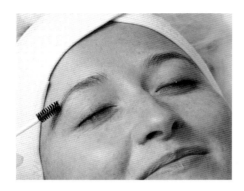

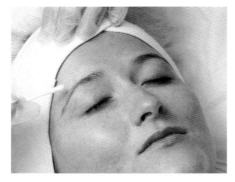

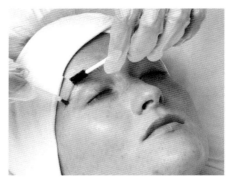

1 Remove some petroleum jelly from its container, using a new disposable spatula.

2 Brush the brow hair away from the skin, using a disposable brow brush (as shown in the picture).

3 Using a disposable brush, surround each eyebrow with petroleum jelly, as close as possible to the brow hair (to avoid skin staining).

4 Mix approximately 5mm of the chosen tint colour with two or three drops of 10-volume (3%) hydrogen peroxide in a tinting bowl. Ensure that the tint is mixed thoroughly to a creamy consistency, according to the manufacturer's instructions.

5 Wipe excess tint off the brush onto the inside of the tinting bowl. Apply the tint neatly and economically to the brow hair of the first eyebrow; ensuring that the brow hairs, from the base to the tips, are evenly covered (as shown in the picture).

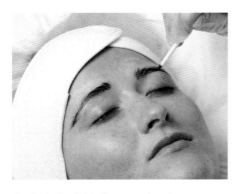

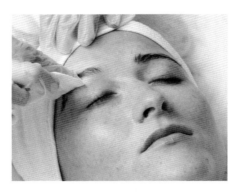

6 Apply the tint to the second eyebrow; following the same procedure.

7 Immediately after application of the tint to the second eyebrow, remove the tint from the first eyebrow. Use a clean dampened cotton wool pad. Place it on the eyebrow, then wipe it across the eyebrow in an outward sweep, removing the excess tint. Ensure that all traces of excess tint have been removed, to prevent skin staining.

Never leave tint on the eyebrows for longer than two minutes. Eyebrow hair colour develops much more quickly than lash hair.

TOP TIP

Application brow hair

To ensure even coverage of brow hair, use a brush to lift the hair to enable application at the roots of the hair to mid-length of the hair shaft.

The effect of tinting depends on the natural colour:

- **Blonde hair** develops colour rapidly – if the tint is left on the eyebrow too long, a harsh, unnatural appearance will be created.

- **Red/grey hair** is more resistant to the tint, and developing will take a little longer – allow 15 minutes' processing time when tinting lash hair.

- **Dark hair** requires tinting to increase the intensity of the natural eyebrow colour, giving a glossy, conditioned appearance.

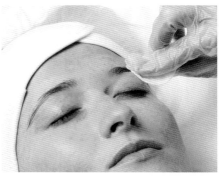

8 Remove the tint from the second eyebrow in the same way.

Show the client the effect of the tinted eyebrows. If the brow hair is not dark enough, reapply the tint to the eyebrow hair; following the same application and removal procedure. Note this on the client's record card.

When you are both satisfied with the colour of the tinted eyebrows, complete the client's record card by recording details of the service.

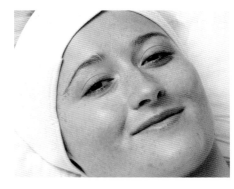

9 The completed effect, showing both eyelash and eyebrow tint.

HEALTH & SAFETY

Skin stains

If skin staining accidentally occurs, use a professional skin stain remover designed for this purpose. Afterwards, use plenty of clean, dampened cotton wool pads to avoid skin irritation.

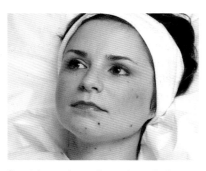

Special occasion make-up is applied before application of artificial eyelashes

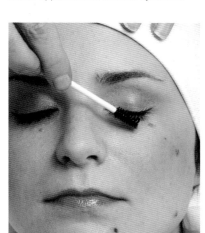

Brushing natural lashes before application

Apply artificial lashes

How to prepare the client

Show the client through to the prepared work area after the record card has been completed. Consult the record card and check the area for any contra-indications to treatment.

1. Position the client comfortably on the treatment couch or beauty chair (which should be slightly elevated). If the client wears contact lenses, these must be removed before the treatment begins.

2. Drape a clean towel across the client's chest and shoulders. Protect their hair with a clean headband.

3. Wash your hands, which indicates to the client that treatment is beginning and in a hygienic and professional manner.

4. It is usual to carry out a full facial cleanse (rather than cleansing only the eye area), as make-up is usually applied to complement the false eyelashes. Use a cleansing milk to dissolve facial make-up, followed by a non-oily eye make-up remover to cleanse the eye area. Both products should be removed with clean, damp cotton wool.

5. To ensure that the eye tissue and eyelashes are thoroughly clean and grease-free, apply a mild oil-free toning lotion: stroke this over the skin using clean, damp cotton wool.

6. Blot the lashes dry, using a fresh facial tissue for each eye. (Any moisture left on the natural lashes will reduce the effectiveness of the eyelash adhesive.)

7. Apply make-up to complement the effect achieved. Brush the natural lashes to separate them before application.

Outcome 5: Apply artificial lashes

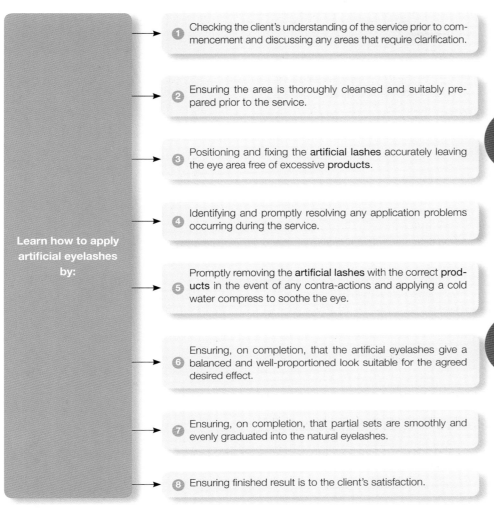

Learn how to apply artificial eyelashes by:

① Checking the client's understanding of the service prior to commencement and discussing any areas that require clarification.

② Ensuring the area is thoroughly cleansed and suitably prepared prior to the service.

③ Positioning and fixing the **artificial lashes** accurately leaving the eye area free of excessive **products**.

④ Identifying and promptly resolving any application problems occurring during the service.

⑤ Promptly removing the **artificial lashes** with the correct **products** in the event of any contra-actions and applying a cold water compress to soothe the eye.

⑥ Ensuring, on completion, that the artificial eyelashes give a balanced and well-proportioned look suitable for the agreed desired effect.

⑦ Ensuring, on completion, that partial sets are smoothly and evenly graduated into the natural eyelashes.

⑧ Ensuring finished result is to the client's satisfaction.

ALWAYS REMEMBER

Do not prepare the lash adhesive until you are ready to use it. It tends to dry on contact with air.

TOP TIP

When applying the individual flare lashes to the inner portion of the eyelid, hold the skin taut, stretching the skin slightly. This will enable you to position the artificial lash more easily.

TOP TIP

Use a clean pair of tweezers to remove the individual flare lashes from their container when required. Holding the tweezers firmly, grip each lash near its base (this avoids misshaping the outer lash hairs).

How to apply individual flare lashes

1 Check that everything you need is on the trolley.

2 Check that the back of the couch or beauty chair is slightly raised, at a height that is comfortable for you.

3 Discuss the service procedure with the client. Explain that she will be required to keep her eyes open during the service. Reassure her that she may blink during application. Very often clients feel that they shouldn't, and their eyes begin to water.

4 Ask her to tilt her head downwards very slightly. This tends to lower the upper eyelids, making application easier.

5 Depending on the effect required, you may start application of the individual flare lashes at different positions along the natural lash line. In general, apply shorter lashes to the inner corners of the eyelid, and longer lashes to the outer corners; this creates a realistic effect and ensures client comfort. If you are applying individual flare lashes to the entire upper lid, it is practical to start application at the

BEST PRACTICE

To ensure efficient application, don't get adhesive on the points of the tweezers.

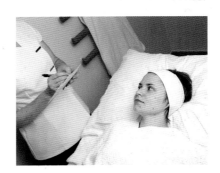

Explaining the service procedure

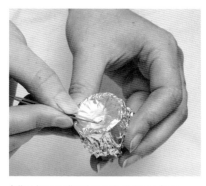

Adhesive application to individual flare artificial eyelashes

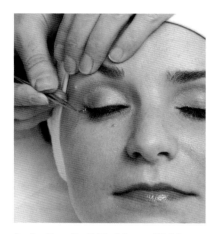

Application of individual flare artificial eyelash to outer eyelash hair

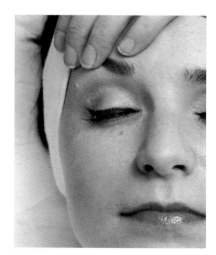

Artificial eyelash positioned

inner corner of the eyelid and work outwards: this follows the natural contour of the eye.

6 With the sterile tweezers, select a lash from the package, holding it near its centre. Brush the underside of the individual flare lash, at the root, through the adhesive. The adhesive should extend slightly beyond the root. You need sufficient adhesive, but not too much – excess adhesive should be removed by wiping the lash against the inside of the adhesive container.

7 Working from behind the client, hold the tweezers at the angle at which the artificial lashes will be applied to the natural lash line. Hold the brow tissue with your other hand to steady the eyelid.

TOP TIP

Positioning the individual flare lashes correctly requires experience. It is a good idea initially to practise application without adhesive.

Using a stroking movement, place the underside of the artificial lashes on top of the natural lash. Stroke the adhesive along the length of the natural eyelash. Guide the artificial lashes towards the base of the natural lash, so that the artificial lashes rests along the length of the natural lash. Wait a few seconds to allow the adhesive to dry (to prevent the lashes from sticking together). Continue placing further artificial lashes side by side until the desired effect is achieved.

During application, keep checking your work. If a lash is out of line, remove it while the adhesive is still soft. If the adhesive has set, the lash will need to be removed using adhesive solvent – see illustration on page 269.

8 Apply the artificial lashes one at a time, to each eye alternately. This avoids sensitizing the eye, and makes it easier for you to create a balanced effect.

9 If the client requires artificial lashes to be applied to the *lower* lid, the application technique is slightly different.

Work facing the client, with the client looking upwards, her eyes slightly open. Follow the same general procedure for applying the false eyelashes; here, however, the lashes curve downwards and the adhesive is applied to the *upper* surface of the lash.

Lashes applied to the lower eyelid are usually shorter than those chosen for the upper lid, and more adhesive is required for the lashes to be secure and have maximum durability.

10 When you have completed the lash application, ask the client to sit up, and show her the completed effect.

11 If the client is satisfied with the result, you can apply a water- or powder-based eye make-up at this stage if desired. Do not apply mascara, as this will reduce the adhesion to the natural lash. Mascara also clogs the lashes together; and is difficult to remove without affecting the eyelash adhesive. On completion, the lashes can be gently brushed – using a disposable brush – to remove particles of eye shadow.

ALWAYS REMEMBER

Tell the client that artificial lashes applied to the lower lashes tend to fall off after one week. (This is probably due to the natural watering of the eye affecting the adhesive.)

How to apply strip lashes

Strip false eyelashes may be applied *before* carrying out the eye make-up – this avoids the eye make-up being spoilt if the eyes water slightly during application.

1 Check that everything required for the false eyelash application is available on your trolley.

2 Carefully apply moisturiser and foundation, taking care not to get any cosmetic products on the lashes. (If you do, gently wipe over the lashes with the non-oily eye make-up remover, and blot the eyelashes dry again with a clean facial tissue.)

3 Brush the lashes to separate them, using a clean disposable mascara brush. This makes artificial lashes application easier, and removes any fine particles of loose powder.

4 Remove the strip lashes from their container; and place them on a clean, disinfected palette. Each strip is designed to fit either the left or the right eye: remember which is which when placing them on the palette.

5 Check the length of the strip against the client's eyelid. The strip should never be applied directly from one corner of the eyelid to the other; but should start about 2mm from the inner corner of the eye, and end 2mm from the outer corner. This ensures a natural effect and maximizes the durability of the artificial lashes.

When you remove the strip lash from the package you will find that there is adhesive on the backing strip, which fixes the lash in the container: this adhesive is sufficient to hold the lash onto the client's natural lash while you measure the length.

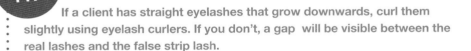

TOP TIP

If a client has straight eyelashes that grow downwards, curl them slightly using eyelash curlers. If you don't, a gap will be visible between the real lashes and the false strip lash.

6 To trim the artificial lashes you require a sharp pair of scissors. First correct the length of the *strip* if necessary. Hold the lashes securely with one hand, and then trim the strip at the outer edge. Then trim the lashes themselves, if necessary. Never reduce the length of the lashes by cutting straight across them: the result would not look natural. Natural eyelashes are of varying lengths, due to the nature of the hair growth cycle; it is this effect that you must simulate. To shorten the lash, 'chip' into the lash. Use the *points* of the scissors to shorten the lash length. Cut the lashes so that the shorter lashes are at the inner corner of the eyelid, gradually increasing toward the outer corner.

7 The couch or beauty chair should be in a slightly raised position. During the treatment you will be working from behind the client: the height must be comfortable for you.

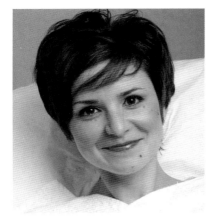
Short individual flare lashes applied to thicken the natural lashes

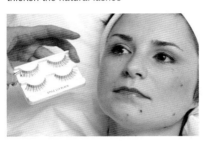
Removal of strip artificial lash from container

HEALTH & SAFETY

Lash length
If the lashes were not shorter at the inner corner of the eyelid, they would irritate the client's eye.

BEST PRACTICE

With individual flare lashes, do not apply adhesive directly from the tube to the eyelash base – you would apply too much adhesive.

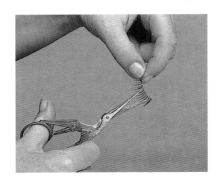
Trimming the lashes

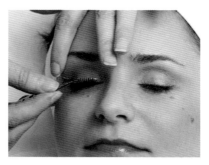

Applying to strip lash to the eye

8 Discuss the treatment procedure with the client. Explain to her that she will be required to keep her eyes open during the application. Ask her to tilt her head downwards very slightly – this lowers the upper eyelids, making application easier.

9 Using the sterile tweezers, remove one of the eyelash strips from the palette. Handle it very carefully, as it can easily become misshapen.

Remembering that the strip is designed to fit either the right or the left eye, place it against the appropriate eyelid and check the length (with the client's eyes closed).

10 Once satisfied that the length of the strip lash is correct (see step 5 for reducing the length), remove the adhesive tape used to hold it in the container.

11 Place a small quantity of strip lash adhesive on the disinfected palette.

12 Ask the client to look down slightly, with her eyes half open. With one hand lift her brow to steady the upper eyelid.

Holding the strip lash with the sterile tweezers at its centre, drag it at its base through the adhesive. (The adhesive must be moist.) It is usually white, but when it dries it becomes colourless.

Position the base of the strip lash as close as possible to the base of the natural eyelash, ensuring that it is about 2mm in from the inner and outer corners of the eye. *Gently* press the false and natural eyelashes together with your fingertips, along the length of the lash and at the outer corners.

TOP TIP

Extra glue (although not excessive) may be applied to the ends of the lashes to prevent lifting while wearing them.

TOP TIP

CPD

As part of your progression you may develop your skills further in the application of artificial lashes by learning the Level 3 Unit Single lash extensions.

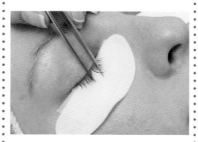

Single lash extensions

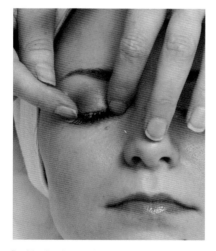

Positioning base of strip lash on the base of the natural lash line

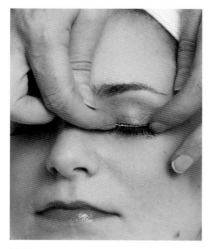

Making sure the strip lash is secure

TOP TIP

Retail opportunity

Mascaras are available formulated to be worn with individual flare lashes. The product is more easily removed than regular non-waterproof mascaras.

13 When you are sure that the first strip lash is secure, apply the second in the same way.

14 If strip lashes are to be applied to the bottom lashes also, apply these now, in the same way as the upper lashes. (Strip lashes for the lower lids are fine, with an extremely thin base. These lashes should be trimmed as before to ensure comfort and durability in wear.)

15 Allow three to five minutes for the adhesive to dry.

16 Gently brush the lashes from underneath the natural lash line, using a clean disposable mascara brush. This will blend the natural and artificial lashes together Check that both sets of lashes are correctly positioned, and that a balanced look has been achieved.

17 Artificial lashes look more realistic if eyeliner is applied to the client's eyelid: this disguises the base of the strip lash.

18 Show the client the finished effect.

19 When you are satisfied, record the details on the client record card.

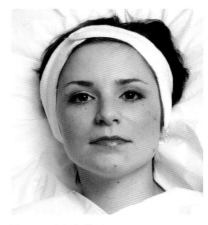

The completed effect

Outcome 6: Provide aftercare advice

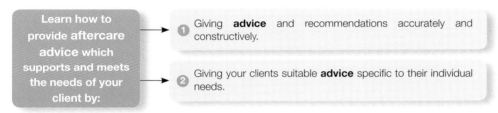

Learn how to provide aftercare advice which supports and meets the needs of your client by:

1 Giving **advice** and recommendations accurately and constructively.

2 Giving your clients suitable **advice** specific to their individual needs.

HEALTH & SAFETY

Client comfort

Check the eyelash application as you work. Ensure that the lower and upper lashes are not stuck together, and that the eyelashes are accurately and evenly applied.

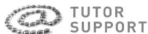

TUTOR SUPPORT

Activity 2: Eye treatments wordsearch

Advise the client on skincare preparations to use at home to enhance the appearance of the eyebrows and lashes.

The following aftercare advice should be given to client's specific to the eye service received.

Eyebrow shape aftercare advice Advise the client to receive the service as follows:

- eyebrow maintenance every 1–2 weeks

- eyebrow re-shaping every 3–4 weeks

While a client receives an eyebrow shape it is an ideal opportunity to promote an eyebrow/eyelash tint.

An eyebrow pencil powder cosmetic can be recommended to disguise bald patches, e,g. scars. Sparse eyebrows can be made to appear thicker. It can also be used to stimulate hairs, when the length needs to be increased.

Explain how to care for the area following the service to avoid an unwanted reaction – a contra-action. Advise the client not to wear eye make-up for at least six hours following the eyebrow-shaping service. The hair follicle has been damaged where the hair has been torn out: it will be susceptible to infection unless the area is cared for while it heals. It should not be necessary for the client to continue using antiseptic lotion at

HEALTH & SAFETY

Cross-infection

Remind the client to avoid touching the area immediately following an eyebrow shaping treatment. This is because the area is susceptible to infection and the fingers may transfer dirt, causing secondary infection.

HEALTH & SAFETY

Avoiding infection

If excess antiseptic lotion or cream is left on the area, this may attract small particles of dust, which could cause infection.

HEALTH & SAFETY

Solvents

Although solvents are formulated to remove artificial lashes from the natural lash, great care must be taken to avoid skin/eye irritation. Ideally this solution should be used to clean the artificial lashes after removal. Removal of artificial lashes should be with an oil-based eye make-up remover product.

TOP TIP

Disposable cotton buds may be used to apply eyelash adhesive solvent.

---

home, but they should be advised to carry out these instructions if discomfort or continued reddening occurs:

1   Explain to the client the action to take in the event of a contra-action.

2   Cleanse the eyebrow area using a mild antiseptic lotion or witch hazel, applied with a small piece of clean, dampened cotton wool.

3   Apply an antiseptic soothing lotion, cream or gel with clean, dry cotton wool.

4   Gently remove excess antiseptic lotion, cream or gel using a clean, soft facial tissue or clean damp cotton wool.

5   Repeat as necessary, approximately every four hours. **If the reddening does not subside in the next 24 hours, contact the salon**.

6   Eye make-up may be worn as soon as the redness has gone – usually after eight hours.

Tint eyebrow and lash aftercare advice

If an unwanted reaction occurs, a contra-action, ie irritation or redness, apply cool water damp cotton wool pad compress to the area.

If reddening continues after 24 hours contact the salon.

Advise the client to receive the service as follows:

- eyelash tinting every 4–6 weeks
- eyebrow tinting every 3–4 weeks

Artificial eyelash aftercare advice

- Provide advice on the action to take it an unwanted reaction, a contra-action, occurs.
- Avoid rubbing the eyes, or the lashes may become loosened.
- Do not use an oil-based eye make-up remover as its cosmetic constituents will dissolve the adhesive.
- Use only dry or water-based eye make-up (as these may readily be removed with a non-oily eye make-up remover).
- If the lashes are made of a synthetic material, heat will cause them to become frizzy. Advise the client to avoid extremes of temperature, such a hot sauna.
- Do not touch the eyes for 1½ hours after application, while the adhesive dries thoroughly.

If the client has had *individual* artificial flare lashes applied, the following homecare advice should be given on caring for the lashes:

- Use a non-oily eye make-up remover daily to cleanse the eyelids and eyelashes. Avoid contact with oil-based preparations in the eye area, such as moisturisers and cleansers – the oil content will dissolve the adhesive, and the lashes would become detached.
- Do not attempt to remove the artificial lashes – pulling at artificial lash will also pull out the natural eyelashes.
- After bathing or swimming, gently *pat* the eye area dry with a clean towel.
- A disposable spiral applicator brush may be used to comb through the lashes to separate.

Clients with individual false eyelashes should have the artificial lashes maintained by regular visits to the salon. Lost individual flare lashes can be replaced as necessary; this is often described as an eyelash *infill* service. Schedule this for every 10–14 days.

If the client wishes to have the individual artificial lashes removed, this should be done professionally.

How to remove individual eyelashes

1 Position the client lying on the couch.

2 Wash your hands.

3 Remove make-up from the eye area, cleansing the skin with a suitable eye make-up remover.

4 While the client's eyes are open, place a pre-shaped eye shield underneath the lower lashes of each eye. (This will protect the eye tissue from the solvent.) Position the eye shields so that they fit snugly to the base of the lower lashes.

5 Ask the client to close her eyes gently, and not to open them again until you tell her to do so.

6 Prepare a new disposable orange stick by covering it at the pointed end with clean, dry cotton wool.

7 Moisten the cotton wool with the artificial eyelash adhesive solvent.

8 Treating one eye at a time, gently stroke down the false eyelashes with the adhesive solvent until the adhesive dissolves and the false eyelash begins to loosen.

9 When you are satisfied that the eyelash adhesive has dissolved, gently attempt to remove the false eyelash. Support the upper eyelid with the fingers of one hand, using the other hand to remove the artificial lash with a sterile pair of manual tweezers. If the adhesive has been adequately dissolved, the eyelash will lift away easily from the natural eyelash. If there is any resistance, repeat the solvent application until the eyelash comes away readily.

10 As the artificial eyelashes are removed, collect them on a clean white facial tissue or a clean pad of cotton wool.

11 Having removed all of the artificial eyelashes from one eye, soothe the area by applying damp cotton wool pads soaked in cool water. (This will also remove any remaining solvent.) A damp cotton wool pad may be placed over the eye, while you remove the artificial lashes from the other eye.

How to remove strip lashes

If a client wears strip eyelashes they will need instructions on how to remove and care for the artificial lashes themselves.

1 Use the fingertips of one hand to support the eyelid at the outer corner. With the other hand, lift the lash strip base at the outer corner of the eye. Gently peel the strip away from the natural lash, from the outer edge towards the centre of the eyelid.

2 Peel the adhesive from the backing strip, using a clean pair of manual tweezers. Take care to avoid stretching the strip lash.

HEALTH & SAFETY

Eye care
Do not allow eyelash adhesive solvent to come into excessive contact with the eye tissue – it could cause irritation of the skin. Ensure that there is sufficient solvent only on the cotton wool: it should be moist but not dripping wet or the solvent might enter the eye.

HEALTH & SAFETY

Client comfort
Never attempt to remove the artificial eyelashes until they have begun to loosen – if you do, the client's natural eyelashes will also be removed, causing them discomfort.

HEALTH & SAFETY

Client comfort
When removing the strip lash, avoid pulling the natural lashes with the artificial lashes.

HEALTH & SAFETY

Semi-permanent lashes
The client should be advised to return to the salon for semi-permanent lashes to be removed professionally.

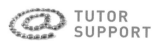

TUTOR SUPPORT

Activity 3: Re-cap and revision evaluation

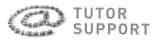

TUTOR SUPPORT

Activity 4: Multiple choice tests

3 Clean the strip lash in the appropriate way.

- **Strips made from human hair** Clean with a commercial lash cleaner or 70% alcohol. This removes the remaining adhesive and the eye make-up.

- **Synthetic strips** Place in warm, soapy water for a few minutes, to clean the lashes and remove the remaining adhesive. Rinse in tepid water.

4 After cleaning the strip lashes should be recurled.

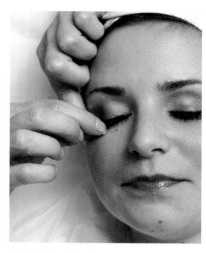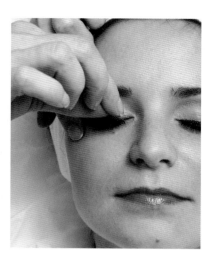

Removing strip lashes

How to recurl strip lashes

For reasons of hygiene and because of the time involved, this service will not be offered by the salon. The client, however, will need advice on how to recurl the lashes at home.

1 On removal from the water, place the lashes side by side, ensuring that the inner edges are together inside a clean facial tissue.

2 Wrap a tissue around an even, barrel-shaped object such as a felt-tip pen, and secure it with an elastic band.

3 The artificial lashes, inside the facial tissue, should then be rolled around this object. Keep the base of the lash straight, so that the whole lash length curls around the object.

Once recurled, the strip lashes can be returned to the contoured shelves in their original container and stored for further use.

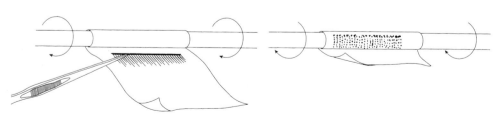

Recurling strip lashes

GLOSSARY OF KEY WORDS

Adhesive specialized glue used to attach artificial lashes to the natural lashes. This glue differs in formulation according to the lash type strip or individual flare lashes.

Aftercare advice recommended advice given to the client following service to continue the benefits of the service.

Artificial lashes threads of nylon fibre which are attached to the natural hair. These are referred to as strip lashes, individual artificial lashes and single lash extensions.

Blepharitis inflammation of the eyelid caused by an infection or an allergic reaction.

Client Groups this term is used in a number of the units and it refers to client diversity. The CRE (Commission for Racial Equality) ethnic group classification is used in the range for these units. These cover white, mixed, Asian, black and Chinese.

Colouring characteristics the client's natural hair colouring, i.e. fair, red, dark and white.

Conjunctivitis a bacterial infection. Inflammation of the mucous membrane that covers the eye and lines the eyelid. The skin of the inner conjunctiva of the eye becomes inflamed, the eye becomes very red, itchy and sore, and pus may exude from the eye area.

Consultation assessment of client's needs using different assessment techniques, including questioning and natural observation.

Contact dermatitis a skin disorder caused by intolerance of the skin to a particular substance, or a group of substances. On exposure to the substance the skin quickly becomes irritated and an allergic reaction occurs.

Contra-action an unwanted reaction occurring during or after service application.

Contra-indication a problematic symptom that indicates that the service may not proceed.

Cortex the thickest layer of the hair structure.

Cyst localized pocket of sebum that forms in the hair follicle or under the sebaceous glands in the skin. Semi-globular in shape, either raised or flat, and hard or soft. Cysts are the same colour as the skin, or red if bacterial infection occurs.

Eyebrow shaping involves the removal of eyebrow hair to create a new shape (reshape) or to remove stray hairs to maintain the existing brow shape (maintenance). Small metal tools, called tweezers, are use to remove the hairs.

Eyelash adhesive used to apply strips and individual eyelashes

Eyelash and eyebrow tinting definition of the brow and lash hair, achieved by the application of a permanent dye especially formulated for use around the delicate eye area.

Hair a long slender structure that grows out of, and is part of, the skin. Each hair is made up of dead skin cells, which contain the protein called keratin.

Hair follicle an appendage (structure) in the skin formed from epidermal tissue. Cells move up the hair follicle from the bottom (the hair bulb), changing in structure to form the hair.

Hydrogen peroxide (H_2O_2) an *oxidant*, a chemical that contains available oxygen atoms and encourages chemical reactions.

Negative skin sensitivity test a test where result produces no skin reaction. in this case you may proceed with the service.

Positive skin sensitivity test an allergic reaction to the skin test. The skin appears red, swollen and feels itchy.

Service plan after the consultation, suitable service objectives are established to treat the client's conditions and needs.

Skin sensitivity test method used to assess skin tolerance/sensitivity to a substance or service.

Solvent a product designed to remove and clean artificial lashes without causing eye irritation.

Stye bacterial infection. Infection of the sebaceous glands of the eyelash hair follicles. Small lumps appear on the inner rim of the eyelid and contain pus.

Toluenediamine small molecules of permanent dye used in tinting service.

Tweezers small metal tools used to remove body hair by pulling it from the bottom of the hair follicle (small opening in the skin where the hair grows from). There are two types: *automatic* – designed to remove the bulk of the hair and *manual* – designed to remove the stray hairs.

Watery eye over-secretion of tears from the eyes, which would normally drain into the nasal cavity.

ASSESSMENT OF KNOWLEDGE AND UNDERSTANDING

Having covered the learning objectives for **Enhance the appearance of eyebrows and eyelashes**, test what you need to know and understand answering the following short questions below. The information covers:

- organizational and legal requirements
- how to work safely and effectively when performing eyebrow and eyelash services
- client consultation, service planning and preparation

- shaping the eyebrows
- tinting the eyebrows and lashes
- applying artificial lashes
- contra-indications and contra-actions
- equipment, materials and products
- aftercare advice for clients

Organizational and legal requirements

1 How should records be stored to comply with the Data Protection Act (1998)?

2 What details should be recorded on the client's record card?

3 Why is it important to keep a record of the service carried out?

4 How should the client be positioned for the eye service to avoid discomfort and ensure effective service application of artificial lashes?

5 Why is it important that the eye service is given in the allocated time?

6 How long would you allocate to carry out an eyebrow shaping service?

7 How long would you allocate to carry out an eyelash and eyebrow tint?

8 Why is the quantity of tint applied to the area important in relation to both efficiency and the final result?

9 At what age is a person classed as a minor? What would you need to obtain for a minor to receive an eye service?

How to work safely and effectively when performing eyebrow and eyelash services

1 What are the acceptable methods of sterilization for tweezers?

2 How would you prepare the service area to ensure general client comfort during service application?

3 How should consumables used during a brow shape be disposed of?

4 What hygiene and safety precautions should be followed when performing the services:
- an eyebrow shape?

- permanent tinting?
- artificial lash application?

5 What should you check on completion of an eye service work area to maintain products in optimum condition?

6 What Personal Protective Equipment (PPE) may be worn and when performing which eye services?

7 What environmental conditions should you check are adequate to work safely and effectively when performing eye services?

8 What is contact dermatitis and how can this be caused as a result of working practice when performing eye services?

Client consultation, service planning and preparation

1 Why is it important to have a thorough consultation before you commence the service?

2 Why is it important to discuss the service plan with the client before service commences?

3 If the client is having an eyelash/brow tint why is it important to check the results of the skin sensitivity test before you proceed?

4 Why is a skin sensitivity test needed before every tinting/artificial individual flare flash service?

5 If the client wished to have their fair brows tinted, but had a positive reaction to the skin test what could you recommend as an alternative?

6 How should the brows be prepared to minimize discomfort and the risk of infection, before shaping commences?

7 What should be considered in the choice of artificial eyelash for a client?

8 How should the eye area be prepared to ensure that the false eyelashes adhere securely to the natural lashes?

Shaping the eyebrows

1 What factors should you consider when deciding the correct eyebrow shape for a client?

2 How can you determine the length of a client's eyebrows that will best suit their facial features?

3 How can you ensure that hairs are removed at their root?

4 What factors should you consider in your approach to eyebrow shaping with the following clients:
- a client with excessively thick eyebrows who requests a thin eyebrow shape?
- a client who has close set eyes?
- a client with a round face?
- a client who has a few stray long, coarse hairs?
- a client with sensitive skin?

5 Why is soothing antiseptic lotion applied following an eyebrow shaping service?

Tinting the eyebrows and lashes

1 How should the lash and brow area be prepared to avoid skin staining and to ensure effective tinting?

2 How do you select the colour when carrying out a permanent tinting service?

3 How would permanent tinting be performed when treating the following clients:
- a very nervous client, to ensure a safe, efficient eyelash tinting service?
- a client who requires an eyebrow shape and an eyebrow tint?

In which order would these services be given and why?

4 What is the difference in processing time between a brow tint and an eyelash tint?

5 How long would you allow the tint to process when treating a client with:
- blonde hair?
- grey hair?
- red hair?
- dark hair?

Applying artificial lashes

1 What safety precautions should be taken during the application of false eyelashes?

2 When applying false eyelashes along the length of the eyelid, how can you avoid irritating the corners of the eye?

3 What is the difference between the application of strip and individual eyelashes?

4 Why should the manufacturer's instructions be referred to when applying artificial eyelashes?

5 What may result in poor adhesion of the artificial lash to the natural lash?

Contra-indications and contra-actions

1 When observing the area for eye services, what conditions would contra-indicate service?

2 What eye disorders would contra-indicate service?

3 At consultation you notice that the client has what you think is conjunctivitis. What action should you take?

4 Give two examples of contra-actions that may occur following eyebrow shaping.

5 What action would you take if a skin contra-action occurred following individual flare artificial lash application?

6 If a client complained of irritation during an eyelash tinting service, what action would you take?

Equipment, materials and products

1 It is important to select the correct and most suitable equipment and materials for the service. When would you select and in what occasions would you recommend:
- automatic tweezers?
- manual tweezers?
- strip lashes?
- individual flare lashes?
- permanent tint?
- temporary brow colour?

Aftercare advice for clients

1 What aftercare advice should be given to a client following an eyebrow shaping service?

2 What aftercare advice should be given to a client following a permanent tinting service?

3 What aftercare advice should be given to a client following:
- artificial strip lash application?
- artificial individual flare lash application?

4 Explain the correct removal of:
- strip eyelashes
- individual flare eyelashes

5 When would you recommend that a client returns to the salon for an eyebrow trim, following an eyebrow shape?

6 When would you recommend that a client returns to the salon for permanent tinting service:

- to the lashes?
- to the eyebrows?

7 How long should a client be advised to wear:
- strip eyelashes?
- individual flare eyelashes?

9 Make-up Services (B8)

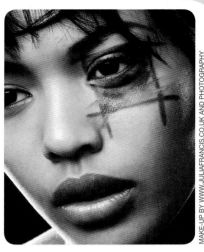

B8 Unit Learning Objectives

This chapter covers **Unit B8 Provide make-up services**.

This unit is about how to provide make-up services for a variety of occasions including day, evening and special occasions. The choice and application of make-up product and technique will be applied to suit the client's skin type, tone, colouring, condition and age.

There are **four** learning outcomes for Unit B8 which you must achieve competently:

1 **Maintain safe and effective methods of working when providing make-up services**

2 **Consult, plan and prepare for make-up services**

3 **Apply make-up products**

4 **Provide aftercare advice**

Your assessor will observe you **on three occasions involving three different clients**, on a range of different skin tones.

From the **range** statement, you must show that you have:

- used all **consultation techniques**

- taken the **necessary action** where a contra-action, contra-indication or service modification occurs

- treated all three **age group** categories

- treated all **skin types**

- applied make-up for all **occasions**

- applied all **make-up products**

- provided **relevant** advice

(continued on the next page)

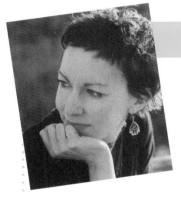

ROLE MODEL

Julia Francis

Make-up artist and body painter
www.juliafrancis.co.uk

" I have been a make-up artist for over ten years working with some of the industry's leading photographers, advertising agencies, directors, musicians, and actors. For film and TV my credits include *Star Wars*, *Hitchhikers Guide to the Galaxy*, *Wimbledon* and *Eastenders*. My Celebrity clients include Sir Tom Jones, Colin Firth, and Jonathan Ross. Agencies and brands that I have worked with include Bacardi, Pantene, Olay, Gillette and Saatchi & Saatchi.

I am also an experienced teacher and make-up consultant and have been conducting workshops for many years. The monthly workshops offer students a unique opportunity to find out how to move forward in a career as a make-up artist. Topics covered include:

- understanding the industry and the role of a freelance make-up artist

- areas of specialization – fashion, body painting, bridal, special effects, wigs, etc.

- advice on choosing make-up courses and qualifications required

- building up a make-up kit

- how to gain work experience, get work and make contacts

- how to create a portfolio, a show reel and a CV

To find out more about these workshops, please email me at: workshops@juliafrancis.co.uk.

(continued)

However, you must prove that you have the necessary knowledge. understanding and skills to be able to perform competently across the range.

When providing make-up services it is important to use the skills you have learnt in the following units:

Unit G20 Make sure your own actions reduce risks to health and safety

Unit G18 Promote additional products or services to clients

Unit G8 Develop and maintain your effectiveness at work

Essential anatomy and physiology knowledge requirements for this chapter, **B8**, are identified on the checklist chart in Chapter 2, page 16.

Make-up services

Make-up is used to enhance and accentuate the facial features to make us appear more attractive – which in turn makes us feel more confident. Make-up is used to create balance in the face, by skilful application of different cosmetic products to reduce or to emphasize facial features.

Each client is unique, so each requires an individual approach for their make-up. The overall effect should be attractive, complementing the client's personality, lifestyle, and the context for which the make-up is to be worn.

Make-up products can also improve the appearance and condition of the skin. Products should be selected to suit the client's skin type, colouring, condition and age.

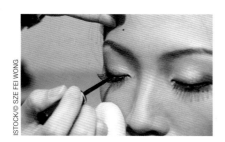

ISTOCK/© SZE FEI WONG

Outcome 1: Maintain safe and effective methods of working when providing make-up services

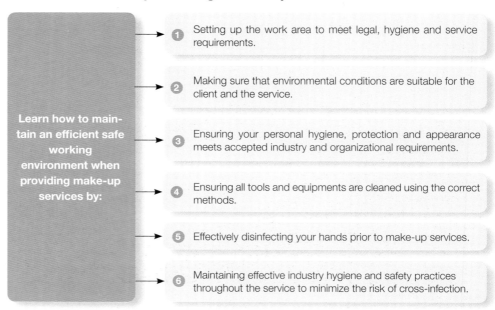

> ## Know your brands
> You will always be asked advice on the best products for people. Although you can't know everything that is available, it is essential that you have a good knowledge of products and have enough variation of different brands to hand. Where possible, try to check in advance if an actor/model is allergic to anything.
>
> Julia Francis

Learn how to maintain an efficient safe working environment when providing make-up services by:

1. Setting up the work area to meet legal, hygiene and service requirements.

2. Making sure that environmental conditions are suitable for the client and the service.

3. Ensuring your personal hygiene, protection and appearance meets accepted industry and organizational requirements.

4. Ensuring all tools and equipments are cleaned using the correct methods.

5. Effectively disinfecting your hands prior to make-up services.

6. Maintaining effective industry hygiene and safety practices throughout the service to minimize the risk of cross-infection.

7 Positioning equipment and materials for ease and safety of use.

8 Ensuring your own posture and position minimizes fatigue and the risk of injury while working.

(continued)
Learn how to maintain an efficient safe working environment when providing make-up services by:

9 Respecting your client's appearance sensitivities and privacy at all times.

10 Disposing of waste materials safely and correctly.

11 Ensuring that the service is cost effective and is carried out within a commercially viable time.

12 Leaving the work area in a condition suitable for further services.

13 Ensuring the client's records are up to date, accurate, easy to read and signed by the client and practitioner.

HEALTH & SAFETY

The chair must offer head support, or the client's neck will become strained during the make-up; also the head needs support if it is to be steady during the application of eye and lip make-up.

The height should be correct for you to avoid stretching and straining to avoid repetitive strain injury

Preparing the work area

The make-up room should be decorated in light, neutral colours to avoid the creation of unnecessary shadows. The area where the make-up is to be applied should be well lit, ideally with the same kind of light as that in which the make-up will be seen.

Place all the **equipment** and materials required on the trolley or work surface, in front of a make-up mirror. If you are displaying the make-up on a trolley, place the cosmetic products on a lower shelf until required, when they can be moved to the top shelf. This avoids cluttering the working area.

> ## Pack your kit well
> The make-up artist's role is not only to apply make-up to actors, models, presenters, performers, etc. but also to look after people and have available anything from plasters to safety pins if you are asked for it. Your kit is very heavy and a suitable case on wheels is a good idea, especially if you don't drive to work.
>
> Julia Francis

> ## Be calm under pressure
> Always remain calm and professional even in situations where you are running out of time or are compromised in some way. There is often a tight schedule that you have to fit in to and you don't want the whole production to be waiting for you. An employable make-up artist is always a calm make-up artist.
>
> Julia Francis

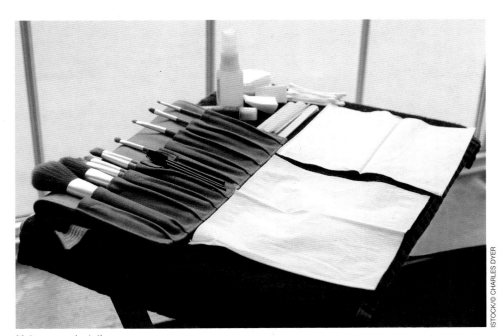

ISTOCK/© CHARLES DYER

Make-up work station

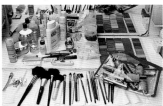
> ### Understand the brief
>
> It is essential that a make-up artist is able to create a look based on the context required and that the choice of products meets the client's requirements. For instance, it needs to be appropriate for the director's vision. You will need to know how long certain looks will take and what you need to have available in order to make them happen.
>
> Julia Francis

HEALTH & SAFETY

Ventilation

Good ventilation is important so that the client's skin does not become too warm. It is easier to apply make-up effectively to cool skin, and the make-up will be more durable.

Keeping the work area tidy promotes an organized and professional image, and prevents time being wasted as you try to find materials and the work area should always be in a condition to provide further make-up services.

Lighting   You need to know the *type* of light in which the proposed make-up will be seen: this is important when deciding upon the correct choice of make-up colours, because the appearance of colours may change according to the type of light. Is the make-up to be seen in daylight, in a fluorescent-lit office, or a softly lit restaurant?

White light (natural daylight) contains all the colours of the rainbow. When white light falls on an object, it absorbs some colours and *reflects* others: it is the reflected colour that we see. Thus, an object that we see as red is an object that absorbs the colours in white light except red. A *white* object reflects most of the light that falls upon it; a *black* object absorbs most of the light that falls on it.

If the make-up is to be worn in natural light, choose subtle make-up products in neutral colours as daylight intensifies colours.

If the make-up is to be worn in the office, it will probably be seen under **fluorescent light**. This contains an excess of blue and green, which have a 'cool' effect on the make-up: the red in the face does not show up and the face can look drained of colour. Reds and yellows should be avoided, as these will not show up; blue-toned colours will. This light also sharpens colours. Don't apply dark colours, as fluorescent light intensifies these. Choose lighter textured products in natural and neutral colours.

Evening make-up is usually seen in **incandescent light** – light produced by a filament lamp. This produces an excess of red and yellow light, which creates a warm, flattering effect. Almost all colours can be used in this light, except that browns and purples will appear darker. Choose a lighter foundation than normal to reflect the light, and use frosted highlighting products where possible for the same reason.

Because it is necessary to choose brighter colours and to emphasize facial features using contouring cosmetics, evening make-up will appear very obvious and dramatic in daylight. Explain to the client the reasons for the effect created, so that when she leaves the salon in daylight she won't feel that the make-up is inappropriate.

Equipment and materials

Before beginning the make-up, check that you have the necessary equipment and materials to hand and that they meet the legal hygiene and industry requirements for make-up service.

EQUIPMENT AND MATERIALS LIST

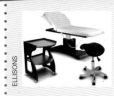

Couch or beauty chair
With sit-up and lie-down positions and an easy-to-clean surface

Trolley
Or other surface on which to place everything

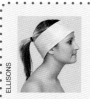

Headband (Clean)
To protect the client's hair while cleansing the skin. Alternatively if the hair has been styled it will be necessary to secure the hair away from the face with a large hair clip

Cleansing lotion
To clean and prepare the skin for make-up application

Eye make-up remover
To remove eye make-up and prepare the skin for make-up application

Toning lotion
To remove excess cleanser and restore the skin's pH balance

Lightweight moisturiser or primer
To facilitate make-up application and create a barrier between the skin and make-up

Dry cotton wool
Stored in a covered jar, to apply loose face powder

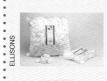

Large white facial tissues
To blot the skin after facial toning, and to protect the skin during make-up application

Make-up (a range)
To suit different skin types, tones and age groups

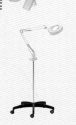

Bright lighting and magnifying lamp
To inspect the skin after cleansing and check for areas requiring special attention, e.g. broken capillaries that require concealer

Make-up brushes (assorted-at least three sets)
To allow for disinfection after use

Disposable applicators and brushes
Where possible for example for mascara and the application of eye shadow and lipstick

Non-latex cosmetic sponges
For applying foundation

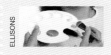

Make-up palette
For preparing and dispensing cosmetic products prior to application

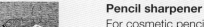

Pencil sharpener
For cosmetic pencils

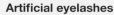

Artificial eyelashes
To enhance the eyes as required

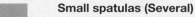

Small spatulas (Several)
For removing make-up products from their containers

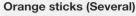

Orange sticks (Several)
For removing make-up products from their containers

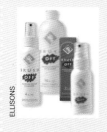

Brush cleanser
A proprietary brand cleaner to care for and maintain brushes hygienically

Eyelash curlers
Tool used to temporarily curl the eyelashes

YOU WILL ALSO NEED:

Disposable tissue (such as bedroll) To cover the work surface and the couch or beauty chair

Towels (2) Freshly laundered for each client – one to be placed over the head of the couch or chair, the other over the client's chest and shoulders to protect their clothing

Hairclips To protect the client's hair during make-up application

Damp cotton wool Prepared for each client and used during skin cleansing

Bowls To hold the prepared cotton wool

Bowls and lined metal pedal bin For waste materials

Hand mirror (clean) To show client the make-up during and after application to ensure satisfaction

Client record card To record the client's personal details, products used and details of the service

Clean your brushes
"Always turn up to a job with clean brushes and a clean kit. Never use the same brushes on more than one person and always maintain high levels of health and hygiene standards.

Julia Francis

You will need to have to hand a good range of make-up, suitable for clients with known skin allergies to cosmetics, for contact-lens wearers, for different skin types, conditions, ages and skin colours including:

- concealing and contouring cosmetics (shaders, highlighters and blushers)
- foundations
- translucent powders
- eye shadows
- eyeliners
- brow liners
- mascara
- lipsticks
- lip glosses
- lip liners

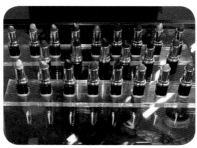
Professional lipstick products

BEST PRACTICE

Positive promotion
Where possible, use make-up that you also sell in the salon, so that the client can buy the products for home use if they wish. Use attractive posters and displays to raise awareness and interest in the products.

Range of brushes

Name	Description
Large face powder dusting brush	To remove excess face powder or to apply specialized powders such as bronzing and shimmer powders.
Foundation brush	To apply foundation to specific areas.
Contouring blush brush	To apply facial contouring products to highlight and shade areas of the face.

Blusher brush (large to medium)	To apply powder colour to the face and for blending.
Small flat angle-edged eye shadow brush	To apply and blend powder eye make-up products in the socket area of the eye.
Small rounded-edged eye shadow brush	To apply eye shadow, blend and shade.
Medium firm eye shadow blending brush	To blend powder eye colours and soften harsh lines and colour.
Small concealer brush	For exact placement of concealing product in areas such as around the nose and mouth.
Eyebrow brush	To remove excess make-up from the brow hair and to add colour, blend eyebrow pencil and groom the brow hair into shape.
Eyeliner brush	A fine brush used to apply make-up eye liner colour to contour the eyes, creating a precise line. A line and define brush is shown.
Mascara wand/comb	To apply mascara and remove excess mascara to separate the lashes.
Lip brush	To apply lip products and ensure a definite, balanced outline to the lips.

BEAUTY EXPRESS LTD

HEALTH & SAFETY

Avoiding cross-infection

To avoid cross-infection, don't use the applicators supplied with cosmetic products directly on a client, i.e. mascara brush. Use disposable applicators.

Make-up brushes These are prepared from different fibres, which may be synthetic or animal including camel, sable, squirrel, pony and goat.

Powder and blusher brushes may be produced from softer hair, but for the purpose of contouring and blending, brushes must be firmer.

BEST PRACTICE

Name badges

Have a clean cotton bud available so that you can remove the powder from any minor mistakes during application.

TOP TIP

Make-up brushes

When buying make-up brushes, make sure that the hairs are secure at the base of the brush. Test the comfort of the bristles, stroke against the skin.

Have more than one set of brushes. To avoid cross-infection they must be cleaned after use.

TOP TIP

Make-up case

If you intend to apply make-up at different locations, buy a large make-up case so that you can transport the make-up easily and hygienically.

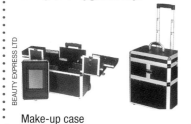

BEAUTY EXPRESS LTD

Make-up case

BEST PRACTICE

Make-up sponges

Keep a store of spare make-up sponges – they soon crumble with repeated cleaning.

HEALTH & SAFETY

Maintaining hygiene

If you drop a make-up tool on the floor, discard it – don't use it again until it has been disinfected and sterilized.

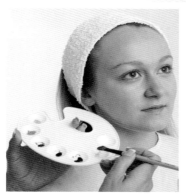

Make-up pallete

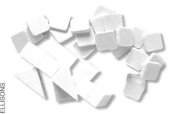

ELLISONS

Make-up sponges

BEST PRACTICE

False eyelashes

False eyelashes should be available if you are applying an evening or special occasion make-up – you may wish to apply these to enhance the final effect.

Transporting make-up

If you are transporting your make-up in a box, keep the box clean. Clients won't be impressed if they see soiled, dirty make-up containers.

TOP TIP

An *alcohol-based cleanser* may be used to clean make-up brushes. The brushes are first cleaned with a solution of warm water and detergent, then thoroughly rinsed in clean water and allowed to dry. They are then briefly immersed in the alcohol solution and again allowed to dry.

TOP TIP

When you give a make-up lesson, do so in front of a large mirror so that the client can watch the various stages of make-up application.

Record the make-up used and the advice given on a separate record, for the client to take away with them.

Sterilization and disinfection

Hygiene must be maintained in a number of ways:

- ensure that tools and equipment are sterile before use
- disinfect work surfaces after every client
- always follow hygienic work practices
- maintain a high standard of personal hygiene

Where possible, use disposable applicators during make-up application, costing these into the service price. Disinfect make-up brushes after each use: wash them in warm water and detergent, rinse them thoroughly in a disinfecting solution and then rinse in clean water, and allow them to dry naturally. Once dry, place the brushes in an ultra-violet light cabinet ready for use.

All cosmetic products should be removed from their containers using a clean spatula or orange stick, and placed on the clean plastic make-up palette before application. (This avoids contamination of the make-up with bacteria from unclean make-up applicators.)

The make-up palette should be cleaned with warm water and detergent, then wiped with a disinfectant solution applied using clean cotton wool. It should be stored in the ultra-violet cabinet.

Mascara should be applied using a disposable brush applicator, fresh for each client. Sharpen cosmetic pencils with a pencil sharpener before each use.

Make-up sponges should be disposed of after use, or washed in warm water and detergent; then placed in a disinfectant solution and rinsed. Allow them to dry, then place them in the ultra-violet cabinet, with each side being exposed for at least 20 minutes.

Outcome 2: Consult, plan and prepare for make-up service

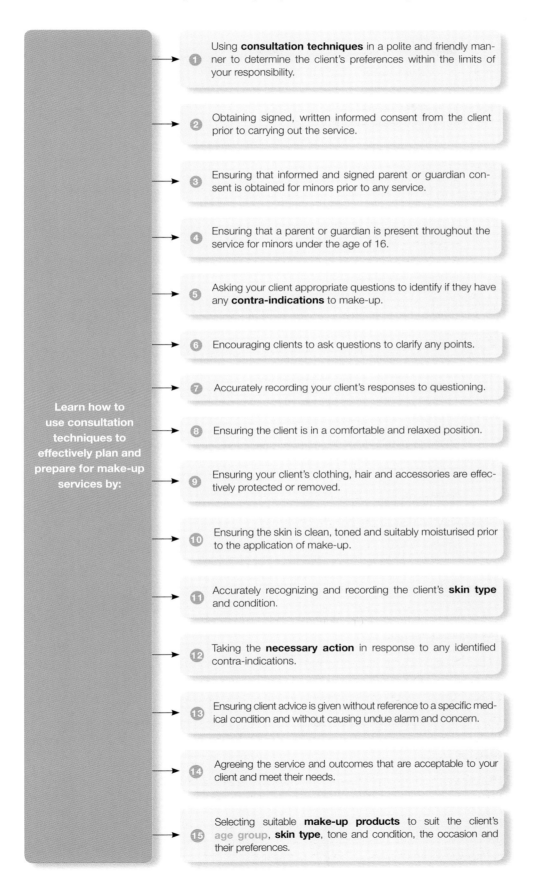

Learn how to use consultation techniques to effectively plan and prepare for make-up services by:

1. Using **consultation techniques** in a polite and friendly manner to determine the client's preferences within the limits of your responsibility.

2. Obtaining signed, written informed consent from the client prior to carrying out the service.

3. Ensuring that informed and signed parent or guardian consent is obtained for minors prior to any service.

4. Ensuring that a parent or guardian is present throughout the service for minors under the age of 16.

5. Asking your client appropriate questions to identify if they have any **contra-indications** to make-up.

6. Encouraging clients to ask questions to clarify any points.

7. Accurately recording your client's responses to questioning.

8. Ensuring the client is in a comfortable and relaxed position.

9. Ensuring your client's clothing, hair and accessories are effectively protected or removed.

10. Ensuring the skin is clean, toned and suitably moisturised prior to the application of make-up.

11. Accurately recognizing and recording the client's **skin type** and condition.

12. Taking the **necessary action** in response to any identified contra-indications.

13. Ensuring client advice is given without reference to a specific medical condition and without causing undue alarm and concern.

14. Agreeing the service and outcomes that are acceptable to your client and meet their needs.

15. Selecting suitable **make-up products** to suit the client's age group, **skin type**, tone and condition, the occasion and their preferences.

TOP TIP

Lighting

If working under artificial light, use warm white fluorescent light for day make-up, as this closely resembles natural light.

A diffuser may be used to cover the fluorescent tube. This softens the cool effect on the make-up and reduces the effects of shadows.

BEST PRACTICE

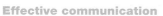

Effective communication

When applying make-up it is important that you fully understand the effect to be achieved. Good communication is essential. Ask the client/photographer what the final result should look like.

It is also important that you check that the client does not have allergies to any products to avoid a contra-action.

ALWAYS REMEMBER

Service timings

Make-up lesson: allow 1 hour.

Special occasion make-up: allow 45 minutes to hour.

Straight make-up: allow 45 minutes.

Reception

When a client makes an appointment for a make-up service, the receptionist will need to check the purpose of the make-up application.

Make-up application is offered for different purposes, called a make-up occasion.

- **A make-up lesson** A chance for the client to learn from a professional how to apply make-up that suits them.

- **Special occasion make-up** that is applied to suit the occasion for which it is to be worn, such as a wedding. If the make-up is for a bride, advise the client to visit the salon for a consultation and a practice session so that you can decide together on appropriate make-up. Ask the client if possible to bring a swatch of the dress material with her, so that you can select colours to complement this and to co-ordinate with the accessories.

- **Evening make-up** will be seen under artificial lighting. The effect this has on the appearance of the make-up will depend upon the light source, which must be considered when applying evening make-up. Generally evening make-up is heavier in application and stronger colours may be applied. Products to emphasize and highlight, such as frosted eye shadows and lip glosses, may be introduced.

- **Remedial make-up** may be applied for remedial purposes, to cover facial disfigurements or birthmarks, and the client can be taught how to do this themselves.

- **Photographic make-up** is applied for many reasons including magazine shoots, portrait work and fashion shows. Make-up application must be skilful to achieve the right end-result as the location may be a photographic studio or outdoors on location.

- **A professional job** Some clients simply wish to have their make-up professionally applied.

All staff, especially the staff communicating with clients at reception should be familiar with the different pricing structures for the range of make-up services and products available for retail.

In the salon advise the client that if they intend to have their hair washed and styled, this should be done before they have the make-up applied.

If a client requests a deep cleansing facial followed by make-up application, suggest that they have the facial at least five days prior to the make-up. The facial will stimulate the skin, increasing its normal physiological functioning. This will affect how long the make-up lasts; it may even cause the colour of the foundation to change.

Do not reshape the eyebrows at the same service as make-up application – secondary infection could occur; also the skin in the area will be very pink, altering the colour and thus the effect of eye shadow.

The consultation If the client is new, complete a record card noting the client's personal details, this will be used to record details of the make-up applied. A sample record card for make-up is found on page 286.

If the client is a minor under the age of 16, it is necessary to obtain parent/guardian permission for the make-up service. The parent/guardian will also have to be present when the service is received.

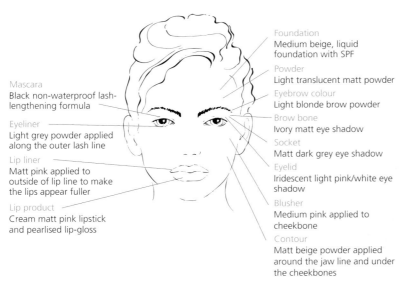

Mascara
Black non-waterproof lash-lengthening formula

Eyeliner
Light grey powder applied along the outer lash line

Lip liner
Matt pink applied to outside of lip line to make the lips appear fuller

Lip product
Cream matt pink lipstick and pearlised lip-gloss

Foundation
Medium beige, liquid foundation with SPF

Powder
Light translucent matt powder

Eyebrow colour
Light blonde brow powder

Brow bone
Ivory matt eye shadow

Socket
Matt dark grey eye shadow

Eyelid
Iridescent light pink/white eye shadow

Blusher
Medium pink applied to cheekbone

Contour
Matt beige powder applied around the jaw line and under the cheekbones

Sample make-up record card showing examples of information to record following a make-up service

ALWAYS REMEMBER

Examples of make-up service modification include:

- choice of make-up products and application techniques for corrective work
- choice of make-up to suit the client's skin type and condition
- disguising minor skin imperfections
- using hypo-allergenic products for a client with cosmetic sensitivity
- age of client, using light-reflecting make-up products for a mature skin or one showing signs of premature aging

HEALTH & SAFETY

Hygiene at home

Advise clients to keep their own make-up clean. Dirty brushes spoil effective make-up application, and offer breeding grounds for bacteria.

Make-up generally has a shelf life of two years and is then past its best and becomes unhygienic. It is recommended that mascara be replaced every six months.

Discuss your make-up plan with the client to ensure that the make-up will meet their requirements. You may need to ask questions such as those that follow, but of course the questions depend on the purpose of the make-up application.

- 'Do you normally wear make-up?'
- 'For what occasion is the make-up to be worn?'
- 'What colour are the clothing and accessories to be worn on this occasion?'
- 'Are there any colours that you particularly like or dislike?'
- 'What effect would you like the make-up to create?' (This question may be asked in many contexts – the client/photographer may wish to achieve a natural or a glamorous effect, or to emphasize or diminish certain facial features.)

Provide the opportunity for your client to ask any questions relating to the make-up service.

The record card should be signed and dated following the consultation to confirm the suitability and consent with the agreed make-up service.

It is important that accurate records are kept and stored in compliance with the Data Protection Act for future reference.

ALWAYS REMEMBER

Accurately record your client's answers to necessary questions to be asked at consultation on the record card.

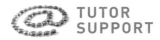

TUTOR SUPPORT

Activity 6: Client record card task

A sample client record card

Date	Beauty therapist name	
Client name	Date of birth (Identifying client age group.)	
Home address	Postcode	
Email address	Landline phone number	Mobile phone number
Name of doctor	Doctor's address and phone number	
Related medical history (Conditions that may restrict or prohibit service application.)		
Are you taking any medication? (This may affect skin sensitivity.)		

CONTRA-INDICATIONS REQUIRING MEDICAL REFERRAL
(Preventing the application of make-up.)

- ☐ bacterial infections (e.g. impetigo, conjunctivitis)
- ☐ viral infections (e.g. herpes simplex)
- ☐ fungal infections (e.g. tinea corporis)
- ☐ parasitic infestations (e.g. pediculosis and scabies)

SKIN TYPE
☐ oily   ☐ dry   ☐ combination

CONCEALER
☐ cream   ☐ stick   ☐ liquid

FOUNDATION
- ☐ liquid   ☐ compact
- ☐ stick   ☐ cream
- ☐ mineral   ☐ tinted moisturiser

POWDER
☐ loose   ☐ compact   ☐ mineral

BRONZING PRODUCTS
☐ powder   ☐ gel   ☐ liquid

EYE PRODUCTS FOR EYE AREA
- ☐ cream eye shadow   ☐ liquid eyeliner
- ☐ pencil eyeliner   ☐ powder eye shadow
- ☐ kohl eyeliner   ☐ mineral and pigment eye shadows
- ☐ cake eyeliner   ☐ gel eye shadow

EYE PRODUCTS FOR BROW AREA
- ☐ pencil   ☐ liquid
- ☐ shadow   ☐ eyebrow mascara

EYE PRODUCTS FOR EYELASHES
- ☐ waterproof mascara   ☐ non-waterproof mascara
- ☐ false lashes   ☐ lash curling

CONTRA-INDICATIONS WHICH RESTRICT SERVICE
(Service may require adaptation.)

- ☐ cuts and abrasions   ☐ bruising and swelling
- ☐ recent scar tissue   ☐ eczema
- ☐ skin allergies   ☐ vitiligo
- ☐ styes   ☐ hyper keratosis
- ☐ watery eyes

MAKE-UP CONTEXT
- ☐ day   ☐ evening
- ☐ special occasion   ☐ make-up instruction

CHEEK PRODUCTS
- ☐ highlighter   ☐ shader
- ☐ blusher

LIP PRODUCTS
- ☐ pencil lip liner   ☐ lip gloss
- ☐ lipstick   ☐ lip balm

Record of make-up products applied

Beauty therapist signature (for reference)
Client signature (confirmation of details)

A sample client record card (continued)

SERVICE ADVICE
Make-up service – allow 45 minutes

SERVICE PLAN
Record relevant details of your service and advice provided for future reference.
Ensure the client's records are up to date, accurate and fully completed following service. Non-compliance may invalidate insurance.

DURING
Find out:
- what products the client is currently using to cleanse and care for the skin of the face and neck

Discuss:
- the importance of a good skincare routine in relation to make-up application
- current satisfaction with the client's make-up technique
- tips and explain each stage of the make-up application to enhance the client's understanding

Note:
- any adverse reaction, if any occur

AFTER
Record:
- any modification to make-up service application that has occurred
- what products have been used in the make-up service
- the effectiveness of the make-up result
- any samples provided (review their success at the next appointment)

Advise on:
- how to reapply products to achieve/maintain the result
- correct make-up removal technique

RETAIL OPPORTUNITIES
Advise on:
- products that would be suitable for the client to use at home to care for their skin
- the benefits of each make-up product clearly and logically during application
- recommendations for further make-up services
- further products or services that the client may or may not have received before

Note:
- any purchase made by the client

EVALUATION
Record:
- comments on the client's satisfaction with the service
- if poor results are achieved, the reasons why

HEALTH AND SAFETY
Advise on:
- avoidance of activities or product application that may cause a contra-action
- appropriate **necessary action** to be taken in the event of an unwanted skin reaction

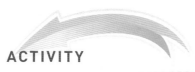

ACTIVITY

Recognizing contra-indications
What skin disorders can you think
of that would contra-indicate make-
up application?

Contra-indications

Certain **contra-indications** prevent make-up application. These include bacterial, fungal, parasitic and viral infections which are described in more detail in Chapter 3, where contra-indications are illustrated and discussed. Check for these at the consultation, and if any of the following are present on inspection of the skin, do not proceed with make-up application.

Remember that not all contra-indications are visible – a current bone fracture, for example would not be. The following disorders may contra-indicate or restrict make-up service. If you suspect the client has any disorder from the list below, do not attempt a diagnosis but refer the client tactfully to their GP without causing concern.

- **pediculosis capitis (head lice)** for full details see Chapter 3, page 94
- **pediculosis corporis (body lice)** for full details see Chapter 3, page 94
- **acne vulgaris (active)** for full details see Chapter 3, page 96
- **herpes simplex (cold sore)** for full details see Chapter 3, page 92
- **impetigo** for full details see Chapter 3, page 91
- **styes or hordeola** for full details see Chapter 3, page 92
- **conjuncitivitis (pink eye)** for full details see Chapter 3, page 91
- **watery eye or epiphora** for full details see Chapter 8, page 242
- **bepharitis** for full details see Chapter 8, page 242

The following conditions also contra-indicate make-up application:

- **skin disorders** including those not listed in the above list, such as bacterial infections (e.g. boils), viral infections (herpes zoster), and fungal infections (e.g. tinea corporis)
- **active psoriasis** and **eczema**
- **bruising** in the area
- **recent haemorrhage**
- **swelling and inflammation** in the area
- **recent scar tissue**
- **sensory nerve disorders**
- **cuts or abrasions** in the area
- **a recent operation** in the area
- **eye disorders** including those not listed in the chart
- **parasitic infestation** such as pediculosis and scabies

Ask the client whether they have any known allergies to cosmetic preparations. Note the answer on the record card. Care must be taken to avoid contact with an allergen.

Remember—never name a contra-indication, you may be wrong. Refer the client to their GP, this is their role.

In the case of the skin disorder herpes simplex, the make-up service may be received when the skin is healed and clear.

Contra-actions

Certain cosmetic ingredients are known to provoke allergic reactions in some people. These allergens may cause irritation, excessive erythema, inflammation and swelling. This is known as a **contra-action**. This may occur during or following service.

Known cosmetic allergens include the following:

- **Lanolin** This is similar to sebum, and is obtained from sheep's wool. It is added to many cosmetics as an emollient.

- **Mineral oils** Examples are oleic acid and butyl stearate.

- **Eosin (bromo-acid dye)** A staining **pigment**, used in some lip cosmetics and perfumes.

- **Paraben** An antiseptic ingredient, used as a preservative in facial cosmetics.

- **Certain colourants** One example is carmine.

- **Perfume** This is added to most cosmetics, and is a common sensitizer.

Products should be selected without the allergen where identified.

Other contra-actions include:

- **Watery eyes** The client's eyes water excessively. If the client has watery eyes a tissue may be placed at the corners until the irritation has ceased. If the client's eyes continue to water, remove eye make-up and discontinue service.

- **Excessive perspiration** Some clients may perspire, which will affect adherence of the make-up and its finished result. Blot the skin with soft facial tissue and apply more loose face powder to absorb perspiration. If the client continues to perspire, discontinue treatment.

External contact with an allergen may cause urticaria (hives or nettle rash), eczema or dermatitis. If an allergy occurs, the product should be removed from the skin and a soothing substance applied. The client should be advised not to use the product again. Always record any allergies on the client's record card so that the offending product may be avoided in the future.

Preparing the client

Take the client through to the make-up work area. Make-up application may take place either at the make-up chair, in front of a mirror, or at the service couch. Before you start the make-up, discuss and plan the make-up with the client, recording significant details on their record card.

Before preparing the client for the service, clean your hands using an approved hand cleansing technique in front of your client who will observe hygienic procedures being carried out. The client need remove only their upper outer clothing, to their underwear. Offer the client a gown, or drape a clean towel or make-up cape across their chest and shoulders. Place a headband or hairclip around the hairline, to protect the hair and keep it away from the face. Any jewellery in the service area should be removed. Refer to the record card to check for any known allergies to cosmetic products.

Ensure that the client is comfortable.

After preparing the client, and before touching the skin, clean your hands again. Now cleanse and tone the skin, using products appropriate to their skin type. Just as skincare

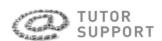

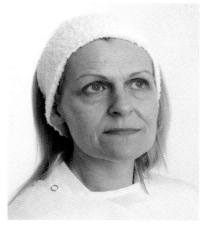

Client preparation

BEST PRACTICE

Headbands

If a headband is used, remove it directly after the facial cleanse so that it doesn't flatten and spoil the hair.

HEALTH & SAFETY

Contact lenses

If the client wears contact lenses, ask them whether they wish to remove them before the skin is cleansed. (The need for this will depend on the sensitivity of the eyes.)

products vary in their formulation to suit the various skin types, so make-up products are designed for different skins. Record all relevant details on the record card.

Inspect the skin using a magnifying lamp. Identify any areas that require specific attention, i.e. broken capillaries, pustules, papules, dark circles, hyper-pigmentation, hypo-pigmentation and scarring.

Apply a light-textured **moisturiser** before make-up application. This has the following benefits.

- it prevents the natural secretions of the skin changing the colour of the foundation
- it seals the surface of the skin, and prevents absorption of the foundation into the skin
- it facilitates make-up application by providing a smooth base

Remove excess moisturiser by blotting the skin with a facial tissue.

Special lotions may be applied to improve the skin texture and increase make-up durability these include skin **primers** and oil control lotions.

Skin primers are silicone-based creating a film on the skin surface. It refines the skin's appearance minimizing open pores and the appearance of fine lines. The formulations can vary to suit the client's skin type and main contain pigments to correct **skin tone**. The primer provides a base and acts as a barrier preventing absorption of the make-up products into the skin. Primers are applied as moisturiser but less is required.

Oil control lotions contain powder ingredients which absorb the skin's natural oil, reducing shine and producing a matt finish. They are ideal to prepare an oily or combination skin before make-up application.

Outcome 3: Apply make-up products

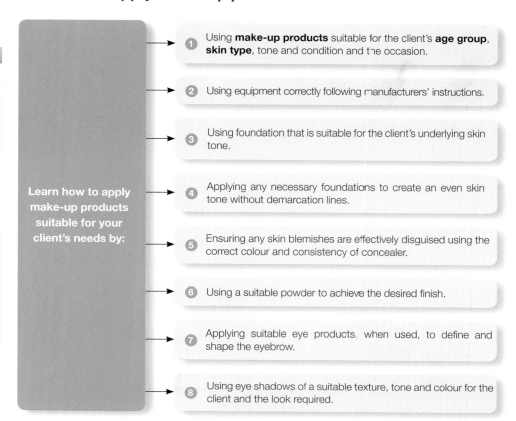

Learn how to apply make-up products suitable for your client's needs by:

1. Using **make-up products** suitable for the client's **age group, skin type,** tone and condition and the occasion.

2. Using equipment correctly following manufacturers' instructions.

3. Using foundation that is suitable for the client's underlying skin tone.

4. Applying any necessary foundations to create an even skin tone without demarcation lines.

5. Ensuring any skin blemishes are effectively disguised using the correct colour and consistency of concealer.

6. Using a suitable powder to achieve the desired finish.

7. Applying suitable eye products. when used, to define and shape the eyebrow.

8. Using eye shadows of a suitable texture, tone and colour for the client and the look required.

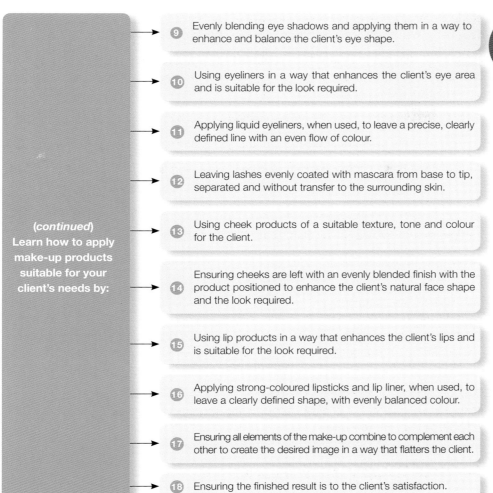

9 Evenly blending eye shadows and applying them in a way to enhance and balance the client's eye shape.

10 Using eyeliners in a way that enhances the client's eye area and is suitable for the look required.

11 Applying liquid eyeliners, when used, to leave a precise, clearly defined line with an even flow of colour.

12 Leaving lashes evenly coated with mascara from base to tip, separated and without transfer to the surrounding skin.

(continued)
Learn how to apply make-up products suitable for your client's needs by:

13 Using cheek products of a suitable texture, tone and colour for the client.

14 Ensuring cheeks are left with an evenly blended finish with the product positioned to enhance the client's natural face shape and the look required.

15 Using lip products in a way that enhances the client's lips and is suitable for the look required.

16 Applying strong-coloured lipsticks and lip liner, when used, to leave a clearly defined shape, with evenly balanced colour.

17 Ensuring all elements of the make-up combine to complement each other to create the desired image in a way that flatters the client.

18 Ensuring the finished result is to the client's satisfaction.

TOP TIP

Removing eyeliner
Existing cosmetic eyeliner is sometimes difficult to remove. Use a cotton bud soaked in eye make-up remover: gently stroke this along the base of the lower eyelashes, in towards the nose.

ALWAYS REMEMBER

Erythema
Avoid excessive pressure and stimulation of the skin while cleansing and preparing the skin for make-up application.

The skin will become too warm, affecting durability and erythema of the skin will occur – skin reddening requires correction.

Applying make-up products

The make-up sequence

The correct sequence for applying make-up is as follows.

1 Conceal any blemishes.

2 Apply foundation.

3 Contour the face (with cream liquid products).

4 Apply powder.

5 Contour the face (with powder products).

6 Apply blusher.

7 Apply eye shadow.

8 Make up the eyebrows.

9 Apply mascara.

10 Make up the lips.

11 Contour products, used to shade and highlight the face and features, can be applied in powder or cream formulation. Application sequence for contouring will depend upon product formulation chosen.

ALWAYS REMEMBER

Order of application
Make-up is applied in a specific sequence to ensure:

- a balanced look is achieved

- products are applied effectively, i.e. cream on cream, powder on powder, which allows products to be blended and set appropriately

- the client's understanding, e.g. when carrying out a make-up lesson or demonstrating how to achieve a certain look

- durability and the optimum look of the make-up is maintained

Concealing may be completed before or after foundation application.

Use all products following manufacturers' instructions to ensure the optimum make-up is achieved.

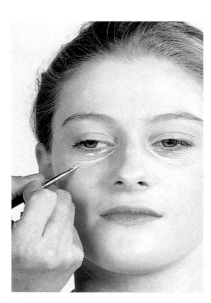

Applying concealer

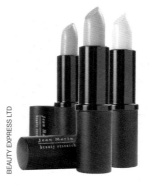

BEAUTY EXPRESS LTD

Concealing products

Age of the client

When applying make-up consider how skin changes with age. This will influence the imperfections and skin conditions that may be present and require correction.

Appearance and age table

Age	Appearance
<15	Nearly perfect skin. Smooth texture, pores small.
15–25	Acne key factor in surface texture. Fine lines start to appear, pore size increasing.
24–45	More fine lines and appearance of first wrinkles (photodamage). Early signs of sagging near the eye. Some loss of elasticity. Adult acne.
45–55	More wrinkles, rough texture. Sallow yellow colour begins to appear. Pores and age spots enlarge and define. Sagging near eye and cheek.
55+	Wrinkles and fine lines in abundance. Uneven colour, pigmentation. Sagging worsens. Dark circles under eye.

DR. JOHN GRAY, THE WORLD OF SKIN CARE

Concealer

Concealing blemishes

Before you begin to apply make-up to the face, inspect the skin and identify any areas that require concealing, such as blemishes, uneven skin colour, dark circles under the eyes or shadows.

Foundation may be used to disguise minor skin imperfections, but where extra coverage is required it is necessary to apply a special concealer, a cosmetic designed to provide maximum skin coverage. The concealer may be applied directly to the skin after skin moisturising, or following application of the foundation.

Choose a concealer that is one to two shades lighter than the client's skin tone.

Concealers designed for use around the eye area are light in texture, lighter in colour than the foundation with a yellow tone to minimize the appearance of dark circles. Concealers designed for covering blemishes are unsuitable for application around the eyes.

Concealer can contain pigment to help correct skin tone.

- **Green** helps to counteract high colouring, and to conceal dilated capillaries.
- **Lilac or pink** counteracts a sallow skin colour.

- **Peach and pink** counteracts dark circles around the eyes and is suitable for darker skin tones.

- **White or cream** helps to correct unevenness in the skin pigmentation.

- **Yellow** helps to counteract the appearance of dark circles around the eyes.

Concealers come in a range of colours and consistencies, to suit all skins and differences in skin texture. Mix different colours together to obtain the required colour.

Colour correctors target problem areas and contain pigments which balance skin tone. Select lighter shades, e.g. light pink for lighter skins, if the skin is darker select shades of peach. Peach is particularly effective to counteract bluish under-eye shadows. Green correctors counteract areas of redness. Yellow counteracts pink tones.

Correctors are applied like concealer and may be followed with concealer or foundation.

Applying concealer Remove a small quantity of the concealer from its container, using a clean disposable spatula. If it has a brush applicator attached to the product, for reasons of hygiene this cannot be used.

Apply the concealer to the area to be disguised, using either a clean make-up sponge or a soft make-up brush. Blend the concealer to achieve a realistic effect. Reapply concealer as necessary until correction is achieved.

TOP TIP

Avoid rubbing the product while blending it, or it will wipe off.

ALWAYS REMEMBER

Asian clients very often have darker skin underneath the eye area, and this may require concealing.

ALWAYS REMEMBER

Common racial skin problems:

- Caucasian – easily damaged by exposure to high temperatures and ultra-violet light, leading to broken veins and pigmentation disorders.

- Oriental – prone to uneven pigmentation on ultra-violet light exposure.

- Asian – often has uneven pigmentation skin tones; darker skin is often found around the eyes.

- African-Caribbean – melanin is present in all layers of the epidermis; this can cause scarring following skin damage, possibly leading to uneven pigmentation, vitiligo and keloids.

Using concealer to camouflage

Specialist techniques are required to conceal problem areas; this is called camouflage. Areas that may be required to be camouflaged include:

- **Scars** caused by injury, post-operative, keloids (lumpy scar tissue forming at the site of wounds), acne vulgaris, burns which can cause the skin to become ridged or discoloured.

- **Birthmarks** Darker pigmented areas.

- **Pigment disorders** Hypopigmentation (reduced melanin production, e.g. vitiligo) and hyperpigmentation (increased melanin production, e.g. chloasmata – brown patches), moles, dermatosis papulosa nigra, (a benign or non-malignant skin condition common among adult black-skinned people characterized by multiple small, hyperpigmented (dark brown to black) papules on the face, neck, upper back and chest).

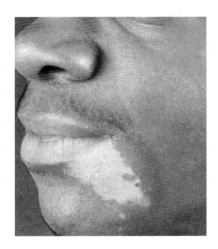

Vitiligo

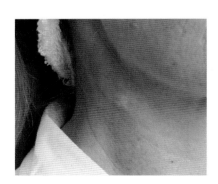

A) Hypopigmentation in the neck area

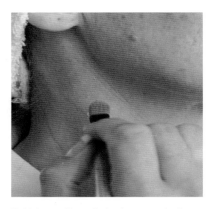

B) Make-up is applied using a synthetic brush to cover the blemish

TOP
TIP

It is preferable to build up several layers to achieve the desired effect, rather than applying a thick layer.

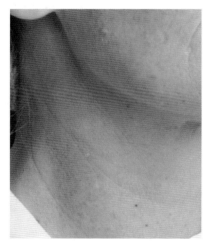

C) The area is disguised

HEALTH & SAFETY

Medicated concealers
Advise clients to avoid medicated 'lipstick'-type concealers – these are too thick for general concealing. They are also unhygienic, as they are designed to be directly applied to a blemish: this means that the product becomes a breeding ground for bacteria.

● **Vascular disorders** Rosacea (chronic inflammation of the skin on the nose and cheeks caused by the dilation of the blood capillaries) and telangiectasia (dilated capillaries appearing on the face).

How to apply concealer to camouflage

Always check the manufacturer's instructions on how to apply the camouflage/concealing product. Brands vary and some may require different preparation and setting techniques.

1 Select the chosen colour or colour mixture that best matches the skin tone surrounding the area to be treated.

2 Using your ring and middle fingers in a patting motion, or using a dry sponge, blend the make-up thinly over the problem area, extending it approximately 2cm past the edge. If disguising scars, a brush may be used to feather the make-up at the edges to create a natural effect. The sponge may be dampened if needed to facilitate extra blending.

3 Build up the colour depth to ensure the blemish is completely covered, thinning the colour at the edge to blend in. A small make-up brush can be used to blend in the edges of the make-up.

4 Once the required result has been achieved, apply the fixing powder generously with a large powder puff.

5 Leave the make-up to set for five to ten minutes.

6 Entirely brush off any excess fixing powder with a large, soft make-up brush, e.g. blusher/powder brush. Blot off excess powder if required with damp cotton wool. The make-up is now waterproof and rub-resistant, and should not be detectable.

7 If the camouflage has been applied to the face, full make-up may now be applied. The foundation colour selected should match the colour of the camouflage make-up.

8 Apply foundation up to the area of camouflage make-up and blend so that an invisible finish is created. Putting an oily cream foundation over the camouflage make-up will move or remove the camouflage make-up; it is best to use a non-oily or liquid foundation.

9 Record on the client record card the make-up products selected and application technique used.

TOP
TIP

● *Covering a deep red mark*: use a green pigmented make-up first, then apply make-up which matches the skin tone over the top.
● *Covering a dark brown mark*: use white, opaque make-up first, then apply make-up which matches the skin tone over the top.
● *Covering a lighter mark*: commence with a darker foundation and apply make-up which matches the skin tone over the top.

Foundation

Foundation is applied to produce an even skin tone, to disguise minor skin blemishes, and as a contour cosmetic. Black skin in particular often has an uneven skin tone, requiring certain parts of the face to be lightened and others darkened to produce an even skin tone.

Foundation is available as cream, liquid, compact stick, gel, cake, mousse, mineral-based and tinted moisturiser.

Foundations can contain **'anti-ageing' ingredients** such as vitamins A, C and E. These are to neutralize **free radicals**, natural chemicals thought to be responsible for damaging the skin and producing the signs of ageing – the lines and wrinkles! Sunscreens and moisturisers are commonly included in foundations to protect the skin from the environment.

Silica beads can be included in the formulations, especially for combination/oily skin, to absorb the skin's natural sweat and oil.

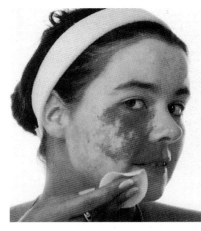

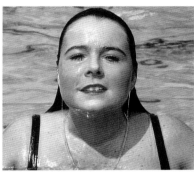

Covering a deep red mark: before and after

ACTIVITY

Comparing foundations
Compare the proportions of ingredients contained in foundations for each skin type. How, and why, are they different?

Kinds of foundations

Each foundation differs in its formulation to suit a particular skin type. The correct choice will guarantee that the foundation lasts throughout the day.

ACTIVITY

Selecting a foundation
Name a suitable foundation for each of the following skin types:

- normal
- dry
- oily
- combination
- sensitive
- blemished

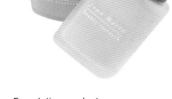

BEAUTY EXPRESS LTD

Foundation products

Cream foundations **Cream foundations** are oil-based and blend easily on application. They provide a heavy coverage, and have these specific service uses:

- dry skin
- normal skin
- mature skin

TOP TIP

To achieve a light, healthy, natural appearance, the client may apply a tinted moisturiser.

HEALTH & SAFETY

Choosing a foundation

- If the skin is oily and blemished, a *medicated* foundation may be used.
- If the client suffers from acne vulgaris, it is preferable not to apply foundation at all – bacterial infections might be aggravated.
- If the skin is sensitive, select a *hypoallergenic* foundation.

ALWAYS REMEMBER

Foundation colour

The skin's natural oils can change to colour of the foundation making it appear darker.

A tester if available should be provided to ensure the correct colour is chosen.

Liquid foundations

Liquid foundations are oil- or water-based, providing light to medium coverage. Oil-based liquid foundations have these specific uses:

- dry skin
- normal skin
- mature skin
- combination skin (apply the foundation to the *dry* areas)

Water-based liquid foundations have the following uses:

- normal skin
- oily skin
- combination skin (apply the foundation to the *oily* areas)

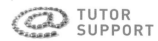

TUTOR SUPPORT

Activity 3: Foundation and concealer handout

Liquid foundations are composed of water, powder, oil, humectant (such as glycerol), pigments and additives.

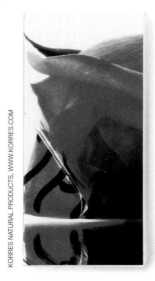

KORRES NATURAL PRODUCTS, WWW.KORRES.COM

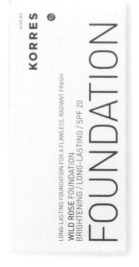

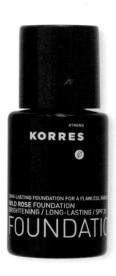

Oil-based liquid foundation

Water-based foundations do not spread very easily because the water content rapidly evaporates, so these foundations must be applied quickly.

Gel foundations

Gel foundations provide sheer, oil-free non-greasy coverage. Provides a matte finish. Light reflective properties are achieved through the addition of pigments. They have these specific uses:

- black, unblemished skin
- tanned skin
- skin on which a natural effect is required

Compact skin or cake foundation

Compact skin or cake foundations may have an oil, wax or powder base. They give a heavy coverage, and have these specific uses:

- dry skin
- normal skin
- badly blemished or scarred skin

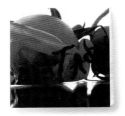 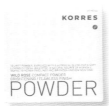 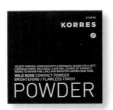 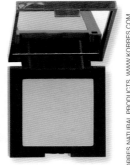

Compact foundation

KORRES NATURAL PRODUCTS, WWW.KORRES.COM

HEALTH & SAFETY

Product formulation MSDS sheets

Legally the manufacturer must produce a list of ingredients used in their product.

Request a Material Safety Data Sheet to refer to and ensure safe product selection.

Mousse foundations

Mousse foundations provide light to medium coverage depending on application technique. They have a mineral oil base. Their specific uses are:

- normal skin
- combination skin

Care must be taken to apply the mousse foundation to an area of the skin and blend quickly or it may start to dry on the face, creating a chalky appearance.

Mineral-based foundation

Mineral liquid foundation This contains the natural light-reflecting properties of micro-minerals. It provides a low to medium coverage, with a skin enhancing, slightly luminous look.

- It helps make the skin appear healthy and fresh.
- It is suitable for all skin types, especially normal to dry skin.

Mineral powder foundation containing micro-minerals in a solid powder with a binding ingredient such as algae. Again, suitable for all skin types providing a heavier coverage through layer application.

Mineral make-up is created from finely ground minerals, a process called micronization. Pure mineral make-up allows the skin to breathe as it does not contain synthetic powders and oils.

The make-up may contain a selection of the following minerals which all contribute an effect to the finished look of the make-up:

- Titanium oxide, a natural white mineral powder providing opacity – titanium is also an ingredient used in cosmetics for its sun protection factor (SPF) effect.
- Zinc oxide, a natural white mineral powder which enhances the appearance of the crystallized minerals; mica, a natural mineral which has light-reflecting properties showing a range of colours. (It also affects the finished formulation providing slip to facilitate make-up application.)
- Bismuth oxychloride, a synthetic white mineral with a silvery metallic sheen providing coverage to the make-up; iron oxide, a synthetic mineral iron used to add colour.

Tinted foundation provides a moist, light to medium coverage available in a range of shades. It offers protection from the environment with added sunscreen and skin moisturisers.

- It helps make the skin appear natural, healthy and fresh.
- It is suitable for all skin types in oil or oil free formulation.

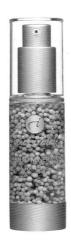

Liquid mineral

TOP TIP

Mineral make-up

Mineral make-up can be applied following a facial as the blend of minerals and pigments form microscopic flat crystals due to their formulation which allows the skin to breathe and function.

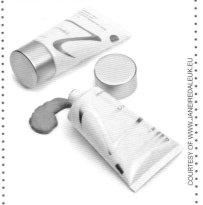

Mineral make-up products

COURTESY OF WWW.JANEIREDALEUK.EU

TOP TIP

A client may be advised to apply tinted foundation with the fingers which provides a sheer coverage. Instruct the client they must wash their hands before application.

TOP TIP

Using a palette
The make-up palette is useful when mixing foundations to match the colour of your client's skin.

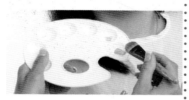

TOP TIP

Selection of foundation colour
If the foundation is too light it will appear ashen.

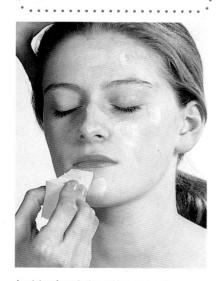

Applying foundation with a cosmetic sponge

Foundation colour

The colour or shade of the foundation should match the client's natural skin colour. Test the foundation for compatibility on the client's jaw line or forehead. If an incorrect colour is selected, or if the foundation is insufficiently blended on application, there will be a noticeable **demarcation line**.

Skin tones may vary on the face with lighter and darker areas, especially on black skin. If the lighter tones are to be emphasized, a lighter coverage foundation product should be selected allowing the skin's natural tone to show. Multi-ethnic skin will require mixing products and shades to create a balanced look. Remember products can be layered to increase coverage.

Skin colour	Foundation colour
Fair	Ivory or light beige, with warm tones of pink or peach.
Olive	Dark beige or bronze.
Suntanned	Bronze.
Florid	Matt beige with a green tint.
Sallow	Beige with a pink tint.
Light brown	Light brown foundation with a warm tone.
Medium brown	Light brown with a yellow/orange tone.
Dark brown	Deep bronze foundation with a yellow/orange tone.
Black	Dark golden bronze (usually a gel).

Applying the foundation

If the foundation is in a jar, remove some from its container using a clean disposable spatula. Put it on a clean make-up palette.

Foundation may be applied using either a large soft foundation brush, which is stroked over the surface of the skin, or a cosmetic sponge. It should be applied to one area of the face at a time, with an outward stroking movement.

Also use a cosmetic sponge to blend the foundation. Take care that you blend it at the hairline and at the jaw line. Avoid clogging the eyebrows with foundation. The **cosmetic make-up wedge** is designed to apply varying amounts of pressure to the different areas of the face, and to ensure even coverage of the foundation.

When applying foundation around the eye area, use a small soft brush or the angular edge of a cosmetic sponge. This will help you achieve accuracy in application.

The extent of coverage can be controlled by the method of application. If the cosmetic sponge is damp, coverage is light and sheer. To achieve a heavier coverage, use a dry latex-free sponge.

Apply foundation to cover the entire face, including the lips and the eyelids. Do not extend the make-up past the jaw line unless the occasion requires this – for example, if a bride's dress exposes part of the upper chest – because the foundation will mark clothes at the neckline.

Trouble spots such as areas of pigmentation should be concealed with a concealing product.

Contouring

Contour cosmetics

Changing the shape of the face and the facial features can be achieved with the careful application of **contour cosmetics**. These products draw attention either towards or away from facial features, and can create the optical illusion of perfection.

Each face differs in shape and size, so each requires a different application technique.

Contour cosmetics include **highlighters**, **shaders** and **blushers**. They are available in powder, liquid and cream forms.

- *Highlighters* Draw attention towards – they emphasize.
- *Shaders* Draw attention away – they minimize.
- *Blushers* Add warmth to the face and emphasize the facial contours.

Some blushers appear very vibrant in the container, yet when they are applied to the skin they are subtle.

Before applying these products, decide on the effect you wish to achieve. Study the client's face from the front and side profiles, and determine what facial corrective work is necessary.

The colour should brighten the face. Hold different blusher shades next to the face to identify a suitable colour. Consider the age of the client, natural shades are preferable rather than bright fashion colours.

Blushers are available in powder, cream and liquid formulations.

Powder blushers Mineral powder blusher is formulated using pigments to add colour and warmth to the skin. Alternatively, synthetic or natural pigments are formulated with a face powder with a talc base to add bulk, and zinc stearate to bind the ingredients together with various skin conditioning agents. A softer look is achieved with powder blusher.

Cream blushers A cream or wax base holds the pigment colour. Silicone is added to cream blushers to facilitate application.

Liquid blusher Pigment providing the tint shade is suspended in a liquid containing water, glycerine, silica and alcohol.

If liquid or cream cosmetics are used, these must be applied on top of a liquid or cream foundation before powder application. (If powder contour products are used, these should be applied after the application of the loose face powder. The rule of contour cosmetic application is: powder on powder; cream on cream.)

Mineral powder blush Minerals are refined to a light-weight, sheer application where colour is achieved by layering. Its ideal usage is for a mature skin.

TOP TIP

Professionally, avoid applying foundation with the fingers. Apart from being less hygienic, with this method the warmth of your hands may cause streaking.

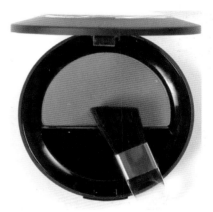

Blusher contour product

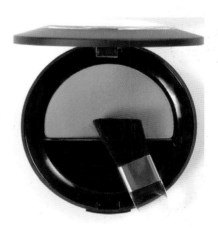

Shader/blusher contour product

TOP TIP

Blusher can be applied to the cheeks and temples to add warmth to the face.

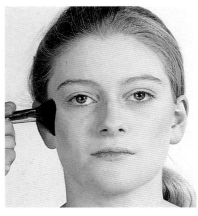

Applying blusher

How to apply powder blushers

Stroke the contour brush over the powder blusher. Tap the brush gently to dislodge excess blusher.

Apply the blusher to the cheek area, carefully placing the product according to the effect you wish to create. The direction of brush strokes should be upwards and outwards, towards the hairline. Keep the blusher away from the nose, and avoid applying blusher too near the outer eye. Ensure the edges of the blusher application are blended and softened.

Apply more blusher if necessary. The key to successful blusher application is to build up colour slowly until you have achieved the optimum effect.

If too much blusher is applied, tone down with the application of a loose face powder.

How to apply cream blushers

Remove the cream blusher hygienically from its container.

Apply the cream blusher after foundation application. Using the fingertips dot the cream blush colour sparingly onto the fullness of the cheek area and blend towards the hair line. Cream blusher is suited to all skin types except oily. Place a loose translucent powder over the cream blusher to set if required. Alternatively it can be left unpowdered for a 'dewy' effect.

Applying mineral powder blush

How to apply liquid blushers

Liquid blusher provides a sheer to strong, stained look, dependent upon product usage. It is best to apply to a normal skin as it is difficult to blend and would be generally unsuitable on a dry skin type.

Dot the liquid blush on the cheek area and blend well. Remember is must be worked with quickly, if left in an area too long it will stain and remain.

TOP TIP
Check blusher result after each application. Look at the client from the front and from each side of the face to check depth of colour and balance in application.

TOP TIP
Foundation may be suitable as a contour cosmetic. Choose a foundation either two shades lighter (as a highlighter) or two shades darker (as a shader) than the base foundation.

ALWAYS REMEMBER

Remember – it is easier to apply more blusher than to remove excess, which disturbs the foundation!

ACTIVITY

Facial bone structure
Draw and label the main facial bones. It is the differing sizes and proportions of these bones that give us our individual features.

To discover the size of each facial feature, feel the bony prominences of your own face with your fingers.

Face shapes

To assess the client's **face shape**, take the hair away from the face – hairstyles often disguise the face shape. Study the size and shape of the facial bone structure. Consider the amount of excess fat and the muscle tone.

Oval *Bone structure* This is regarded as the perfect face shape.

Corrective make-up Corrective make-up application usually attempts to create the *appearance* of an oval face shape. Draw attention to the cheekbones by applying shader beneath the cheekbone, and highlighter above. Blusher should be drawn along the cheekbone and blended up towards the temples.

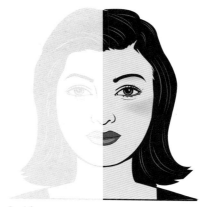
Oval face

Round *Bone structure* Broad and short.

Corrective make-up Apply highlighter in a thin band down the central portion of the face to create the illusion of length. Shader may be applied over the angle of the jaw to the temples. Apply blusher in a triangular shape, with the base of the triangle running parallel to the ear.

Square *Bone structure* A broad forehead and a broad, angular jaw line.

Corrective make-up Shade the angles of the jawbone, up and towards the cheekbone. Apply blusher in a circular pattern on the cheekbones, taking it towards the temples.

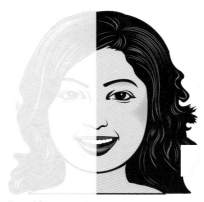
Round face

Heart *Bone structure* A wide forehead, with the face tapering to a narrow, pointed chin, like an inverted triangle.

Corrective make-up Highlight the angles of the jawbone and shade the point of the chin, the temples and the sides of the forehead. Apply blusher under the cheekbones, in an upward and outward direction towards the temples.

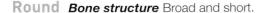

TOP TIP

Blusher
Keep blusher away from the centre of the face to avoid accentuating the breadth of the face.

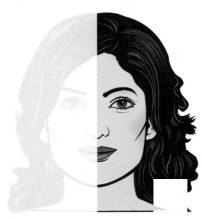
Square face

Diamond *Bone structure* A narrow forehead, with wide cheekbones tapering to a narrow chin.

Corrective make-up Apply shader to the tip of the chin and the height of the forehead, to reduce length. Highlight the narrow sides of the temples and the lower jaw. Apply blusher to the fullness of the cheekbones to draw attention to the centre of the face.

Oblong *Bone structure* Long and narrow, tapering to a pointed chin.

Corrective make-up Apply shader to the hairline and the point of the chin to reduce the length of the face. Highlight the angle of the jawbone and the temples to create width. Blend blusher along the cheekbones, outwards towards the ears.

Pear *Bone structure* A wide jaw line, tapering to a narrow forehead.

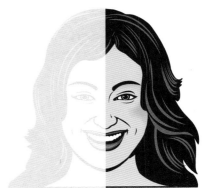
Heart face

Corrective make-up Highlight the forehead and shade the sides of the chin and the angle of the jaw. Apply blusher to the fullness of the cheeks, or blend it along the cheek-bones, up towards the temples.

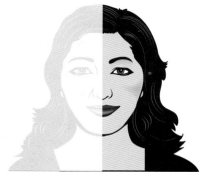

Diamond face

Oblong face

Pear face

Features

Noses

- **If the nose is too broad:** apply shader to the sides of the nose.
- **If the nose is too short:** apply highlighter down the length of the from the bridge to the tip.
- **If the nose is too long:** apply shader to the tip of the nose.
- **If there is a bump on the nose:** apply shader over the area.
- **If there is a hollow along the bridge of the nose:** apply highlighter the hollow area.
- **If the nose is crooked:** apply shader over the crooked side.

ACTIVITY

Contouring
Study three different clients or colleagues. Identify their face shapes. Where would you apply the contouring cosmetics for each face shape, and why?

ACTIVITY

Correcting nose shapes
Think of the different nose shapes you may encounter, such as Roman, turned up, bulbous, or with a long tip. Which contour cosmetics would you select to correct each? Where would you apply them?

Foreheads

- **If the forehead is prominent:** apply shader centrally over the prominent area, blending it outwards toward the temples.
- **If the forehead is shallow:** apply highlighter in a narrow band below the hairline.
- **If the forehead is deep:** apply shader in a narrow band below the hairline.

Chins

- **If the jaw is too wide:** apply shader from beneath the cheekbones and along the jaw line, blending it at the neck.
- **If the chin is double:** apply shader to the centre of the chin, blending it outwards along the jawbone and under the chin.

TOP TIP

An Asian face may appear as a flat plane: the skilful application of shading and highlighting products can create highs and lows.

- *If the chin is prominent:* apply foundation to the tip of the chin.
- *If the chin is long:* apply shader over the prominent area.
- *If the chin recedes:* apply highlighter along the jaw line and at the centre of the chin.

Necks

- *If the neck is thin:* apply highlighter down each side of the neck.
- *If the neck is thick:* apply shader to both sides of the neck.

Face powder

Face powder is applied to set the foundation, disguising minor blemishes and making the skin appear smooth and oil-free. It protects the skin from the environment by acting as a barrier. It also allows the application and smooth blending of other powder products such as blusher and eye shadow.

Most powders are based on **talc** as the main ingredient, but talc particles are of uneven size, and substitutes such as **mica** are now becoming popular. These give a more natural, flattering appearance to the skin.

Powder adheres to the foundation through the addition of **zinc, magnesium stearate** or **fatty esters**. These chemicals set the make-up and remove tackiness. Further powder products can then be applied to the skin.

Face powder contains absorbent materials such as **precipitated chalk, rice powder** or **nylon derivatives**. These absorb sweat and sebum throughout the day, reducing shine and giving the foundation greater durability.

Light-reflecting ingredients such as mica and moisturising ingredients are popular to reduce and soften the signs of ageing such as fine lines.

Shine control ingredients or 'blot powder' is created for use in professional situations and for touch-ups. Blot powder contains crystallized minerals and silica to absorb excess oils and reduce shine on the skin's surface.

Kinds of face powders

There are two basic products: loose powders and compact powders.

Loose powders **Loose powders** do not contain any oils or gums to bind the powder together. They are available in a range of shades, with different pastel pigments added to counteract skin imperfections. Colours include pink and lilac, which are flattering when viewed under artificial lights; yellow, which enhances a tanned skin; and green, which counteracts a red skin. Iridescent ingredients may be included to produce shimmering and highlighting effects.

Many cosmetic products contain **titanium dioxide**, an opaque white pigment, to provide coverage. When applied to black skin, this can give the skin a chalky appearance. When selecting products for black skin, bear in mind not just the shade but also the ingredients.

Compact powders **Compact powders** contain a gum, mixed with the ingredients to bind them together. These powders provide a greater coverage, especially if

TOP TIP

Foreheads
Foreheads can be improved by a flattering hairstyle:
- *Prominent forehead*: choose soft, flat, textured fringes.
- *Shallow forehead*: choose a shorter, soft fringe. Height will make the forehead appear longer.
- *Deep forehead*: choose a longer, soft fringe

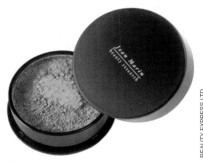

Face powder

BEAUTY EXPRESS LTD

HEALTH & SAFETY

Avoiding contamination
Before application, always remove sufficient loose powder from the container. This minimizes the chances of bacteria entering the powder.

they contain titanium dioxide. Pressed powders should be recommended mainly for a client's personal use, and then only to remove shine from the skin during the day, as required.

TOP TIP

Don't apply face powder to excessively dry skin, as it would aggravate and emphasize the dry skin condition.

Beware of applying powder if a client has superfluous facial hair, as it may emphasize this.

If the skin appears too pale apply a facial bronzer to correct.

Oily skin can make the powder darker. If this occurs apply a lighter powder to correct.

TOP TIP

Powders
Some powders reflect light while appearing subtle and non-shiny. These are most flattering for mature skin, as wrinkles appear less obvious.

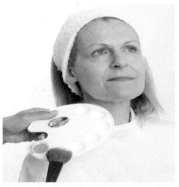

Light-reflecting mineral loose powder

How to apply powder

Face powder is applied **after** the foundation, unless a water-based foundation or a combination powder foundation has been selected. Select a matt powder for a daytime make-up, and an iridescent shimmer powder for an evening make-up.

Loose face powder

1 Remove the loose powder from its container, using a clean spatula or, if the powder is in a shaker, by sprinkling it out. Place the powder on a clean facial tissue.

2 Ask the client to keep their eyes closed. Using a clean piece of cotton wool or velour sponge, press into the powder and then press the powder all over the face.

3 Remove excess powder using a large, disinfected facial powder brush. Direct the brush strokes first up the face, which dislodges the powder, then down the face, which flattens the facial hair and removes the final residue of excess powder.

Compact powder   Apply powder with a brush or velour powder puff.

Facial contouring using powder products may now be carried out.

Bronzing products

Bronzing products are applied to create a healthy, natural or subtle tanned look. They are formulated to create a matt or shimmer effect and are also suitable as a highlighting contouring product.

Kinds of bronzing products

Bronzing products are available in powder, gel and liquid formulation. Powder bronzer, a tinted powder in different shades, gives skin natural colour effects and highlights. Ideal for enhancing a client's skin tone or tan and suitable for all skin types, although they can emphasize a dry or mature skin. Gel bronzer contains gel and glycerine in which the pigment is suspended. Gel bronzer is preferable for a dry, mature skin type and can be applied to the whole face or specific areas. Liquid bronzer is suitable for all skin types and contains a pearlized, light-reflective micro – fine powder with an oil-free formulation. Silicone enhances its application.

Apply bronzing products according to the effect you want to achieve after powder application or in the case of gel and liquid after foundation application. Remember you can use bronzers as a contour product also.

Powder   Using a large powder brush apply the bronzer powder. Stroke the brush over the cheek area, followed by nose, chin and neck area.

Gel   As for liquid blusher you need to blend the gel bronzer quickly over each area. Apply with the fingers or a damp sponge. Commence at the cheek area, forehead, nose and chin.

Liquid   Apply as for gel bronzer.

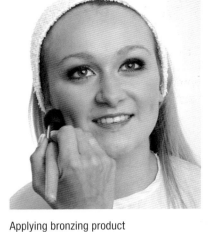

Applying bronzing product

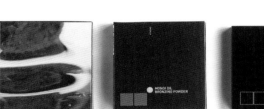

Bronzing products

> **TOP TIP**
>
> **Bronzers for males**
> A bronzing powder has been designed especially for males which is matt and natural.

The eyes

Make-up is applied to the eye area to complement the natural eye colour, to give definition to the eye area, and to enhance the natural shape of the eye.

> **HEALTH & SAFETY**
>
> **Eye cosmetics**
> The eye tissue is particularly sensitive. Eye cosmetic products should be of the highest quality, and be permitted for use according to the Cosmetics Products (Safety) Regulations (2008).

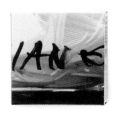 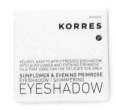 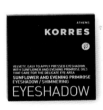 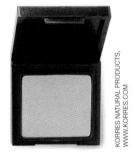

Eye shadows

Eye shadow

Eye shadow adds colour and definition to the eye area. The different types include matt, pearlized, metallic and pastel. They are available in cream, crayon or powder form. Eye shadows are composed of either oil-and-water emulsions or waxes containing inorganic pigments to give colour.

- **Powder eye shadows** have a talc base, mixed with oils to facilitate application. Lighter shades are produced by the addition of **titanium dioxide** – avoid

> **TOP TIP**
>
> **Cream eye shadows**
> Cream eye shadows are less popular – they are difficult to blend and quickly settle into creases. They are usually used by clients who have dry, mature skin.

HEALTH & SAFETY

Contact lenses

It is preferable for the client not to be wearing contact lenses during eye shadow application.

ALWAYS REMEMBER

When applying powder colours, always tap the brush before application to remove excess eye shadow. If too much colour is deposited on the applicator, stroke it over a clean tissue to remove the excess.

Remember it is better to apply more product in stages until you create the look you want to achieve.

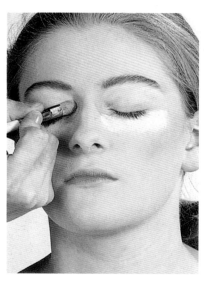

Applying eye shadow

HEALTH & SAFETY

Eye pencil

A good-quality eye pencil will be quite soft when applied to the skin, to avoid dragging the delicate eye tissue.

these on dark skin as they contrast too harshly with the natural skin colour.

- **Cream eye shadows** contain wax, oil and silica.
- **Liquid eye shadows** contain water, mica, glycerine and butylene glycol to achieve the correct viscosity.
- **Crayon eye shadows** are composed of wax and oil, and are similar in appearance and application to an eye pencil.

Pearlized mineral eye shadows are created by the addition of **bismuth oxychloride**, a fine crystalline powder or **mica,** a light-reflecting mineral powder; a *metallic* effect is created by the addition of fine particles of **gold leaf, aluminium** or **bronze**.

How to apply eye shadow

Eye shadow application will differ according to the eye shape of the client and the look to be achieved.

Powder eye shadow

1 Protect the skin beneath the eye with a clean tissue or loose powder as shown – this is to collect small particles of eye shadow that may fall during application.

2 Lift the skin at the brow slightly to keep the eye tissue taut, enabling you to reach the skin near to the base of the eyelashes.

3 Apply the selected eye shadow to the eyelid, using a sponge or a brush applicator.

4 Highlight beneath the brow bone.

5 Using a brush, apply a darker eye shadow to the socket area, beginning at the outer corner of the eye. Blend the colour evenly, to avoid harsh lines.

6 Ask your client to open her eyes during application so that you can look at the effect created.

Cream eye shadow Apply over a base to hold the cream shadow in place. It may be applied with a brush and blended with the finger or brush.

Liquid eye shadow Apply the liquid shadow pearly colour with a brush stroking and blending over the eyelid where required.

ACTIVITY

Eye shadow application techniques

There are many different looks that can be created by the placement of eye shadow. Consider 'smoky' and 'winged'. Collect different images of techniques and practise their application.

Eyeliner

Eyeliner defines and emphasizes the eye area. It is available in pencil, liquid or powder form.

- **Eye pencil** Made of wax and oil, and contains different pigments which give it its colour.

- **Liquid and gel eyeliner** A gum solution, in which the pigment is suspended.

- **Powder eyeliner** A powder base with the addition of mineral oil.

Powder eyeliner is the most suitable choice for a client who is exposed to a warm environment, as it will not smudge.

How to apply eyeliner
If you are using a powder or liquid eyeliner, apply it with a clean eyeliner brush.

1 Lift the skin gently upwards at the eyebrows, to keep the eyelid firm and make application easier.

2 Draw a fine line along the base of the eyelashes (as close to the lashes as possible), as required.

3 If using an eye pencil or powder line, lightly smudge the eyeliner to soften the effect of the line. (This is not effective with liquid liner.) If required, a further application may be applied for a thicker line.

4 Eyeliner may be applied to the inner eye, usually accompanying a 'smoky' eye shadow look. This technique is unsuitable on small eyes as it would make them appear smaller.

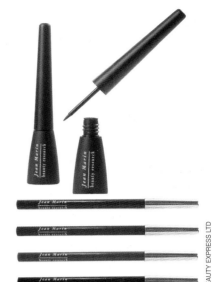

Eyeliners

BEAUTY EXPRESS LTD

BEST PRACTICE

Have a clean cotton bud available so that you can remove the powder from any minor mistakes during application.

TOP TIP

Kohl eyeliner
Kohl was used by the Ancient Egyptians, a black cosmetic containing stibium. This is now banned. Iron oxide is a mineral ion commonly used today.

TOP TIP

Powder eye shadow may be applied over the eye pencil application to increase its durability, as heat and moisture can disturb the wax/oil content of a pencil.

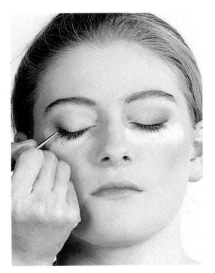

Applying eyeliner to the upper lashline

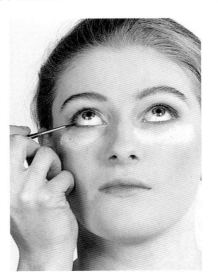

Applying eyeliner to the base lashline

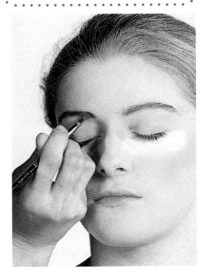

Applying eyebrow colour

WWW.SHAVATA.CO.UK

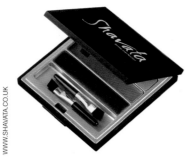

Brow perfector

COURTESY OF WWW.JANEIREDALEUK.EU

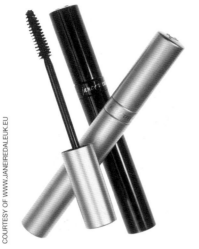

Mascara

Eyebrow colour

Eyebrow colour emphasizes the eyebrow, darkens the hair, alters their shape, disguises bald patches and can make sparse eyebrows look thicker. It is available in pencil, liquid or powder form.

- **Eyebrow pencil** Firmer than an eye pencil, and is composed of waxes that hold the inorganic pigments.

- **Powder brow colour** Composed of a talc base, mixed with mineral oil and pigments.

- **Liquid eyebrow** A fluid, quick-drying eyebrow colour to define the brows.

- **Eyebrow mascara** Composed of mineral oil and waxes with pigment suspended in it. The mascara defines the brows and controls and shapes them.

How to apply eyebrow colour

1 Select an appropriate colour of powder or eyebrow pencil. Brush the eyebrows with a clean brow brush to remove excess face powder and eye shadow. A specialized wax or gel can be applied which aids adherence of powder brow shadow and separates and defines the brow hair.

2 Simulate the appearance of brow hair by using fine strokes of colour, or disguise bald patches with a denser application. Use a pencil or liquid eyebrow to apply feathery strokes or alternatively using a brush apply powder to the prepared brow hair.

3 Brush the eyebrows into shape if necessary without disturbing product application.

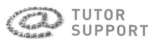

TOP TIP

Eyelash curling
The eyelashes may be temporarily curled before mascara application to open up the eye area.

TUTOR SUPPORT

Activity 4: Make-up techniques wordsearch

ACTIVITY

Brow colour
What brow colour product would you select for the following and how would you apply it:

- fair-haired client, day wear?
- dark-haired client, evening make-up?
- red-haired client, special occasion?
- grey-haired client, sparse brow hair, day make-up?

Mascara

Mascara enhances the natural eyelashes, making them appear longer, changed in colour and thicker. It is available in liquid, cream and block-cake forms. It is composed of waxes or an oil-and-water emulsion, and contains pigments which give it its colour. Other ingredients can be added to increase its durability, making it waterproof which will require a special eye make-up remover for waterproof mascara.

- **Liquid mascara** – a mixture of gum in water or alcohol; the pigment is suspended in this. It may also contain short textile filaments that adhere to the lashes and have a thickening, lengthening effect. Water-resistant mascara contains resin instead of gum, so that it will not run or smudge.

- **Cream mascara** – an emulsion of oil and water, with the pigment suspended in this.

- **Block mascara** – composed of mineral oil, lanolin and waxes, which are melted together to form a block on setting. It must be dampened with water before application.

How to apply mascara Using a disposable mascara brush, apply mascara to the eyelashes:

1 Hold the brush horizontally to apply colour to the length of the lashes. Where the lashes are short and curly, or difficult to reach, hold the brush vertically and use the point of the brush.

2 Place a clean tissue underneath the base of the lower eyelashes, and stroke the brush down the length of the lashes from the base to the tips.

3 Lift the eyelid at the brow bone. Ask the client to look down slightly while keeping their eyes open. From above, stroke down the length of the lashes from the base to the tips.

4 Using a zigzag motion, draw the brush upwards through the upper and lower surfaces of the lashes, from the base to the tips. Apply several coats to create a dramatic evening look.

5 Finally, separate the eyelashes with a clean brush or lash comb.

ALWAYS REMEMBER

Curly lashes will require brushing, using a clean brush, both before mascara application and after each coat, to separate the lashes. A specialized gel may be applied before mascara application which, on drying, separates the lashes.

TOP TIP

Mascara accidents!
If you accidentally get mascara on the skin, remove with a cotton bud. If waterproof you may need a small amount of eye make-up remover on the bud. Apply any corrective make-up to follow and conceal.

Eye make-up for the client who wears glasses

If the client wears glasses, check the function of the lens, as this can alter the appearance and effect of the eye make-up.

- ***If the client is short-sighted, the lens makes the eye appear smaller.*** Draw attention to the eyes by selecting righter, lighter colours. When applying eye shadow and eyeliner, use the corrective techniques for small eyes. Apply mascara to emphasize the eyelashes.

- ***If the client is long-sighted, the lens will magnify the eye.*** Make-up should therefore be subtle, avoiding frosted colours and lash-building mascaras. Careful blending is important, as any mistakes will be magnified!

HEALTH & SAFETY

Mascara
Mascara when purchased is usually provided with a brush applicator. This applicator cannot be effectively cleaned and disinfected, however, so it should not be used. Instead use a disposable mascara brush for each client.

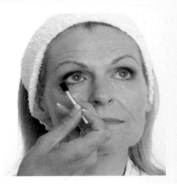

HEALTH & SAFETY

Allergies
If the client has hypersensitive eyes or skin, use hypoallergenic cosmetics that contain no known sensitizers.

Contact lenses
If the client wears contact lenses, don't use either lash-building filament mascaras or loose-particled eye shadows, which have a tendency to flake and may enter the eye.

TOP TIP

Clear mascara makes the lashes appear thicker, while appearing very natural.

ALWAYS REMEMBER

Never pump the mascara wand when loading it with mascara. This encourages air to enter and makes the mascara dry out.

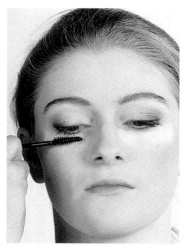

Applying mascara

ACTIVITY

Choosing mascara
What colour mascara should be applied if the client has the following hair colouring: brown, red, black or grey?

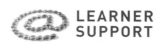

LEARNER SUPPORT

Corrective eye make-up diagram

How to apply corrective eye make-up

Dark circles

1   Minimize the circles by applying a concealing product.

Dark circles

Wide-set eyes

1   Apply a darker eye colour to the inner portion of the upper eyelid.

2   Apply lighter eye shadow to the outer portion of the eyelid.

3   Apply eyeliner in a darker colour to the inner half of the upper eyelid.

4   Eyebrow pencil may be applied to extend the inner bowline.

Wide-set eyes

Close-set eyes

1   Lighten the inner portion of the upper eyelid.

2   Use a darker colour at the outer eye.

3   Apply eyeliner to the outer corner of the upper eyelid.

4   Pluck brow hairs at the inner eyebrow – this helps to create the illusion of the eyes being further apart.

Close-set eyes

Round eyes

1   Apply a darker colour over the prominent central upper-lid area.

2   Elongate the eyes by applying eyeliner to the outer corners of the upper and lower eyelids.

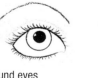

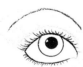

Round eyes

Prominent eyes

1   Apply dark matt eye shadow over the prominent upper eyelid.

2   Apply a darker shade to the outer portion of the eyelid, and blend it upwards and outwards.

3   Highlight the brow bone, drawing attention to this area.

4   Eyeliner may be applied to the inner lower eyelid.

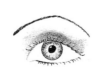

Prominent eyes

TOP TIP

To make the eyes appear less prominent, select matt eye shadows – pearlized and frosted eye shadows will highlight and emphasize the eye.

Overhanging lids

1 Apply a pale highlighter to the middle of the eyelid.

2 Apply a darker eye shadow to contour the socket area, creating a higher crease (which disguises the hooded appearance).

Overhanging lids

Deep-set eyes

1 Use light-coloured eye shadows.

2 Eye shadow may also be applied in a fine line to the inner half of the lower eyelid, beneath the lashes.

3 Apply eyeliner to the outer halves of the upper and lower eyelids, broadening the line as you extend outwards.

Deep-set eyes

Downward-slanting eyes

1 Create lift by applying the eye shadow upwards and outwards at the outer corners of the upper eyelid.

2 Apply eyeliner to the upper eyelid, applying it upwards at the outer corner.

3 Confine mascara to the outer lashes.

Downward-slanting eyes

Small eyes

1 Choose a light colour for the upper eyelid.

2 Highlight under the brow, to open up the eye area.

3 Curl the lashes before applying mascara.

4 Apply a light-coloured eyeliner to the outer third of the lower eyelid.

5 A white eyeliner may be applied to the inner lid, to make the eye appear larger.

Small eyes

Narrow eyes

1 Apply a lighter colour in the centre of the eyelid, to open up the eye.

2 Apply a shader to the inner and outer portions of the eyelid.

Narrow eyes

Oriental eyes

1 Divide the upper eyelid in two vertically. Place a lighter colour over the inner half of the eyelid and a darker colour at the outer half.

2 Apply a highlighter under the eyebrow.

3 White eyeliner may be applied at the base of the lash line, on the lower inner eyelid.

Oriental eyes

MAKE-UP BY WWW.JULIAFRANCIS.CO.UK AND PHOTOGRAPHY BY WWW.PETEWEBB.COM

TOP TIP

False eyelashes may be effective in enhancing the eye's natural shape, or when requiring additional length for the lashes or for a special occasion make-up.

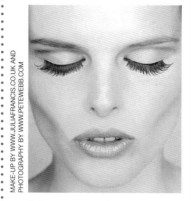

False eyelashes

TOP TIP

Eyelash curling is beneficial for Oriental clients who have short lashes that grow downwards.

The eyelashes

To emphasize the eyelashes, making them appear longer temporarily, curl them using eyelash curlers. If performing after mascara application it must be dry.

How to curl the eyelashes

1 Rest the upper lashes between the upper and lower portions of the eyelash curlers.

2 Bring the two portions gently together with a squeezing action.

3 Hold the lashes in the curlers for approximately ten seconds, then release them.

4 If the lashes are not sufficiently curled, repeat the action.

MAKE-UP BY WWW.JULIAFRANCIS.CO.UK AND PHOTOGRAPHY BY WWW.PETEWEBB.COM

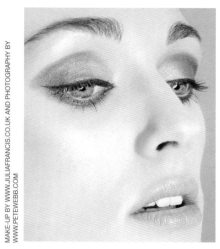

Eye shadow on model

WWW.FOTOSEARCH.COM/PHOTOS-IMAGES/EYELASH-CURLER.HTML

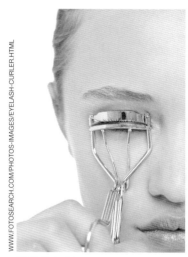

Eyelash curler

HEALTH & SAFETY

Eyelash curling
Repeated eyelash curling can lead to breakage. The technique should therefore be used only for special occasions.

The lips

Lip cosmetics add colour and draw attention to the lips. As the lips have no protective sebum, the use of lip cosmetics also helps to prevent them from drying and becoming chapped.

It is not uncommon for the lips to be out of proportion in some way. Using lip cosmetics and corrective techniques, symmetrical lips can be created. A careful choice of product and accurate application are required to achieve a professional effect.

The main lip cosmetics are lip liner, lipsticks, lip tints, lib balm and lip glosses. Sometimes the lips may be unevenly pigmented. The application of a lip toner or foundation over the lips corrects this.

MAKE-UP BY WWW.JULIAFRANCIS.CO.UK AND PHOTOGRAPHY BY WWW.PETEWEBB.COM

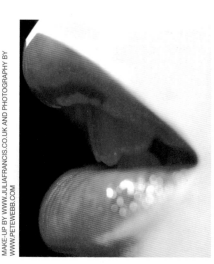

Lip make-up

Lip liner

Lip liner is used to define the lips, creating a perfectly symmetrical outline. This is coloured in with another lip cosmetic, either a lipstick or a lip gloss. The lip liner also helps to prevent the lipstick from 'bleeding' into lines around the lips.

Lip liner has a wax base which does not melt and can be applied easily. It contains pigments which give the pencil its colour.

When choosing a lip liner, select one that is the same colour as, or slightly darker than, the lipstick to be used with it.

Lipstick

Lipstick contains a blend of oils and waxes, which give it its firmness, and silicone, essential for easy application. It also contains pigment, to add colour, an emollient moisturiser, to keep the lips soft and supple and perfume, to improve its appeal. In addition it may include vitamins, to condition the lips, or sunscreens, to protect the lips from ultra-violet rays. Some lipsticks contain a relatively large proportion of water – these moisturise the lips and provide a natural look. The coverage provided by a lipstick depends on its formulation.

Lipsticks are available in the following forms: cream, matt, frosted and translucent. Frosted lipstick has good durability, as it is very dry. Some other lipsticks also offer extended durability, and are suitable for clients who are unable to renew their lipstick regularly.

When choosing the colour of lipstick, take into account the natural colour of the client's lips (it is best if it is the same colour tone), the skin and hair colours, and the colours selected for the rest of the make-up.

Lip gloss

Lip gloss provides a moist, shiny look to the lips. It may be worn alone, or applied on top of a lipstick. Its effect is short-lived. Lip gloss is made of mineral oils, with pigment suspended in the oil.

Note that mature clients often have creases on the lips that extend to the surrounding skin. If lip gloss is used it will often bleed into these lines.

Lip stain

Lip stain adds intense colour to the lips and is made of water, glycerine, skin-conditioning ingredients and mineral pigments. Prepare the lip with lip liner. Apply to lips quickly, using the fingertips or a make-up sponge. Build up the colour to achieve the result required.

Lip balm

Lip balm is a lip moisturiser containing oil and beeswax, vitamins C and E to help prevent dryness and improve skin texture, and pigment to add colour and sheen. Following the lip liner, apply to the lips with a brush. A gloss may then be applied to enhance the lips.

Dry lips Sometimes the lips become dry and chapped. Recommend that the client keeps them moisturised at all times, especially in extremes of heat, cold or wind. Some facial exfoliants can be professionally applied over the lips to remove dead skin.

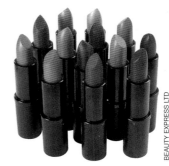

Lip cosmetics

BEAUTY EXPRESS LTD

HEALTH & SAFETY

Lip pencils

Lip pencils are form of lip liner contained in wood. Always sharpen the lip pencil before use on each client, to provide a clean, uncontaminated cosmetic surface.

Lip pencil

COURTESY OF WWW.JANEIREDALEUK.EU

HEALTH & SAFETY

Lipstick

For reasons of hygiene, remove a small quantity of lipstick by scraping the stick with a clean spatula – don't apply the lipstick directly.

HEALTH & SAFETY

Allergies

Lipsticks often contain ingredients that can cause allergic reactions, such as lanolin and certain pigment dyes. If the client has known allergies, use a hypoallergenic product instead.

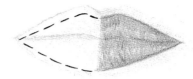

Thick lips

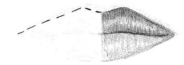

Thick upper lip

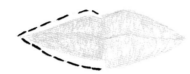

Thick lower lips

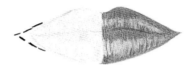

Thin lips

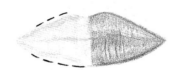

Small mouth

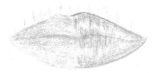

Uneven lips

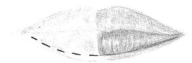

Lines around the mouth

If the client does not like to wear make-up during the day, or if the client is male, recommend that the lips be protected with a lip-care product.

How to apply corrective lip make-up

Thick lips Select natural colours and darker shades, avoiding bright, glossy colours.

1   Blend foundation over the lips to disguise the natural lip line.

2   Apply a darker lip liner inside the natural lip line to create a new line.

Thicker upper or lower lip

1   Use the technique described above to make the larger lip appear smaller.

2   Apply a slightly darker lipstick to the larger lip.

3   If the lips droop at the corners, raise the corners by applying lip liner to the corners of the upper lip, to turn them upwards.

Thin lips Select brighter, pearlized colours. Avoid darker lipsticks, which will make the mouth appear smaller.

1   Apply a neutral lip liner just outside the natural lip line.

Small mouth

1   Extend the line slightly at the corners of the mouth, with both the upper and the lower lips.

Uneven lips

1   Use a lip liner to draw in a new line.

2   Apply lipstick to the area.

Lines around the mouth

1   Apply lip liner around the natural lip line.

2   Apply a matt cream lipstick to the lips. (Don't use gloss, which might bleed into the lines around the mouth.)

How to apply lipstick

1   Select a lip pencil and lipstick to complement the client's colouring and the colour theme of the make-up.

2   Using a pencil sharpener, sharpen the lip pencil to expose a clean surface.

3   Ask the client to open her mouth slightly.

4   Outline the lips, carrying out lip correction as necessary. Begin the lip line at the outer corner of the mouth, and continue it to the centre of the lips. Repeat the process on the other side of the lip, commencing at the outer corner of the mouth.

5   Remove sufficient lipstick using a clean spatula.

6   Using a disinfected lip brush, apply the lipstick to the lips.

7 Apply a clean facial tissue over the lip area, and gently press it onto the lips. This process, known as blotting, removes excess lipstick and fixes the colour on the lips.

8 The application of powder on the first application of lipstick will make the lipstick longer lasting.

9 A second light application of lipstick may then be applied.

10 If desired, lip-gloss may be applied over the lipstick to add sheen, again using a disinfected lip brush.

TOP TIP

To obtain the correct colour of lipstick, you may need to mix different lipstick shades together.

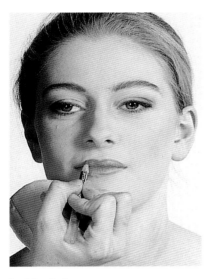

Applying lip liner

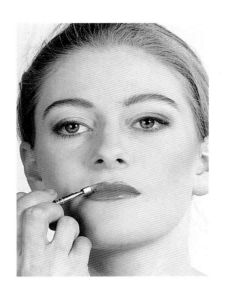

Applying lipstick

HEALTH & SAFETY

Lip brushes
Disposable lip brushes are available to enable lip cosmetics to be applied hygienically.

When you have finished . . .

After applying the make-up, fix the client's hair and then discuss the finished result in front of the make-up mirror.

Wash your hands. Record details of the service on the client's record card. Provide aftercare advice.

Outcome 4: Provide aftercare advice

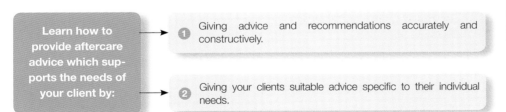

| Learn how to provide aftercare advice which supports the needs of your client by: | ❶ Giving advice and recommendations accurately and constructively. |
| | ❷ Giving your clients suitable advice specific to their individual needs. |

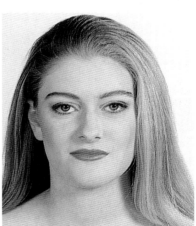

The complete make-up

Aftercare advice

Following make-up application, recommend the correct skincare products to remove the products you have applied.

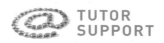

TOP TIP

In poor lighting, face shading should be subtle as it makes shadows appear darker.

Eye cleansing advice

● Cleanse the eye area using a suitable eye make-up remover.

● Remove waterproof mascara usually using an oily eye make-up remover.

● If false lashes have been applied their removal must also be discussed (see Chapter 8, pages 269–270).

Skincare advice

● Apply cleansing preparations to remove facial make-up with an appropriate cleanser in an upwards and outwards direction. Remove with damp cotton wool or clean facial sponges.

● Apply a suitable toner to suit skin type to remove excess cleanser.

● Apply day or night moisturiser, apply in small dots to the neck, chin, cheeks, nose and forehead. Quickly evenly spread a thin film over the face, using light upward, outward stroking movements.

● Blot the skin with a soft facial tissue to remove excess moisture.

Advise the client on application procedures to maintain the effect, e.g. removal of facial shine from the face with pressed powder, lip liner to stop 'bleeding', re-application of blusher to add warmth.

Explain to the client that you can offer a make-up lesson in which you would discuss the reason for the selection of make-up products and colours, and the techniques for applying them. Recommend the correct skincare products to remove the products you have applied.

Have retail products available for the client to purchase. These include the products that you have used during the make-up application and skincare products for preparation and removal of make-up.

Share tips that will ensure that the client gets the best out of any products purchased. Explain how to use the product hygienically and when it should be replaced.

Explain what action to take in the event of a contra-action.

Finally, at the end of the make-up service ensure that the client's records are updated, accurate and signed by the client and beauty therapist.

TUTOR SUPPORT

Activity 2: Case studies project

The client's needs

Day make-up

The effect should be natural. Any corrective work carried out should be very subtle and kept to the minimum, as natural light makes any imperfections appear obvious.

Select a foundation the same colour as the skin – aim to even out the skin tone. Set the foundation with a translucent face powder.

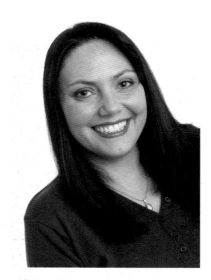

Day make-up

Apply a subtle, warm blusher or bronzing product to add colour to the face. Avoid strong colours of cosmetics, especially on the eyes. The mascara colour should be chosen to complement the client's natural lash and skin colours. Mascara should be used to emphasize, but not exaggerate, the length and thickness of the eyelashes. Eyeliner may be used, but it should be carefully placed and blended.

Line the lips in a colour that will co-ordinate with the lipstick to be applied, which again should be quite natural.

Evening make-up

This should be applied bearing in mind the type of lighting in which the client will be seen. Artificial light dulls the effect, and changes the colour of the make-up: dark shades lose their brilliance, appearing 'muddy', so you need to use brighter colours. Emphasize the facial features with the careful placement of contouring cosmetics.

Areas where shadows may be created, such as the eyes, should be emphasized using light, bright and highlighting cosmetic products. Add warmth to the face with an intense colour of blusher placed on the cheekbones. A highlighting or shimmer powder in a pearlized or metallic shade may be applied directly on top of or over the blusher. The client may like to try adventurous cosmetics such as metallics and frosted eye products.

Curl the eyelashes with eyelash curlers or apply false eyelashes to emphasize the eyes. Fashion shades of mascara may be selected, in purples, greens and blues, to complement the make-up and produce the effect required. Light shades of eyeliner may be used to frame the eyes and to 'open' them up.

Add a lip gloss to the lips, or apply a frosted lipstick to emphasize the mouth.

Colour the eyebrows, and carefully groom them to frame the eye area.

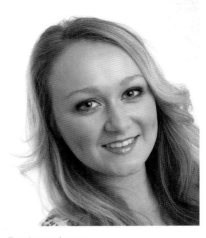

Evening make-up

Special occasion make-up

A special occasion is usually an important event such as a wedding, day at the races, graduation ceremony or New Year's Eve party.

Whatever the occasion, whether daytime or evening, indoors or outdoors, you will need to consider the type of lighting the make-up will be viewed in – natural or artificial – and any other factors, such as how long it is to be worn for.

The selection of colours should co-ordinate with what the client will be wearing, and finally you need to know the effect they wish the make-up to create – should it be subtle or glamorous? Make-up products can then be selected and appropriately applied to suit the occasion.

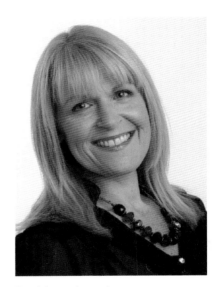

Special occasion make-up

Photographic make-up

If applying make-up for photographic purposes, it is important to consider the effect to be created. This should be planned with the photographer in advance of the make-up application.

Consider the brightness of the lighting used. The brighter the lighting is the lighter the make-up pigment will appear. Make-up will therefore need to be applied more strongly. Lighting can be hot and may affect the make-up application making it melt, especially with oil-based make-up. Therefore, avoid oily make-up and regularly apply powder to remove shine.

Generally, matt colours are used, as the lighting will emphasize any shine.

For black and white photography remember dark colours will appear darker when photographed. Therefore, it may be necessary to apply lighter shades in preference to dark – for example, a dark shade of cheek colour would create a dark shadow.

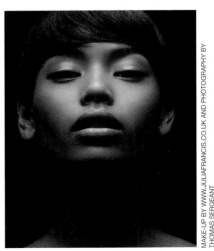

Photographic make-up

Avoid lip gloss unless you wish the lips to appear full.

It is important to define facial features using shading and highlighting techniques, as photographic make-up removes natural shades and highlights.

Care should be taken to blend all make-up to avoid any demarcation lines, which will be emphasized in the photograph.

ALWAYS REMEMBER

Make-up considerations for photographic make-up

Pearlized colours used on the eyes will draw attention to the eyes and emphasize problem areas such as fine lines, so be subtle in their application. Areas that you do not wish to emphasize should be matt as powder minimizes flaws.

Oily face make-up will emphasize open pores.

Thick lashes, if required, can create shadows under the eye area. The lighting would have to be adjusted to avoid shadowing.

Photographic make-up may be applied in a photographer's studio or on location. Ensure you are able to transport your make-up safely.

Make-up to suit skin and hair colouring

Fair skin and blonde hair If the client has fair hair and fair skin, keep the skin colour natural. Apply a blusher in rose pink or beige.

Define the eyes with soft tones of browns and pinks. Apply a brown-black mascara.

Colour the lips with a rose-pink or peach lip-colour. Avoid lip colours lighter than the natural skin tone.

Oriental skin and black hair For creamy, sallow skin with dark hair, use blusher to add warmth and to brighten the skin, in either pink or brown.

The eyes are dark, with a prominent brow bone. Emphasize the socket of the eye with careful shading; extend this upwards and outwards. Place highlighter along the brow bone.

Pastel colours complement the eye colour. Select black mascara to emphasize the eyes. Deep pinks and orangey-reds suit the lips.

Fair skin and red hair Redheads usually have fair skin with freckles. The skin will flush and colour easily, probably requiring the application of a green-tinted moisturiser, concealer or face powder. Apply blusher in a warm rose or peach colour. Browns, rusts, greens and peach eye shadow colours suit this skin and complement the eyes. Brown mascara is preferable, to avoid making the eyes appear hard.

For the lips, select a lipstick in peach, golden rust or pink.

Black skin and black hair A yellow-toned foundation is required: it may be necessary to blend foundations to obtain the correct colour. Avoid pink-toned foundations, which make the skin appear chalky.

Women with dark skin tend to have dark brown to brown-black eyes, and can use a wide range of heavily pigmented colours, especially browns and bronzes. Dark shades

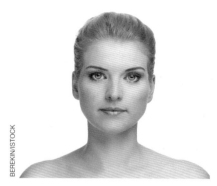

BEREKIN/ISTOCK

Fair skin

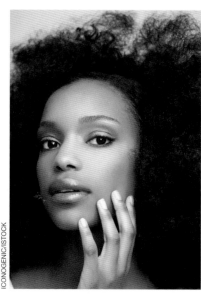

ICONOGENIC/ISTOCK

Black skin

of blusher in red and plum may be chosen; eyeliner and mascara can be black, or any other dark shade.

Avoid lip colours lighter than the skin tone. A lip liner darker than the lip colour may be used.

Olive or fair skin and dark hair Select a foundation to suit the basic skin tone. If the skin is fair, choose an ivory base; if it is sallow, select a foundation with a rusty, yellow tone. (With a sallow skin, avoid the use of pinks on the eyes – they make the eyes look sore.)

A beige blusher suits this skin colour, and is complemented by the selection of brown or green shades for the eyes. Black mascara should be used for the eyelashes.

For the lips, choose warm reds or beige.

Make-up for the mature skin

As the skin ages it becomes sallow in colour and appears thinner. Small capillaries can be seen, commonly on the cheek area, and small veins may appear around the eyes. Pigment changes in the skin become obvious, and remain permanently.

At the make-up consultation, discuss your ideas with your client. Very often a mature client will have been using the same colours and the same cosmetics for many years, and they may not even be complementary. You will need to advise them tactfully on a fresh approach.

Select a foundation that matches the skin colour yet enhances the skin's appearance. An oil-based foundation is appropriate for use on mature skin: it keeps the skin supple and prevents the foundation from settling into the creases and emphasizing the lines and wrinkles.

A concealer may be applied to cover obvious capillaries and small veins, or a foundation may be selected which provides adequate coverage.

A lighter foundation may be applied over wrinkled areas, to make them less obvious. These areas include:

- around the eyes (crow's feet)
- between the brows
- across the forehead
- between the nose and the mouth (nasolabial folds)
- around the mouth (the lip line)

With age, the contours of the face lose their firmness as the fat cells that plump the face reduce, and the facial muscles lose tone and sag. Poor muscle tone can be seen in the following areas:

- the cheek area
- loose skin along the jaw line
- loose skin under the brow and overhanging the lid
- loose skin on the neck

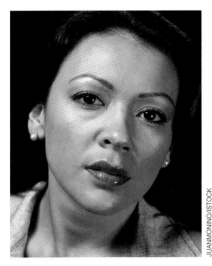
Olive skin

ALWAYS REMEMBER

Dark circles under eyes

Dark circles under the eyes can be minimized with concealer. Select a concealer lighter than the foundation to be applied.

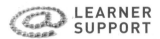
LEARNER SUPPORT

Make-up wordsearch

ACTIVITY

Shading
Where would you place the shading product in order to correct poor muscle tone in the areas discussed opposite?

ALWAYS REMEMBER

Cream eye shadow

Cream eye shadow settles into creases, which emphasize a crepey eyelid. Frosted or pearlized eye shadows also emphasize a crepey eyelid.

TOP TIP

Positive promotion

If the client is visiting the salon for make-up, you could recommend that they have a professional make-up lesson – at which you could discuss a fresh approach to their make-up.

The application of a shader, subtly blended, can improve the appearance of such areas. Apply translucent powder. It may be preferable to avoid doing so in the eye area as it can emphasize lines around the eyes. To reduce the powdery effect, which may make the skin appear dry, you may direct a fine water spray from a suitable distance to set the make-up.

Apply a blusher with a warm tone – avoid harsh, bright shades. A cream blusher may be applied after the foundation. Place it high on the cheekbone and blend it upwards at the temples, drawing attention upwards rather than downwards.

The lip line becomes less obvious as one grows older, and lines often appear along it. Lip liner should be applied to redefine the lips and to prevent the lipstick from 'bleeding' into the lines. Select a lip liner that is the same colour as, or slightly lighter than, the lip colour. (A darker lip colour would create an unwanted shadow.) A special lip fixative may be recommended, and a durable cream lipstick applied. Avoid the use of a gloss lipstick, which emphasizes lines around the mouth.

The angle of the mouth may droop. Corrective techniques may be used to disguise this.

Powder matt eye shadows should be selected for use on the eyelid: these soften the appearance of any lines in the area. Choose natural, light shades. Dark colours can make the eyes appear small and tired.

Eyeliner should be used in neutral shades of brown and grey – avoid harsh, bright colours, which will give a hard appearance.

Eyebrows should be perfectly groomed, and arched to give lift to the eye. Bushy eyebrows give the eyes a hooded appearance. If eyebrow colour is required, select a colour that is slightly lighter than the brow colour, or a blend of two colours. If the client has grey hair, use grey and charcoal to provide a natural effect.

Eyelashes should be emphasized with a natural-looking shade of mascara, lightly applied. (If the eyelashes lose their colour, you can recommend that the client has their lashes professionally – and permanently – tinted. Individual false eyelashes may be recommended for corrective purposes.)

Step-by-step: Mature client special occasion make-up application

Make-up is to be applied to a Caucasian client to achieve a glamorous appearance for a social evening. We allowed 45 minutes to achieve this look.

The client has dry skin as the sebaceous and sudoriferous glands have become less active as part of the ageing process. Noticeable facial **skin characteristics** include the following.

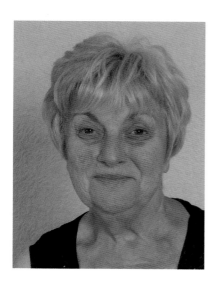

The client's skin has been cleansed, toned, moisturised and blotted to remove excess moisturiser.

- Dark circles appear around the eyes area.

- Thin, delicate tissue is found around the eyes with small veins and capillaries showing through the skin.

- Habitual frown lines occur.

- Poor muscle tone has resulted in slack facial contours, e.g. double chin.

- Poor skin tone exists because the skin loses its elasticity, resulting in wrinkling and loss of firmness.

- Sallow skin colour is due to poor blood circulation.

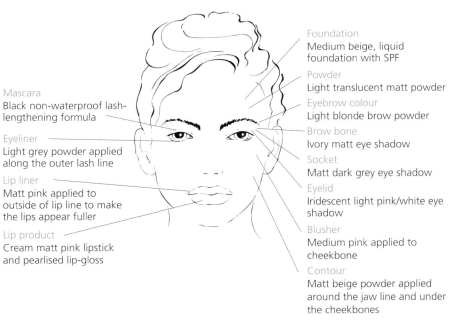

Mascara
Black non-waterproof lash-lengthening formula

Eyeliner
Light grey powder applied along the outer lash line

Lip liner
Matt pink applied to outside of lip line to make the lips appear fuller

Lip product
Cream matt pink lipstick and pearlised lip-gloss

Foundation
Medium beige, liquid foundation with SPF

Powder
Light translucent matt powder

Eyebrow colour
Light blonde brow powder

Brow bone
Ivory matt eye shadow

Socket
Matt dark grey eye shadow

Eyelid
Iridescent light pink/white eye shadow

Blusher
Medium pink applied to cheekbone

Contour
Matt beige powder applied around the jaw line and under the cheekbones

Mature client special occasion retail advice make-up record card

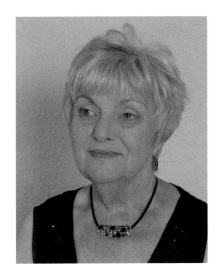

The finished special occasion make-up

Step-by-step: Asian client day make-up application

Corrective work completed is subtle, as natural daylight makes any imperfections seem more obvious.

The client's skin has been cleansed, toned, moisturised and blotted to remove excess moisturiser. Thirty minutes were allowed to achieve the look.

This is an oily skin type, where over-activity of the sebaceous glands in the skin is creating a shiny, sallow appearance. Darker skin underneath the eye area requires concealer correction.

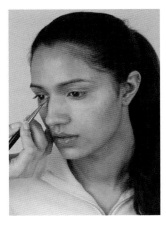

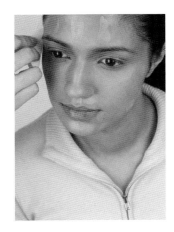

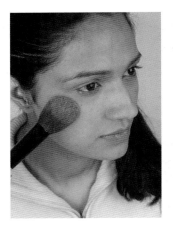

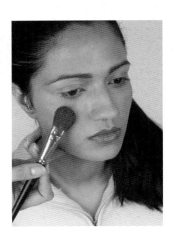

1 A concealer is applied with a brush underneath the eyes to disguise the darker skin tone.

2 A liquid foundation matched to the client's skin tone is applied. Application is over the whole face, including the eyelids and lips, as this gives an even skin tone.

3 Following the application of loose powder, again matched to the client's skin tone, excess powder is removed using a large powder brush. Application is upwards and outwards.

4 Blusher colour is applied to accentuate the cheek area and add colour to the face.

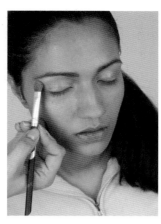

5 Colour applied to the eye emphasizes the eye area. We used complementary colours in a purple range. A highlighting colour accentuates the brow bone.

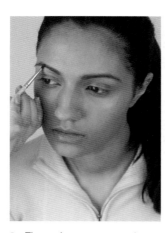

6 The eyebrows are accentuated using a dark matt brown colour applied with a stiff eyebrow brush. This gives definition to the eyebrow, disguising sparse hair and gaps.

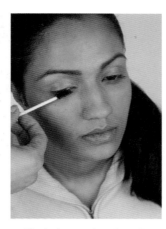

7 The lashes are lengthened using a lash-building mascara in black.

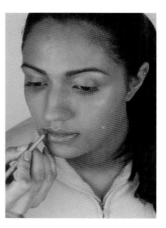

8 Lip liner colour is applied to define the desired lip contour. A co-ordinating lip colour is selected to match the lip liner and complement the eye make-up colour.

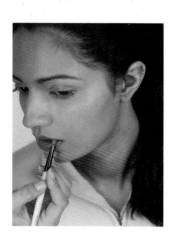

9 The lip colour is applied using a lip brush.

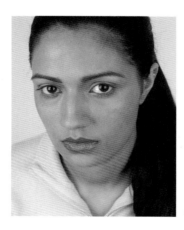

10 The final day make-up look.

Step-by-step: African–Caribbean client evening make-up application

Make-up which will be seen under artificial lighting is applied. Stronger pigmented make-up colours have been selected, and the make-up effect emphasizes facial features through the choice and application of make-up products. Forty-five minutes were allowed to achieve the look.

The client's skin has been cleansed, toned, moisturised and blotted to remove excess moisturiser.

This is a combination skin type and the sebaceous glands are overactive in the T zone – forehead, nose and chin – and the pores appear larger in this area. The sebaceous glands are less active in the cheek, which results in dry skin with tight pores.
Other noticeable facial characteristics include the following:

- the skin tone of the face has uneven pigmentation

- the face shape requires balance, which can be achieved using shaded contour colour

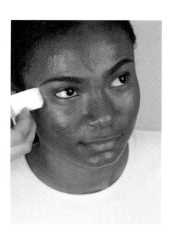

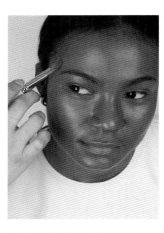

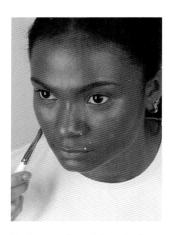

1 Foundation is selected to match the client's skin type and even the skin tone. A mousse foundation has been used to provide a medium coverage and has been blended quickly to avoid a chalky appearance.

2 A cream formulation shading product, in a darker shade than the foundation, is applied underneath the cheekbone and at the temples to accentuate the cheekbones and reduce the width of the face at the temples.

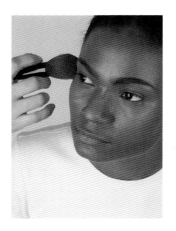

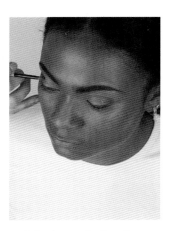

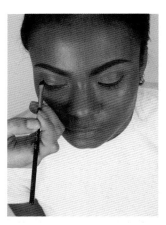

3 Loose powder matching the client's skin tone is applied to set the foundation and facilitate application of further powder products. Powder blusher is applied to the cheekbone.

4 Following application of a neutral eye shadow matt colour, a darker shading product is used to emphasize the eye socket.

5 The natural lash line is accentuated by eyeliner application. A steady hand is required!

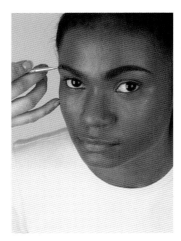

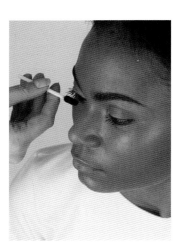

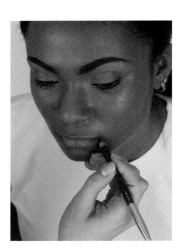

6 The brows are defined.

7 Mascara application draws attention to the eyes.

8 Lip liner is applied to define the perfect lip line.

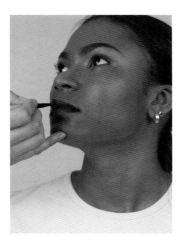

9 The lips are coloured in using a matt lipstick co-ordinated to suit the lip liner. Lip gloss achieves a final touch which will focus attention and add emphasis in darker lighting.

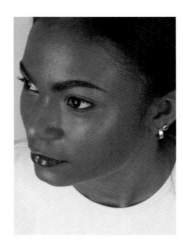

10 The final evening make-up look.

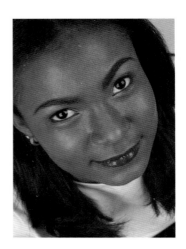

Chapter 10 instructs clients in the use and application of skincare products and make-up, and discusses in detail the application of make-up to the different age groups and skin types.

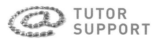 **TUTOR SUPPORT**

Activity 5: Re-cap, revision and evaluation

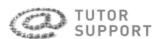 **TUTOR SUPPORT**

Activity 7: Multiple choice quiz

GLOSSARY OF KEY WORDS

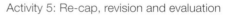

Aftercare advice recommendations given to the client following service to continue the benefits of the service.

Age groups the different classification of age groups to be covered: 16–30, 31–50 and over 50 years.

Blusher cosmetic applied to add warmth to the face and emphasize the facial contours.

Bronzing products make-up product applied to create a healthy, natural or subtle tanned look. They are formulated to create a matt or shimmer effect and are also suitable as a highlighting contouring product.

Cleanser a skincare preparation that removes dead skin cells, excess sweat and sebum, make-up and dirt from the skin's surface to maintain a healthy skin complexion. These are formulated to treat the different skin types, skin characteristics and facial areas.

Client groups this term is used in a number of the units and it refers to client diversity. The CRE (Commission for

Racial Equality) ethnic group classification is used in the range for these units. These cover white, mixed, Asian, black and Chinese.

Colour corrector make-up product applied to target problem areas. It contains pigments which balance skin tone.

Concealer cosmetic product used to disguise minor skin imperfections such as blemishes, uneven skin colour or shadows.

Consultation assessment of client's needs using different assessment techniques, including questioning and natural observation.

Contour cosmetics applied to cosmetically change and enhance the shape of the face and facial features.

Contra-action an unwanted reaction occurring during or after service application.

Contra-indication a problematic symptom that indicates that the service may not proceed or may restrict service application. Contra-indications identified

for facial services are discussed in more detail in Chapter 3.

Equipment tools used within a make-up.

Eyebrow colour cosmetic applied to emphasize the eyebrows, alter their shape, and which can make sparse eyebrows look thicker.

Eyeliner cosmetic applied to define and emphasize the eye area.

Eye shadow cosmetic applied to the eye to complement the natural eye colour, to give definition to the eye area and enhance the natural shape of the eye.

Face shape the size and shape of the facial bone structure. Face shapes include oval, round, square, heart, diamond, oblong and pear.

Facial features the size of a person's nose, eyes, forehead, chin, neck, etc. When applying make-up products, make-up application can emphasize or minimize the appearance of facial features.

False eyelashes threads of nylon fibre or real hair attached to the natural eyelash hair. There are two main types: individual or strip.

Foundation a make-up product applied to produce an even skin tone, to disguise minor skin blemishes and as a contour cosmetic.

Highlighter a make-up product that draws attention to and emphasizes features.

Hyperpigmentation increased pigment production.

Hypopigmentation loss of pigmentation.

Lip balm a lip moisturiser which may contain pigment.

Lip gloss cosmetic applied to the lips to provide a moist, shiny look.

Lip liner cosmetic used to define the lips, creating a perfectly symmetrical outline.

Lip stain make-up product which adds intense colour to the lips.

Lipstick cosmetic applied to the lips to add colour and keep the lips soft and supple.

Make-up cosmetics applied to the skin of the face to enhance and accentuate, or to minimize facial features. Make-up products create balance in the face.

Make-up occasion the context the make-up is to be applied for, i.e. day, evening and special occasion.

Make-up products different cosmetics available to suit skin type, colour and condition, i.e. sensitive or mature. Make-up products include concealing and contour cosmetics, foundations, translucent powders, eye shadows, eyeliners, brow liners, mascaras, lipsticks, lip glosses, lip liners, etc.

Mascara cosmetic that enhances the natural eyelashes, making them appear longer, changed in colour and/or thicker.

Mineral make-up is created from finely ground minerals (a process called micronization). It is used in the formulation of different make-up products.

Minor a person classed as a child who requires by law to have a guardian or adult present.

Moisturiser a skincare preparation whose formulation of oil and water helps maintain the skin's natural moisture by locking in moisture, offering protection and hydration. The formulation is selected to suit the skin type, facial characteristics and facial area.

Necessary action the action taken to deal safely with a contra-action or contra-indication.

Pigment the colour of skin and hair, called melanin. The amount of pigment varies for each client, resulting in different skin and hair colour.

Powder cosmetic applied to set the foundation, disguise minor skin blemishes and make the skin appear smoother and oil-free.

Primer provides a base for make-up and acts as a barrier preventing absorption of the make-up products into the skin.

Promotion ways of communicating products or services to clients to increase sales.

Record cards confidential records recording personal details of each client registered at the salon.

Service plan after the consultation, suitable service objectives are established to treat the client's conditions and needs.

Shader a make-up product that draws attention away from and minimizes certain facial features.

Skin characteristics while looking at the skin type, additional characteristics may be seen. These include skin that may be sensitive, dehydrated, moist or oedematous (puffy), in addition to dry, oily or combination.

Skin tone the strength and elasticity of the skin.

Skin type the different physiological functioning of each person's skin dictates their skin type. There are four main skin types: normal (balanced), dry (lack of oil), oily (excessive oil) and combination (a mixture of two skin types, i.e. dry and oily).

Toning lotion a skincare preparation formulated to treat the different skin types: and facial characteristics. It is applied to remove all traces of cleanser from the skin. It produces cooling and skin-tightening effects.

ASSESSMENT OF KNOWLEDGE AND UNDERSTANDING

Having covered the learning objectives for **Provide make-up services**, test what you need to know and understand answering the following short questions below.

The information covers:
- organizational and legal requirements
- how to work safely and effectively when performing make-up services
- client consultation, service planning and preparation
- contra-indications and contra-actions
- make-up application
- aftercare advice for clients

Anatomy and physiology questions required for this unit are found in Chapter 2, page 16.

Organizational and legal requirements

See Chapter 4 for details of legislation.

1 What are your responsibilities under the relevant health and safety legislation?

2 What actions must be taken before a client under 16 years of age receives make-up?

3 How can you ensure you comply with the legislation of the Disability Discrimination Act when completing make-up services?

4 Why must a clients signature be obtained before commencing a make-up service?

5 Taking into account health and safety hygiene requirements, how would you prepare yourself for service?

6 How should all client records be stored when completing make-up services to comply with the Data Protection Act (1998)?

7 How long would you allow to complete a make-up service?

8 Why is it important for staff to be familiar with the make-up pricing structures?

9 What details should be recorded on the client's record card and why is it important to keep accurate records which are maintained?

10 How can repetitive strain injury be avoided when performing make-up services? Give three examples.

How to work safely and effectively when performing make-up services

1 How can you ensure that the make-up environment is suitable for the application of make-up?

2 What do you understand by the terms disinfection and sterilization? State two methods used in a facial service and when.

3 How should the make-up brushes be prepared for each client to avoid cross-infection?

4 Why is it important to have a variety of make-up products available?

5 How should the client be positioned when performing make-up?

6 Why is it important to match lighting with the occasion for which the make-up is to be worn?

7 Give five examples of how the work area should be prepared ready for the next client following a make-up service. Why is this important?

Client consultation, service planning and preparation

1 How can you ensure that you fully understand the effect to be achieved with the make-up application?

2 In order to select the correct skincare and make-up products to complement the client's skin, it is necessary to identify the skin type. What are the facial characteristics of the following skin types that you learnt about in Chapter 7 (Unit B4 Provide facial skincare treatment):
   - oily?
   - dry?
   - combination?

3 How should the skin be prepared before the application of make-up?

4 What should be considered when planning a make-up with a client?

5 Why should you encourage the client to ask questions about the planned make-up?

6 Why is it important to check if the client wears contact lenses or glasses and check the function of the lens?

7 The client should be comfortable and relaxed following the consultation and preparation for the service. How could you tell is the client was relaxed or tense through their body language?

8 What is the legal relevance of client questioning and recording the client's responses?

9 Why is it important that you never diagnose a contra-indication?

10 When would you perform a skin sensitivity test before make-up application?

Contra-indications and contra-actions

1 Name three skin disorders and three eye disorders that would contra-indicate make-up service.

2 What product ingredients are known to cause allergic reactions, and should therefore not be used on a client with a sensitive skin?

3 Name three contra-actions that could occur during or after make-up application. What action should be taken?

Make-up application

1 What is the difference in application technique for the following make-up contexts:
   - day?
   - evening?
   - special occasion?

2 How is the correct colour of foundation selected for your client?

3 Why is it important that make-up is applied in a suitable sequence?

4 How can you ensure hygienic practice when applying the following products:
   - foundation?
   - face powder?
   - mascara?
   - lipstick?

5 For what purpose would you apply a concealer?

6 Why does the age of the client influence make-up product selection and application technique?

7 What is a colour corrector? Why is it pigmented?

8 What is the purpose of:
   - shader?
   - highlighter?

9 What corrective make-up techniques would you apply for each of the following:
   - square face?
   - high forehead?
   - narrow eyes?
   - hyperpigmentation?
   - hypopigmentation?

10 When would you apply a bronzer product?

Aftercare advice for clients

1 What aftercare advice should be given to a client following make-up application?

2 How can you promote the sale of skincare and make-up products during make-up application?

3 From a magazine, collect a photographic image from the client group below where make-up has been applied:
   - African Caribbean
   - Asian
   - Caucasian
   - Oriental

   Describe how each look has been created, explaining the make-up application and products used.

4 What reapplication make-up tips could you recommend to a client to increase the durability of their make-up?

5 Clients should be advised of suitable make-up removal techniques. Explain the skincare products required and how they should be used.

6 How can clients maintain the hygiene of their make-up products?

10 Instruction and Application of Skincare Products and Make-up (B9)

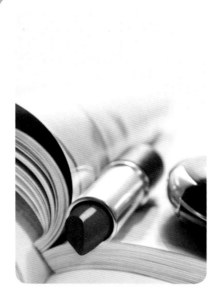

B9 Unit Learning Objectives

This chapter covers **Unit B9 Instruct clients in the use and application of skincare products and make-up**.

This unit is about how to provide skincare and make-up product advice and instruction. The choice and application of skincare and make-up products will be recommended and applied to suit the client's skin type, tone, colouring, condition, age and make-up context, i.e. day, evening and special occasion.

There are **four** learning outcomes for Unit B9 which you must achieve competently:

1   Maintain safe and effective methods of working when providing skincare and make-up instruction

2   Consult, plan and prepare for skincare and make-up instruction

3   Deliver skincare and make-up instruction

4   Evaluate the success of skincare and make-up instruction

Your assessor will observe you **on at least three occasions**, each involving instruction for a different look on a different client.

From the **range** statement, you must show that you have:

● used all **consultation techniques**

● treated all **skin types**

(continued on the next page)

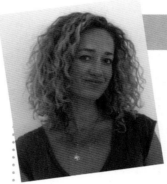

(continued)

- treated all three **age group** categories
- taken the necessary action where a contra-action, contra-indication or **service modification occurs**
- applied **instruction** to cover all skincare and make-up requirements
- used all **instructional techniques**
- used all **resources**

However, you must prove that you have the necessary knowledge, understanding and skills to be able to perform competently across the range.

When instructing clients in the use and application of skincare products it is important to use the skills and knowledge you have learnt in the following units:

Unit G20 Make sure your own actions reduce risks to health and safety

Unit G18 Promote additional products or services to clients

Unit G8 Develop and maintain your effectiveness at work

Unit B4 Provide facial skincare service

Unit B8 Provide make-up services

The beauty therapist has the professional expertise to advise each client on how to improve the appearance and condition of their skin by the application of appropriate cosmetic skincare products and services.

When correctly selected and applied, make-up increases a person's confidence while accentuating their best features and correcting their worst.

Professional instruction including skincare and make-up lessons and demonstrations can be delivered in an individual or group context. The instructional session should enable the client to develop the skills, learn tips and gain the knowledge to apply skincare and make-up confidently themselves.

The work environment should be prepared to meet legal hygiene and service requirements for skincare and make-up.

Outcome 1: Maintaining safe and effective methods of working when providing skincare and make-up instruction

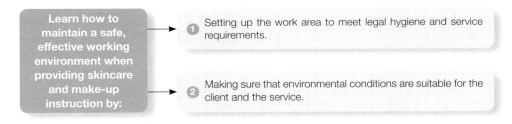

Learn how to maintain a safe, effective working environment when providing skincare and make-up instruction by:

1. Setting up the work area to meet legal hygiene and service requirements.

2. Making sure that environmental conditions are suitable for the client and the service.

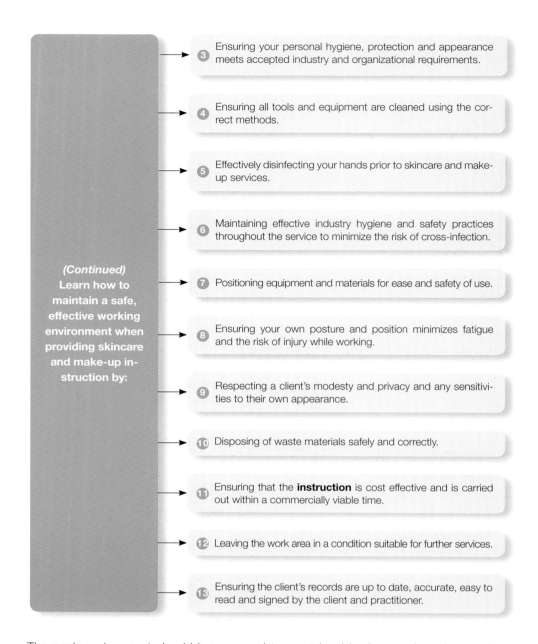

(Continued) Learn how to maintain a safe, effective working environment when providing skincare and make-up instruction by:

3 Ensuring your personal hygiene, protection and appearance meets accepted industry and organizational requirements.

4 Ensuring all tools and equipment are cleaned using the correct methods.

5 Effectively disinfecting your hands prior to skincare and make-up services.

6 Maintaining effective industry hygiene and safety practices throughout the service to minimize the risk of cross-infection.

7 Positioning equipment and materials for ease and safety of use.

8 Ensuring your own posture and position minimizes fatigue and the risk of injury while working.

9 Respecting a client's modesty and privacy and any sensitivities to their own appearance.

10 Disposing of waste materials safely and correctly.

11 Ensuring that the **instruction** is cost effective and is carried out within a commercially viable time.

12 Leaving the work area in a condition suitable for further services.

13 Ensuring the client's records are up to date, accurate, easy to read and signed by the client and practitioner.

The work environment should be prepared to meet legal hygiene and service requirements for skincare and make-up.

Skincare and make-up instruction may take place in a private or public area at the workplace or in the client's home environment. Check suitability with the client beforehand and to ensure client modesty and privacy is considered in location selected. The client's seat should offer adequate support, the mirror should be facing and close enough to observe practical application techniques. The height should be correct for you to avoid stretching and straining and to avoid repetitive strain injury.

Ensure that lighting is adequate to show each stage of the skincare or make-up instruction application (removal) effectively. The area where the make-up instruction takes place should be well lit.

Consider all health and safety issues especially any potential hazards. A hazard is something with potential to cause harm; this may range from using a product on a client who has an allergy to an ingredient, to tripping over clients' bags that are in the work area.

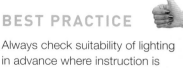

BEST PRACTICE

Always check suitability of lighting in advance where instruction is to be delivered. You may need to request additional lighting, i.e. if working as a freelance beauty therapist or make-up artist.

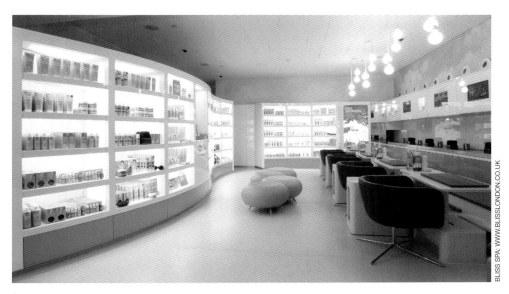

Salon area

Equipment, materials and products

Before beginning the skincare or make-up instruction make sure that you have the necessary equipment and materials to hand and that they meet the legal hygiene and industry requirements.

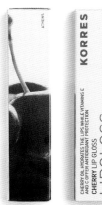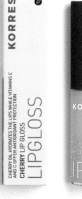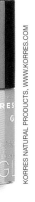

Make-up products

EQUIPMENT AND MATERIALS LIST

Chair

Headband (clean) or large hair clip To protect the clients hair while cleansing the skin

Skincare range To suit different skin types, tones and ages

Consumables Such as cotton wool dry and damp, tissues and cotton buds

Small bowl To hold water

Make-up range To suit different skin types, tones and ages

Bright lighting To inspect the skin after cleansing and to check for areas requiring special attention, e.g. dark circles, areas of pigmentation

Make-up brushes (assorted) Several sets required to allow for disinfection after use

Brush cleaner A proprietary brand cleaner to care for and maintain brushes hygienically

Disposable applicators These are used wherever possible during make-up application to ensure hygiene and prevent cross-infection

Cosmetic sponges For applying foundation

Pencil sharpener For cosmetic pencils

Small spatulas For dispensing products from their containers

Mirror To instruct the client in step-by-step application technique

Record card To record the clients personal details, products used and details of the service

Written instruction leaflet For the client to take away with them and refer to for guidance

Bowls and lined waste Bin for waste materials

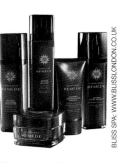

Skincare products

> You have to be prepared to think on your feet and to come up with a solution fast. My kit bag contains some unusual items such as dental floss, eye drops or an energy drink, but it is things like this that can sometimes make the difference and save the day.
>
> **Wendy Turner**

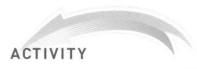

ACTIVITY

Hand disinfection

What is the correct hand washing technique as recommended by Habia to minimize cross-infection?

Which parts of the hands harbour microorganisms add?

Sterilization and disinfection

Ensure all tools are disinfected using the correct method. All products and consumables for skincare and make-up instruction should be available for you to choose from.

Hygiene must be maintained in a number of ways:

- Ensure that tools and equipment are sterile/disinfected before use. Use disposable applicators wherever possible.

- Disinfect work surfaces after every client.

- Always follow hygienic work practices for skincare and make-up application.

- Maintain a high standard of personal hygiene.

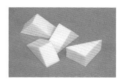

Mascara

Disposable tools

Where possible use mascara

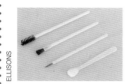

Brush
Lip product applicator
Eyeliner brush
Mascara brush

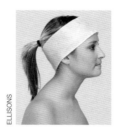

Headband

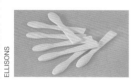

Spatulas

Make-up sponges

> First impressions really count so try to be open, friendly and relaxed so that you put your clients at ease. Photo shoots start early in the morning and I am usually the first person they meet on set so it is important we get off on the right foot, no matter how tired we all are!
>
> **Wendy Turner**

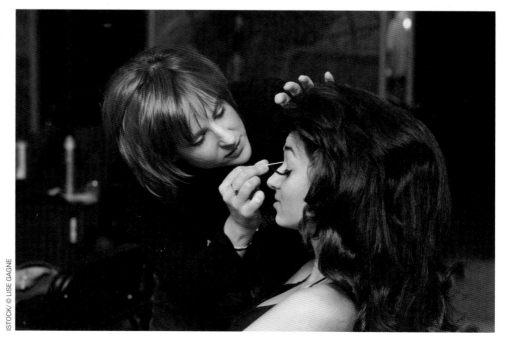

Professional make-up artist at work

Preparation of the beauty therapist Remember your own personal appearance is important to gain client confidence in you and the products – look your best! Many employers will provide workwear which must be worn as directed to promote the correct image. It is best practice to use the skincare products yourself and wear the make-up as a positive promotion and to show your confidence and loyalty to the product.

Before carrying out any skincare and make-up instruction it is essential that you are familiar with the products you are working with. It is important to complete regular Continuous Professional Development (CPD) to ensure your skills and expertise are current. Instruction must be cost effective, avoiding unnecessary wastage and completed in a commercially viable time. Allow 75 minutes for a make-up instruction session and 75 minutes for skincare instruction.

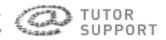

TUTOR SUPPORT

Activity 4: Job description task

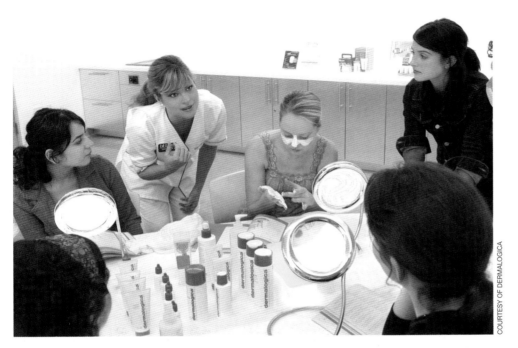

COURTESY OF DERMALOGICA

Facial skincare consultant

Outcome 2: Prepare and plan for skincare and make-up instruction

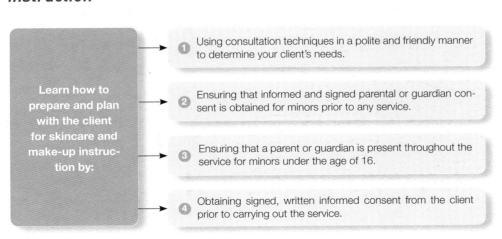

Learn how to prepare and plan with the client for skincare and make-up instruction by:	① Using consultation techniques in a polite and friendly manner to determine your client's needs.
	② Ensuring that informed and signed parental or guardian consent is obtained for minors prior to any service.
	③ Ensuring that a parent or guardian is present throughout the service for minors under the age of 16.
	④ Obtaining signed, written informed consent from the client prior to carrying out the service.

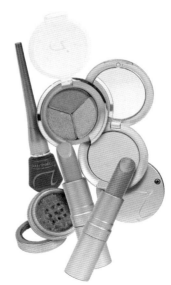

COURTESY OF WWW.JANEIREDALEUK.EU

Make-up products

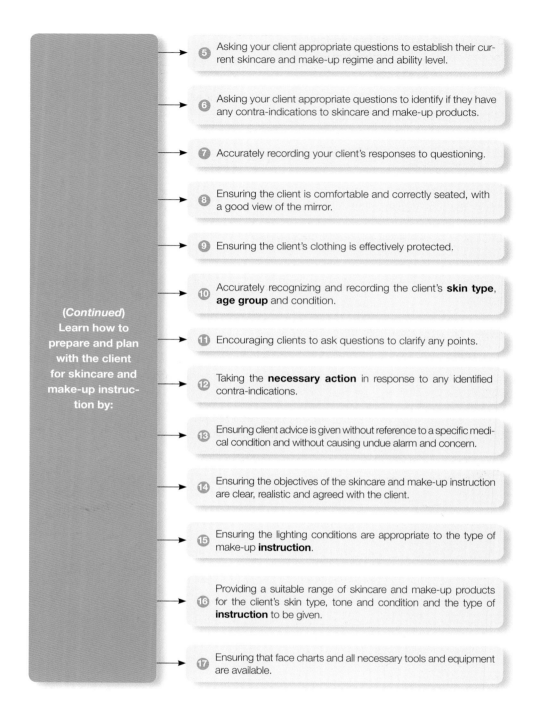

(Continued) Learn how to prepare and plan with the client for skincare and make-up instruction by:

5. Asking your client appropriate questions to establish their current skincare and make-up regime and ability level.

6. Asking your client appropriate questions to identify if they have any contra-indications to skincare and make-up products.

7. Accurately recording your client's responses to questioning.

8. Ensuring the client is comfortable and correctly seated, with a good view of the mirror.

9. Ensuring the client's clothing is effectively protected.

10. Accurately recognizing and recording the client's **skin type**, **age group** and condition.

11. Encouraging clients to ask questions to clarify any points.

12. Taking the **necessary action** in response to any identified contra-indications.

13. Ensuring client advice is given without reference to a specific medical condition and without causing undue alarm and concern.

14. Ensuring the objectives of the skincare and make-up instruction are clear, realistic and agreed with the client.

15. Ensuring the lighting conditions are appropriate to the type of make-up **instruction**.

16. Providing a suitable range of skincare and make-up products for the client's skin type, tone and condition and the type of **instruction** to be given.

17. Ensuring that face charts and all necessary tools and equipment are available.

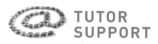

TUTOR SUPPORT

Activity 6: Client record card task

ALWAYS REMEMBER

It is important to defer to your client's needs during consultation. Consider the client's cultural, religious background, age, disability and gender and how this may influence the service planning and delivery. Research and attend CPD workshops to attain the necessary skills to be able to instruct all clients.

Consultation

At consultation identify what it is the client wishes to achieve. Client preference must always be considered. Many clients requesting make-up instruction have tired of their usual make-up application and require inspiration; some are unaccustomed to wearing make-up but recognize its potential to enhance. Other clients will request make-up instruction service for special occasions, e.g. bridal. Skincare clients may be experiencing a particular skin problem or would like professional recommendation on how to maintain or improve their skin. Ensure the objectives for the skincare and make-up instruction are realistic and agreed with the client. If the client is a minor under the age of 16, it is necessary to obtain parent/guardian permission for service. The parent/guardian will also have to be present when the service is received.

Skincare and make-up instruction presentations are a great way to launch a company's new products or season colours.

Sometimes the client may have received the make-up instruction as a gift so you will need to use effective questioning techniques to ensure you understand and achieve a result the client will be confident with.

If you have a promotion campaign this is usually advertised. The instruction session may include the demonstration of products and the client will be aware of what to expect.

foundations

Makeover or Make-up Lesson Voucher

Name : ....

To make your booking please contact ....

Professional make-up lesson gift voucher

foundations

Pamper yourself for the party season!
10% off your first visit for a professional makeover - ask inside the salon for details.

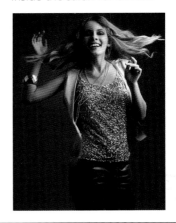

Promotional campaign flyer

Identifying the client's needs

Gaining an understanding of the client's requirements is important to achieve client satisfaction. Engage the client in conversation to establish their needs, concerns, likes and dislikes. Never presume; let the client tell you!

Use open questions which may not be answered with yes or no, during the consultation. Open questions usually start with *why*, *how*, *when*, *what* and *which*.

An effective consultation will have gathered important information such as the information in the table below.

> " You have to be prepared to get on with lots of people you might not know very well. It helps to be lively and chatty but also maintain your professionalism and know when to just be a good listener. I work with a lot of celebrities so it is important to be discreet.
>
> **Wendy Turner**

Make-up instruction consultation	Skincare consultation
Is the client used to wearing make-up?	What is the client's current skincare routine?
What is the make-up instruction for?	What products do they use? How often are specialist products used, e.g. facemasks?
Does the client normally wear make-up? (If not, try and find out why – they may not be confident in techniques of application). If not, a more subtle effect should be aimed for.	How long have they been using the products?
Are the client happy with the durability of their current make-up products – does it last?	What are the client's main service requirements? What would they like to improve on – their concerns?
Consider client preferences with regard to colours selected and the overall effect to be achieved.	Particular preferences, e.g. using water on the face when cleansing the skin?
Does the client have any known allergies?	Does the client have any known allergies?
Does the client were contact lenses? If a glasses wearer check the function of the lens, as this can alter the effect of the make-up.	Does the client wear contact lenses?

TOP TIP

Promotions

Promotions are a useful method to generate further revenue and interest in other areas of the business that a client has not experienced.

ACTIVITY

It is a good idea to observe an experienced, qualified practitioner delivering a client instruction session so you can gain best practice tips and gain insight into what works well. This will increase your professional confidence.

I always tell my clients that it is good to start with a clean, toned and moisturised face. I recommend you start with a good make-up base or primer before applying any foundation. That way the foundation will last longer and be more flawless.

Wendy Turner

HEALTH & SAFETY

ACTIVITY

If you were unsure as to the suitability of the client to receive the service what action should you take?

The answers provided will indicate the level of experience and confidence the client has so you can pitch your instruction at the correct level, e.g. beginners or advanced. You will also be able to comment on the suitability of the home products that are currently being used. If the client is wearing contact lenses these will need to be removed before the instructional activity. If the client wear glasses check of she is short- or long-sighted as this will influence make-up application, see make-up Chapter 9, page 309.

Agree all details of the skincare or make-up instruction with the client. Encourage the client to ask questions to clarify any points.

Identify the client's skin type, condition and age group to select the suitable products.

Check client suitability

Certain contra-indications will prevent skincare and make-up application. Check for these at the consultation. See a list of facial contra-indications page 188 and make-up contra-indications page 288. Remember, not all contra-indications are visible and you will need to ask, e.g. allergies to skincare and make-up products.

Explain to the client that in some instances the skin may have an undesirable reaction – skin irritation and a burning sensation indicating an allergy. This can also lead to swelling of the skins tissues. Explain you will check client comfort during the skincare/make-up application. If an unwanted reaction – a contra-action occurs the products must be removed immediately and a soothing compress and skincare product applied. A note should be made on the client record card. Alternative products may be sourced and trialled for suitability.

Record all client details accurately on their client record card. Record cards that can be used for facial instruction see pages 186–187 and make-up instruction see pages 286–287.

Preparing the client

The client's outer clothing, i.e. coat/jacket should be removed. Also, if there is any obstructive clothing in the neck area this too should be removed. The client should be offered a gown/towel or make-up cape as appropriate for protection. Place a headband or hair clip around the hairline, to protect the hair and keep it away from the face. Any jewellery in the area should be removed as appropriate. Ensure that the client is comfortable.

Outcome 3: Deliver skincare and make-up instruction

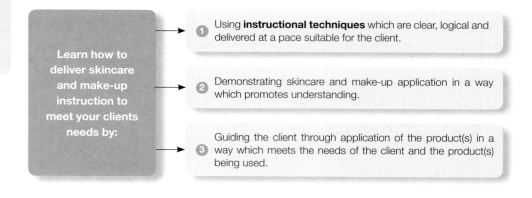

Learn how to deliver skincare and make-up instruction to meet your clients needs by:

1. Using **instructional techniques** which are clear, logical and delivered at a pace suitable for the client.

2. Demonstrating skincare and make-up application in a way which promotes understanding.

3. Guiding the client through application of the product(s) in a way which meets the needs of the client and the product(s) being used.

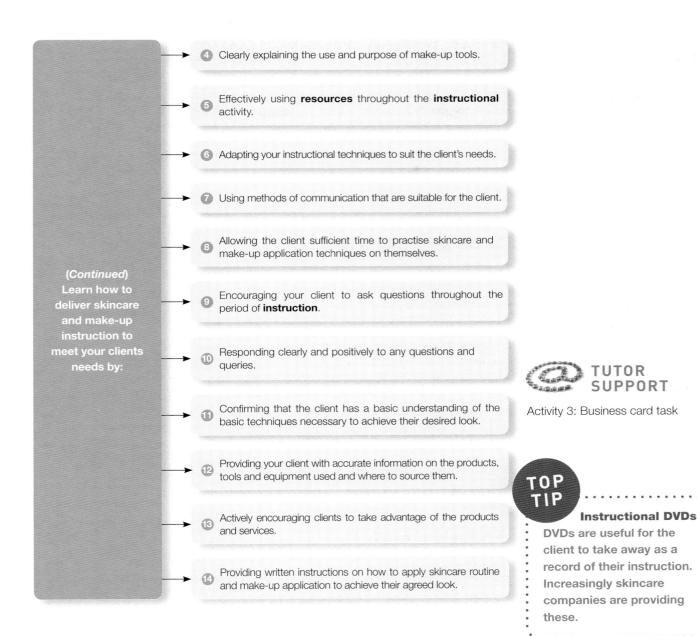

(Continued)
Learn how to deliver skincare and make-up instruction to meet your clients needs by:

4 Clearly explaining the use and purpose of make-up tools.

5 Effectively using **resources** throughout the **instructional** activity.

6 Adapting your instructional techniques to suit the client's needs.

7 Using methods of communication that are suitable for the client.

8 Allowing the client sufficient time to practise skincare and make-up application techniques on themselves.

9 Encouraging your client to ask questions throughout the period of **instruction**.

10 Responding clearly and positively to any questions and queries.

11 Confirming that the client has a basic understanding of the basic techniques necessary to achieve their desired look.

12 Providing your client with accurate information on the products, tools and equipment used and where to source them.

13 Actively encouraging clients to take advantage of the products and services.

14 Providing written instructions on how to apply skincare routine and make-up application to achieve their agreed look.

TUTOR SUPPORT

Activity 3: Business card task

TOP TIP

Instructional DVDs
DVDs are useful for the client to take away as a record of their instruction. Increasingly skincare companies are providing these.

Skincare and make-up instruction should be demonstrated in such a way that it enhances client understanding and showing cost effectiveness of the product usage. Observe body language during instruction. This will usually indicate satisfaction. If the client is exhibiting negative body language try and resolve this through questioning to involve the client, listen actively and adapt the instruction to meet their needs.

Clients will have a preferred way of learning new skills. These include visual, auditory (listening) or kinaesthetic (practical, hands-on). Many clients will be a mixture of all three learning styles. It is good practice to use all these learning styles in your instruction. How they may be used is discussed below:

Skincare and make-up instruction

Remember to use all products following manufacturer's instructions to ensure the optimum result is achieved. Explain these techniques to the client.

> You have to understand the contours of the face and how light, shadows and bright lights affect the look of the skin. Direct daylight can be harsh and flash photography will emphasize any shine so you must counteract this with more powder to reduce the effect.
>
> **Wendy Turner**

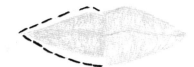

TUTOR SUPPORT

Activity 1: Corrective make-up task

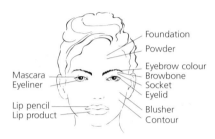

Making thin lips look thicker

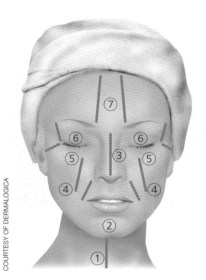

Make-up diagram

Make-up application sequence	Skincare application sequence
Concealing any blemishes.	Eye and lip make-up removal.
Applying foundation.	Applying cleanser.
Contouring the face (with cream liquid products).	Applying toning lotion.
Applying powder.	Exfoliation (specialist used once or twice a week dependent upon skin type and condition).
Contouring the face (with powder products).	Applying mask to cleanse or replenish.
Applying blusher.	Applying moisturiser.
Applying eye shadow.	Applying eye gels.
Making the eyebrows up.	Applying specialist serums.
Applying mascara.	
Making the lips up.	

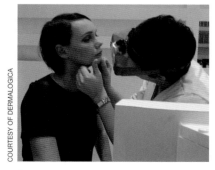

COURTESY OF DERMALOGICA

Facial diagram – face chart

Face mapping: identifying facial characteristics to diagnose skin type and condition and its specific treatment needs

COURTESY OF DERMALOGICA

Skill demonstration

Position the client in front of a mirror with all products and equipment to hand. Use a logical practical sequence that the client will be able to remember. Take the client through the instruction slowly. Support client participation in the instruction activity. She should be encouraged to copy what you have demonstrated. For example you may demonstrate application on one half of the face and she completes the other using the same technique. You will be able to correct her technique as necessary, explaining why.

Tools of the trade are important, and the client must be shown which make-up/skincare tool/brush is selected to achieve a particular result. Supportive advice should be given to the client during this process, while responding positively to any questions with recommendations.

Use of diagrams

Diagrams are good for visual learners these can be referred to during instruction, recording the application techniques to achieve the desired result. Tips can be recorded, e.g. how to make the lips thinner.

Diagrams have been used to record the products used during instruction for the day, evening and special occasion make-up shown. For make-up, the colours used can be placed on the make-up charts. A face chart diagram can be used to show what areas of the skin require attention and the products to be applied for correction.

Diagrams can be used to show how to apply and remove skincare products.

Verbal explanation

It is important that the client can hear and clearly follow all stages of the skincare/make-up instruction. If there is music in the work area ensure that it is not too loud for the client to hear instructions. Confirm at the start of the instruction that the client can hear you.

Avoid unnecessary technical vocabulary which the client will not be familiar with, otherwise the client will 'switch off'. Check the pace is not too fast when explaining instructional techniques.

Explain the features and benefits of the products used personalized to your client's service objectives. A feature is the skincare or make-up products specialist ingredients and the effects their application can achieve. A benefit is what the client could expect from using the product. You can use link statements for features and benefits such as "this means that …", and "the benefit of this is …". Be enthusiastic about the products you are using; this will inspire the client.

Knowledge will sell not only your products but yourself as well.

Use of written instructions

Written instructions are useful to ensure that client does not get confused when she completes the skincare/make-up routines at home independently. Skincare companies usually provide these in pad form with a tear-off prescription listing suitable products and their order of application.

TOP TIP

Colour blind clients receiving make-up instruction

If a client were colour blind they could have the colours numbered on their make-up chart and their make-up products numbered for easy reference.

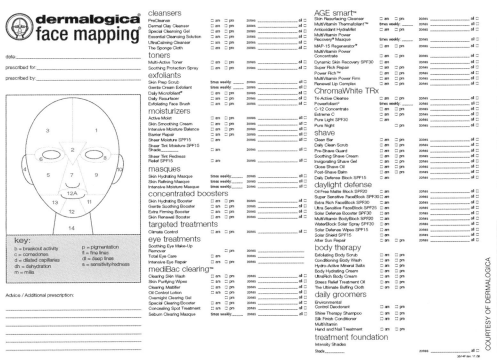

Skincare prescription

BEST PRACTICE

Product use

Product usage it is important to show the client the correct amount of product to dispense to avoid wastage and so that the product is effective.

Remember to also explain safety and hygiene in product use.

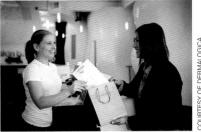

Providing a client with skincare application instructions

A booklet may be provided that lists the products and their recommended application. These often contain useful diagrams which show application techniques.

Following instruction provide the opportunity for the client to look at and handle the products or tools, such as make-up brushes, further. If possible give the client a complimentary gift of samples and information on suitable products. If you do not supply retail products provide the client with information on where they can be purchased.

At all stages of the instruction ask questions to assess and confirm client understanding. During the demonstration keep the work area, clean and tidy. On completion of the session the work area should be in a condition to provide further services.

Deliver make-up instruction: step-by-steps

The following make-ups were delivered as a make-up lesson explaining the choice and application of make-up products. The products used and where they have been applied to are recorded on a make-up chart.

Using shimmer is a great way to emphasize a certain look. Shimmer on the edge of the bows of the lip will make the lips appear bigger. A lovely liquid shimmer (soft pink) on the upper cheek bone and eyebrow bone will create a dewy, soft and natural look.

Wendy Turner

Client 1

Combination skin type.
Age group 16–30 years.
Evening make-up.

Explain to the client that the make-up will be applied considering the type of lighting the make-up will be seen in. (See page 278 for further guidance.)

The client's skin has been prepared using skincare preparations to balance the skin for a teenage, combination skin type. An oil control product has been used in the oily areas.

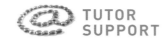

TUTOR SUPPORT

Activity 2: Make-up techniques wordsearch

18. Lip liner in 'nude' with glitter applied.

19. Pink lip gloss applied for finishing effect.

20. After.

1. Before.

2. Under-eye concealer in yellow tone applied to minimize bluish grey circles under the lower eyelid.

3. Blemishes are concealed.

4. Areas of redness around the nose are concealed.

17. Bronzing powder is applied to emphasize the cheekbones.

16. Powder blush is applied to apples of cheeks in a pinkish shade for a youthful effect.

15. Cotton bud may be used to correct any mistakes or as a tool for blending. Eye shimmer applied to 'open' the eye area.

5. Liquid mineral foundation in medium colour with warm undertones, is applied with damp brush for lighter application.

6. The make-up is tested on the client's jaw line to select the correct tone.

7. Pressed powder is applied with flat brush to give matt finish, suitable for the oily areas.

14. Black mascara is applied to upper and lower lashes.

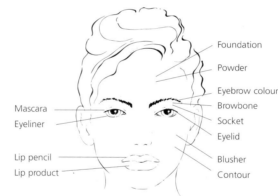

Make-up diagram

Foundation
Powder
Eyebrow colour
Browbone
Socket
Eyelid
Blusher
Contour

Mascara
Eyeliner

Lip pencil
Lip product

11. Protective powder is applied around the eyes to prevent eye shadow pigment damage to the foundation. Matt eye shadows applied to give smoky effect.

10. Powder highlighter is applied to inner corner of eye.

9. Powder highlighter is applied to brow bone.

8. Blonde brow gel is applied to enhance and define the brows.

13. Gel/liquid eyeliner applied to bottom eyelid lash line.

12. Gel/liquid is eyeliner applied top eyelid lash line.

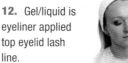

Client 2

Dry skin type.

Age group over 50 years.

Special occasion make-up.

For special occasion make-up you will need to find out the type of event and lighting considerations. (See pages 317 and 278 for further guidance.)

The client's skin has been prepared using collagen-boosting skincare preparations and botanical ingredients to encourage cellular renewal, increase skin firmness and protect against free radicals. The dry lips have been conditioned with the application of a lip balm. A skin primer has been applied as a base to smooth the skins surface.

Under-eye concealer, concealing pen applicator applied to dark circles and shadows to lighten and lift mature skin.

18. Finishing spray is applied all over face to set make-up and soften look.

19. After.

1. Before.

2. The highlighting pen is hygienically dispensed from container.

3. Application to dark circles.

17. Moisturising rose lip colour applied.

4. Application to naso-labial folds (lines that deepen with aging from the nose to the outer corner of the mouth) to minimize their appearance.

16. Lip pencil is used to define the lips – with age the lip line becomes less distinct.

5. Liquid mineral foundation, light to medium colour with warm tones, is applied with damp brush for lighter application.

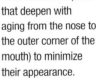

15. Contouring powder is applied along jaw line to sharpen the contour of the face.

Foundation

Powder

Eyebrow colour

Mascara
Eyeliner

Browbone

Socket

Eyelid

Lip pencil
Lip product

Blusher

Contour

Make-up diagram

6. Finished foundation application providing an even skin tone.

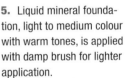

7. Loose mineral powder is applied with large powder brush in circular movements to give light reflecting glow.

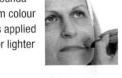

14. A highlighter contour product may be placed along the upper cheekbone to draw attention to the area, keeping away from fine lines around the eye area.

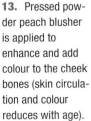

13. Pressed powder peach blusher is applied to enhance and add colour to the cheek bones (skin circulation and colour reduces with age).

12. Brown-black lash-lengthening mascara is applied as less harsh than black.

11. Soft pencil brown eyeliner is applied top and bottom.

10. Eyeshadows applied in natural tones to accentuate eye colour.

9. Eyeshadow base is applied to lids to even out tone and texture before applying eyeshadows.

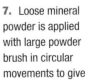

8. Brunette powder and gel is applied to eyebrows to give definition.

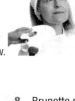

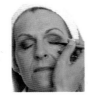

Client 3

Oily skin type.
Age group 31–50 years.
Day make-up.
The client's skin has been prepared using oil-free skincare preparations.
For day make-up the effect should be natural. (See pages 316–317 for further guidance).

15. Strong dark rose lip colour applied.

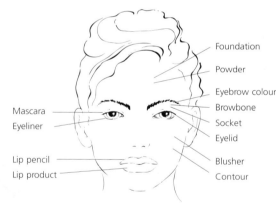

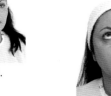

16. After.

1. Before.

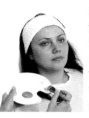

2. Under-eye concealer applied.

3. Liquid mineral foundation, golden brown colour with neutral under-tones, is applied with dry brush to give coverage.

14. Selection and preparation for hygienic application of lip product.

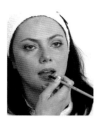

4. Pressed powder is applied with brush or powder puff to give matt effect.

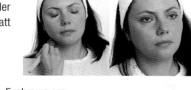

13. Lip pencil in dark pink applied to outline the lips.

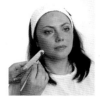

5. Eyebrows are groomed and defined with brush and powder.

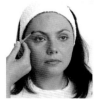

Foundation
Powder
Eyebrow colour
Mascara
Eyeliner
Browbone
Socket
Eyelid
Lip pencil
Lip product
Blusher
Contour

Make-up diagram

12. Soft shade rose blush applied to cheeks.

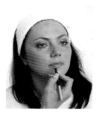

6. Highlighter is applied to brow bones.

11. Mascara applied to lower lashes.

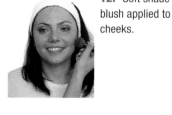

9. Eye pencil in black-grey applied to lower eyelid along lash line.

8. Eye pencil in black-grey is applied to the upper eyelid.

7. Natural shades are applied to lids to open up eyes.

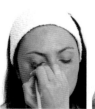

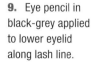

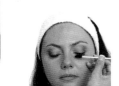

10. Mascara in black applied to upper lashes.

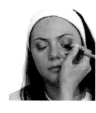

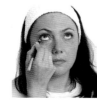

> Get to know what make-up looks work best. Four individual false lashes on the outer corner of the eye will create a fantastic and flirtatious look. A dark colour eyeliner on the upper lid helps create an almond shaped eye and a soft pink on the inside bottom of the eye will open it up and make it appear larger.
>
> Wendy Turner

ALWAYS REMEMBER

Make-up for mature skin
Considerations to be taken when applying a make-up for a mature skin can be found on page 319.

TOP TIP

Group demonstration of make-up activity

It is important that the audience can see and hear all stages of the skincare product/make-up application. A large screen and a microphone that does not restrict your movement (such as a headpiece microphone) may be useful. Recording the demonstration is a useful marketing tool to present in the future and to evaluate for effectiveness.

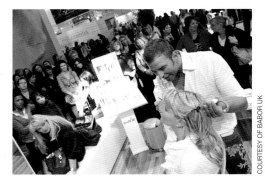

COURTESY OF BABOR UK

Make-up demonstration

TOP TIP

Client instruction for confidence

- Be organized.
- Look your best.
- Complete a thorough consultation.
- Practice your instruction style to meet the needs of all clients.

TUTOR SUPPORT

Activity 7: Planning a make-up demonstration

Outcome 4: Evaluate the success of instruction

Learn how to evaluate the success of instruction and client satisfaction by:

1. Asking your client to make an evaluation of their own learning and then providing additional support to meet their needs.

2. Asking your client suitable questions on the effectiveness of the instruction process and recording their feedback.

3. Using client feedback to make improvements to your own skincare and make-up **instructional techniques**, if necessary.

TOP TIP

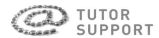

Discounted prices could be offered for clients who book a service or purchase products following the instruction session.

A successful instruction session should defer to the needs of your clients. Each client will be enthusiastic about the products and services offered for their own individual reasons. If the client purchases a product or books a service following your instruction it will be because they want to or feel they need to.

Ensure that the client is satisfied with the professional instruction provided and that it has met their needs.

Evaluate the effectiveness of the instruction:

- Where the training objectives met? Did the instruction answer the client's questions identified at consultation?

- Was your instruction clear? Ask the client specific questions to check understanding. If unsure you may need to further develop your communication techniques.

- What specifically did the client learn?

- Will the client feel confident applying and using the products in the future?

Evaluation is useful for the clients too as it enables them to reflect and confirm their knowledge and confidence following the instruction.

Allow time for the client to ask further questions about the products discussed and applied. The skincare prescription or make-up record chart is useful to list products used and how the make-up look has been achieved. Give this to the client to reinforce the discussion that has taken place and is invaluable if the client returns to purchase any of the products you have used.

Record evaluative comments on the client record card.

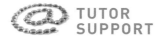

TUTOR SUPPORT

Activity 5: Re-cap, revision and evaluation

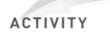

ACTIVITY

Evaluation

A simple series of questions may be provided for the client to complete following the instructional activity which are scored according to satisfaction level:

O Poor   O Fair   O Good   O Excellent

One question could be how the client rated the instruction provided. What other evaluative questions may you ask the client?

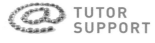

TUTOR SUPPORT

Activity 8: Multiple choice quiz

GLOSSARY OF KEY WORDS

In addition to the glossary shown below also refer to the glossary provided for the facial chapter (see Chapter 7, pages 227–228) and the make-up chapter (see Chapter 9, pages 324–325).

Age groups the different classification of age groups to be covered: 16–30, 31–50 and over 50 years.

Client groups this term is used in a number of the units and it refers to client diversity. The CRE (Commission for Racial Equality) ethnic group classification is used in the range for these units. These cover white, mixed, Asian, black and Chinese.

Consultation techniques methods used to identify the client's needs using differing assessment techniques, including questioning, manual and natural observation.

Evaluation method used which measures the value of the instructional activity.

Instructional activity the method used to teach a skill or develop a person's knowledge and understanding in a new area of learning.

Instructional techniques educational methods to teach a person a skill or develop their knowledge and understanding in a new area of learning. These include demonstration, use of instructional diagrams, verbal explanation and use of written instructions.

Necessary action the action taken or service modification required to deal safely with a contra-action or contra-indication.

Resources the different products, equipment and other things needed to complete an activity.

ASSESSMENT OF KNOWLEDGE AND UNDERSTANDING

Having covered the learning objectives for **Instruct clients in the use and application of skincare products and make-up**, test what you need to know and understand answering the following short questions below.

The information covers:

- organizational and legal requirements

- how to work safely and effectively when providing skincare and make-up services

- client consultation, instruction planning and preparation

- instructional skills

- planning and preparing for skincare and make-up instruction

- evaluation

Organizational and legal requirements

For full legislation details, see Chapter 4.

1 What are your responsibilities under the relevant health and safety legislation?

2 What actions must be taken before a client under 16 years of age receives skincare or make-up instruction?

3 Why is it important to keep records of the instruction services provided? And why should the client's signature always be obtained?

4 To comply with health and safety hygiene related requirements, how would you prepare yourself for instructional service?

5 How should all client records be stored to comply with the Data protection Act (1998)?

6 How long would you allow to complete a skincare/make-up instructional service?

7 Why is it important for staff to be familiar with the skincare/make-up instruction pricing structures?

8 What details should be recorded on the client's skincare/make-up face chart and why is it both useful and important to keep these client records?

9 What factors should be considered when positioning the client for make-up services? Why is this important?

How to work safely and effectively when providing skincare and make-up instruction

1 How can you ensure that the lighting is suitable for the application of make-up?

2 What do you understand by the terms disinfection and sterilization? State two methods for each used in a facial and make-up instruction service?

3 Why is it important to have a variety of skincare/make-up products available for an instructional activity?

4 What must be considered and questions asked when planning a make-up lesson for a special occasion make-up?

5 How should you maintain the area during a skincare/make-up instructional activity? Why is this important?

Client consultation, service planning and preparation

1 How can you ensure that you fully understand the client's requirements for the skincare/make-up instructional activity?

2 In order to select the correct skincare and make-up products to complement the client's skin, it is necessary to identify the skin type. What are the facial characteristics of the following skin types:

- oily?

- dry?

- combination?

3 Why should you encourage the client to ask questions about the planned skincare/make-up instructional activity?

4 Why is it important to check if the client wears contact lenses or glasses and check the function of the lens before make-up application?

5   The client should be comfortable and relaxed following the consultation and preparation for the service. Give three examples of both positive and negative body language.

6   What is the legal relevance of client questioning and recording the client's responses?

7   If a contra-indication were diagnosed during the consultation, what action would you take and recommend the client to take?

8   How can you ensure that the client is comfortable with the location where the instructional activity is to take place? Why is it important to check this?

Planning and preparing for skincare and make-up instruction

1   If you did not retail the skincare or make-up products for client purchase what would you advise the client?

2   Why is it essential to have a reputable range of skincare and make-up products to select from? What must you consider to ensure these products will be suitable for all clients?

3   State the main resources you will need to provide skincare/make-up instruction.

Instructional skills

1   What should be considered when planning your delivery for a skincare/make-up instruction session?

2   What instructional methods and resources can be used to present information and instructions to the client?

3   Why is it important to present information to the client in a logical sequence?

4   How can you check that the client fully understands the instructions that you have given?

5   How can you ensure that the skincare/make-up instruction is personalized to each client and their preferred method of learning?

6   How can a client's confidence in practical application be developed during instruction?

Evaluation

1   Why is it important to evaluate the success of each instructional activity in terms of meeting the client's needs?

2   How can feedback be obtained from the client?

3   Where would you record evaluative comments for future reference?

11 Skin Camouflage (B10)

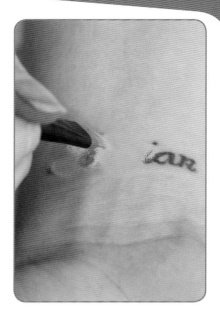

B10 Unit Learning Objectives

This chapter covers **Unit B10 Enhance appearance using skin camouflage**.

This unit describes how to return the appearance of the skin colouration temporarily to the surrounding skin tone, using specialized cosmetics. The different skin conditions to be corrected that do not involve medical consultation include hyperpigmentation and hypopigmentation or previous skin adornment procedures such as permanent tattooing. The products and application procedures will be modified according to the area of service including the head, limbs or trunk.

There are **four** learning outcomes for Unit B10 which you must achieve competently:

1   Maintain safe and effective methods of working when providing skin camouflage

2   Consult, plan and prepare for skin camouflage

3   Carry out skin camouflage

4   Provide aftercare advice

Your assessor will observe you **on four occasions**, each involving a different client.

(continued on the next page)

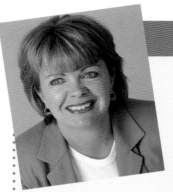

ROLE MODEL

Pamela Linforth
Head of Human Resources Ellisons

❝ My whole career has been in the beauty therapy industry. I started out by qualifying as a beauty therapist in the late 1970s when it was a very specialist and narrow field. I have been so lucky to have been part of the growth, expansion and acceptance of beauty therapy as a professional industry and valued career. My career has moved through working in a salon, electrolysis clinic, spa and into teaching. I have worked in the FE sector and industry and am now Head of Human Resources at Ellisons, suppliers to the professional hair and beauty industry. The beauty industry has been the best choice of career, allowing me to grow and develop my own skills and qualifications. It is always interesting, changing and challenging with so many opportunities. I have met, worked with and trained so many people in the industry over the years and it is these dedicated and enthusiastic professionals who make my day every day.

(continued)

From the **range** statement, you must show that you have:

- used all **camouflage products**

- used all **application tools**

- used all **consultation techniques**

- treated all **camouflage needs**

- taken the **necessary action** where a contra-action, contra-indication or service modification occurs

- have used camouflage techniques for different body **areas**

- provided relevant **aftercare advice**

However, you must prove that you have the necessary knowledge, understanding and skills to be able to perform competently across the range.

When providing skin camouflage it is important to use the skills you have learnt in the following units:

Unit G20 Make sure your own actions reduce risks to health and safety

Unit G18 Promote additional products or services to clients

Unit G8 Develop and maintain your effectiveness at work

ALWAYS REMEMBER

Photo-sensitivity of racial skin groups

- Caucasian – easily damaged by exposure to high temperatures and ultraviolet light, leading to broken veins and pigmentation disorders

- Oriental – prone to uneven pigmentation on ultraviolet light exposure

- Asian – often has uneven pigmentation skin tones; darker skin is often found around the eyes

- African-Caribbean (black) – greater protection against ultraviolet light as melanin is present in all layers of the epidermis; but tends to scar easily, possibly leading to uneven pigmentation, vitiligo and keloids

Essential anatomy and physiology knowledge requirements for this unit, **B10**, are identified on the checklist in Chapter 2, page 16. This chapter also discusses anatomy and physiology specific to this unit.

Camouflage make-up

Specialist application techniques are required for **camouflage** make-up. People asking for this service require an area of their skin to be disguised they are often distressed about this aspect of their appearance. The camouflage application requirements vary according to the skin imperfection to be disguised.

Camouflage make-up application techniques are carried out using products specifically made for the purpose. This make-up is opaque; you cannot see through it and is used to conceal and disguise an area completely. It should blend easily and be easy to apply.

Skin camouflage needs

Skin imperfections that may be camouflaged:

- **Scars:** injury, post-operative, burns, keloid (lumpy scar tissue forming at the site of wounds), acne vulgaris, raised or discoloured.

- **Burns:** scars which are ridged or discoloured.

- **Skin grafts:** where the skin is a different colour from the surrounding area and may also be hairy.

- **Birthmarks:** strawberry naevus, capillary naevus (port wine stain), darker pigmented areas.

- **Bruising:** temporary post-operative or post-injury bruising.

- **Pigmentation disorders:** hypopigmentation (reduced melanin production), e.g. vitiligo (white patches); hyperpigmentation (increased melanin production), e.g. chloasmata, also known as melasma (brown patches).

- **Vascular disorders:** acne rosacea (chronic inflammation of the skin on the nose and cheeks caused by dilation of the blood capillaries), telangiectasia (dilated capillaries appearing on the face, body or legs), varicose veins (deep blue and purple veins on the legs), erythema and redness possibly caused by acne rosacea or general high colour.

- **Tattoos:** these may be professional or amateur but both are permanent.

- **Age spots:** darker areas of pigmentation on the face, body and hands.

- **Moles:** large brown naevi on the face and body.

- **Dark skin around eyes:** dark circles due to illness, stress, lack of sleep, hereditary causes.

ALWAYS REMEMBER

Skin graft
A skin graft is where skin is moved from one part of the body to another for skin repair. This may result in differing skin tones and scarring.

TOP TIP

Vitiligo and chloasmata
Vitiligo is commonly seen around the eyes, mouth and hands; chloasmata are commonly seen on the forehead, cheek area and around the lips.

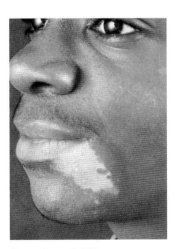

Skin before camouflage

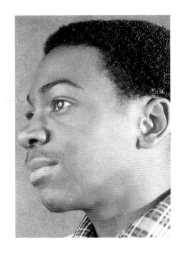

After skin colouration has been restored

TUTOR SUPPORT

Activity 3: Corrective make-up spidergram task

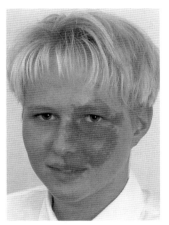

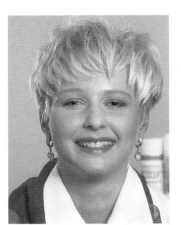

Camouflage of vitiligo

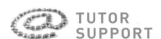

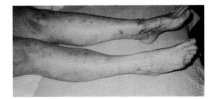

Camouflage of varicose veins

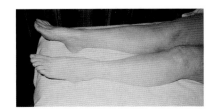

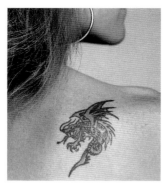
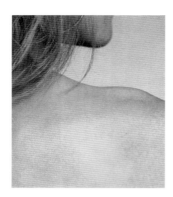
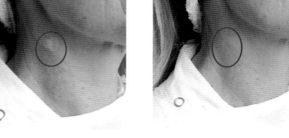

Camouflage of tattoo to the back

Concealing minor hypopigmentation

Outcome 1: Maintain safe and effective methods of working when providing skin camouflage

Learn how to maintain an efficient safe working environment when providing skin camouflage by:

1. Setting up and monitoring the service area to meet organization procedures and manufacturers' instructions.

2. Making sure that environmental conditions are suitable for the client and the skin camouflage.

3. Ensuring your personal hygiene, protection and appearance meets accepted industry and organizational requirements.

4. Effectively disinfecting your hands prior to service.

5. Ensuring your own posture and position minimizes fatigue and risk of injury while working.

6. Ensuring all tools are cleaned using the correct methods.

7. Positioning skin camouflage products and **application tools** for ease and safety of use.

8. Ensuring the client is in a comfortable and relaxed position suitable for the skin camouflage.

9. Maintaining accepted industry hygiene and safety practices throughout the skin camouflage application.

10. Adopting a positive, polite and reassuring manner towards the client throughout the service.

11. Respecting the client's modesty, privacy and any sensitivities to their personal appearance.

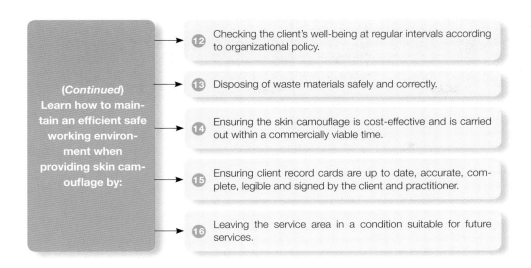

(Continued)
Learn how to maintain an efficient safe working environment when providing skin camouflage by:

12 Checking the client's well-being at regular intervals according to organizational policy.

13 Disposing of waste materials safely and correctly.

14 Ensuring the skin camouflage is cost-effective and is carried out within a commercially viable time.

15 Ensuring client record cards are up to date, accurate, complete, legible and signed by the client and practitioner.

16 Leaving the service area in a condition suitable for future services.

Equipment and materials

Before beginning the skin camouflage, check that you have the necessary equipment and materials to hand and that they meet the legal, hygiene and industry requirements for skin camouflage services.

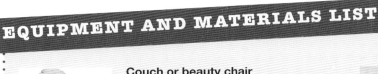

EQUIPMENT AND MATERIALS LIST

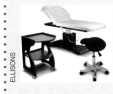

Couch or beauty chair
With reclining back and headrest and an easy-to-clean surface

ELLISONS

Trolley or other surface
On which to place everything

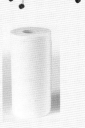

Disposable tissue (such as bedroll)
To cover work surface and the couch or beauty chair

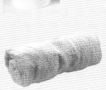

Towels (two)
Freshly laundered for each client – one to be placed over the head of the couch, the other to protect the client's garments

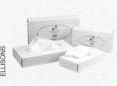

Specialized cleansing and toning preparations
Efficient at removing waterproof make-up

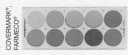

ELLISONS

Large white facial tissues
To blot the skin after cleansing and moisturiser application

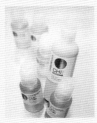

COVERMARK®, FARMECO®

Range of concealing and camouflage make-up products
To treat a variety of skin types and colours

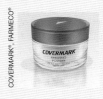

COVERMARK®, FARMECO®

Camouflage setting or fixing powder
Essential for a matt finish, which absorbs skin oils and perspiration, giving the make-up durability

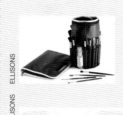

Make-up application brushes (assorted)

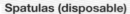

Spatulas (disposable)

To remove products from containers while preventing contamination

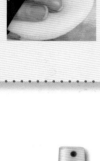

Sponges

To apply the camouflage make-up to larger areas or dampened sponge may be provided for a lighter effect

Velour puff

To apply fixing powder to set the camouflage make-up

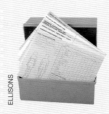

Client record card

To record the client's personal details, products used and details of the service

YOU WILL ALSO NEED:

Moisturiser To prepare the skin

Magnifying lamp To inspect the area after cleansing

Cotton wool Dry and damp, prepared for each client

Bowls To hold the prepared cotton wool

Mirror To show the client camouflage make-up application throughout the service

Disinfecting solution For all surfaces

Waste container Lined bin with lid

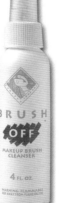

Brush cleaner

Preparation of the work area

The service area should have good ventilation so that the client's skin does not become too warm. The service couch or make-up chair should be clean and covered with fresh towels, and/or disposable bedroll as required. The trolley should display all the required make-up, applicators (including sponges, spatulas and brushes), skin cleansers, toners and moisturisers ready to use. Cotton wool, tissues and protective make-up capes are normally used. A lined waste bin must be available for disposal of waste.

The work area should remain in a condition suitable for further skin camouflage services throughout the working day.

Sterilization and disinfection

Make-up must be removed from containers using clean, disinfected or disposable spatulas. Colours can be mixed on a disinfected or disposable colour-mixing palette. Applicators such as brushes and sponges can either be disposable, or alternatively should be thoroughly washed using a soap-free antibacterial cleanser, rinsed in cold, clean water, allowed to dry and then stored in an ultraviolet cabinet.

Professional make-up brush cleaner can be sprayed onto the brushes, dried and then removed onto tissue along with the make-up. The quick antibacterial action allows the brushes to be used again almost immediately.

Short nails are important when applying the make-up by hand to avoid make-up collecting underneath the nails during application.

Commercial brush cleaner can be used to maintain hygiene of your brushes.

ACTIVITY

Research which types of camouflage make-up are available and how you would buy them. Compare the costs of setting up a range for the salon.

Suitable lighting

Lighting should be considered when applying camouflage make-up because it will make a difference to how it looks.

Lighting

You need to know the *type* of light in which proposed make-up to the face will be seen. This is important when deciding on the correct choice of make-up colours, because the appearance of colours may change according to the type of light. For further details about lighting, see Chapter 9, page 278.

Preparation of the beauty therapist

Complete a record card during the consultation, or if this is a repeat visit, have the client's record card ready. Hands must be sanitized before treating the client.

The beauty therapist's presentation must meet the organization's and the industry's professional standards. A clean, fresh uniform and smart appearance, and, if female, preferably wearing make-up, will make the client feel relaxed and reassured that they are in capable hands.

Outcome 2: Consult, plan and prepare for skin camouflage

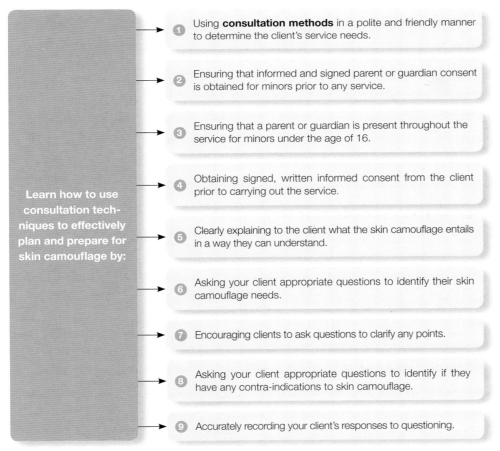

Learn how to use consultation techniques to effectively plan and prepare for skin camouflage by:

1. Using **consultation methods** in a polite and friendly manner to determine the client's service needs.

2. Ensuring that informed and signed parent or guardian consent is obtained for minors prior to any service.

3. Ensuring that a parent or guardian is present throughout the service for minors under the age of 16.

4. Obtaining signed, written informed consent from the client prior to carrying out the service.

5. Clearly explaining to the client what the skin camouflage entails in a way they can understand.

6. Asking your client appropriate questions to identify their skin camouflage needs.

7. Encouraging clients to ask questions to clarify any points.

8. Asking your client appropriate questions to identify if they have any contra-indications to skin camouflage.

9. Accurately recording your client's responses to questioning.

HEALTH & SAFETY

Brushes and sponges

Brushes and sponges kept damp will encourage bacterial growth, possibly resulting in skin irritation and cross-infection. Wash thoroughly and store dry, preferably in an ultraviolet cabinet.

TOP TIP

Brushes

Fine brushes are required when disguising small scars and blemishes.

ALWAYS REMEMBER

Artificial light

If applying the make-up under artificial light, use warm fluorescent light for day make-up, as this closely resembles natural light.

BEST PRACTICE

Further consultations

Further consultations may be recommended to select differing cosmetic colours, as skin colour changes on exposure to ultraviolet light, e.g. sun tanning.

ALWAYS REMEMBER

Skin tones

Skin tones vary from person to person and body to face.

There are yellow, red and olive tones.

ALWAYS REMEMBER

Assessing skin type

The **Fitzpatrick Classification System** is a scale developed to assess the amount of melanin pigment in the skin providing your skin colour and how your skin will react to sun without protection (photo-sensitivity). There are six skin type classifications from Caucasian (skin type I) to African-Caribbean (skin type VI). The higher up the scale the more pigmented the skin. Certain skin conditions and disorders are more prevalent to each skin type.

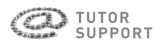

TUTOR SUPPORT

Activity 1: Client record card task

BEST PRACTICE

Before and after photographs
Photographs of 'before' and 'after' make-up are useful at the consultation to illustrate the obtainable results.

ACTIVITY

Contra-actions can sometimes occur when applying camouflage make-up or make-up for enhancing the appearance. What form would these contra-actions take? What actions would you need in order to help prevent the contra-actions or to help alleviate them if they occur?

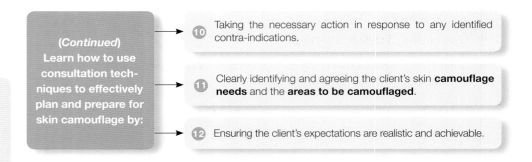

(Continued) Learn how to use consultation techniques to effectively plan and prepare for skin camouflage by:

10 Taking the necessary action in response to any identified contra-indications.

11 Clearly identifying and agreeing the client's skin **camouflage needs** and the **areas to be camouflaged**.

12 Ensuring the client's expectations are realistic and achievable.

Consultation

The **consultation** should be confidential and relaxed, in order for the client to feel comfortable in discussing the area requiring attention. Often the client may be psychologically upset and as such the consultation and questions asked should be tactful and reassuring.

Explain what the camouflage service involves, its benefits and limitations. Identify the client's **camouflage needs** by asking the client why they want the area to be corrected – it may be for a special occasion, often a wedding, photograph or for disguise during normal day wear. It is important to establish whether the client's expected outcomes from the service are realistic.

A case history of the skin imperfection is required. Ask questions such as:

● How long has the imperfection been there? Congenital abnormalities, i.e. capillary haemangioma (port wine stain) are present at birth. Pigmentation abnormalities, e.g. chloasmata (brown patches) or vitiligo (white patches) will have developed with age.

● If scars are present, what was their cause? They may be due to accidental or self-harm injury, e.g. cuts, burns or surgery.

● If tattoos are present, ask when and how the tattoo completed. Tattoos may be professionally done or self-applied; both are permanent, although non-professional tattoos will fade and blur.

● Is surgery or laser service being carried out in the area? When was the last service done?

● How long has healing been taking place for?

● Is there any soreness or lack of sensitivity in the area?

Contra-indications

If, while completing the record card, or on visual inspection of the skin, the client is found to have any of the following in the service area, specialist make-up should not be applied. If in doubt, then the client must be referred to their GP to confirm their suitability for service.

● Broken skin, unhealed wounds.

● Eye infections (e.g. conjunctivitis).

- Skin disorders or disease.
- Skin swelling, irritation, soreness.
- Suspicious moles (showing signs of growing, changing colour, itching, soreness or weeping).

If camouflage make-up is to be used to cover post-operative bruising (e.g. after face lifting), then the client must provide evidence of the surgeon's permission before service.

Contra-actions

Camouflage products are formulated to be used on sensitive and delicate skin types, so allergic reaction is rare. However, allergic reactions can occur in some people. This is known as a contra-action and may occur during or following service.

Irritation, soreness, erythema If skin irritation occurs, cleanse all traces of make-up from the skin and advise the application of a cool compress and soothing lotion. If skin irritation continues, ask the client to seek their GP's advice.

Blocked pores, pustules The client may not be following the aftercare advice. Discuss how to cleanse the skin thoroughly and advise against wearing the make-up for longer than 24 hours at a time.

HEALTH & SAFETY

Prevention of cross-infection
Three sets of make-up brushes are required to allow for effective disinfection between clients. Remove products from containers using a disposable spatula. Never apply make-up over broken skin, and only over scar tissue when it is completely healed.

Contamination
Do not put any applicators that have been in contact with the client's skin directly in the make-up containers. The make-up may become contaminated with bacteria, resulting in cross-infection.

Make-up containers
If using make-up in containers, always remove it with a clean spatula.

Examine the area carefully, noting the extent of the camouflage need, as well as the colours and skin tones around it.

Record all responses to questions asked and related notes on the client record card.

Clients who have unrealistic expectations should be accurately and tactfully advised of achievable outcomes.

Following consultation, ensure the client fully understands the aims of the service to be received. Question the client to confirm understanding.

ALWAYS REMEMBER

Manufacturer's instructions

Check the manufacturer's instructions on how to apply the camouflage make-up. Brands vary and some may require different preparation or setting techniques.

ALWAYS REMEMBER

Examples of camouflage service modification includes:

- changing the brand of make-up to one that suits the client better
- improving the skin condition with facials or skin services before make-up application

ACTIVITY

The type of light under which camouflage make-up is seen makes a difference to how it will look. Experiment with three different light sources, e.g. daylight, fluorescent light, incandescent light, to see how the make-up will look in each.

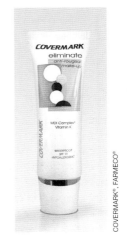

Camouflage cosmetics

Sample client record card

Date	Beauty therapist name	
Client name	Date of birth	
Address	Postcode	
Email address	Landline phone number	Mobile phone number
Name of doctor	Doctor's address and phone number	
Related medical history (Conditions that may restrict or prohibit service application.)		
Are you taking any medication? (Especially antibiotics, steroids, the pill.)		

CONTRA-INDICATIONS REQUIRING MEDICAL REFERRAL
(Preventing cosmetic camouflage make-up.)

- ☐ skin disorders
- ☐ skin infections
- ☐ eye infections
- ☐ swelling, irritation or soreness
- ☐ suspicious moles (showing signs of growing, changing colour, itching, soreness or weeping)

SERVICE AREAS

- ☐ face
- ☐ neck
- ☐ chest
- ☐ shoulders
- ☐ back
- ☐ arms
- ☐ legs
- ☐ other

CAMOUFLAGE NEEDS
Pigment disorders

- ☐ hyperpigmentation
- ☐ hypopigmentation

Vascular disorders

- ☐ erythema
- ☐ tattoos

SPECIAL NOTES AND CONSIDERATIONS
(e.g. skin very sensitive, imperfection very dark and difficult to conceal)

CONTRA-INDICATIONS WHICH RESTRICT SERVICE
(Service may require adaptation.)

- ☐ any condition adjacent to the camouflage area which is sore or tender e.g. post-operative swelling and bruising

LIFESTYLE

- ☐ active exercising and swimming
- ☐ active exercise only
- ☐ no specific exercise
- ☐ generally busy, e.g. family and job

OBJECTIVES OF SERVICE

- ☐ to be used daily
- ☐ to be used when needed
- ☐ to be used for a special occasion

PRODUCTS USED

- ☐ camouflage cream – colour
- ☐ camouflage powder – colour
- ☐ setting or fixing product – colour

APPLICATION TOOLS

- ☐ brushes
- ☐ fingers
- ☐ sponges
- ☐ velour puffs

Beauty therapist signature (for reference)
Client signature (confirmation of details)

Sample client record card (continued)

SERVICE ADVICE
Camouflage make-up lesson for any area – *allow 1 hour*
Camouflage application   large area – *allow 1 hour*
                 medium sized area – *allow 1/2 hour*
                            tattoo – *allow 1/2 hour*

SERVICE PLAN
Record relevant details of your service, lesson and advice provided for future reference. Ensure the client's records are up to date, accurate and fully completed following service. Non-compliance may invalidate insurance.

DURING
- Take a photo of the area to be camouflaged with the client's permission.
- Explain the skin preparation and why it is important.
- Explain each stage of choosing the right colour of make-up and mixing it to match the skin tone.
- Demonstrate the application and then encourage the client to do it themselves with your help.
- Note any adverse reaction, or evidence of skin sensitivity if any occurs.

AFTER
- Record the results of the make-up application.
- Take a photo of the result.
- Record which products and colours have been used for future reference.
- Discuss the best way for the client to keep the camouflage make-up looking good.
- Instruct the client on the removal of the products.
- Instruct the client on the hygiene necessary for make-up application.

RETAIL OPPORTUNITIES
The client will need to buy all the products you have used in order to successfully apply/remove the camouflage at home.
- Recommend skincare products for home use to maintain the skin in good condition of the face and body.
- Advise if there are any other services which may help the condition e.g. facials, eye services, airbrush tanning.

EVALUATION
- Record comments of the client's satisfaction with the service and the result.
- If the camouflage effect is not what the client wanted, then record this and why.
- Record how you may change the make-up application next time to achieve a better result.

HEALTH AND SAFETY
- Advise the client how to look after the area after the service to avoid any unwanted reaction.
- Advise the client of the appropriate necessary action to take if there is an unwanted skin reaction.

Service plan

The content of the service plan discussed should be agreed by the client and their signature recorded on the service record card prior to carrying out the camouflage service.

If the client is a minor under the age of 16 it is necessary to obtain parent/guardian permission for service. The parent/guardian will also have to be present when the service is received.

Reception

Camouflage make-up sessions will often take the form of a lesson. This will enable the client to apply make-up in the future for the purpose of correction and concealment.

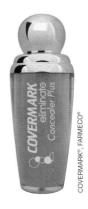
COVERMARK®, FARMECO®

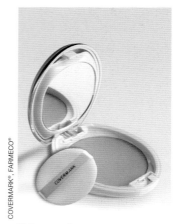

Fixing powder

TOP TIP

Dry areas

Do not use moisturiser on an area that is to be camouflaged, unless it is very dry. It may change the colour of the make-up or prevent it from setting properly.

ALWAYS REMEMBER

Camouflage make-up can help to disguise:

- facial shapes and features
- scars
- burns
- skin grafts
- tattoos
- birthmarks
- dark circles under eyes
- bruising
- pigmentation disorders
- vascular disorders

The client will have her camouflage make-up applied by the beauty therapist, showing each step of the procedure. One hour is booked for this, which allows for instruction to be conducted in a relaxed manner. It is not always possible for the beauty therapist immediately to match the client's skin tone, so time must be allowed for experimentation. Once successfully completed, should the client then want to return to the salon to have professional application for a special occasion, then 30 to 45 minutes is normally allocated. Service times will vary according to client's needs, size of area and service requirements.

If the client has sensitive skin, a skin test must be recommended to test for allergy to the camouflage make-up.

The projected costs and service duration should be agreed beforehand with the client.

All staff, especially the staff communicating with clients at reception should be familiar with the different pricing structures for the range of skin camouflage services and products available for retail.

Preparation of the client

The client must be made to feel relaxed and confident on the service couch or make-up chair. Protect the client's clothing with tissue, towel or a make-up cape and remove jewellery from the area of application.

- When working on the face, have the client sitting up so that the face is viewed resting in its natural shape and contours. Protect and cover collars and clothing and, if necessary, hair.

- When working on the arms and shoulders, have the client sitting up with the area to be worked on free of clothing. Protect and cover any clothes nearby with large tissue or a towel to avoid spillage or marking.

- When working on the abdomen, have the client lie on their back, support the head and under the knees to ensure client comfort.

- When working on the back, the client can either sit up with their back towards you or lie flat on their front – whichever is best for them and for you.

- When working on the legs, have the area to be camouflaged exposed and have the client lying comfortably either on their back (for the fronts of the legs) or on their side or front (for the backs of the legs).

BEST PRACTICE

Prevention of cross-infection

- Use disposable applicators where possible.
- Clean and disinfect brushes, sponges and applicators that are not disposable after every client.
- Wash your hands before every service.
- Do not treat areas that appear inflamed or infected.
- Do not dip your applicators or fingers into the make-up.

Ensure the client is relaxed and comfortable before the service proceeds. The area to be treated should be cleansed and toned with the appropriate skincare preparations.

If moisturiser is to be used, it must be lightweight and absorbed before make-up is applied. This usually takes about ten minutes. Before make-up application, any excess moisturiser may be blotted off using a clean tissue. Oily creams will interfere with the make-up consistency.

For facial services have a mirror ready to use through the stages of the camouflage make-up application, so that the client can see what it looks like as you progress, and how to apply it.

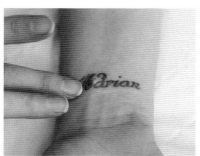

Cleansing the skin

Plan and prepare for the camouflage make-up application

Outcome 3: Carry out skin camouflage

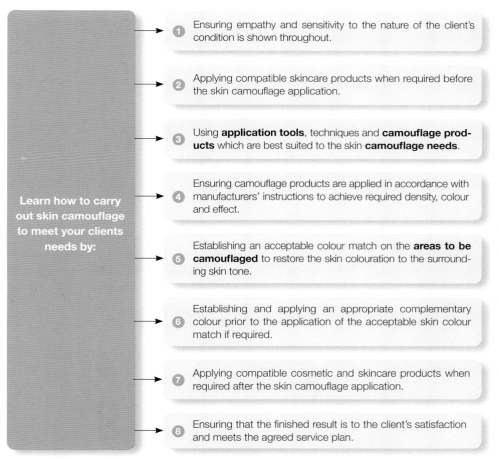

Learn how to carry out skin camouflage to meet your clients needs by:

1. Ensuring empathy and sensitivity to the nature of the client's condition is shown throughout.

2. Applying compatible skincare products when required before the skin camouflage application.

3. Using **application tools**, techniques and **camouflage products** which are best suited to the skin **camouflage needs**.

4. Ensuring camouflage products are applied in accordance with manufacturers' instructions to achieve required density, colour and effect.

5. Establishing an acceptable colour match on the **areas to be camouflaged** to restore the skin colouration to the surrounding skin tone.

6. Establishing and applying an appropriate complementary colour prior to the application of the acceptable skin colour match if required.

7. Applying compatible cosmetic and skincare products when required after the skin camouflage application.

8. Ensuring that the finished result is to the client's satisfaction and meets the agreed service plan.

Moisturiser application

> " Areas that need to have skin camouflage are often more sensitive than the surrounding skin. Be gentle and scrupulously clean and hygienic in your work.
>
> **Pamela Linforth**

Carry out and instruct the client on skin camouflage

In order to select the correct colours for camouflage make-up it is important to understand the principles of colour. During the skin type analyzis, you need to identify the undertones of the client's skin.

ALWAYS REMEMBER

Posture

Always position the client and work station ensuring that your working posture is correct, minimizing the risk of injury and tiredness caused by muscle fatigue.

HEALTH & SAFETY

Hygiene recommendations

The department of health has issued strict hygiene recommendations in the application of skin camouflage products. Research these recommendations.

> When applying skin camouflage make-up you must be considerate about the client's sensitivity to their problem area. Don't let this make you nervous; be relaxed, friendly, calm and matter of fact and you will make it a good experience for your client and you.

Pamela Linforth

ACTIVITY

Colour theory

Research the principles of colour theory and make a colour wheel. Experiment to see which colours best suit which skin conditions.

> Make sure that you offer your camouflage make-up for sale and have it available in your retail displays for your clients. They will want to buy it to carry on the camouflage work at home so don't miss the chance of good sales.

Pamela Linforth

Colour theory

- **Primary colours** are red, yellow and blue. All other colours are made up from these colours.

- **Secondary colours** are formed by mixing primary colours and are green, orange and purple.

- **Tertiary colours** are formed by mixing primary and secondary colours, and include blue-green, red-violet and yellow-orange.

- **Analogous colours** – any three harmonious colours that are side by side on a 12-part colour wheel (shown below), for example, orange, orange-red, orange-brown.

Complementary colours are any two colours opposite each other on the colour wheel. Opposite colours neutralize each other, therefore, if a colour is hard to conceal look at the opposite colour on the colour wheel, e.g. green neutralizes red for vascular imperfections. Select yellow tones to neutralize blue or purple imperfections. This neutralizing colour should only be applied to the affected area.

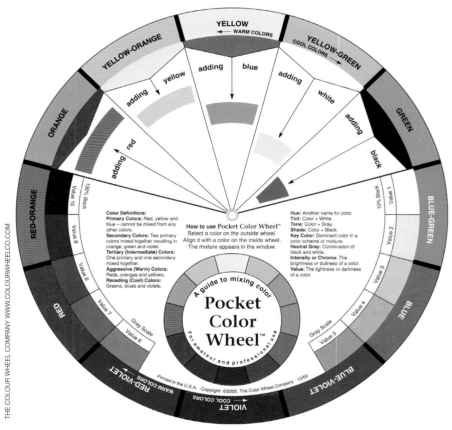

Colour wheel

How to apply camouflage make-up

1 Select the chosen colour or colour mixture which best matches the skin tone surrounding the area to be treated. This will normally need to be a mixture of colours

TOP TIP

Layering

It is preferable to build up several layers to achieve the desired effect, rather than applying a thick layer.

- **Covering a deep red mark:** use a green pigmented make-up first to neutralize, then apply make-up that matches the skin tone over the top.
- **Covering a dark brown mark:** use white, opaque make-up first to disguise, then apply make-up that matches the skin tone over the top.
- **Covering a lighter mark:** commence with a darker foundation and apply make-up that matches the skin tone over the top.
- **Covering yellow marks:** use a lilac pigmented make-up, then apply make-up that matches the skin tone over the top.

ALWAYS REMEMBER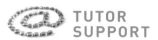

Using counteracting colours to neutralize

If the counteracting colour can be seen you have used too much. Always mix sparingly until you get the required result.

@ TUTOR SUPPORT

Activity 4: Skin camouflage word puzzle

as one colour is rarely an exact match. Mix the colours together on one palette and then test them on a small area of normal skin near the blemish to get the right colour. Keep it simple: remember the client needs to be able to do the mixing for herself at home.

2 Using your ring and middle fingers in a patting motion, or using a dry sponge, blend the make-up thinly over the problem area, extending it approximately two centimetres past the edge. If disguising scars, a brush may be used to feather the make-up at the edges to create a natural effect. The sponge may be dampened if needed to facilitate extra blending. A fine brush as shown may be used to disguise small scars and blemishes or, as in this case, a tattoo.

3 Build up the colour depth to ensure the blemish is completely covered, thinning the colour at the edge to blend in. A small make-up brush can be used to blend in the edges of the make-up.

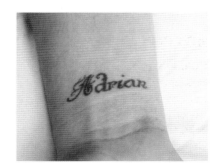

The tattoo to be camouflaged

4 Once the required result has been achieved, apply the fixing powder generously with a large powder puff. Fixing powder may be applied between applications where counter-acting procedures are not used.

5 Leave the make-up to set for 5–10 minutes.

6 Gently brush off any excess fixing powder with a large, soft make-up brush, e.g. blusher/powder brush. Blot off excess powder if required with damp cotton wool. The make-up is now waterproof and rub-resistant, and should not be detectable.

7 If the camouflage has been applied to the face, full make-up may now be applied. The foundation colour selected should match the colour of the camouflage make-up.

8 Apply foundation up to the area of camouflage make-up and blend so that an invisible finish is created. Putting an oily cream foundation over the camouflage make-up will only move or remove the camouflage make-up: it is best to use a non-oily or liquid foundation.

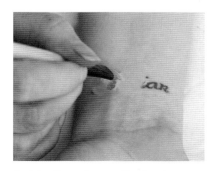

Applying the make-up with a brush

9 Ensure the finished result is to the client's satisfaction.

10 Record on the client record card the make-up products selected and application technique used.

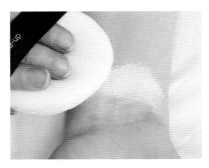

Applying fixing powder

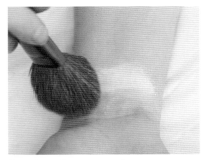

Brushing off excess powder

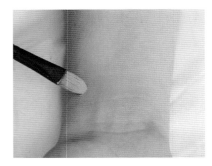

The finished cosmetic camouflage make-up

A successful skin camouflage will match the surrounding skin tone while disguising the imperfections.

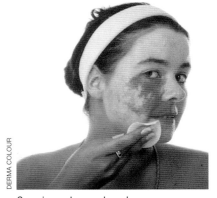

DERMA COLOUR

Covering a deep red mark

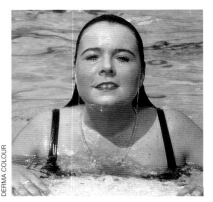

DERMA COLOUR

Camouflage make-up is waterproof

Minor skin camouflage

Concealing Before you begin to apply make-up to the face, inspect the skin and identify the areas that require concealing, such as blemishes, uneven skin colour or shadows.

Foundation may be used to disguise minor skin imperfections, but where extra coverage is required it is necessary to apply a special **concealer** – a cosmetic designed to provide maximum skin coverage. The concealer may be applied directly to the skin after skin moisturising, or following application of the foundation.

Choose a concealer that matches the client's skin tone as closely as possible. If the concealer is to be applied *after* the foundation, it should match the colour of the *foundation*.

Concealer can contain pigment to help correct skin tone:

- **Green** helps to counteract high colouring, and to conceal dilated capillaries.
- **Lilac** counteracts a sallow skin colour and disguises dark circles.
- **White** or **cream** helps to correct unevenness in the skin pigmentation and is light-reflecting and line concealing.

How to apply concealer Remove a small quantity of the concealer from its container, using a clean, disposable spatula. Apply the concealer to the area to be disguised, using either a clean make-up sponge or a soft make-up brush. Blend the concealer to achieve a realistic effect.

Airbrushing

Airbrushing techniques are used for all types of camouflage and corrective make-up. The technique involves using an air-powered (by compressor) airbrush which sprays extremely tiny droplets of make-up in a water suspension over the area. Several sweeps of the airbrush are used to carefully build up the colour and amount needed. The make-up is especially formulated for the airbrush.

Preparation The skin is prepared by cleansing, toning and blotting with a tissue. Moisturiser is not normally used as it may interfere with the result of the airbrushing. Very dry skins that need moisture have a fine layer of jojoba oil airbrushed onto the make-up when it is completed.

The order of work is the same as normal for the application of make-up. Mascara and lipstick are applied in the normal way once the airbrushing is complete.

Airbrushing has the following benefits:

- A sheer, flawless coverage can be achieved.

- It is hygienic as the skin is not touched with brushes or sponges.

- The seamless blending and long-lasting properties make it suitable for covering blemishes and tattoos.

- It is suitable for all skin types and colours.

- The application is very quick.

- It is both rub and water resistant.

- It sets on contact with the skin.

> **TOP TIP**
>
> **Experiment!**
> It is important to experiment with different applications to ensure the best result.

> **TOP TIP**
>
> **Skin tone**
> Copy the surrounding skin tone carefully to ensure the most natural effect, i.e. add freckles or shade the camouflage make-up to match darker or lighter areas.

How to apply camouflage make-up with an airbrush

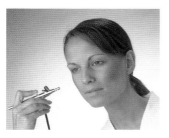 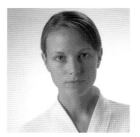 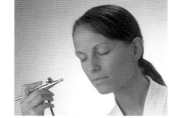

Applying camouflage make-up with an airbrush

Outcome 4: Provide aftercare advice

Learn how to provide aftercare advice which supports and meets the needs of your client by:

1. Giving **advice** and recommendations accurately and constructively.

2. Giving your clients suitable **advice** specific to their individual needs.

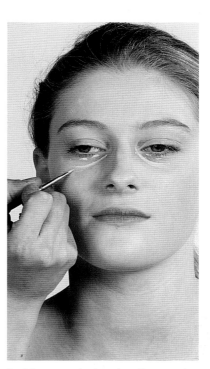

Applying concealer to reduce the appearance of dark shadows under the eyes

TOP TIP

Titanium dioxide

Concealing products containing large quantities of titanium dioxide should be avoided on black skin because they will make the skin look grey.

TUTOR SUPPORT

Activity 2: Product research task

TOP TIP

Retail

As well as the camouflage products, have all application tools available for retail so the client will be using the correct tools to achieve the required result.

" Always be on the look out for chances to offer skin camouflage make-up. Clients will often complain about an imperfection that they have. Show your initiative by telling them about the service that you offer, you'll be surprised at how many will take up the chance to get their problem area concealed.

Pamela Linforth

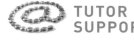

TUTOR SUPPORT

Activity 5: Re-cap, revision and evaluation

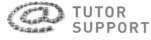

TUTOR SUPPORT

Activity 6: Multiple choice quiz

Offering aftercare advice at the end of the camouflage service will ensure the client knows how to maintain the make-up and ensure its durability. They will also know correct removal techniques to maintain the health and appearance of the skin. Aftercare advice will basically be as follows:

- All the make-up must be thoroughly removed using the appropriate cleansers and toners. Camouflage make-up manufacturers normally specify their own brands. These are often oily, in order to help remove the waterproof make-up effectively. The client must have the right cleanser and toner for use at home. Recommend a good skincare routine and stress the importance of hygiene and keeping make-up and applicators clean to avoid contamination.

- Camouflage make-up initially will take longer to apply than normal make-up products. This must be allowed for. With experience and confidence application will become quicker.

- Avoid a heavy application; gradually layer the product until you achieve the required result using appropriate tools including brushes, fingers, sponges and velour puffs.

- If wearing the make-up in a hot environment the make-up will be less durable and will require regular attention.

- Care should be taken if the area covered becomes wet. Advise the client to pat the area dry gently with a soft towel.

- Corrective make-up should not be left on for longer than 24 hours at a time as it may clog the skin and cause irritations and blemishes.

- Once you have shown the client how to apply the make-up, they can apply it for themself at home. Recommend that the client applies the make-up in the proper light, preferably daylight.

- Explain to the client that the camouflage make-up should be treated gently in order to keep it looking effective. Rubbing, for example from clothes or straps, may remove or smudge it.

- Oily products such as body lotions will remove the make-up, so must not be put onto the skin in close proximity.

- The client's current skincare routine should be discussed because incorrect skincare routines can affect the condition of the skin.

- The client should be advised to wear regular sun protection in the case of pigmentation disorders.

- Provide aftercare instructions and details of application procedures in written format, but encourage the client to contact you if they have any further questions about the result achieved.

- It is also necessary to advise the client what to do in the event of a contra-action.

TOP TIP

Camouflage product formulations

Many camouflage products contain sun protection factors (SPF) to protect the skin from UV damage, plus other beneficial ingredients, such as anti-oxidants and silica to absorb the skin's natural oils.

GLOSSARY OF KEY WORDS

Aftercare advice recommendations given to the client following service to maintain the finished result and enable the benefits to be continued at home.

Camouflage needs identifying the area and skin imperfection requiring camouflage, e.g. tattoos, hyperpigmentation, hypopigmentation and erythema (redness).

Camouflage products cosmetic make-up products designed to conceal skin imperfections including creams, powders and setting products for the face and body.

Client groups this term is used in a number of the units and it refers to client diversity. The CRE (Commission for Racial Equality) ethnic group classification is used in the range for these units. These cover white, mixed, Asian, black and Chinese.

Colour theory the colour wheel places the three primary colours with the secondary colours in-between. These result from mixing the two adjacent primary colours. In-between these are the tertiary colours achieved by mixing the primary and secondary colours. Colour is reduced or removed by mixing colours that are directly opposite each other in the colour wheel.

Consultation assessment of client needs using different assessment techniques including questioning and natural observation.

Contra-action an unwanted reaction occurring during or after service.

Contra-indication a problematic symptom that indicates the service may not proceed.

Fitzpatrick Classification System a scale developed to assess the amount of melanin pigment in the skin providing your skin colour and how your skin will react to sun without protection (photosensitivity). There are six skin type classifications from Caucasian (skin type I) to African-Caribbean (skin type VI).

Necessary action the appropriate action to take in the event of a contra-action or contra-indication to ensure the welfare of the client.

Service plan after the consultation, suitable service objectives are established to treat the client conditions and needs.

ASSESSMENT OF KNOWLEDGE AND UNDERSTANDING

Having covered the learning objectives for **Enhance appearance using skin camouflage**, test what you need to know and understand answering the following short questions below. The information covers:

- organizational and legal requirements
- how to work safely and effectively when providing skin camouflage
- client consultation, planning and preparation
- anatomy and physiology
- contra-indications and contra-actions
- skin camouflage
- aftercare advice for clients

Organizational and legal requirements

For full legislation details, see Chapter 4.

1 Which health and safety legislation is relevant to skin camouflage service?

2 Why is it essential to keep service records of your skin camouflage services and how does the Data Protection Act affect this?

3 What details should be recorded on the client's record card?

4 Why is it important that the skin camouflage is provided in the allocated commercial time?

5 How long would you allocate to carry out a skin camouflage to a large tattooed area on the back?

How to work safely and effectively when providing skin camouflage

1 It is important to maintain standards of hygiene and to avoid cross-infection. How would you do this?

2 Why is it important to position your clients in a comfortable and suitable way? How is it possible to injure yourself if this is not done?

3 What environmental conditions should you consider when planning for skin camouflage?

4 Research two different ranges of camouflage make-up and what are the features and benefits of each. Where could these be obtained from and is there a retail range for client purchase?

5 How would you make sure you were properly prepared for a camouflage make-up lesson?

Client consultation, planning and preparation

1 Why would you only offer camouflage service to a client once they have asked about it?

2 When going through the consultation procedure with a new client, how can you make sure you are using effective communication and consultation techniques?

3 How would you encourage your client to seek medical advice about a possible contra-indication to skin camouflage?

4 It is necessary to maintain the client's modesty and privacy at all times. How can you make sure this is done?

5 How would you prepare the plan for the skin camouflage?

Anatomy and physiology

For anatomy and physiology details, see Chapter 2.

1 Draw and label a detailed diagram to show the skin structure.

2 Describe the functions of the skin.

3 Describe how skin structure differs in different racial groups.

4 How can photo-sensitivity of skin in different skin groups be classified?

5 State five skin conditions that may be camouflaged and discuss their cause.

Contra-indications and contra-actions

1 Name three contra-indications that may be seen at consultation and which would contra-indicate service.

2 Why is it important not to name specific contra-indications when asking clients to seek medical advice?

3 Name three contra-indications that would restrict camouflage application.

4 What sort of contra-action could you observe during service? How can you minimize the possibility of contra-actions?

Skin camouflage

1 Each camouflage application is very different. How would you select the right products and colours for the service?

2 How can you demonstrate the methods of application to your clients and how can you make sure the clients understand and are able to perform it for themselves?

3 What are the main principles of colour theory?

4 How would you colour match and why is this important?

5 During a camouflage instruction why is it useful to show the client the difference between the made-up area and untreated area? How could you do this during the service?

6 Why should suitability of the client's current skincare routine be checked for compatibility with camouflage products?

Aftercare advice for clients

1 What advice should you give the client about keeping the camouflage make-up on and then removing it in the correct way with the right products?

2 Why is a further consultation follow-up beneficial for the client and beauty therapist?

12 Manicure Services (N2)

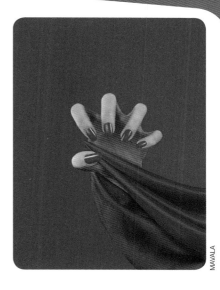

MAVALA

N2 Unit Learning Objectives

This chapter covers **Unit N2 Provide manicure services**.

This unit is all about improving and maintaining your client's hands, nails and surrounding skin. A manicure includes filing the nails to shape, buffing the nail plate surface, using specialized nail products, cuticle products and treatments, massaging the lower arm and hand and providing a complementary nail finish to suit the client.

There are **four** learning outcomes for this chapter which you must achieve competently:

1 **Maintain safe and effective methods of working when providing manicure services**

2 **Consult, plan and prepare for the manicure services**

3 **Carry out manicure services**

4 **Provide aftercare advice**

Your assessor will observe you on at least **three occasions** (each occasion must involve a different hand and nail service from the range).

From the **range** statement, you must show that you have:

- used all **consultation techniques**

- taken the necessary action where a contra-indication or treatment modification occurs

- applied all **hand and nail services**

(continued on the next page)

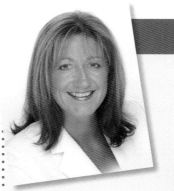

ROLE MODEL

Jacqui Jefford
Consultant and freelance session nail technician

" I have been in the nail and beauty industry for over 25 years, and am one of the leading figures in the industry in the UK and internationally. My work has taken me to many countries as a consultant in education, competitions (winning, designing and judging them), taking educational seminars and working in PR, TV and with the consumer press. I also have my salon, school and distribution company, and work with many FE colleges as a tutor, assessor and internal verifier. I have particularly enjoyed working at London and Paris Fashion Weeks as well as decorating the covers of top magazines such as Vogue. I have written four successful books and been involved in five DVDs. My passion has always been good education and I have worked alongside Habia on many projects over the last ten years.

(continued)

- applied all **nail finishes**

- provided relevant service **advice**

However you must prove that you have the necessary knowledge, understanding and skills to be able to perform competently across the range.

When providing manicure services it is important to use the skills you have learnt in the following units:

Unit G20 Make sure your own actions reduce risks to health and safety

Unit G18 Promote additional products or services to clients

Unit G8 Develop and maintain your effectiveness at work

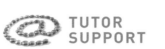

TUTOR SUPPORT

Activity 1: label the nail structure

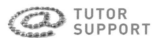

TUTOR SUPPORT

Activity 2: label the bones of the arm and hand

Essential anatomy and physiology knowledge requirements for this unit, **N2**, are identified on the checklist chart in Chapter 2, page 16.

The purpose of a manicure

The word manicure is derived from the Latin words *manus*, meaning 'hand', and *cura*, meaning care'. A manicure therefore cares for the hands for the following reasons:

- to improve the hands' appearance

- to keep the nails smooth

- to keep the cuticles attractive and healthy

- to keep the skin soft

Preparing for the manicure

Outcome 1: Maintain safe and effective methods of working when improving manicure services

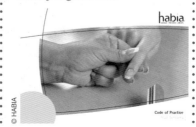
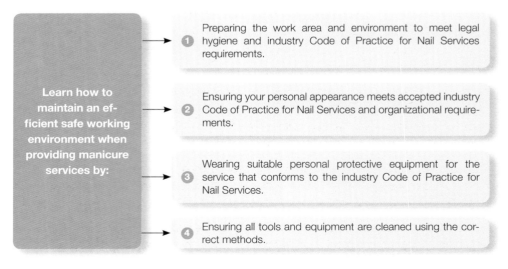

Learn how to maintain an efficient safe working environment when providing manicure services by:

1. Preparing the work area and environment to meet legal hygiene and industry Code of Practice for Nail Services requirements.

2. Ensuring your personal appearance meets accepted industry Code of Practice for Nail Services and organizational requirements.

3. Wearing suitable personal protective equipment for the service that conforms to the industry Code of Practice for Nail Services.

4. Ensuring all tools and equipment are cleaned using the correct methods.

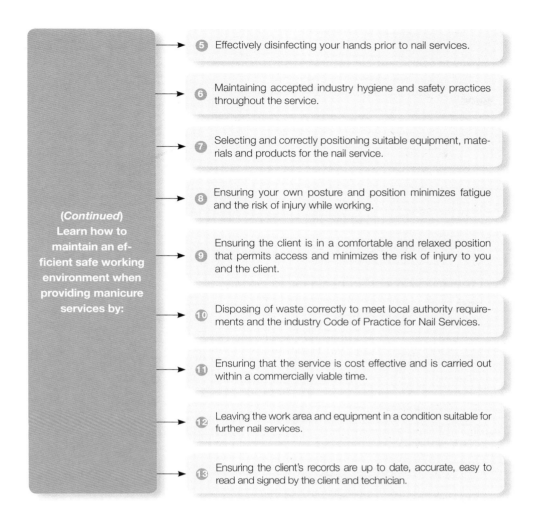

(Continued) Learn how to maintain an efficient safe working environment when providing manicure services by:

⑤ Effectively disinfecting your hands prior to nail services.

⑥ Maintaining accepted industry hygiene and safety practices throughout the service.

⑦ Selecting and correctly positioning suitable equipment, materials and products for the nail service.

⑧ Ensuring your own posture and position minimizes fatigue and the risk of injury while working.

⑨ Ensuring the client is in a comfortable and relaxed position that permits access and minimizes the risk of injury to you and the client.

⑩ Disposing of waste correctly to meet local authority requirements and the industry Code of Practice for Nail Services.

⑪ Ensuring that the service is cost effective and is carried out within a commercially viable time.

⑫ Leaving the work area and equipment in a condition suitable for further nail services.

⑬ Ensuring the client's records are up to date, accurate, easy to read and signed by the client and technician.

Preparing the work area Ensure that all manicure tools and equipment are clean, sterilized and disinfected, as appropriate, and that all necessary materials are neatly organized on the work station which is suitably positioned.

Repetitive Strain Injury (RSI) is experienced when movements are highly repeated. This results in injury to the skeleton and muscle of the upper body and limbs. A height adjustable chair with back support should be used ensuring that this is the correct height for the work station. Foot rests should be used for therapists who cannot place their feet flat on the floor. All equipment, products and tools should be easily accessible between knee and shoulder height. Regular breaks should be taken to avoid fatigue.

Keeping the working area tidy promotes an organized and professional image, and prevents time being wasted as you try to find materials. It should always be left in a condition suitable for further nail services.

Place a towel over the work surface, then fold another towel into a pad and place it in the middle of the work surface. The pad helps to support the client's forearm during service. Place the third towel over the pad, with more of the towel on the manicurist's side – this is used to dry the client's hands during service.

A tissue or disposable manicure mat may then be placed on top of the towels, to catch any nail clippings or filings. This can be thrown away later, avoiding irritation to the client from filings. All towels should be replaced with freshly laundered ones following each service.

Before beginning the manicure, check that you have the necessary equipment and materials to hand and that they meet legal hygiene and industry requirements for nail services.

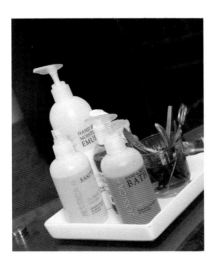

Manicure equipment

EQUIPMENT AND MATERIALS LIST

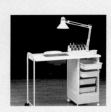

Manicure table or trolley
On which to place everything

Emery boards
Used to shorten and shape the nail free edge

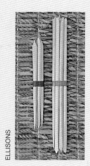

Orange sticks
Tipped at either end with cotton wool. (Orange sticks should be disposed of after each client, as they cannot be effectively sterilized.) Used to remove products from containers, to ease the cuticle back and clean under the free edge

Hand cream or oil
Use hand cream or oil to massage the skin of the hand and arm

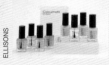

Base coat
To prevent nail staining and provide an even surface to improve nail polish application and adherence

Coloured nail polish
A selection for the client to choose from

Top coat
To provide shine and strength to the nail polish. Reduces peeling and chipping and increases durability of the nail polish

Nail polish remover
To remove nail polish and excess nail care and skincare preparations

Hoof stick
To gently push back the softened cuticles

Cuticle nippers
To remove excess cuticle and dead, torn skin surrounding the nail

Nail scissors
To shorten nail length

Disinfectant solution
To store small stainless steel sterilized tools

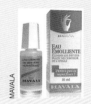

Cuticle remover
Used to soften the skin cells and the cuticle before service so excess skin can be easily removed

Cuticle oil or cream
Used to condition the skin of the cuticle; especially beneficial for dry nails and cuticles

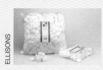

Cotton wool
To remove nail polish and excess nail preparations

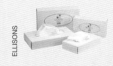

Tissues
To protect client's clothing in the area, etc.

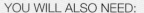

YOU WILL ALSO NEED:

Medium-sized towels (3) To dry the skin, nails, etc.

Small bowls (3) Lined with tissues for storage etc.

A finger bowl To place the hand into a nail cleansing agent to soak, soften and cleanse the skin

Cuticle knife To remove excess eponychium and periony-chium from the nail plate

Buffers Buffers are used to improve nail shine, stimulate blood circulation and remove surface ridges when used with a buffing paste

Buffing paste Used to reduce the appearance of ridges on the nail plate surface

Disinfecting solution For all surfaces

Skin disinfectant To cleanse and disinfect the client's skin. Specialized sprays and gels are available for this purpose

Four-sided buffer To impart shine and improve nail appearance

Client record card To record the client's personal details, products used and details of the service

Nail polish drier An aerosol or oil preparation applied to speed up the drying process of nail polish

Hand and nail service Equipment including:
paraffin wax
Hand masks
thermal mitts
Exfoliators and warm oil

Waste container This should be a lined metal bin with a lid to contain vapours from solvents

Products used in both manicure and pedicure services

Product	Ingredients	Uses
Nail polish remover	Acetone or ethyl acetate – solvent. Perfume. Colour. Oil – emollient to reduce drying effect of solvent.	To remove nail polish. To remove grease from the nail plate prior to applying polish.
Hand/foot lotion/oil	Vegetable oils (e.g. almond oil). Perfume. Emulsifying agents (e.g. beeswax or gum tragacanth). Emollients (e.g. glycerine or lanolin). Preservatives.	To soften the skin and cuticles. To provide slip during hand/foot massage.
Nail bleach	Citric acid or hydrogen peroxide – bleaches the nail. Glycerine – emollient. Water.	To whiten stained nails and the surrounding skin.
Nail polish	Formaldehyde – film-forming plastic resin, improving adherence and flexibility. Solvent – creates a suitable consistency when applying, and to help polish dry at a controlled rate. Colour pigments – create nail polish colour. Resin – improves adhesion of polish to nail plate and flexibility.	To colour nail plates. To provide some protection.

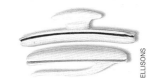

Buffers

ELLISONS

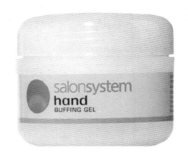

Buffing paste

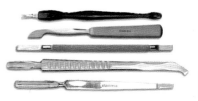

Cuticle knives

ELLISONS

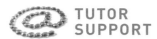

TUTOR SUPPORT

Activity 3: benefits of a manicure handout

Product	Ingredients	Use
	Toluene – solvent which dissolves ingredients in nail polish. Nitrocellulose – film-forming plastic which holds colour. Plasticizers – to provide flexibility after the polish has dried, reducing chipping. Pearlized particles – create a pearlized effect.	
Cuticle cream	Emollients (e.g. lanolin or glycerine). Perfume. Colour.	To soften the cuticles.
Cuticle oil	Emollient oils such as lanolin and organic oils such as almond oil.	To condition the nail and surrounding skin.
Nail strengthener	Formaldehyde – film-forming plastic resin.	To strengthen weak nails.
Cuticle remover	Potassium hydroxide – a caustic alkali. Glycerine – a humectant added to reduce the drying effect on the nail plate.	To soften the skin of the cuticles.
Buffing paste	Perfume. Colour. Abrasive particles (e.g. pumice, talc or silica) to remove surface cells.	To provide a shine to the nail plate (used with a buffer).
Nail polish drier	Mineral oil – assists drying. Oleric acid or silicone – lubricant.	Increases the speed at which the polish hardens.
Nail polish solvent	Ethyl acetate – thins nail polish consistency. Toluene – solvent which dissolves nail polish ingredients.	Thins nail polish that has thickened, restoring consistency.

ALWAYS REMEMBER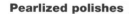

Pearlized polishes

Pearlized polishes are created by the addition of sparkling, reflective particles such as mica, a synthetic product.

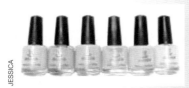

JESSICA

Pearlized polish

Sterilization and disinfection Hygiene must be maintained in a number of ways:

- ensure that tools and equipment are clean and sterile before use
- dispense products from containers, e.g. creams and lotions, with a disposable spatula
- disinfect work surfaces after every client
- use disposable products wherever possible
- always follow hygienic working practices
- maintain a high standard of personal hygiene

Manicure and pedicure tools and equipment can be disposable or can be sterilized or disinfected by the following methods:

Tool/Equipment	Method	Term used
Cuticle knife	Autoclave	Sterilization
Cuticle nippers	Autoclave	Sterilization
Orange stick	Throw away after use	Disposable
Callus file	Autoclave	Sterilization
	Chemical (e.g. disinfectant)	Disinfection
Bowl	Chemical (e.g. disinfectant)	Disinfection
Emery board	Throw away after use	Disposable
Buffer	Wipe handle with surgical spirit or disinfectant	Disinfection
	Wash buffing cloth in hot (60°C) soapy water	Cleansed
Towel	Wash in hot soapy water (60°C)	Cleansed
Spatula	Throw away after use	Disposable
Nail clippers	Autoclave	Sterilization
Scissors	Autoclave	Sterilization
Hoof stick	Immerse in chemical (e.g. disinfectant)	Disinfection
Trolley	Wipe with chemical (e.g. disinfectant)	Disinfection

Metal tools when ready for use should be placed in a disinfecting solution. After the manicure service they must be replaced and re-sterilized.

Outcome 2: Consult, plan and prepare for manicure service

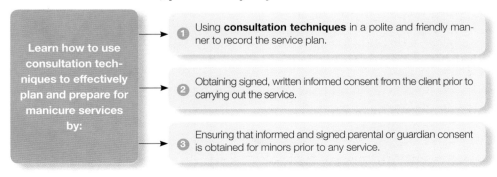

Learn how to use consultation techniques to effectively plan and prepare for manicure services by:

1. Using **consultation techniques** in a polite and friendly manner to record the service plan.

2. Obtaining signed, written informed consent from the client prior to carrying out the service.

3. Ensuring that informed and signed parental or guardian consent is obtained for minors prior to any service.

ALWAYS REMEMBER

UV stabilizers

UV stabilizers are additives which prevent the polish changing colour on exposure to UV sunlight.

HEALTH & SAFETY

Disinfecting sprays

You can buy disinfecting sprays to disinfect the surface of the tools that the chemical agent comes into contact with. Any debris must first be removed using a detergent before the use of a disinfecting spray. Use in a well-ventilated area and avoid contact with flame and excessive heat.

HEALTH & SAFETY

Any metal to be placed in the autoclave should be of a high-quality stainless steel, to prevent rusting. Always dry immediately to prevent damage.

> No one knows everything or can be everything, so teamwork is really important. We learn from those around us.
>
> **Jacqui Jefford**

ACTIVITY

Making appointments

What questions could the receptionist ask when booking a client for manicure in order to make the appointments run more efficiently? Write down your answers.

ACTIVITY

Stretching exercises to avoid RSI

Perform regular, daily stretching exercise to reduce tension and improve flexibility for the fingers, wrists, hands, arms, shoulder, neck and upper back.

Design simple stretching exercises for each of the above body area.

> " Never stop learning. Education is the key to knowledge. Knowledge is power.
>
> **Jacqui Jefford**

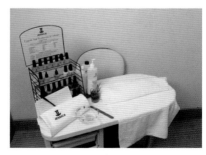

Work area

> " An employer will always want someone who shows passion and initiative in all they do.
>
> **Jacqui Jefford**

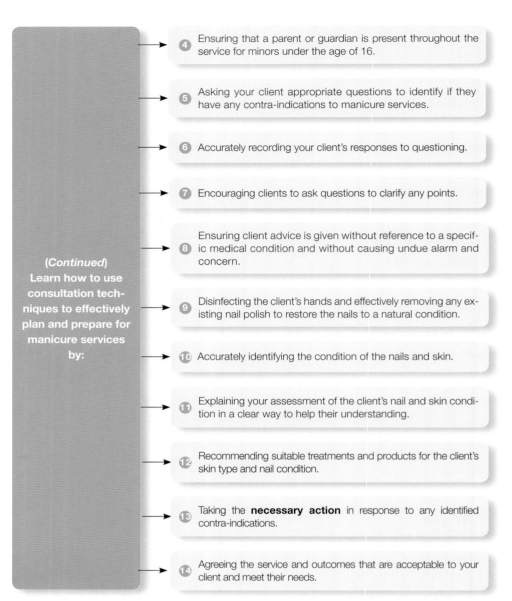

(Continued) Learn how to use consultation techniques to effectively plan and prepare for manicure services by:

4. Ensuring that a parent or guardian is present throughout the service for minors under the age of 16.

5. Asking your client appropriate questions to identify if they have any contra-indications to manicure services.

6. Accurately recording your client's responses to questioning.

7. Encouraging clients to ask questions to clarify any points.

8. Ensuring client advice is given without reference to a specific medical condition and without causing undue alarm and concern.

9. Disinfecting the client's hands and effectively removing any existing nail polish to restore the nails to a natural condition.

10. Accurately identifying the condition of the nails and skin.

11. Explaining your assessment of the client's nail and skin condition in a clear way to help their understanding.

12. Recommending suitable treatments and products for the client's skin type and nail condition.

13. Taking the **necessary action** in response to any identified contra-indications.

14. Agreeing the service and outcomes that are acceptable to your client and meet their needs.

Reception

When a client makes an appointment for a manicure service, the receptionist should ask a few simple questions that will help guide how long the service will take.

- Do they require nail polish? With drying time, this part of the service can last up to 20 minutes, so the client should be made aware of this.

- Are any nails damaged or in need of repair? Again extra time will need to be allowed for this work.

- Do they require any **hand and nail treatments** in addition to the manicure, such as exfoliation or paraffin wax? Allow extra time accordingly.

- Has the client had artificial nails applied previously which require removal? Allow approximately 20 minutes for this process.

Allow 45 minutes for a manicure.

Allow up to one hour for a specialist hand-nail service.

All staff, especially the staff communicating with clients at reception should be familiar with the different pricing structures for the range of manicure services and products available for retail.

The receptionist should also check the age of the client. If the client is a minor under the age of 16, it is necessary to obtain parent/guardian permission for treatment. The parent/guardian will also have to be present when the treatment is received.

Consultation

Before carrying out a manicure service, it is necessary to assess the condition of the client's skin, nails and cuticles. This is done in order that the most appropriate hand and nail treatments and products may be chosen. Also, by correctly assessing and analyzing the client's hand condition and writing this on their record card, you will be able to see over a period of time how the condition is progressing.

Assess the condition of the following:

- **The cuticles** Are they dry, tight or cracked, or are they soft and pliable?

- **The nails** Are they strong or weak, brittle or flaking? Are they discoloured or stained? What shape are they – square, round, oval? Are they long or short? Are they bitten?

- **The skin** Is the skin dry, rough or chapped, or is it soft and smooth? Is the colour even?

While assessing the client's hands for service, you should also be looking for any *contra-indications* to service.

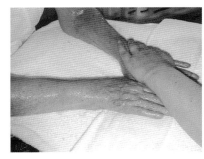

Specialist hand and nail treatment: warm oil application

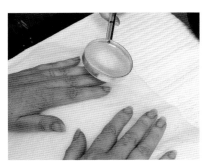

Assessing the nails and skin

ALWAYS REMEMBER

Artificial nails

If the client has had several new sets of artificial nails applied this will damage the natural nail.

The nail plate may be thin, ridges may appear upon the nail plate and the removal technique, using acetone, will cause dehydration. All of these effects will need to be discussed with your client at consultation and an appropriate service plan discussed.

Skin and nail disorders of the hands

When a client attends for a manicure service, as part of the consultation and assessment of the client's needs, the therapist should always look at the client's skin and nails to check that no infection or disease is present which might contra-indicate service. These include bacterial, fungal, viral and parasitic infections. These are described in more detail in Chapter 3, where **contra-indications** are illustrated and discussed.

If the client is wearing nail polish, this must be removed before checking.

Contra-indications The following disorders may contra-indicate or restrict manicure service. If you suspect the client has any disorder from the chart below, do not attempt a diagnosis, but refer the client tactfully to their GP without causing unnecessary concern.

ACTIVITY

Assessing the hands

Look closely at your own hands. Assess their condition and make notes about everything you see.

Then assess the hands of a colleague. How do they differ from your own?

Complete a record card and record the condition of the nails and surrounding skin. Design a suitable service plan for your client to meet their needs.

ALWAYS REMEMBER

Accurately record your client's answers to necessary questions to be asked at consultations on the record card.

Disorder	Description
Broken bones 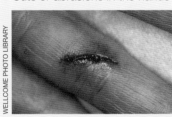	Injury resulting in a broken bone can often not be seen; confirm at consultation that there is no known injury in the service area.
Cuts or abrasions in the hands 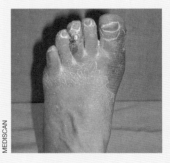	Broken skin. Any cut or abrasion could lead to secondary infection and the area should not be treated until healed.
Diabetes	If a client has diabetic foot or hand condition, they are vulnerable to infection as they have slow skin healing. This could be problematic if the skin was accidentally broken during a pedicure service. Permission must be obtained from the client's GP before service can be received.
Paronychia 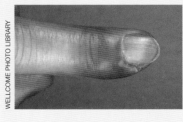	Infectious bacterial infection. Swelling, redness and pus appears in the cuticle area of the skin of the nail wall.
Scabies or itch mites 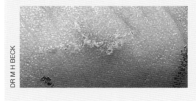	An infestation of the skin by an animal parasite. The animal parasite burrows beneath the skin and invades the hair follicles. Papules and wavy greyish lines appear, where dirt enters the burrows. Secondary bacterial infection may occur as a result of scratching.

WELLCOME PHOTO LIBRARY

WELLCOME PHOTO LIBRARY

MEDISCAN

WELLCOME PHOTO LIBRARY

DR M H BECK

Severe **eczema of the nail**

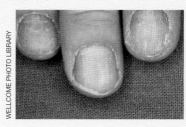

WELLCOME PHOTO LIBRARY

Inflammation of the skin occurs. Differing changes to the nail may occur, including the appearance of ridges, pitting, **onycholysis** or nail thickening (hypertrophy).

Severe eczema of the skin

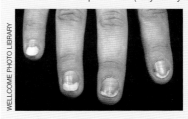

DR A L WRIGHT

Inflammation of the skin caused by contact internally or externally, with an irritant.
Reddening of the skin occurs with swelling and blistering; the blisters leak tissue fluid, which later hardens and forms scabs.

Severe nail separation (onycholysis)

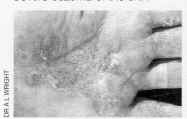

WELLCOME PHOTO LIBRARY

Lifting of the nail plate from the nail bed, may be caused by trauma or infection to the nail or surrounding area; where separation has occurred this appears as a greyish-white area on the nail as the pink undertone of the nail bed does not show.

Severe **psoriasis of the nail**

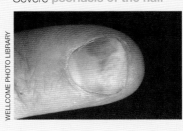

WELLCOME PHOTO LIBRARY

An inflammatory condition where there is an increased production of cells in the upper part of the skin.
Pitting occurs on the surface of the nail plate.
Separation (onycholysis) may also occur.

Severe psoriasis of the skin

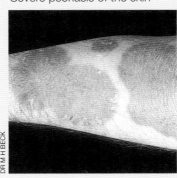

DR M H BECK

Red patches of skin appear covered in waxy, silvery scales.
Bleeding will occur if the area is scratched and the scales are removed.
The cause is unknown.

Tinea corporis (body ringworm)

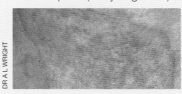

DR A L WRIGHT

Fungal infection of the skin, which may occur on the limbs. Small scaly red patches, which spread outwards and then heal from the centre, leaving a ring.

Tinea unguium

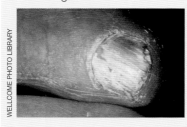

WELLCOME PHOTO LIBRARY

Fungal infection of the fingernails. The nail plate is yellowish-grey.
Eventually the nail plate becomes brittle and separates from the nail bed.

Verrucae or warts

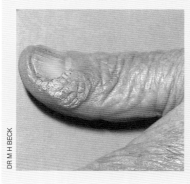

DR M H BECK

A viral infection.
Small epidermal skin growths. Warts may be raised or flat depending upon their position. Warts vary in size, shape, texture and colour. Usually they have a rough surface and are raised. Plane wart – found on the surface of the hand.

Below is a list of common disorders that may be seen on the hands. Not all of these contra-indicate service.

Disorder	Cause	Appearance	Salon service	Homecare advice
Blue nail	Poor blood circulation in the area. Heart disease.	The nail bed does not appear a healthy pink colour but has a blue tinge.	Permission to treat to be received from the client's GP. Regular manicure, including hand service to improve circulation.	General manicure advice. Hand exercises and massage to improve circulation.
Bruised nails	Trauma to the nail (e.g. trapping it in a door); severe damage can result in loss of the nail.	Part of the nail plate may appear blue or black where bleeding has occurred on the new bed.	Although this disorder does not contra-indicate service, it is advisable to postpone manicuring the nails until the condition is no longer painful. Nail polish may be used to disguise the damaged nail.	Seek medical advice if swelling is present or if pain persists.

WELLCOME PHOTO LIBRARY

DR A L WRIGHT

Eggshell nail WELLCOME PHOTO LIBRARY	Illness.	Thin, fragile, white nail plate, curving under at the free edge.	Permission for treatment to be received from the client's GP. Regular manicure.	General manicure advice. Strengthening base coats.
Hangnail 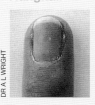 DR A L WRIGHT	Biting the skin around the nails. Cracking of a dry skin or cuticle condition.	Epidermis around the nail plate cracks and a small piece of skin protrudes between the nail plate and the nail wall, sometimes accompanied by redness and swelling: this condition can become extremely painful.	Warm-oil services to soften the skin and cuticles. Remove the protrusion of dead skin with cuticle nippers: do not cut into live tissue.	Regular use of a rich hand cream. Wear rubber gloves when cleaning and washing up. Wear warm gloves in cold weather. Ensure a balanced diet.
Leuconychia DR A L WRIGHT	Trauma to the nail plate or matrix, due to pressure or hitting the nail with a hard object. Air pockets form between the nail plate and nail bed	White spots or marks on the nail plate: will grow out with the nail.	General manicure service. Coloured nail polish application will disguise their appearance until the damaged area disappears as it grows towards the free edge.	Be careful with the hands. Wear protective gloves when doing housework or gardening. Do not use the nails as tools!
Longitudinal ridges in the nail plate (corrugated nails)  DR A L WRIGHT	Illness. Damage to the matrix. Age, associated with the ageing process.	Grooves in the nail plate running along the length of the nail from the cuticle to the free edge: may affect one or all nails.	Abrasive buffing paste applied to smooth out the ridges. Use of a ridge-filling base coat prior to nail polish application.	General manicure advice. Use of a ridge-filling base coat polish. Ensure a balanced diet.
Minor nail separation (onycholysis)  WELLCOME PHOTO LIBRARY	Lifting of the nail plate from its bed. Can accompany a medical condition such as eczema or psoriasis or a fungal infection in the area.	Where separation has occurred this appears as a greyish-white area as the pink undertone of the nail bed does not show through the nail plate.	It is advisable to postpone manicuring for this nail until the condition is corrected. Refer the client to their GP to confirm cause.	Be careful to avoid infection of the nail bed. Protect the nail with a protective dressing.

Disorder	Cause	Appearance	Salon service	Homecare advice
Onychophagy DR A L WRIGHT	Excessive nail-biting.	Very little nail plate; bulbous skin at the fingertip; nail walls often red and swollen, due to biting of the skin surrounding the nails.	Regular weekly manicures. Cuticle service to maximize the visible nail-plate area. Nail conditioning services to prevent dry cuticles and hangnails.	Bitter-tasting preparations painted onto the nail plate. Wear gloves to avoid biting in bed.
Onychorrhexis DR A L WRIGHT	Using harsh detergents without wearing gloves. Poor diet. Not wearing gloves in cold weather.	Split, flaking nails.	Warm-oil manicures on a weekly basis.	Regular use of a rich hand cream. Always wear rubber gloves when cleaning or washing up. Always wear warm gloves in cold weather. Ensure a balanced diet. Prescribe nail base coat to protect split, flaking nails.
Pitting WELLCOME PHOTO LIBRARY	Eczema. Psoriasis.	Pitting resembling small irregular pin pricks appear on the nail plate.	Refer the client to their GP for permission to treat if required. Regular manicure with gentle buffing.	General manicure advice. Ridge-filling base coat polish.
Pterygium DR A L WRIGHT	Neglect of the nails.	Overgrown thickened cuticles, often tightly adhered to the nail plate: if left untreated, this may lead to splitting of the cuticle and subsequent infection.	Warm-oil or paraffin wax services weekly. Once softened, remove excess cuticle with cuticle nippers. If overgrown cuticle is excessive, refer client to their GP.	Regular use of a rich cuticle cream. Wear rubber gloves when cleaning and washing up. Gently push back the cuticles with a soft towel when softened, e.g. after bathing.
Transverse furrows in the nail plate (Beau's lines) DR A L WRIGHT	Temporary arrested development of the nail in the matrix, due to illness or trauma of the nail.	Groove in the nail plate, often on all nails simultaneously, running from side to side: this will grow out with the nail.	Regular manicure until normal cells replace the damaged cells.	General manicure advice. Ensure a balanced diet.

Contra-actions

Certain cosmetic ingredients are known to cause allergic reactions in some people. This is known as a **contra-action**, this may occur during or following treatment.

The client – or the manicurist – may at some time develop an allergy to a manicure product that has been successfully used previously. This could be for a number of reasons, including new medication being taken or illness.

The symptoms of an allergic reaction could be:

- redness of the skin (erythema)
- itching
- swelling
- raised blisters

The symptoms do not necessarily appear on the hands. In the case of nail polish allergy, the symptoms often show up on the face, which the hands are continually touching.

In the case of an allergic reaction:

- Remove the offending product immediately, using water or, in the case of polish, nail polish solvent.
- Apply a cool compress and soothing agent to the skin to reduce redness and irritation.
- If symptoms persist, seek medical advice.

Always record any allergies on the client's record card, so that the offending product may be avoided in future.

Further contra-actions may occur as a result of poor manicure techniques, e.g. failing to check the temperature of **paraffin wax** before application, which if too hot could cause skin sensitivity, even burning!

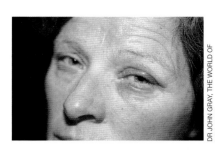

DR. JOHN GRAY, THE WORLD OF SKIN CARE

Client with an allergic reaction that has affected the eyes causing redness and swelling

HEALTH & SAFETY

You are not qualified to diagnose, this is the job of the GP.

Therefore if you are unsure about any nail or skin condition present refer the client to their GP.

Service plan

After analyzing the client's nails and adjacent skin, a **service plan** should be considered and agreed with the client. In order to correct skin and nail problems, the client should attend the salon weekly. They should also be advised of the appropriate service preparations to use at home, so as to support the salon service. Specialist nail services to use will depend upon the nail and skin condition; they include:

- **Nail strengthener** This is used on brittle, damaged nails, to strengthen, condition and protect them against breaking, splitting or peeling.
- **Ridge filler** This is used on nails with ridges to provide a more even surface, creating a bond between the **base coat** and polish, allowing a smoother application of polish.
- **Nail oil** This contains ingredients to rehydrate the nail and soften the cuticle.
- **Cuticle creams** These nourish the skin and restore the condition of the cuticle.
- **Creams and lotions** These nourish the skin preventing the skin becoming dry.
- **Specialist hand and nail services** These may also be recommended within the manicure service to improve the appearance of the skin texture, nail and cuticle condition and provide a number of physiological benefits. These may be offered each time the client has a manicure service to maintain the condition of the nails and hands.

Provide the opportunity for your client to ask any questions relating to the manicure service or treatment plan.

The record card should be signed and dated by the manicurist following the consultation to confirm the suitability and consent with the agreed manicure treatment.

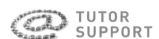

TUTOR SUPPORT

Activity 4: promoting luxury treatments

A sample client record card

Date	Beauty therapist name	
Client name	Date of birth (identifying client age group)	
Home address	Postcode	
Email address	Landline phone number	Mobile phone number
Name of doctor	Doctor's address and phone number	
Related medical history (Conditions that may restrict or prohibit service application.)		
Are you taking any medication? (This may affect the sensitivity of the skin to the service.)		

CONTRA-INDICATIONS REQUIRING MEDICAL REFERRAL
(Preventing manicure service application.)

☐ bacterial infections (e.g. **paronychia**)
☐ viral infections (e.g. plane warts)
☐ fungal infections (e.g. **tinea unguium**)
☐ parasitic infections, (e.g. scabies)
☐ severe nail separation
☐ severe eczema and psoriasis
☐ severe bruising

EQUIPMENT AND MATERIALS

☐ nail and skin service tools
☐ abrasives (e.g. buffing cream)
☐ cuticle softeners
☐ nail and skin products
☐ nail conditioners (e.g. cuticle cream)
☐ skin conditioners (e.g. hand cream)
☐ nail, skin and cuticle corrective services (e.g. paraffin wax)
☐ consumables

HAND AND NAIL SERVICES

☐ warm oil hand mask
☐ paraffin wax
☐ **thermal mitts**
☐ exfoliators

NAIL FINISH

☐ light colour
☐ dark colour
☐ French manicure
☐ buffing

CONTRA-INDICATIONS WHICH RESTRICT SERVICE
(Service may require adaptation.)

☐ minor nail separation
☐ minor eczema and psoriasis
☐ recent scar tissue
☐ severely bitten nails
☐ severely damaged nails
☐ broken bones
☐ minor cuts or abrasions
☐ minor bruising or swelling

COURSE OF SERVICE

	Date	Date	Date
☐ improvement of skin condition products used	___	___	___
☐ improvement of nail condition products used	___	___	___

NAIL, CUTICLE AND SKIN CONDITION

Nails

☐ healthy   ☐ brittle
☐ dry   ☐ weak
☐ ridged

Cuticle

☐ healthy   ☐ dry   ☐ split   ☐ overgrown

Skin

☐ healthy   ☐ dry   ☐ hard

MASSAGE MEDIUMS

☐ creams   ☐ oils

Beauty therapist signature (for reference)
Client signature (confirmation of details)

A sample client record card (continued)

SERVICE ADVICE

Manicure – *allow 45 minutes*

Specialized hand/nail service – *allow up to 60 minutes*

SERVICE PLAN

Record relevant details of your service and advice provided for future reference.

Ensure the client's records are up to date, accurate and fully completed following service. Non-compliance may invalidate insurance.

DURING

Discuss:

- details that may influence the client's nail condition, such as their occupation
- the products the client is currently using to care for the skin of the hands and nails, and the regularity of their use;
- the client's satisfaction with these products
- relevant manicure procedures (e.g. how to file the nails correctly)

Note:

- any adverse reaction, if any occur

AFTER

Record:

- results of service
- any modification to service application that has occurred
- what products have been used in the manicure service
- what hand and nail services have been used
- the effectiveness of service
- any samples provided (review their success at the next appointment)

Advise on:

- product application in order to gain maximum benefit from product use
- specialized products following manicure service for homecare use
- general hand/nail care and maintenance
- the recommended time intervals between services
- the importance of a course of service to improve nail/skin conditions

RETAIL OPPORTUNITIES

Advise on:

- progression of the service plan for future appointments
- products that would be suitable for the client to use at home to care for the skin of the hands and nails
- recommendations for further services
- further products or services that the client may or may not have received before

Note:

- any purchase made by the client

EVALUATION

Record:

- comments on the client's satisfaction with the service
- if poor results are achieved, the reasons why
- how you may alter the service plan to achieve the required service results in the future, if applicable

HEALTH AND SAFETY

Advise on:

- appropriate necessary action to be taken in the event of an unwanted skin or nail reaction

LEVEL 2 BEAUTY THERAPY

HEALTH & SAFETY

Contact dermatitis

Contact dermatitis is a skin problem caused by intolerance of the skin to a particular substance or a group of substances. On exposure to the substance the skin quickly becomes irritated and an allergic reaction occurs. This may occur when a manicurist's skin is exposed to dust and chemicals on a regular basis. Follow all HSE guidelines to reduce the risk of developing this skin disorder which could result in the need for a career change!

Always follow manufacturers' guidelines on the use of products.

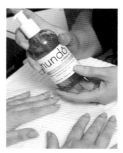

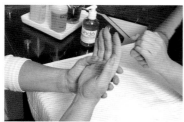

Cleaning the hands

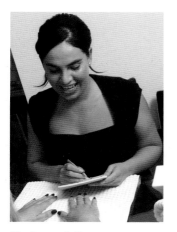

Client consultation

It is important that accurate records are kept and stored in compliance with the Data Protection Act for future reference.

Preparing the client

Ensure that the client is warm and comfortable when preparing them for a manicure.

Lighting must be good to avoid eyestrain and to allow the service to be performed competently. Avoid positioning the work station in direct sunlight however to prevent discomfort to client and manicurist.

A lightweight gown may be offered to the client to cover their clothing. This will prevent damage to their clothes from accidental spillage of products during service. Ask them to remove any jewellery from the area to be treated, to prevent the jewellery being damaged by creams and to avoid obstructing massage movements. Place the jewellery where the client can see it. Alternatively, ask the client to take possession of it for safe-keeping – follow your salon security policy. Ensure that the client is seated at the correct height, and close enough to the manicurist to avoid having to lean forward.

When the client is comfortably seated, clean your hands using an approved hand cleaning technique – preferably in view of the client, who will then observe hygienic procedures being carried out. This will assure them that they are receiving a professional service. The client should also wash their hands before the service commences. The client's skin can also be cleaned with a disinfectant gel of spray.

Consult the client's record card, and begin the service.

TOP TIP

Examples of manicure service

Following your consultation, you may need to adjust your manicure to meet your client's need by modifying:

- the depth of massage pressure when applying hand and arm massage and choice of massage movements applied; an elderly client's skin is thinner and has less elasticity
- the choice of massage medium when client has excessively hairy arms
- the choice of nail polish product to improve the nail condition and appearance

BEST PRACTICE

Removal of artificial nails

These are removed using a solvent containing acetone that softens the product, allowing removal from the natural nail. However, it is particularly drying to the natural nail which will later require rehydrating.

Procedure

- Remove any nail polish, trim any excess length using clippers.
- Soak the nails in acetone for approximately 20 minutes, until the product has thoroughly softened.
- Remove the softened product with an orange stick.
- Wash the hands and nails thoroughly to remove acetone.
- Continue with manicure service.

Carrying out manicure services

Outcome 3: Carry out manicure services

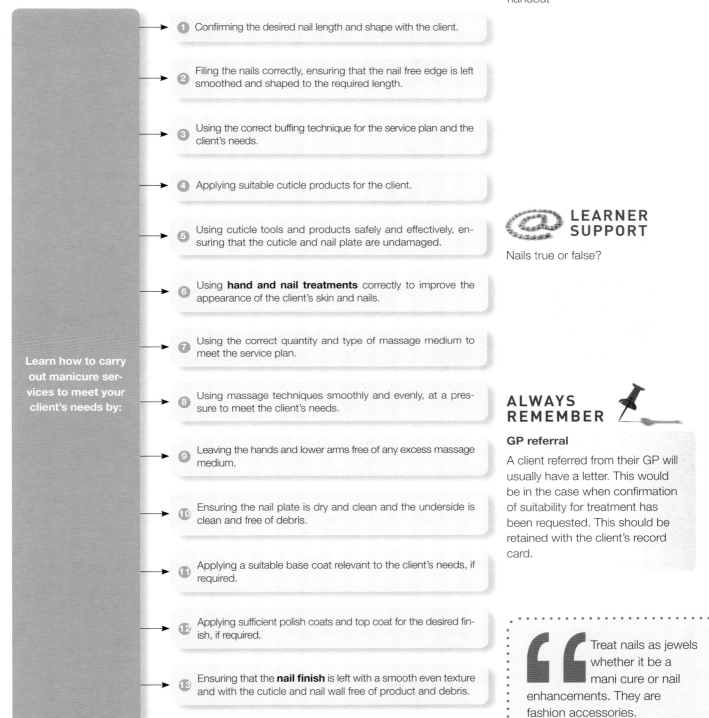

Learn how to carry out manicure services to meet your client's needs by:

1. Confirming the desired nail length and shape with the client.

2. Filing the nails correctly, ensuring that the nail free edge is left smoothed and shaped to the required length.

3. Using the correct buffing technique for the service plan and the client's needs.

4. Applying suitable cuticle products for the client.

5. Using cuticle tools and products safely and effectively, ensuring that the cuticle and nail plate are undamaged.

6. Using **hand and nail treatments** correctly to improve the appearance of the client's skin and nails.

7. Using the correct quantity and type of massage medium to meet the service plan.

8. Using massage techniques smoothly and evenly, at a pressure to meet the client's needs.

9. Leaving the hands and lower arms free of any excess massage medium.

10. Ensuring the nail plate is dry and clean and the underside is clean and free of debris.

11. Applying a suitable base coat relevant to the client's needs, if required.

12. Applying sufficient polish coats and top coat for the desired finish, if required.

13. Ensuring that the **nail finish** is left with a smooth even texture and with the cuticle and nail wall free of product and debris.

14. Ensuring that the finished result is to the client's satisfaction and meets the agreed service plan.

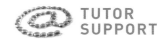

TUTOR SUPPORT

Activity 5: hand and nail treatments handout

LEARNER SUPPORT

Nails true or false?

ALWAYS REMEMBER

GP referral

A client referred from their GP will usually have a letter. This would be in the case when confirmation of suitability for treatment has been requested. This should be retained with the client's record card.

> Treat nails as jewels whether it be a mani cure or nail enhancements. They are fashion accessories.
>
> **Jacqui Jefford**

Step-by-step: Manicure procedure

This procedure briefly shows the stages in the manicure. Each step is discussed in detail later in the chapter. The procedure may start with the right or left hand.

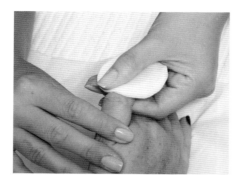

1 Remove any existing nail polish with nail polish remover, using fresh cotton wool for each hand.

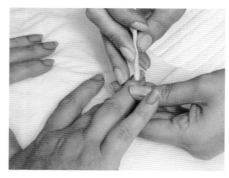

2 Use a cotton wool tipped orange stick to apply nail polish remover around the cuticle area as necessary to remove any excess nail polish. Avoid unnecessary contact with the skin to avoid drying out.

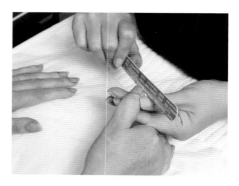

3 File the nails of the right hand to the desired length and shape.

Ensure the free edge is smooth by performing upward strokes with the file often referred to as **bevelling**.

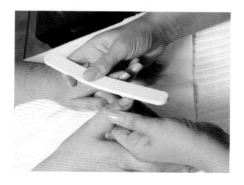

4 Buff the nail plate of the right hand.

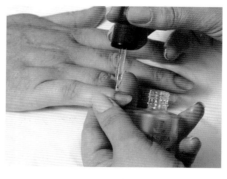

5 Apply cuticle cream or oil to the cuticle area.

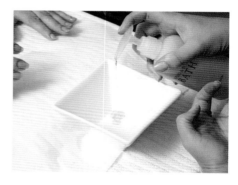

6 Place a small amount of liquid soap formulated for use in manicures and add warm water when ready to use.

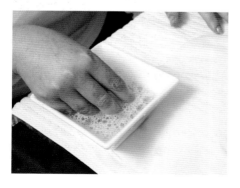

7 Place the right hand in the manicure bowl containing warm water and liquid soap. Repeat steps **3**, **4**, **5** and **7** for the left hand.

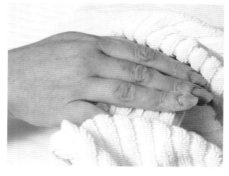

8 Remove the right hand from the manicure bowl and dry with a towel. Place the left hand into the manicure bowl.

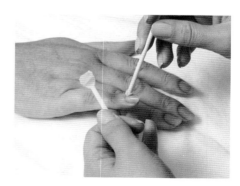

9 Apply cuticle remover to the right hand.

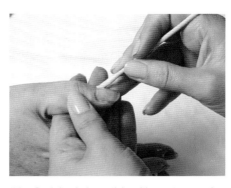

10 Push back the cuticle with a cotton wool-tipped orange stick or **hoof stick**.

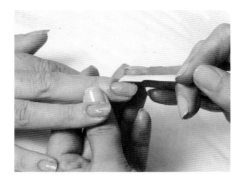

11 Remove excess cuticle with nippers.

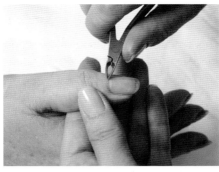

12 Remove excess eponychium with a cuticle knife.

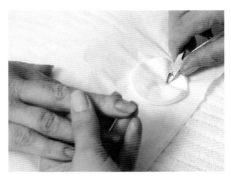

13 Collect excess skin tissue on a clean piece of cotton wool and dispose of it immediately following completion of this stage of the service.

Wipe the nails with damp cotton wool to remove excess cuticle remover.

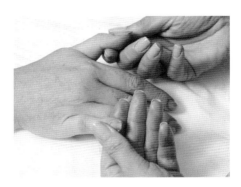

14 Apply cuticle oil and massage it in with your thumbs. Repeat steps **9–13** for the left hand. Apply massage routine to both hands and forearms.

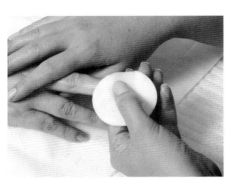

15 Remove grease from the nail plate with a cotton wool pad soaked in nail polish remover.

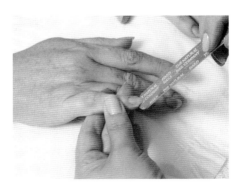

16 Refile the nails as necessary to ensure they are smooth and even.

17 The client may find it convenient to pay for her service at this stage, to avoid smudging her polish later. Also, if jewellery has been removed ask her to replace it to avoid damage to the polish after application.

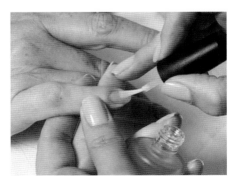

18 Confirm and apply the **nail finish**. If applying the polish, apply: base coat (once); polish (twice); and top coat (once). If a pearlized polish is used, a top coat is not required and a third coat of polish may be applied. If the client doesn't want polish, buff to a shine with buffing paste or use a four-sided buffer.

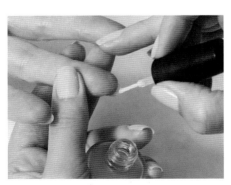

19 Base coat may be applied under the edge of the nail to create a protective seal.

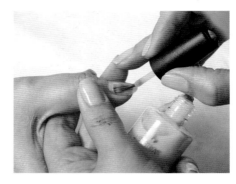

20a French manicure polish application: neutral nail polish applied in soft beige to evenly cover the surface. Apply one or two coats.

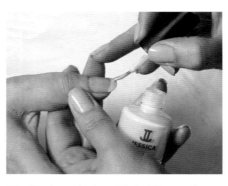

20b The free edge is painted white ensuring that the line is even. Apply one coat. If the nails are particularly stained the reverse of the free edge may be painted also.

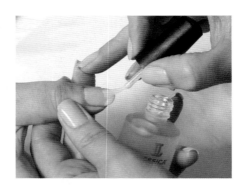

20c Apply a top coat to seal and protect the nail polish.

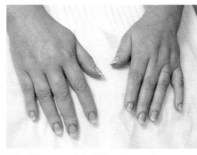

21 The completed French manicure.

BEST PRACTICE

Keep the client's jewellery in full view throughout the service, so that they don't forget it when they leave.

Filing

The part of the nail that is filed is the free edge. This should be filed to complement the nail shape and condition. When filing the natural nail, use a fine emery board. Very often emery boards have different degrees of coarseness on either side, indicated by different colours. Use the darker, rougher side to remove excess length, and the lighter, smoother side for shaping and removing rough edges. A flexible emery board is preferable to a stiff one as it generates less friction.

Always file the nails from the side to the centre, with the emery board sloping slightly under the free edge. Use swift, rhythmical strokes. Avoid a sawing action – this would generate friction and might cause the free edge to split.

Never file completely down the sides of the nail, as strength is required here to balance the free edge. Always allow about 4mm of nail growth to remain at the sides of the nail.

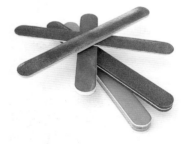

A selection of files

ALWAYS REMEMBER

Nail shapes

When filing the nails ensure that the finished appearance complements the client's nail/hand.

If the fingers are long and thin, select a rounded/square shape and keep the nail length short.

If the fingers are short and fat, the nails should be filed into an oval shape and the nail length should be longer to elongate the fingers.

BEST PRACTICE

Cost the emery board into the manicure service it is a consumable, and cannot be used again. The client can keep the emery board for personal use. Instruct the client on how the nails should be filed to avoid nail damage.

TOP TIP

Nail filing

Some nail product suppliers consider the nails best filed after specialized oil application. It is considered less damaging than when filing the natural nail when dry.

Cutting the nails Where it is necessary to reduce nail length, it is more efficient to do so by cutting the nail free edge. This is performed using nail **scissors** or sometimes nail clippers, which have been sterilized before use on each client. Support the nail wall with one hand on the free edge being cut. This minimizes client discomfort. Dispose of the trimmed nail plate hygienically in the metal lined waste bin.

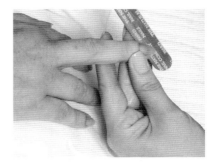

Filing the nails

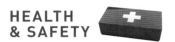

Personal Protective Equipment
When cutting the nail length you may wish to wear safety glasses which protect the eyes from flying debris reducing potential injury.

Deciding nail shape

The nail shape should complement the client's fingers and hand length and size.

Oval The ideal nail shape is oval. This is the shape that offers the most strength to the free edge.

Square A fashionable shape chosen by many clients. The client should be informed, however, that if they have severe corners on the nails they will be more likely to catch and break them.

Pointed One nail shape that should never be recommended is the pointed nail. This leaves the nail tip very weak and likely to break.

Squoval A combination of oval and square nail shape. The nail is filed to a square finish at the free edge and is then gently curved at the corners.

Round The free edge is rounded and is an ideal shape for short nails. This style is popular with male clients.

Fan The nail becomes broader as it grows towards the free edge, appearing as a fan shape. The wider sides of the nail at the free edge should be shaped to achieve an oval shape.

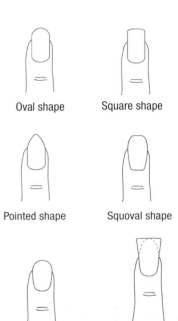

Oval shape   Square shape

Pointed shape   Squoval shape

Round shape   Fan shape

Buffing

In manicure, **buffing** is used for these reasons:

- to give the nail plate a sheen
- to stimulate the blood supply in the nail bed, increasing nourishment and encouraging strong, healthy nail growth
- to smooth any surface irregularities

A buffer should have a handle made of plastic and a replaceable convex pad covered with chamois or soft leather. **Buffing paste** is the cream used to help smooth out surface irregularities, and thereby give the nail a shine. It contains abrasive particles such as pumice, talc or kaolin.

The **four-sided buffer:** this is shaped like a thick emery board and has four types of surface, ranging from slightly abrasive to very smooth. It can be used to bring the nail to a shine without the need for buffing paste. It cannot be effectively sterilized, however, and must therefore be discarded after use on one client.

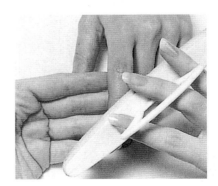

Buffing using a traditional chamois leather covered buffer

HEALTH & SAFETY

If you accidentally cut the skin causing bleeding at the cuticle area, protect you hands with disposable gloves and wipe the skin with an antiseptic wipe. Any waste is classed as clinical waste and should be disposed of in a yellow medical sealed bag in accordance with the **Environment Act 1990**.

See the *Habia Hygiene in Beauty Therapy* booklet for further guidance.

Buffing is carried out after filing to stimulate healthy nail growth and before the nails are soaked in the finger bowl. It could also be used instead of polish at the end of the manicure, or as a nail finish. It is popular when performing a male manicure service as an alternative finish to nail polish application.

If it is being used, **buffing paste** is applied by taking a small amount out of the pot with a clean orange stick and applying this to each nail plate. With the fingertip, use downward strokes from the cuticle to the free edge to spread the paste without getting it under the cuticle (which would cause irritation). With the buffer held loosely in the hand, buff in one direction only from the base of the nail to the free edge, using smooth, firm, regular strokes. Use approximately six strokes per nail. Avoid excessive strokes which would cause friction and heat to the nail plate causing drying.

Cuticle work

Cuticle work is carried out to keep the cuticle area attractive and also to prevent cuticles from adhering to the nail plate, which could lead to splitting of the cuticle as the nail grows forward, and subsequently to infection of the area.

The work is carried out after soaking the nails in warm soapy water. This step loosens dirty particles from the free edge and softens the skin in the cuticle area.

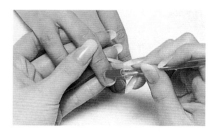

Pushing back cuticles using a hoof stick

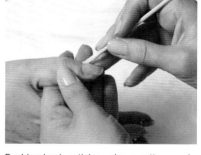

Pushing back cuticles using a cotton wool tipped orange stick

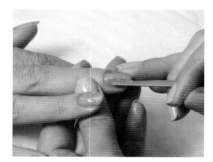

Using a cuticle knife

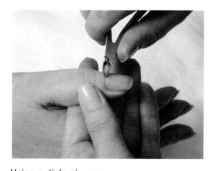

Using cuticle nippers

HEALTH & SAFETY

Hygiene
Use a fresh orange stick for each part of the manicure service, and when working on different hands, to prevent cross-infection. The orange stick is disposed of after use.

How to provide cuticle work

1   Take the fingers from the soapy water and pat them dry with a soft towel.

2   Apply cuticle remover to the cuticle and nail walls, using the applicator brush. (Cuticle remover is a slightly caustic solution that helps soften and loosen the cuticles and the eponychium from the nail plate.)

3   Gently push back the cuticle with a cotton wool-tipped orange stick or hoof stick. (The cotton wool is to avoid splinters from the wood, and also may be easily replaced if necessary.) Use a gentle, circular motion to push back the cuticle, holding the orange stick like a pen.

4   Hold the cuticle knife at 45° to the nail plate and stroke it in one direction only, gently loosening any eponychium that has adhered to the nail plate: do not scratch it backwards and forwards. The cuticle knife should have a fine-ground

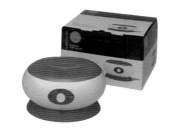

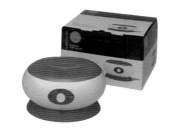

An oil wax heater

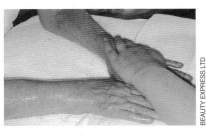

Warm oil application

flat blade which can be re-sharpened when necessary. Dampen it regularly in the manicure bowl to prevent scratches occurring on the nail plate.

5 Hold the nippers comfortably in the palm of the hand, with the thumb resting just above the blades – this gives firm control over what can be a dangerous instrument. Use the cuticle nippers to remove any loose or torn pieces of cuticle, and to trim excess dead cuticle. **Do not cut into live cuticle:** if you do, it will bleed profusely and will be very uncomfortable for the client. Not every client will require the use of cuticle nippers – use them only when needed. (Cuticle nippers should have finely ground cutting blades to give a clean cut and to avoid tearing the cuticle.)

Hand and nail services

In addition to a manicure, further hand and nail services may be included as appropriate to achieve the service plan aims.

Hand and nail services include:

Warm-oil service

- Warm-oil service involves gently heating a small amount of organic oil (such as almond oil) and soaking the cuticles in it for ten minutes. This nourishes the nail plate, softens the cuticles and the surrounding skin, and is an excellent service for clients with dry, cracked cuticles.

- Warm oil may also be applied to the skin of the hand and forearm to improve skin texture, colour and blood circulation in the area.

Exfoliating service

Exfoliating service is carried out as part of the massage routine. The massage is performed as usual, using an exfoliant a mildly abrasive cream. It may be applied prior to hand and arm massage also to expose new cells and aid the absorption of the massage oil/cream. This service offers the following benefits:

- the removal of dead skin cells
- improvement of the skin texture
- improvement of the skin colour
- increased blood circulation

The abrasive particles must be thoroughly removed with hot, damp towels before continuing with the rest of the manicure.

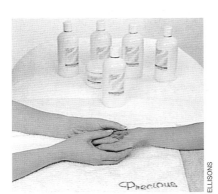

An exfoliating service

Hand service mask

An appropriate service mask may be applied, according to the client's service requirements. This may be either stimulating and rejuvenating, or moisturising. The hands may be placed inside warm mittens or hand gloves for ten minutes to enable the mask to penetrate the epidermis. Several layers are applied. The mask is then removed, and followed with service massage cream.

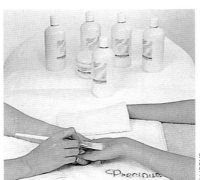

A hand service mask

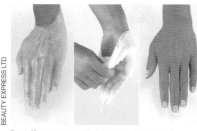

BEAUTY EXPRESS LTD

Paraffin wax application and removal

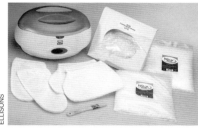

ELLISONS

Paraffin wax resources

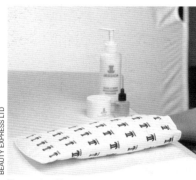

BEAUTY EXPRESS LTD

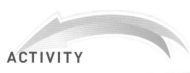

Thermal mitts

ACTIVITY

Researching services

Research other types of hand and nail services. Write down the details of your research, and try out the services on clients.

Paraffin wax service

The wax is heated in a special bath to a temperature of 50–55°C. It is then applied to the hands with a brush, covered with a plastic protective covering and left to set for 10–15 minutes before removal. Several layers are applied. This offers the following benefits:

- the heating effect stimulates the blood circulation
- eases discomfort of arthritic and rheumatic conditions
- softens the skin; improving the appearance and condition of the nails and dry skin

After use the wax is disposed of.

Thermal mitts

These are electrically heated gloves in which the hands are placed for approximately 15 minutes.

They are usually used following the application of a service within the manicure routine. The hands are prepared by wrapping them in a plastic protective covering.

The service has the following benefits:

- decreases joint stiffness in the case of a client suffering from arthritis
- improves the condition of dry skin of the cuticles and hands by increasing the absorption of moisturising products
- improves skin colour and blood circulation

Always follow manufacturers' guidelines in the application procedure for hand and nail services.

Step-by-step: Specialist hand and arm service

Specialist services should be offered to your client when there is a specific service need or if they feel they would like to benefit from such a service.

Specialist training in these advanced techniques is usually offered by major product companies.

The model for this specialist hand and arm service is a mature client who suffers from the medical condition rheumatoid arthritis where the joints become inflamed and painful.

The following hand and arm service will:

- stimulate the blood circulation
- have a skin cleansing action
- remove dead skin cells (desquamation)
- improve the moisture content of the skin
- minimize discomfort caused by an arthritic, rheumatic condition

Your services should be adapted the meet the service objectives for the client.

Allow 30 minutes for this specialist hand and arm service.

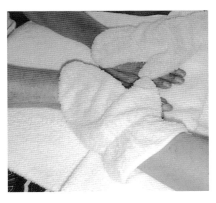

1 The hands and arms are cleansed using warm towelling mitts infused with lime oil for its therapeutic, refreshing and energizing properties.

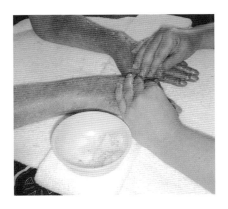

2 The hands are exfoliated to remove all dead skin cells and brighten the skin. A salt-based preparation with emollient, skin-softening ingredients is applied to the skin of each hand and is rubbed gently over the skin's surface.

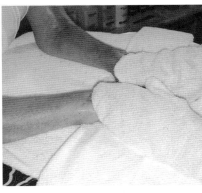

3 Towelling mitts are used to remove the exfoliating service. These have been steamed and are warm when used.

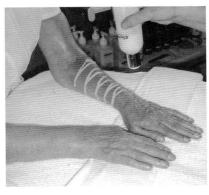

4 A skin-nourishing milk lotion is applied to each arm using a 'drizzling' technique. The milk is particularly beneficial for dry, sensitive skin.

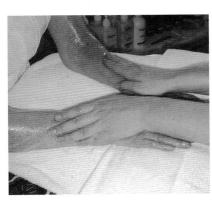

5 Massage movements are applied using effleurage and petrissage massage manipulations.

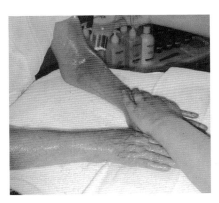

6 A further skin treatment product, warm oil, is applied and massaged into the skin. This will act as a treatment mask for the skin.

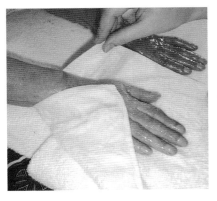

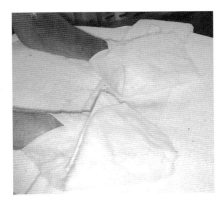

7 The hands are then placed in steamed towels and encased in a plastic bag and dry towelling mitten for 10–15 minutes. Remove mittens and continue with nail polish application if desired.

> " You can only sell if you believe in what you are selling.
>
> **Jacqui Jefford**

Hand and forearm massage

Hand massage is generally carried out near the end of the manicure service, just prior to nail polish application. It can also be carried out on its own if the client wants the effects of the massage but does not need or want service to their nails.

The massage incorporates classic massage movements, each with different effects:

- **Effleurage** – a stroking movement, used to begin the massage as a link manipulation, and to complete the massage sequence.

- **Petrissage** – movements including **kneading** where the tissues are lifted away from the underlying structures and compressed. Pressure is intermittent, and should be light yet firm.

The beauty therapist can adapt the massage application according to the needs of the client. Either the **speed of application** or **depth of pressure** can be altered.

The reasons for offering a hand massage during a manicure are as follows:

- to moisturise the skin with hand cream
- to increase blood circulation to the lower arm and hand
- to help maintain joint mobility
- to ease discomfort from arthritis or rheumatism
- to relax the client
- to help remove any dead skin cells (desquamation)

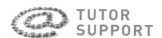

TUTOR SUPPORT

Activity 6 & 7: manicure wordsearches

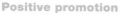

BEST PRACTICE

Positive promotion

Hand massage can be included during a facial while the mask is applied, maximizing service benefits and client relaxation. It also gives you the opportunity to promote another product or service to the client.

Step-by-step: Hand and forearm massage

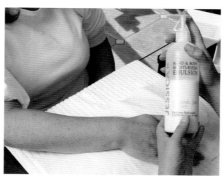
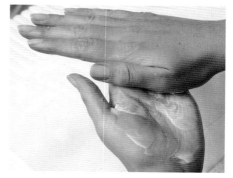

1 Dispense the massage medium into the hands, warm the product over the palms and apply to the client's skin using effleurage technique.

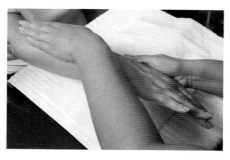
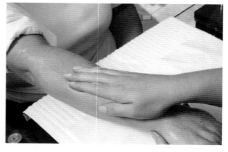

2 **Effleurage to the whole hand and forearm** Use long sweeping strokes from the hand to the elbow, moving on both the outer and the inner sides of the forearm.

Repeat step 2 a further 5 times.

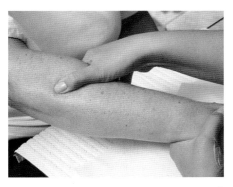
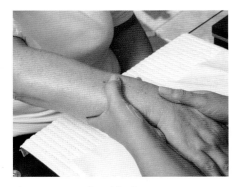

3 Using a **petrissage movement** pick up the flexor and extensor muscles of the lower arm.

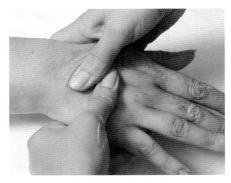
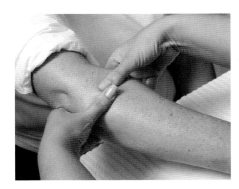

4 **Thumb kneading to the back of the hand and the forearm** Use the thumbs, one in front of the other, and move backwards and forwards in a gently kneading action. Move from the hand to the elbow, then slide the thumbs back down to the hands.

Repeat step 4 a further 2 times.

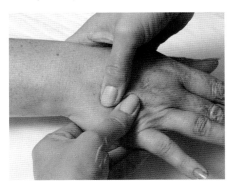
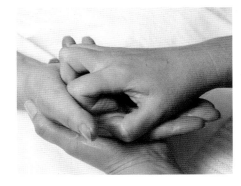

5 **Perform a scissoring, friction movement** using both thumbs between each metacarpal bone in the hands.

6 **Perform a 'knuckling' petrissage movement** rotating the fingers in a small fist shape against the muscles in the palms of the hand.

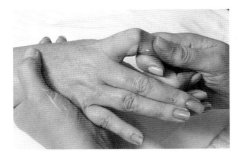
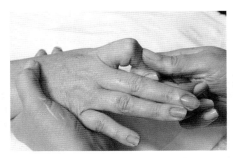
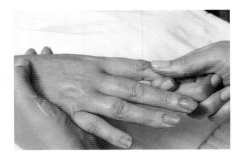

7 **Move the phalange bones of each finger**, bending the finger at each joint and then straightening in a resistance movement.

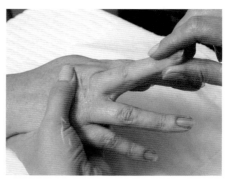

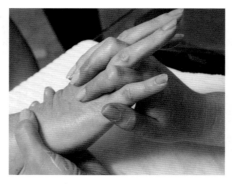

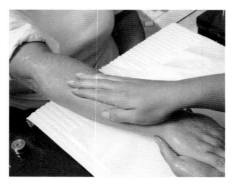

8 Finger circulations, supporting the joints
Supporting the knuckles with one hand, hold the fingers individually and gently take each through its full range of movements, first clockwise and then anticlockwise. Move from the little finger to the thumb.

Repeat step 8 a further 2 times.

9 Wrist circulations, supporting the joints
Support the wrist with one hand and put your fingers between the client's, gently grasping his/her hand. Move the wrist through its full range of movement, first clockwise and then anticlockwise.

Repeat step 9 a further 2 times.

10 Effleurage to the whole hand and forearm
Use the same movement as in step 2.

Repeat step 10 a further 5 times.

HEALTH & SAFETY

Joint mobility
If the client has any joint mobility restrictions, e.g. arthritis, you will need to modify your massage technique and application accordingly.

Nail polish application

Nail polish is used to coat the nail plate for a number of reasons:

- to adorn the nail
- to disguise stained nails
- to add temporary strength to weak nails
- to improve the condition or appearance of the natural nail
- to co-ordinate with clothes or make-up
- to create designs and effects, called 'nail art'

Before nail polish is applied, the client's hand jewellery may be replaced, to avoid smudging afterwards.

Styles of polish application

- ***Traditional application*** This style is the one most commonly requested by clients: the entire nail plate is covered with polish.

- ***French application*** This style involves painting the nail plate of the nail bed pink or pale beige, and the free edge white.

- ***Free lunula application*** This style involves applying polish over the whole nail plate except the area of the lunula.

- ***Painted lunula application*** This style involves painting the lunula a contrasting colour.

- ***Application to give the appearance of longer nails*** This style creates an optical illusion that the nails are longer than they really are. The whole nail plate is painted, leaving a slightly larger gap than usual along the nail walls.

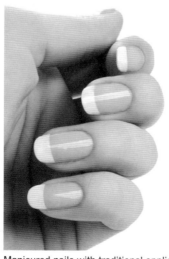

Manicured nails with traditional application

Tips for nail painting

- Ensure the surface of the nail is grease-free. If grease is present this will result in nail polish peeling or chipping.

- Select colours that suit the client's nail length and skin colour.

- Dark colours will draw attention to the nails, and will make small/short nails appear smaller/shorter.

- If the nails are very broad leave a margin at the sides of the nail's wall free of polish, this will help them to appear slimmer.

- Avoid pearlized polish if the client's nail surface is uneven or ridged. The polish will emphasize the imperfection.

- Always apply a good quality base coat suited to the client's nail condition. This helps to prevent staining from pigment in the polish, and may strengthen the nail or smooth ridges depending on its formulation.

- When applying nail polish colour, apply two coats, allowing the nails to dry between each coat to prevent the appearance of brush marks.

- Ensure good colour coverage.

- Allow nail polish to dry before **top coat** application.

- Always follow manufacturer recommendations for their nail polish application.

Reasons for peeling and chipping nail polish

Chipping may be explained by any of the following:

- The nail polish was not thick enough because of over-thinning with solvent.

- No base coat was used.

- Grease was left on the nail plate prior to painting.

- The nail plate is flaking.

- The polish was dried too quickly by artificial means.

Peeling polish may have the following explanations:

- No top coat was used.

- Successive coats were not allowed to dry between applications.

- The nail polish was too thick, due to evaporation of the solvent.

- Grease was left on the nail plate prior to painting.

Nail polish storage Nail polish should be stored in a cool, dark place, to avoid separation and fading. The caps and the rims of bottles **must** be kept clean, not only for appearance but also to ensure that the bottle is airtight.

If polish does thicken, **solvent** may be added to restore the correct consistency. This should be done 20 minutes prior to use to ensure an even consistency.

TOP TIP

Fast-drying products
A nail 'fast-drying' product may be applied to reduce the time taken for the polish to dry.

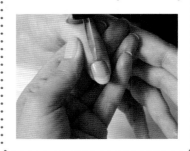

BEST PRACTICE

Choosing colours

For short nails, select a pale, neutral colour. Darker, more dramatic colours suit healthy, long nails, especially on clients with darker skin tones.

ALWAYS REMEMBER

Essential nail polish qualities
Nail polish should:

- adhere to the nail plate and be flexible to resist peeling and chipping

- have good durability on exposure to water, detergents and other chemicals it may come into contact with

- not stain the nail plate

- flow freely onto the nail plate and be easy to apply

HEALTH & SAFETY

Stock storage
Always check MSDS recommendations that stock is stored safely and to maintain its quality.

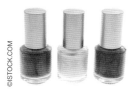

©ISTOCK.COM

Pearlized nail polish

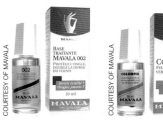

COURTESY OF MAVALA

Base coat   **Top coat**

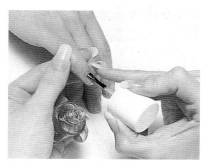

Types of polish The following types of polish may be used:

- *Cream* This has a matt finish, and requires a top coat application to give a sheen.

- *Pearlized* This has a frosted, shimmery appearance due to the addition of natural fish scales or synthetic ingredients such as bismuth oxychloride.

- *Base coat* This protects the nail from staining by a strong-coloured nail polish; it also gives a good grip to polish, and smooths out minor surface irregularities. Many base coats are formulated using ingredients to treat different nail problems such as weak, brittle, peeling or ridged nails.

- *Top coat* This gives a sheen to cream polish, and adds longer wear as it helps to prevent chipping.

Contra-indications to nail polish Do not apply polish in these circumstances:

- if there are diseases and disorders of the nail plate and surrounding skin

- if the client is allergic to nail polish

In addition, pearlized nail polish should not be applied to excessively ridged nails as it may appear to exaggerate the problem. Short or bitten nails should be painted only with pale polishes, to avoid attracting attention.

Step-by-step: Dark polish application

Confirm the client's choice of nail colour. A cream formulation has been demonstrated.

Ensure the free edge is smooth and the cuticles are neat and smooth.

> **TOP TIP**
>
> **Cleaning the nail plate before polish application**
> Use a lint-free pad as cotton wool may leave fibres, which may spoil the application of nail polish.

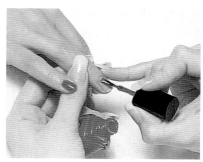

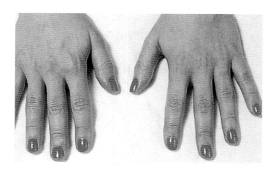

1   Ensure that the nail plate is free from grease. Starting with the thumb, apply three brush strokes down the length of the nail from the cuticle to the free edge, beginning in the centre, then down either side close to the nail wall.

Take care to avoid touching the cuticle or the nail wall. If flooding occurs, remove the polish immediately with an orange stick and polish remover.

Apply one coat of base coat.

2   Apply the coloured polish, two coats are applied, followed by one coat of top coat.

3   The complete dark polish application.

Confirm with the client that the finished result is to their satisfaction.

Complete details on the client's record card.

HEALTH & SAFETY

Ensure the area is well ventilated to avoid inhalation of excessive fumes. Lighting should be good to enable you to avoid eyestrain. It is a good idea to use a table lamp when painting the nails.

Manicure for a male client

A man's hands differ slightly from a woman's so some adaptations to the basic manicure are necessary if the service is to be effective:

- File the nails to a shorter length.
- Usually coloured nail polish is omitted.
- Shape the nails square rather than oval.
- Buff the nails with paste, if a shine is required.
- Use unperfumed lotion for massage.
- Use a lotion or an oil rather than cream for massage, to avoid dragging body hair.
- Use deeper movements during hand and arm massage.

Step-by-step: Male manicure

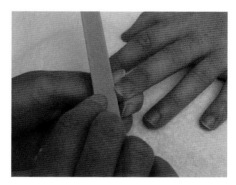

1 File the nails to a shorter length. The nails are usually filed to a square shape rather than oval.

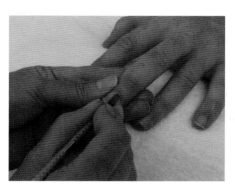

2 Improve the appearance of the cuticles. Push back the cuticles gently.

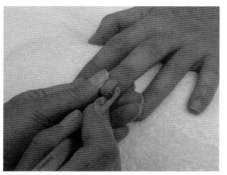

3 A cuticle knife is used to remove the excess eponychium from the cuticle area. Remember to keep the blade dampened to avoid scratches to the nail plate.

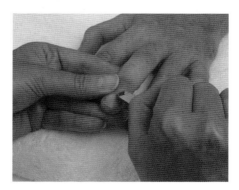

4 Remove excess cuticle using cuticle nippers.

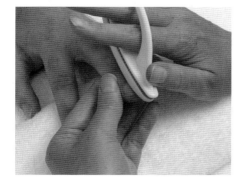

5 Buff the nails to improve blood circulation to the nail bed, giving a healthy appearance to the nail. Buff the nails with a buffing paste if a shine is required.

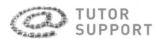

TUTOR SUPPORT

Activity 9: Manicure evaluation task

Step-by-step: Hand and arm massage

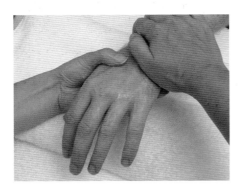

1 Effleurage to the hand and forearm. This movement starts and concludes the hand and arm massage. Use long, sweeping strokes from the hand to the elbow, moving on both the outer and inner sides of the forearm.

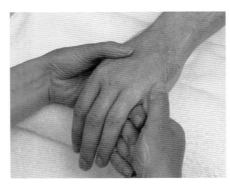

2 Finger twists movement. Gently apply a rotary petrissage movement to each finger.

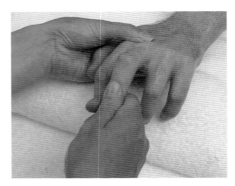

3 Finger resistance movement. Move each finger backwards through its range of movement to exercise the joints.

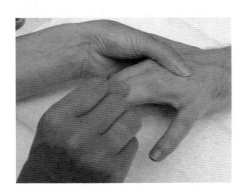

4 Finger rotary movement. Circle each finger in a rotary movement clockwise and then anticlockwise. Move the little finger to the thumb.

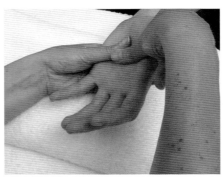

5 Thumbs kneading movement to the palm of the hand.

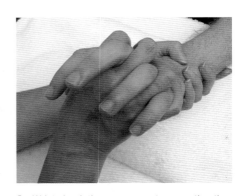

3 Wrist circulations movement, supporting the joints. Support the wrist with one hand and put your fingers between the client's, gently grasping their hand. Move the wrist through its full range of movement, first clockwise and then anti-clockwise. Repeat Step **1** effleurage to conclude the massage.

Outcome 4 : Provide aftercare advice

"Always know the features and benefits of what you are trying to sell whether it be a product or a treatment.

Jacqui Jefford

Learn how to provide aftercare advice which supports and meets the needs of your client by:

1 Giving **advice** and recommendations accurately and constructively.

2 Giving your clients suitable **advice** specific to their individual needs.

Aftercare and advice

It is important when carrying out a manicure that the client knows how to care for their nails at home. It is your duty as a therapist to ensure that the correct aftercare advice is given. If it isn't, the client may unwittingly undo all the good work you have done during the service.

When giving aftercare advice you have a good opportunity to recommend retail products, such as nail service, polish or hand cream, thereby enhancing retail sales and the salon's profit.

Aftercare advice will differ slightly for each client, according to individual needs, but generally it will be as follows:

- Wear rubber gloves when washing up.

- Wear protective gloves when gardening or doing domestic chores.

- Always wear gloves in cold weather.

- Dry the hands thoroughly after washing, and apply hand cream. Some hand creams contain UV filters which reduce hyperpigmentation to the backs of the hands occurring.

- Avoid harsh soaps when washing hands.

- Advising the client on how to file their nails.

- Do not use the fingernails as tools (for instance, to prise lids off tins).

- Advising on appropriate nail/skincare products to remedy the problems present, e.g. dry skin, weak nails.

- Advising the client on what other professional services you could recommend.

- Advising the client on a service plan to improve the nail/skin condition and the time intervals recommended between each service.

It is also necessary to tell the client what to do in the event of a contra-action.

Have retail products available for the client to purchase. These include emery boards, coloured nail polishes, nail polish remover and nail/skin treatment products.

It is a good idea to have available the nail polish colours that you have used. The client can then touch up any accidental chips themselves.

Recommend the use of top coat applied every three to four days to protect the nail polish, increase its durability and impart shine.

Finally, at the end of the manicure service ensure the clients records are updated, accurate and signed by the client and manicurist. Ensure that the finished result is to the client's satisfaction and meets the agreed service plan.

Exercises for the hands

Hand exercises play an important role in the homecare advice given to clients, for the following reasons:

- They keep the joints supple, allowing greater movement.

- Circulation is increased, encouraging healthy nail and skin growth.

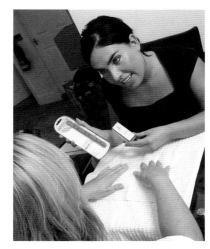

Recommending aftercare products to meet the client's needs

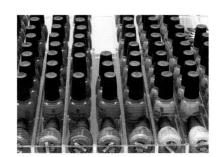

A range of nail polishes for retail

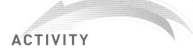

ACTIVITY

Designing an aftercare leaflet
Devise an aftercare leaflet for clients, advising a suitable home-care routine. It is good practice to provide the client with an aftercare leaflet outlining all recommendations following service.

● Good circulation helps to prevent cold hands.

● Exercises keep the client interested in their hands, and so more likely to keep regular salon appointments.

Exercise routine

1 Rub the palms together, back and forth, until warm.

2 Make a tight fist with each hand, then slowly stretch out all the fingers as far as possible.

*Repeat step **2** a further 3 times.*

3 With the fingers extended, rotate the wrists slowly in large clockwise circles.

*Repeat step **3** a further 3 times.*

4 With the fingers extended, rotate the wrists slowly in large anticlockwise circles.

*Repeat step **4** a further 3 times.*

5 Play an imaginary piano vigorously with the fingers for ten seconds.

6 With the hands together as if praying, gently widen the fingers as far as possible, then relax.

*Repeat step **6** a further 3 times.*

TOP TIP

Hand exercises

Remember hand exercises should be performed by the manicurist also to keep the hands supple, reducing the possibility of the effects of RSI in the hands.

TUTOR SUPPORT

Activity 8: Re-cap, revision and feedback

TUTOR SUPPORT

Activity 10: Multiple choice quiz

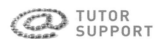

Hand exercises

GLOSSARY OF KEY WORDS

Aftercare advice recommendations given to the client following service to continue the benefits of the service.

Base coat a nail polish product applied to protect the natural nail and prevent staining from coloured nail polish.

Bevelling a nail filing technique used at the free edge of the nail to ensure it is smooth.

Blue nail nail condition where the nail bed has a blue tinge rather than a healthy pink colour due to poor blood circulation in the area.

Bruised nail nail condition where the nail appears blue/black in colour where bleeding has occurred on the nail bed following injury.

Buffer a manicure tool with a handle made of plastic and a pad with a replaceable cover, used on the nail to give a sheen, increase blood supply to the area and, if used with the gritty cream buffing paste, to help smooth out nail surface irregularities.

Client groups this term is used in a number of the units and it refers to client diversity. The CRE (Commission for Racial Equality) ethnic group classification is used in the range for these units. These cover white, mixed, Asian, black and Chinese.

Consultation techniques assessment of client's needs using different assessment techniques, including questioning and natural observation.

Contact dermatitis a skin disorder caused by intolerance of the skin to a particular substance, or a group of substances. On exposure to the substance the skin quickly becomes irritated and an allergic reaction occurs.

Contra-action an unwanted reaction occurring during or after service application.

Contra-indication a problematic symptom that indicates that the service may not proceed.

Cuticle cream or oil a cosmetic preparation used to condition the skin of the cuticle.

Cuticle knife a metal tool used on the nail to remove excess eponychium and perionychium (the extension of the skin of the cuticle at the base of the nail).

Cuticle nippers a metal tool used to remove excess cuticle and neaten the skin around the cuticle area.

Cuticle remover a cosmetic preparation used to soften and loosen the skin cells and cuticle from the nail.

Eczema of the nail inflammation of the skin, causing changes to the nail including ridges, pitting, nail separation and nail thickening.

Effleurage a stroking massage movement, used to begin the massage, as a link manipulation and to complete the massage sequence.

Eggshell nail nail condition where thin, fragile white nails curve under at the free edge.

Emery board a nail file used to shape the free edge of the nail.

Exfoliant a mild abrasive cream applied and massaged over the skin's surface to remove dead skin cells and improve the appearance and texture of the skin.

Hand and nail treatments specialized products and equipment designed to improve the condition and appearance of different nail and skin conditions.

Hand cream/oil a cosmetic mixture of waxes and oils applied to soften the skin of the hands and cuticles.

Hangnail nail condition where small pieces of epidermal skin protrude between the nail plate and nail wall, accompanying a dry cuticle condition.

Hoof stick a nail tool used to gently push back the softened cuticles.

Leuconychia nail condition where white spots or marks appear on the nail plate.

Longitudinal ridges nail condition where grooves appear in the nail plate, running along the length of the nail from the cuticle to the free edge.

Manicure a service to care for and improve the condition and appearance of the hands and nails.

Mask a service mask applied to the skin of the hands to treat and improve the condition of the skin. This may include properties to stimulate, rejuvenate and moisturise.

Nail finish the product finally applied to the natural nail to enhance its appearance, i.e. buffed nail or nail polish application.

Nail polish a clear or coloured nail product that adds colour/protection to the nail. Cream polish has a matt finish and requires a top coat application. Pearlized polish produces a frosted, shimmery appearance and top coat is not required.

Nail polish drier an aerosol or oil preparation applied following nail polish application to increase the speed at which the polish hardens.

Nail polish remover a solvent used to remove nail polish and grease from the nails prior to applying polish.

Nail polish solvent used to thin nail polish and restore its consistency.

Nail strengthener a nail polish product that strengthens the nail plate, which has a tendency to split.

Necessary action the appropriate action to take in the case of a contra-action or contra-indication to ensure the welfare of the client.

Onycholysis nail condition where the nail plate separates from the nail bed.

Onychophagy nail condition where a person bites their nails excessively.

Onychorrhexis nail condition where the person has split, flaking nails.

Orange stick a disposable wooden tool used around the cuticle and free edge of the nail and to apply products to the nail.

Paraffin wax this is heated and applied to the skin of the hands to provide a warming effect. This improves skin functioning, aids the absorption of products and is beneficial to ease the discomfort of arthritic and rheumatic conditions.

Paronychia bacterial infection where swelling, redness and pus appear in the cuticle area of the nail wall.

Petrissage massage movements, including kneading, where the tissues are lifted away from the underlying structures and compressed. Pressure is intermittent, and should be light yet firm.

Psoriasis of the nail an inflammatory condition where there is an increased production of cells in the upper part of the skin. Pitting occurs on the surface of the nail.

Pterygium nail condition where the cuticle is thickened and overgrown.

Ridge-filler a nail product used on ridged nails that improves the nail's appearance and provides a more even surface.

Scissors nail tools used to shorten the length of the nail before filing.

Service plan after the consultation, suitable service objectives are established to treat the client's conditions and needs.

Thermal mitts electrically heated gloves in which the hands are placed following the application of a skin service product such as a mask. The heat aids the absorption of the product and improves skin functioning.

Tinea unguium fungal infection of the nails. The nail is yellowish-grey in colour.

Top coat a nail polish product applied over another nail polish to provide additional strength and durability to the finish.

Transverse furrows nail condition where grooves appear on the nail, running from side to side.

Verruca or wart a viral infection where small epidermal skin growths appear, either raised or flat depending upon their location, and have a rough surface.

Warm-oil service involves gently heating a small amount of oil and soaking the nails and cuticles in it to nourish the nails and soften the cuticles and surrounding skin.

ASSESSMENT OF KNOWLEDGE AND UNDERSTANDING

Having covered the learning objectives for **Provide manicure services**, test what you need to know and understand answering the following short questions below.

The information covers:

- organizational and legal requirements
- how to work safely and effectively when performing manicure services
- consult, plan and prepare for treatments with clients
- contra-indications and contra-actions
- anatomy and physiology
- manicure services
- aftercare advice for clients

Organisational and legal requirements

For full legislation details, see Chapter 4.

1 What information does the industry Code of Practice for Nail Services provide?

2 What actions must be taken before a client under 16 years of age receives a manicure?

3 How can you ensure compliance with the legislation of the Disability Discrimination Act (2005)?

4 Taking into account health and safety hygiene requirements, how can cross-infection be avoided when carrying out manicure services?

5 How should all client records be stored to comply with the Data Protection Act (1998)?

6 How long would you allow to complete a basic manicure treatment and a specialized manicure including a hand and nail treatment?

7 Why is it important for staff to be familiar with the different manicure pricing structures?

8 What details should be recorded on the client's record card and why is it important to keep accurate records which are maintained?

9 What is the cause of Repetitive Strain Injury and how can this be avoided when performing manicure services?

How to work safely and effectively when performing manicure services

1 What personal protective equipment may be used when performing manicure and explain its purpose?

2 What are the symptoms of the skin disorder contact dermatitis and how can it be caused when performing manicure services? What steps could you take to minimize the risk of developing contact dermatitis?

3 Why is it important that the client is warm and comfortable when receiving a manicure?

4 Why is good lighting important?

5 What is the potential risk of poor positioning of the client and yourself when performing a manicure service?

6 What are the methods of disinfecting and sterilizing tools and equipment? Give three examples of tools and equipment that are sterilized and disinfected.

7 Personal presentation and hygiene is important to create a good impression. Give three examples relevant to the Code of Practice for Nail Services of good personal presentation and hygiene practice.

8 Why is it important to complete your manicure service in the allocated time?

9 How would you dispose of general and contaminated waste in the salon?

Consult, plan and prepare for treatments with clients

1 Communication is important. Give three examples of good communication techniques.

2 Why should the manicurist consult the client's record card prior to treatment?

3 Why is it important to assess the condition of the client's hands and nails before treatment commences?

4 Why is it important to discuss and agree the treatment service and outcomes with your client at the consultation?

5 Why should you record your client's responses to questions asked at consultation?

6 Following the consultation what should be considered in the design of your service plan?

Contra-indications and contra-actions

1 Name three contra-indications observed at consultation that would prevent treatment being carried out.

2 What types of hand and nail disorders would restrict treatment application?

3 Name three contra-actions that could occur during or following a manicure service.

4 If you suspected a client had a contagious contra-indication what actions would you take for the welfare of the client, yourself and others?

5 Contra-indications are not always visible. How can you ensure the client's suitability for manicure service?

Anatomy and physiology

For full anatomy and physiology details, see Chapter 2.

1 How many bones form the hand? Name them.

2 Name the bones of the forearm.

3 Name the main arteries of the arm and hand.

4 Name two muscles of the hand.

5 What are the group of muscles called that bend the wrist, drawing it towards the forearm?

Manicure services

1 How would you recognize each of the following, and what would you recommend to improve the appearance and condition:
  - weak nails?
  - dry nails?
  - brittle nails?
  - ridged nails?
  - dry cuticles?
  - overgrown cuticles?
  - dry skin?
  - hard skin?

2 Why would you choose to include the following hand and nail treatments in your treatment plan:
  - paraffin wax therapy?
  - hand mask?
  - warm oil?
  - thermal mitts?
  - exfoliators?

3 How can buffing improve the appearance of the natural nails?

4 Which manicure tools are used to improve the condition of the cuticles?

5 Describe how a cuticle knife should be used in order to avoid damage to the surface of the nail plate and cuticle.

6 If used incorrectly, cuticle remover can cause drying of the cuticle. Explain how this could occur.

7 What products used on the cuticles help to prevent them from drying and splitting?

8 When filing the nail how is the shape of the client's free edge determined?

9 Why are several treatments often necessary to improve the condition of the nails and skin to their full potential?

10 What are the differences in formulation and treatments benefits of the following massage mediums:
  - cream?
  - oil?

11 How may you adapt your manicure service when treating a male client?

12 What are the terms used for the different types of massage used in a manicure?

13 State four benefits of hand and arm massage.

14 How would you remove excess moisture and general debris created during the manicure from the natural nails before nail polish application?

15 What is the difference between a base coat and a top coat in terms of purpose and application technique?

16 What is the nail polish application technique for a 'French Manicure'?

17 What would you consider when recommending a nail finish for a client?

18 If a client had very short nails, what type of polish would you suggest they chose and why?

19 Which nail polish product would reduce the appearance of ridges on the nail plate?

20 If a client has their nails polished professionally what would be the recommended time interval between treatments?

21 Why is it a good idea to retail the nail polish colours used with the treatment?

22 What is the correct procedure for removing nail polish?

Aftercare advice for clients

1 What general advice should be given to a client on maintaining the condition and appearance of their nails following a manicure?

2 Why is it important to advise the client to avoid a sawing action when filing the nails?

3 What aftercare advice would you give to a client with very dry hands and cuticles?

4 List three retail products that you could recommend to a manicure client.

5 For each of the clients below suggest a treatment routine. Detail the treatment plan to include: cause of the condition, aims of the treatment, products used, treatments recommended, relevant retail sales and aftercare advice.
- A hairdresser with very soft, weak, stained nails.
- An engineer with a bruised nail, overgrown cuticles and cracked skin on the fingers.
- A teenager who has badly bitten nails.
- An elderly client with strong, ridged nails and dry skin on the hands.

13 Pedicure Services (N3)

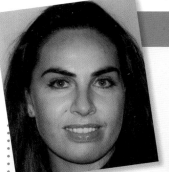

ROLE MODEL

Vicky Ann Kennedy
Paramedical skin practitioner and beauty therapist

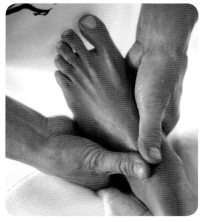

N3 Unit Learning Objectives

This chapter covers **Unit N3 Provide pedicure services**.

This unit is all about improving and maintaining your client's feet, nails and surrounding skin. A pedicure includes filing the nails to shape, using specialized nail, cuticle products and services, massaging the lower leg and foot and providing a complementary nail finish to suit the client.

There are **four** learning outcomes for Unit N2 which you must achieve competently:

1 Maintain safe and effective methods of working when providing pedicure services

2 Consult, plan and prepare for the pedicure service

3 Carry out pedicure service

4 Provide aftercare advice

Your assessor will observe you on at **least three occasions** (each occasion must involve a different foot and nail service from the range).

From the **range** statement, you must show that you have:

● used all **consultation techniques**

● taken the **necessary action** where a contra-action, contra-indication or service modification occurs

● applied all **foot and nail services**

● applied all **nail finishes**

● provided relevant **advice**

However you must prove that you have the necessary knowledge, understanding and skills to be able to perform competently across the range.

(continued on the next page)

" I have been the principal owner of a very successful beauty clinic since 1991. I knew the career path i wanted to take by the age of 12, but had to wait until the age of 19 before it became a reality. I trained at Bolton College under Lorraine Nordmann, and became Student of the Year when I left. I have carried on striving to achieve every day since.

Before starting my own business, I had not worked in many other places, but I already knew how I wanted things to be done and how standards should be followed.

I think that if your heart is in it, working in the beauty industry is very rewarding and a beauty salon is a lovely, happy place to work. I have no regrets and after nearly 20 years, still enjoy every day.

(continued)

When providing pedicure services it is important to use the skills you have learnt in the following units:

Unit G20 Make sure your own actions reduce risks to health and safety

Unit G18 Promote additional products or services to clients

Unit G8 Develop and maintain your effectiveness at work

Essential anatomy and physiology knowledge requirements for this unit, **N3**, are identified on the checklist chart in Chapter 2, page 16.

The purpose of a pedicure

The word **pedicure** is derived from the Latin word *pedis*, meaning 'foot' and *cura*, meaning 'care'. The service is very similar to manicure except that it is carried out on the feet instead of the hands. A pedicure is carried out for many reasons:

- to improve the appearance of the foot
- to reduce the amount of hard skin
- to relax tired, aching feet
- to keep the nails smooth and healthy

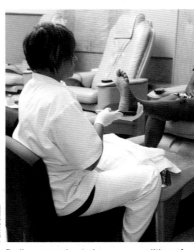

Pedicure service to improve condition of the feet

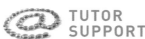

TUTOR SUPPORT

Activity 6: Benefits of foot and nail treatments

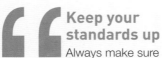

Keep your standards up

Always make sure that you keep your standards high, especially when dealing with hygiene and avoiding cross infection. Remember the good practices that you learnt at college and always use them.

Vicky Ann Kennedy

Outcome 1: Maintain safe and effective methods of working when improving pedicure services

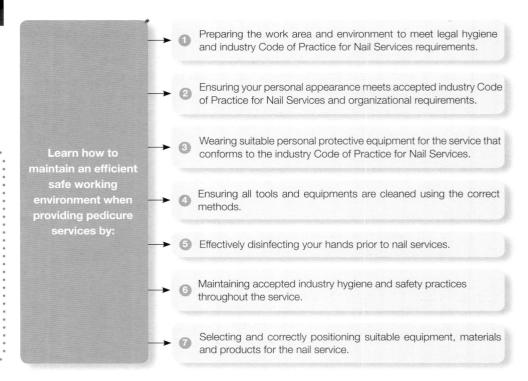

Learn how to maintain an efficient safe working environment when providing pedicure services by:

1. Preparing the work area and environment to meet legal hygiene and industry Code of Practice for Nail Services requirements.

2. Ensuring your personal appearance meets accepted industry Code of Practice for Nail Services and organizational requirements.

3. Wearing suitable personal protective equipment for the service that conforms to the industry Code of Practice for Nail Services.

4. Ensuring all tools and equipments are cleaned using the correct methods.

5. Effectively disinfecting your hands prior to nail services.

6. Maintaining accepted industry hygiene and safety practices throughout the service.

7. Selecting and correctly positioning suitable equipment, materials and products for the nail service.

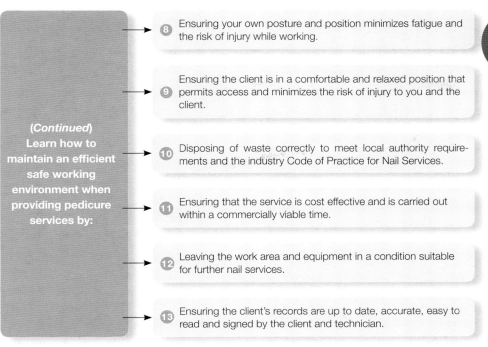

8 Ensuring your own posture and position minimizes fatigue and the risk of injury while working.

9 Ensuring the client is in a comfortable and relaxed position that permits access and minimizes the risk of injury to you and the client.

(Continued) Learn how to maintain an efficient safe working environment when providing pedicure services by:

10 Disposing of waste correctly to meet local authority requirements and the industry Code of Practice for Nail Services.

11 Ensuring that the service is cost effective and is carried out within a commercially viable time.

12 Leaving the work area and equipment in a condition suitable for further nail services.

13 Ensuring the client's records are up to date, accurate, easy to read and signed by the client and technician.

TOP TIP

Advise the client booking a pedicure service that they will have to allow the nail polish to dry thoroughly before replacing footwear. It is a good idea to wear footwear that will enable the toes to dry thoroughly to avoid spoiling the nail polish.

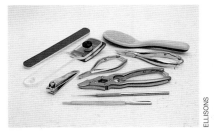

Pedicure equipment

Preparing the working area

All metal instruments should be sterilized in the autoclave prior to use. Non-metal instruments should be disinfected by immersing them in a suitable disinfecting fluid. Prepare the equipment neatly on the work station so that everything you need is to hand and the client need not be disturbed during service.

The work area should remain in a condition suitable for further nail services during the working day.

Place a towel on the floor between you and the client. The foot bowl or foot spa containing warm, soapy water should be placed on this towel.

Towels should be placed on your lap: one is for protection, the other is for drying the client's feet. Keep the other towels close by for wrapping the client's feet. Alternatively, the pedicure may be performed on a beauty couch or at a pedicure station. In this case towels are only required for drying and wrapping up feet.

When cutting the client's nails and removing hard skin, disposable tissue should be placed on your lap and then removed before continuing service.

Personal protective equipment, e.g. safety glasses and synthetic powder-free gloves may be worn for protection from skin and nail debris at this stage.

When the client is comfortably seated, clean your hands using an approved hand cleaning technique, preferably in view of the client, who will observe hygienic procedures being carried out. This will assure them that they are receiving a professional service.

Equipment and materials

Before beginning the pedicure, check that you have the necessary equipment and materials to hand and that they meet the legal hygiene and industry requirements for nail services.

TOP TIP

Foot spa

Foot spas help to relax the feet by a combination of massage provided by an integral vibration feature, aeration of the water, creating a bubbling effect, and heating of the water.

ALWAYS REMEMBER

Beauty services are continuously progressing to meet client needs and improve the service available. The pedicure service featured on page 421 shows specialised pedicure equipment.

EQUIPMENT AND MATERIALS LIST

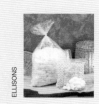

Dry cotton wool
To remove nail polish and excess nail preparations

Nail polish remover
To remove nail polish and excess nail care and skincare preparations

Scissors **or toenail clippers**
To shorten nail length

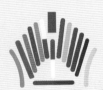

Emery boards
To shorten and shape the nail free edge

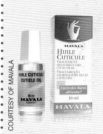

Cuticle oil
Used to condition the skin of the cuticle; especially beneficial for dry nails and cuticles
Cuticle remover
Used to soften the skin cells and the cuticle before service

Cuticle nippers
To remove excess cuticle and dead, torn skin surrounding the nail

Hoof stick **or cuticle pusher**
To gently push back the softened cuticles

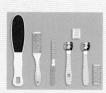

Foot rasp **or callous file**
To remove excess dead skin from the foot

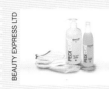

Massage lotion or oil
To massage the skin of the foot and lower leg

Base coat
Provides an even surface to improve nail polish application and adherence and prevent skin staining

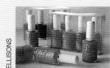

Coloured nail polish
A selection for the client to choose from
Top coat
To provide shine to nail polish. Adds strength and reduces peeling and chipping and increases durability of the polish

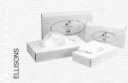

Tissues
To protect client's clothing in the area, etc.

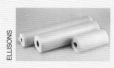

Disposable bedroll tissue
To collect waste and be replaced as necessary during the service

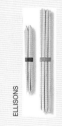

Orange sticks
Tipped at either end with cotton wool. (Orange sticks should be disposed of after each client as they cannot be effectively sterilized.) Used to remove products from containers, to ease the cuticle back and clean under the free edge

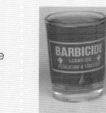

Disinfectant solution
Disinfects small stainless steel sterilized tools

YOU WILL ALSO NEED:

Pedicure bowl or foot spa **(1)** To soak and cleanse the foot. The foot spa also revitalizes and refreshes the skin by stimulation of the blood and circulation

Small towels (5) To protect and dry the client's skin

Small bowls (3) For storage, etc.

Liquid soap Specialized foot cleaning products to cleanse, soften and deodorize the feet

Skin disinfectant To cleanse and disinfect the client's skin. Specialized sprays and gels are available for this purpose

Cuticle knife To remove excess eponychium and perionychium from the nail plate

Client's record card To record the client's personal details, products used and details of the service

Nail polish drier An aerosol or oil preparation applied to speed the drying process of nail polish

Disposable toe separators Used to keep the toes separated during nail polish application. Alternatively, disposable items such as cotton wool or tissues may be used for this purpose

Disposable footwear (optional) Enabling the client to move without smudging the nail polish application

Disinfecting solution For all surfaces

Foot and nail treatment equipment Including: paraffin wax, foot masks, thermal boots and exfoliators

Waste container This should be a lined metal bin with a lid to contain vapours for solvents

Products used in pedicure services

For full details of products used for both manicures and pedicures, their ingredients and uses, see the table in Chapter 12, pages 371–372. In addition to these, an exfoliating pedicure scrub may also be used for the feet (see below).

Product	Ingredients	Use
Exfoliating pedicure scrub	Abrasive ingredients such as pumice, sea salt, detergent, water and water-soluble ingredients, added moisturisers, refreshing agents, e.g. peppermint oil.	To remove dead skin cells, cleanse the skin, condition, soften and refresh the skin, improving blood circulation in the area.

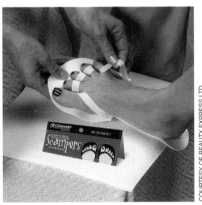

Waste container

Disposable toe separator footwear

Sterilization and disinfection

Hygiene must be maintained in a number of ways:

- ensure that tool and equipment are clean and sterile before use
- dispense products from containers, e.g. creams and lotions, with a disposable spatula
- disinfect work surfaces after every client
- always follow hygienic working practices
- maintain a high standard of personal hygiene

Pedicure tools and equipment can be disposable or can be sterilized and disinfected by the methods shown on page 373.

ELLISONS

COURTESY OF BEAUTY EXPRESS LTD

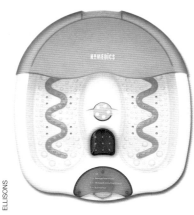

ELLISONS

Foot spa

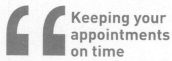

Sterilize your tools

Never use tools that are not completely sterile. Use disposable products where possible.

Vicky Ann Kennedy

ALWAYS REMEMBER

GP referral

A client referred from their GP will usually have a letter. This would be in the case when confirmation regarding suitability for service has been requested. This should be retained with the client's record card.

Keeping your appointments on time

Clients like to be seen promptly so try not to run behind with your appointments. To keep the service area ready for the next client, always ask your clients to bring flip flops with them, then they can leave the service area as soon as you have finished, without having to wait until toenails are dry.

Vicky Ann Kennedy

Service plan

After analyzing the client's nails and adjacent skin, a service plan should be considered and agreed with the client. In order to correct any skin and nail problems the client should attend the salon weekly. They should also be advised of the appropriate service preparations to use at home, so as to support the salon service. Specialist foot services to use will depend upon the skin and nail condition; they include:

- **Revitalizing foot spa agents** These may be in tablet form or as a foaming soak. They are dissolved in warm water, in which the feet are then immersed.

- **Exfoliator** This is used following immersion of the feet in the foot spa. It removes surface dead skin cells, preventing the formation of callus (excess dead tissue) tissue.

- **Massage lotion or cream** This is a massage preparation which includes refreshing essential oils such as peppermint. It is recommended for the relief of tired, aching feet.

- **Foot mask** A **mask** may be applied to cool and to refresh the feet. Booties may be worn while the mask penetrates the epidermis.

- **Foot gel or spray** This may be applied to create an immediate cooling, refreshing effect.

Provide the opportunity for your client to ask any questions relating to the pedicure service or service plan.

The record card should be signed and dated by the client and pedicurist following the consultation to confirm the suitability and consent with the agreed pedicure service.

Reception

When a client makes an appointment for a pedicure service, the receptionist should advise the client how long the service will take. This will include sufficient time for the nail polish to dry before replacing footwear.

To allocate the appropriate length of time ask if they require a specialist foot service with their pedicure

Ask the client whether they are currently receiving service from a chiropodist for conditions such as verrucas or athlete's foot. These would contra-indicate service: the receptionist should advise the client to wait until the condition has cleared.

If the client is a minor under 16 years of age, it is necessary to obtain parent/guardian permission for service. The parent/guardian will also have to be present when the service is received.

Allow 45 minutes for a pedicure.

Allow up to 1hour for a specialist foot service.

All staff, especially the staff communicating with clients at reception should be familiar with the different pricing structures for the range of pedicure services and products available for retail.

A sample client record card

Date	Beauty therapist name
Client name	Date of birth (Identifying client age group.)
Home address	Postcode
Email address	Landline phone number	Mobile phone number
Name of doctor	Doctor's address and phone number
Related medical history (Conditions that may restrict or prohibit service application.)	
Are you taking any medication? (This may affect the sensitivity of the skin to the service.)	

CONTRA-INDICATIONS REQUIRING MEDICAL REFERRAL
(Preventing pedicure service application.)

- ☐ bacterial infections (e.g. paronychia)
- ☐ viral infections (e.g. plantar warts)
- ☐ fungal infections (e.g. tinea unguium, tinea pedis)
- ☐ parasitic infections, (e.g. scabies)
- ☐ severe toenail separation
- ☐ severe eczema and psoriasis
- ☐ severe bruising
- ☐ diabetes

EQUIPMENT AND MATERIALS

- ☐ toenail and skin service tools
- ☐ abrasives (e.g. buffing paste)
- ☐ cuticle softeners
- ☐ toenail conditioners (e.g. **cuticle cream**)
- ☐ skin conditioners (e.g. **foot cream**)
- ☐ toenail, skin and cuticle corrective services (e.g. paraffin wax)
- ☐ consumables

FEET AND TOENAIL SERVICES

- ☐ paraffin wax
- ☐ foot masks
- ☐ thermal boots
- ☐ exfoliators

TOENAIL FINISH

- ☐ light colour
- ☐ dark colour
- ☐ French manicure

CONTRA-INDICATIONS WHICH RESTRICT SERVICE
(Service may require adaptation.)

- ☐ mild toenail separation
- ☐ minor eczema and psoriasis
- ☐ recent scar tissue
- ☐ broken bones
- ☐ minor cuts or abrasions
- ☐ minor bruising or swelling

COURSE OF SERVICE

	Date	Date	Date
☐ improvement of skin condition products used	___	___	___
☐ improvement of toenail condition products used	___	___	___

TOENAIL, CUTICLE AND SKIN CONDITION

Toenails

- ☐ normal   ☐ brittle
- ☐ dry   ☐ weak
- ☐ ridged

Cuticle

- ☐ normal   ☐ dry
- ☐ split   ☐ overgrown

Skin

- ☐ normal   ☐ dry
- ☐ hard

MASSAGE MEDIUMS

- ☐ creams   ☐ oils

Beauty therapist signature (for reference)
Client signature (confirmation of details)

A sample client record card (continued)

SERVICE ADVICE

Pedicure – *allow 45 minutes*

Specialized foot/nail service – *allow up to 60 minutes*

SERVICE PLAN

Record relevant details of your service and advice provided for future reference.

Ensure the client's records are up to date, accurate and fully completed following service. Non-compliance may invalidate insurance.

DURING

Discuss:

- details that may influence the client's toenail condition, such as the client's occupation
- the products the client is currently using to care for the skin of the feet and toenails
- the client's satisfaction with these products
- relevant pedicure procedures (e.g., how to file the toenails correctly)

Note:

- any adverse reaction, if any occur

AFTER

Record:

- results of service
- any modification to service application that has occurred
- what products have been used in the pedicure service
- what foot services have been used
- the effectiveness of service
- any samples provided (review their success at the next appointment)

Advise on:

- product application in order to gain maximum benefit from product use
- specialized products following pedicure service for homecare use
- general foot/toenail care and maintenance
- the recommended time intervals between services
- the importance of a course of service to improve toenail/skin conditions

RETAIL OPPORTUNITIES

Advise on:

- progression of the **service plan** for future appointments
- products that would be suitable for the client to use at home to care for the skin of the feet and toenails
- recommendations for further services
- further products or services that the client may or may not have received before

Note:

- any purchase made by the client

EVALUATION

Record:

- comments on the client's satisfaction with the service
- if poor results are achieved, the reasons why
- how you may alter the service plan to achieve the required service results in the future, if applicable

HEALTH AND SAFETY

Advise on:

- appropriate necessary action to be taken in the event of an unwanted skin or nail reaction

It is important that accurate records are kept and stored in compliance with the Data Protection Act for future reference.

Preparing the Client

Ensure that the client is seated at the correct height, so that you can work comfortably and healthily and the client can enjoy the service without strain to the muscles and joints of the leg.

Ensure that the client is warm and comfortable when preparing for the pedicure. Client privacy and modesty should also be considered. Not all clients would be happy to be on view while receiving the service. Ensure that lighting is good to avoid eye strain and to enable the service to be performed competently. Avoid positioning the work station in direct sunlight however, to prevent discomfort to the client and pedicurist.

Before service begins, ask the client to remove their tights or socks, and any clothing that might restrict their lower leg movement, such as jeans or trousers. Cover their upper legs with a clean towel or provide a gown. This will help them to be more comfortable and allow you to work without restriction.

Ask them to remove any jewellery from the area to be treated, to prevent the jewellery being damaged by creams and to avoid obstructing massage movements. Place the jewellery where the client can see it. Alternatively ask the client to take possession of it for safe keeping – following your salon security policy.

When the client is comfortably seated, clean your hands using an approved hand cleaning technique – preferably in view of the client, who will observe hygienic procedures being carried out. This will assure them that they are receiving a professional service.

Outcome 2: Consult, plan and prepare for the pedicure service

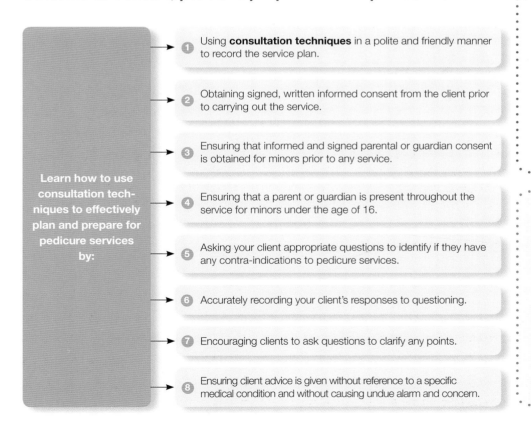

Learn how to use consultation techniques to effectively plan and prepare for pedicure services by:

1. Using **consultation techniques** in a polite and friendly manner to record the service plan.

2. Obtaining signed, written informed consent from the client prior to carrying out the service.

3. Ensuring that informed and signed parental or guardian consent is obtained for minors prior to any service.

4. Ensuring that a parent or guardian is present throughout the service for minors under the age of 16.

5. Asking your client appropriate questions to identify if they have any contra-indications to pedicure services.

6. Accurately recording your client's responses to questioning.

7. Encouraging clients to ask questions to clarify any points.

8. Ensuring client advice is given without reference to a specific medical condition and without causing undue alarm and concern.

HEALTH & SAFETY

Avoiding RSI
Remember to consider your posture and prevent any awkward movements during delivery of the pedicure service. Ensure the work station is at the correct height to avoid stretching and straining your upper body and limbs.

TOP TIP

Pedicure spa chair
Pedicure spa chairs provide comfort and luxury for the client. The client immerses their feet in a tray equipped with hydrotherapy jets to massage the feet, while the chair also features a vibrating massage system.

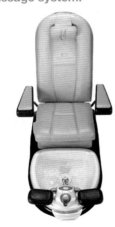

BEAUTY EXPRESS LTD

Keep aware when working
Always check during service that your client is comfortable and not feeling any discomfort. Don't soak feet for too long as they may become too soft making it more likely that you will accidentally remove too much callous.

Vicky Ann Kennedy

THE NATURAL NAIL COMPANY/JESSICA NAILS

TOP TIP

Advise the client to wear open-toed shoes or sandals on the day of the pedicure to allow time for polish to dry completely before putting on shoes.

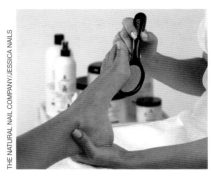

Ensure client is sat at the correct height so they can enjoy the service without strain to the leg

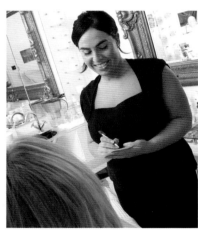

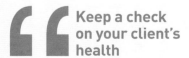

Consultation

"Keep a check on your client's health

Always check for contra-indications before commencing with any part of the pedicure service. Do your consultation thoroughly and especially find out whether your client is diabetic or on any medication.

Vicky Ann Kennedy

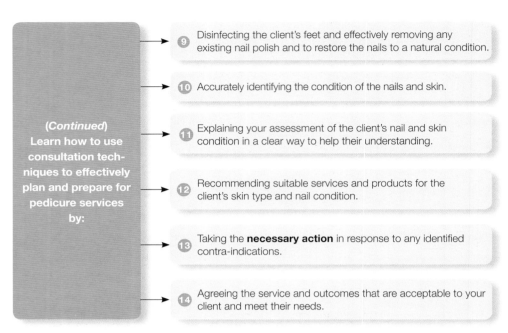

(Continued) Learn how to use consultation techniques to effectively plan and prepare for pedicure services by:

9 Disinfecting the client's feet and effectively removing any existing nail polish and to restore the nails to a natural condition.

10 Accurately identifying the condition of the nails and skin.

11 Explaining your assessment of the client's nail and skin condition in a clear way to help their understanding.

12 Recommending suitable services and products for the client's skin type and nail condition.

13 Taking the **necessary action** in response to any identified contra-indications.

14 Agreeing the service and outcomes that are acceptable to your client and meet their needs.

Consultation

Before carrying out a pedicure service, it is necessary to assess the condition of the client's skin, nails and cuticles. This is done in order that the most appropriate foot and nail services and products may be chosen. Also, by correctly assessing and analyzing the client's foot condition and writing this on their record card, you will be able to see over a period of time how the condition is progressing.

Assess the condition of the following:

● *The cuticles* Are they dry, tight, cracked or overgrown, or are they soft and pliable?

● *The nail* Are they strong or weak, thickened, discoloured or stained? Sometimes this may indicate a nail disorder. The nails of the foot should be filed straight across into a square shape. Shaping the nails at the corners can cause ingrowing toenails.

● *The skin* Is the skin dry, rough or cracked, or is it soft and smooth? Is the colour even? Also check the skin between the toes.

While assessing the client's feet, you should also be looking for any contra-indications to the service.

Skin and nail disorders of the feet

Contra-indications When a client attends for a pedicure service, the therapist should always look at the client's skin and nails to check that no infection or disease is present which might contra-indicate service.

These include bacterial, fungal, parasitic and viral infections, which are described in more detail in Chapter 3, where contra-indications are illustrated and discussed.

If the client is wearing nail polish this must be removed before checking.

The following disorders contra-indicate pedicure services. If you suspect the client has any disorder from the chart below, do not attempt a diagnosis, but refer the client tactfully to their GP or a chiropodist without causing unnecessary concern.

Disorder	Description
Broken bones	For full details, see Chapter 12, page 376.
Cuts of abrasions on the feet	
Diabetes	
Paronychia	
Scabies or itch mites	
Severe eczema of the nail	
Severe eczema of the skin	
Severe nail separation (onycholysis)	For full details, see Chapter 12, page 377.
Severe psoriasis of the nail	
Severe psoriasis of the skin	
Tinea corporis (body ringworm)	
Tinea unguium	

Ingrowing toenail	The sides of the nail penetrates the nail wall: redness, inflammation and pus may be present, depending on the severity of the condition.
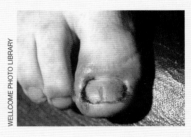	The client should be referred to chiropodist for appropriate service.
	To prevent ingrowing toenails clients should be advised to cut the toenails straight across, and not too short.

WELLCOME PHOTO LIBRARY

Tinea pedis (athletes' foot)	Fungal infection of the foot occurring in the webs of the skin between the toes Small blisters form, which later burst. The skin in the area can become dry, with a scaly appearance.
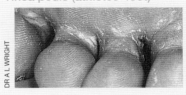	

DR A L WRIGHT

Verrucae or plantar warts on the feet	A viral infection
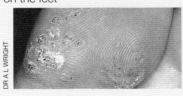	Small epidermal skin growths. Warts occurring on the sole of the foot grow inwards,due to the pressure of body weight. Warts vary in size, shape, texture and colour. Usually they have a rough surface and are raised.
	Plantar wart – found on the sole of the foot.

DR A L WRIGHT

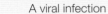

TOP TIP

The role of the chiropodist

A chiropodist is a person who is trained and qualified to treat minor foot complaints. Refer the treatment of non-cosmetic foot conditions to a chiropodist, e.g. conditions such as excessive hard skin.

TUTOR SUPPORT

Activity 1: Label the bones of the leg and foot

TUTOR SUPPORT

Activity 2: Label the nail structure

"Charge the correct fee

When you become self employed, always remember that 'business is business' and start as you mean to carry on. A lot of clients do become your friends, but this should not interfere when charging. You may be happy to set a family discount at the beginning, but don't forget that your time (and your wages) are just as important to you as they are to everyone else.

Vicky Ann Kennedy

Below is a list of common disorders that may be seen on the feet. Not all of these contra-indicate service. See also 'bruised nails', Chapter 12, page 378.

Disorder	Cause	Appearance	Salon service	Homecare advice
Blue nail (shown on the fingernail)	Poor blood circulation in the area. Heart disease.	The nail bed does not appear a healthy pink colour but has a blue tinge.	Permission to treat to be received from the client's GP. Regular pedicure including foot service to improve circulation.	General pedicure advice. Foot exercises and massage to improve circulation.
Bunions	Long-term wear of ill-fitting shoes, especially those with high heels or pointed toe areas. A weakness in the arches of the feet.	The large joint at the base of the big toe protrudes, forcing the big toe inwards towards the other toes.	None – refer the client to a chiropodist if the bunion is painful; gentle massage may help to ease any pain or discomfort.	Try to keep pressure off the affected area.
Calluses	Incorrect footwear.	Thick, yellowish, hardened patches of skin, usually found on prominent areas of the foot such as the heel and the ball of toe: may be painful.	Use a rasp or pumice stone gently to remove any build-up of hard skin: painful calluses should be treated by a chiropodist.	Ensure that shoes fit correctly. Avoid standing for long periods. Alternate style of footwear regularly Keep the skin of the foot moisturised with a specialized skin conditioner for the feet. Use a pumice stone regularly to remove excess skin.
Chilblains	Poor blood supply to the hands and feet, aggravated in cold weather.	Fingers and toes may be red, blue or purple in colour; the client may complain of painful or itchy area.	Regular pedicures, with special attention paid to massage which will help to improve the circulation.	Keep affected areas warm and dry. Avoid tight footwear, which might restrict the circulation. If the condition is severe, seek medical advice.

WELLCOME

MEDISCAN

DR A L WRIGHT

MEDISCAN

Disorder	*Cause*	*Appearance*	*Salon service*	*Homecare advice*
Corns 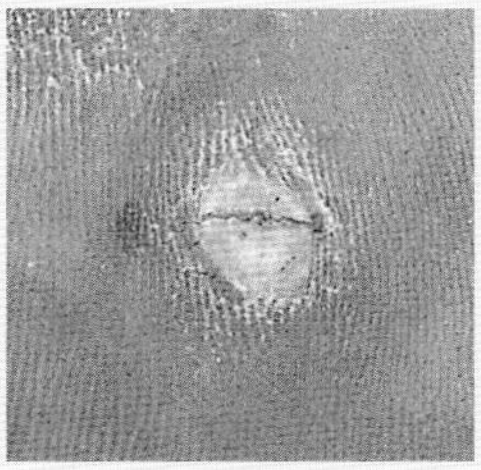 DR A L WRIGHT	Incorrect footwear (corns are often found on toes which have been squeezed together by tight shoes).	Similar to calluses except that the affected area is smaller and more compact; corns often look white, and may be extremely painful.	Small corns may be treated in the same way as a callus, but if the client has large or painful corns she should be treated by a chiropodist.	Ensure that shoes fit correctly. Avoid standing for long periods. Alternate style of footwear regularly.
Pitting (shown on the fingernail) 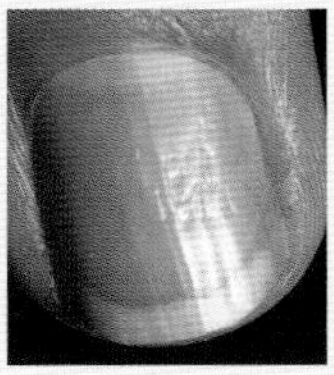 WELLCOME	Eczema and/or psoriasis.	Pitting, resembling small, irregular pin pricks, appear on the nail plate.	Refer the client to their GP for permission to treat if required. Regular pedicure with gentle buffing.	General pedicure advice. Ridge-filling base coat polish.

Contra-actions

Certain cosmetic ingredients are known to cause allergic reactions in some people.

The client – or the pedicurist – may at some time develop an allergy to a pedicure product that has been successfully used previously. This could be for a number of reasons, including new medication being taken or illness. This is known as a **contra-action**. This may occur during or following a pedicure service.

The symptoms of an allergic reaction could be:

- redness of the skin (erythema)
- swelling
- itching
- raised blisters

The symptoms do not necessarily appear on the feet. In the case of nail polish allergy, the symptoms often show up on the face.

In the case of an allergic reaction:

- Remove the offending product immediately, using water or, in the case of polish, nail polish solvent.
- Apply a cool compress and soothing agent to the skin to reduce redness and irritation.
- If symptoms persist, seek medical advice.

Always record any allergies on the client's record card, so that the offending product may be avoided in future.

Other contra-actions could occur as a result of incorrect use of pedicure tools, i.e. sore, sensitized skin following hard skin removal. Sore, reddened skin in the cuticle area due to excessive trimming of the cuticle.

HEALTH & SAFETY

Contact dermatitis

Contact dermatitis is a skin problem caused by intolerance of the skin to a particular substance or a group of substances. On exposure to the substance the skin quickly becomes irritated and an allergic reaction occurs. This may occur when a manicurist's skin is exposed to dust and chemicals on a regular basis. Follow all HSE guidelines to reduce the risk of developing this skin disorder which could result in the need for a career change!

Always follow manufacturers' guidelines on the use of products.

ALWAYS REMEMBER

Accurately record your client's answers to necessary questions to be asked at consultation on the record card.

Outcome 3: Carry out pedicure service

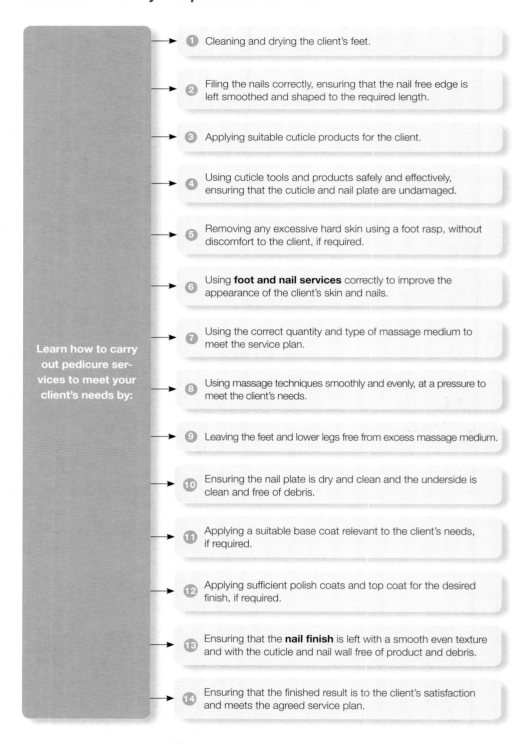

Learn how to carry out pedicure services to meet your client's needs by:

1. Cleaning and drying the client's feet.

2. Filing the nails correctly, ensuring that the nail free edge is left smoothed and shaped to the required length.

3. Applying suitable cuticle products for the client.

4. Using cuticle tools and products safely and effectively, ensuring that the cuticle and nail plate are undamaged.

5. Removing any excessive hard skin using a foot rasp, without discomfort to the client, if required.

6. Using **foot and nail services** correctly to improve the appearance of the client's skin and nails.

7. Using the correct quantity and type of massage medium to meet the service plan.

8. Using massage techniques smoothly and evenly, at a pressure to meet the client's needs.

9. Leaving the feet and lower legs free from excess massage medium.

10. Ensuring the nail plate is dry and clean and the underside is clean and free of debris.

11. Applying a suitable base coat relevant to the client's needs, if required.

12. Applying sufficient polish coats and top coat for the desired finish, if required.

13. Ensuring that the **nail finish** is left with a smooth even texture and with the cuticle and nail wall free of product and debris.

14. Ensuring that the finished result is to the client's satisfaction and meets the agreed service plan.

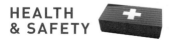

HEALTH & SAFETY

Always remove products hygienically from containers to avoid contamination and cross-infection.

Carrying out pedicure services
Step-by-step: Pedicure procedure

This process briefly shows the stages in the pedicure. Each step is discussed in detail later in the chapter. The procedure may start with either the right or left foot.

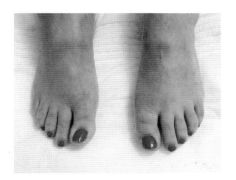

1 Nails before pedicure procedure.

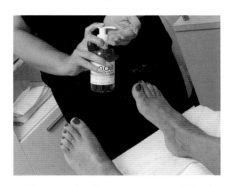

2 Clean your hands using an approved hand cleaning technique.

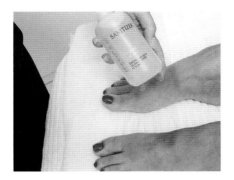

3 Wipe both feet including between the toes with cotton wool soaked in skin disinfectant (product example shown here) or a specialized hygiene spray for the feet. Use separate pieces of cotton wool for each foot.

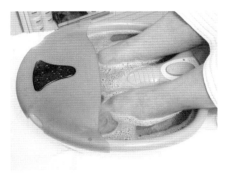

4 Soak both feet in warm water to which a liquid soap or a similar appropriate product has been added. Take out left foot and towel dry it.

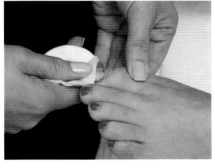

5 Remove any existing nail polish, and check again for contraindications below the nail plate. (If a nail contra-indication is present service must not continue. Tactfully explain why and give appropriate referral advice.)

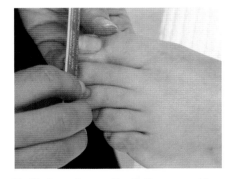

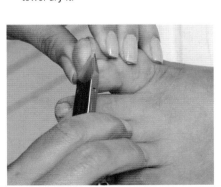

6 Cut the toenails straight across, using toenail clippers or scissors.

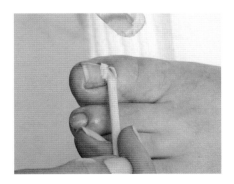

7 File the nails smooth with the coarse side of the emery board. Again do not shape the nails at the sides to avoid ingrowing nails.

8 Apply cuticle massage cream or oil.

9 Place the foot back in the water.

10 Remove the right foot and repeat steps **5–10**.

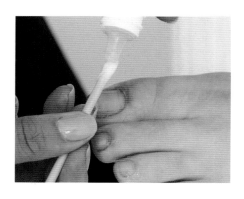

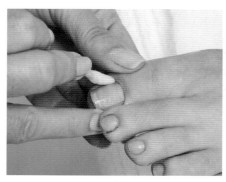

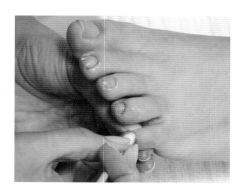

11 Dry the left foot and apply cuticle remover.

To avoid excessive application and contaminating the applicator apply to a cotton wool-tipped orange stick.

12 Push back the cuticles with a cotton wool-tipped orange stick, hoof stick or cuticle pusher.

13 Clean under the free edge with a separate cotton wool-tipped orange stick.

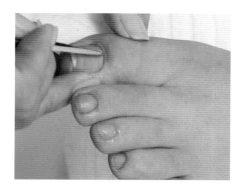

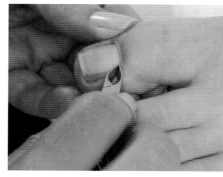

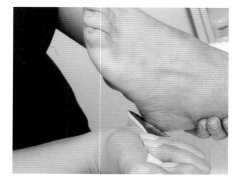

14 Use the cuticle knife where indicated to remove excess eponychium and periony-chium. Collect excess skin in a tissue or a clean piece of cotton wool and dispose of immediately.

15 Wipe off any remaining cuticle remover with damp cotton wool, and file the nails again if necessary. Apply cuticle oil.

16 Use cuticle nippers where necessary to remove excess cuticle.

17 Remove any hard skin. This may be done with exfoliating cream, pedicure callous file or a rasp, depending on the severity of the condition.

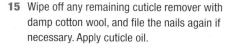

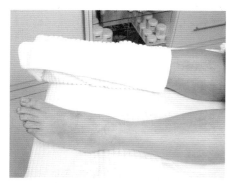

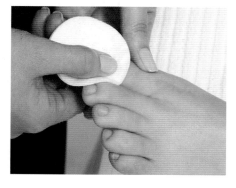

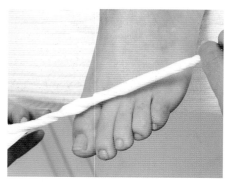

18 Wrap the foot in a dry towel and to keep it warm.

19 Repeat steps **12–19** for the other foot.

20 Remove the foot bowl from the working area.

21 Perform a foot and lower leg massage. (See pp 427–429.)

22 Remove any grease from the nail plates with a cotton wool pad soaked in nail polish remover. Refile the nails as necessary to ensure they are smooth and even.

23 Place disposable toe separators or other hygienic equivalent to separate them and facilitate polish application.

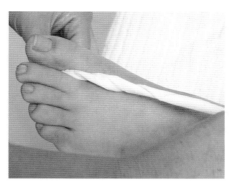

23 Continued.

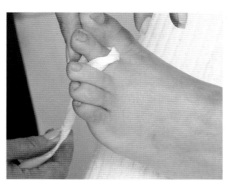

23 Continued.

24 Apply the polish: base coat (once), cream polish (twice) and top coat (once) where indicated. If a pearlized polish is used a top coat is not required and a third coat of polish may be applied.

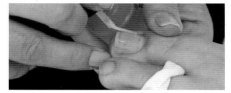

24a Application of base coat.

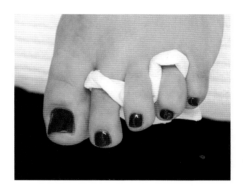

24b Application of first coat of polish

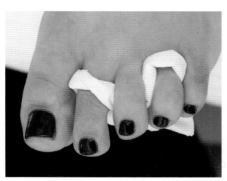

24c Application of second coat of coloured polish.

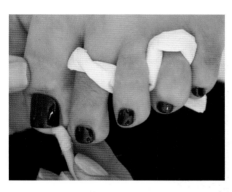

(A cotton wool-tipped orange stick may be used to apply nail polish remover to remove any excess polish from the surrounding skin.)

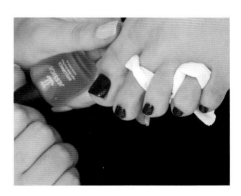

24d Application of top coat as the product is a cream polish, requiring a top coat.

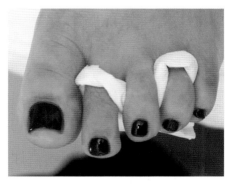

25 The complete dark polish pedicure

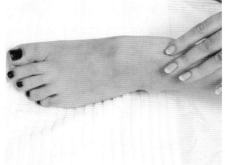

Complete nail service. (French polish application shown as illustrated in the manicure chapter.)

Cutting and filing toenails

Toenails should be cut straight across, using nail clippers or strong sharp scissors, then filed smooth using the coarse side of the emery board. This helps to avoid ingrowing

HEALTH & SAFETY

Disposing of waste

All waste should be disposed of as instructed by your local authority requirements and the Industry Code of Practice for Nail Services.

HEALTH & SAFETY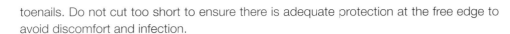

Cutting toenails

Never cut toenails down at the sides. This increases the chance of ingrowing toenails, and may lead to infection.

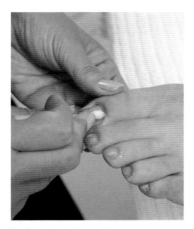

Pushing back the cuticles

toenails. Do not cut too short to ensure there is adequate protection at the free edge to avoid discomfort and infection.

Cuticle work Cuticle work is carried out to keep the cuticle area attractive and also to prevent cuticles from adhering to the nail plate, which could lead to splitting of the cuticle as the nail grows forward, and subsequently to infection of the area.

The work is carried out after soaking the feet in warm soapy water. This step loosens dirty particles from the free edge and softens the skin in the cuticle area.

How to provide cuticle work Cuticle work on the feet follows the same principles and cuticle work on the hands. For a detailed description, see Chapter 12, pages 390–391.

HEALTH & SAFETY

If you accidentally cut the skin causing bleeding at the cuticle area, protect you hands with disposable gloves and wipe the skin with an antiseptic wipe. Any waste is classed as clinical waste or contaminated waste and should be disposed of in a yellow medical bin liner in accordance with the **Environmental Act (1990)** and **Controlled Waste Regulations (1992).**

See Habia *Hygiene in the Beauty Therapy* booklet for further guidance.

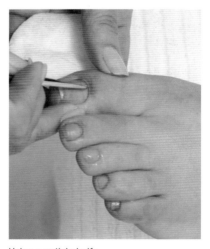

Using a cuticle knife

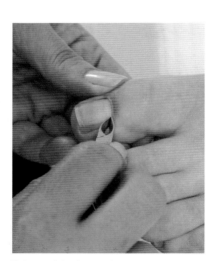

Using cuticle nippers

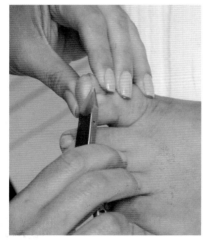

Cutting toenails

Removing hard skin

Hard skin develops on the feet as a form of protection, either from friction from footwear or from standing for long periods of time.

It is therefore not advisable to remove *all* the hard skin from an area, as this would remove the protective pad. Hard skin should be removed only to improve the appearance of the feet. Hard skin build-up that causes pain or discomfort should be referred to a chiropodist for treatment.

Excess hard skin may be removed from the feet in a number of ways, including exfoliators, pumice stones, callus files, chiropody sponges, and corn planes. Exfoliators should be used with a deep circular massage movement: they are ideal when only a very small build-up of hard skin is present. Files, pumice stones and the rest should be used with a

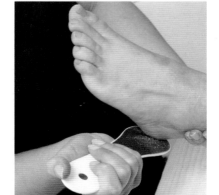

Removing hard skin with a pumice file

swift stroking movement in one direction only (similar to buffing). Sawing back and forth would lead to friction, and discomfort for the client.

Always finish off a hard skin removal procedure with the application of a specialized foot moisturiser or lotion, to soften the newly exposed skin.

Foot and nail services

In addition to the pedicure, further services may be added as appropriate. Here are some examples:

- **Exfoliating service** is carried out prior to massage or as part of the massage routine. An abrasive massage cream is massaged over the skin of the foot in circular movements, concentrating over the ball and heel of the foot. Exfoliation removes dead skin, increases blood circulation and improves the condition and appearance of the skin and the absorption of further service products.

- **Foot service mask** is applied according to the client's service requirements. The mask is applied to the skin, then covered with a plastic protective cover and the feet can then be wrapped in warm thermal booties to aid the absorption of the mask. The mask removes dead skin cells, improves blood circulation and improves the condition of the skin of the feet.

- **Paraffin wax service** – this wax is heated in a special bath to a temperature of 50–55°C. The heating effect stimulates the blood circulation, eases the discomfort of arthritic and rheumatic conditions, and softens the skin, improving the appearance and condition of dry skin.

  After checking the client's tolerance to the wax temperature, the client's whole foot and ankle is covered with paraffin wax. The liquid wax is usually applied with a brush. The initial wax application quickly sets, becoming solid and then further layers of paraffin wax are applied to provide a waterproof covering. Once applied the feet should then be placed in a plastic protective covering and covered with towelling booties. The wax may be removed after 10–15 minutes. It is a good idea to remove the wax with the plastic covering, which is usually in one action. After use the wax is disposed of.

- **Thermal booties** are electrically heated booties. They are used to stimulate, rejuvenate and moisturise the skin of the feet. The feet are prepared with the application of a foot service mask, protected in a plastic covering and placed inside warm booties for ten minutes to enable the mask to penetrate the skin of the epidermis.

Always follow manufacturers' guidelines in the application procedure for feet and nail services.

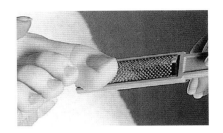
Removing hard skin with a rasp

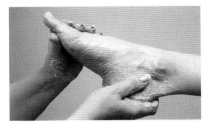
Exfoliating service

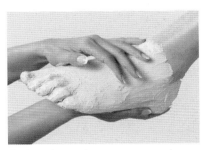
Foot service mask

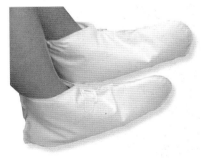
Thermal booties

ELLISONS

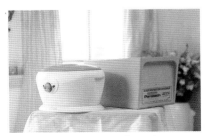
Paraffin wax tools and equipment

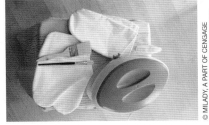

© MILADY, A PART OF CENGAGE LEARNING, PHOTOGRAPHY BY DINO PETROCELLI

TOP TIP

Paraffin wax

Heat the wax at least half an hour before the client arrives to ensure it has melted properly. Paraffin wax may have essential oils added to enhance the therapeutic effects.

Step-by-step: Specialist foot and leg service

Specialist services should be offered to your client when there is a specific need or if they feel they would like to benefit from such a service. Specialist service training in these advanced techniques is usually offered by major product companies.

The model for this specialist foot and leg service is a client who regularly visits the gym and wished to benefit from a spa therapy revitalizing service following a workout.

The following foot and leg service will:

- stimulate the blood circulation
- aid with the removal of toxins and waste products
- have a skin-cleansing action
- remove dead skin cells (desquamation)
- improve the moisture content of the skin
- relax tense/stiff muscles in the foot and leg

Your services should be adapted the meet the service objectives for the client. Allow 30 minutes for the specialist foot and leg service below.

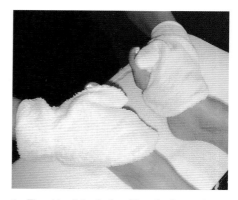

1 The skin of the feet and legs is cleansed using warm towelling mitts infused with lime oil for its therapeutic refreshing and energizing properties.

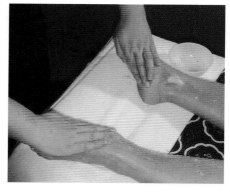

2 The feet and legs are exfoliated to remove all dead skin cells and brighten the skin. A sea salt-based preparation with emollient, skin softening ingredients is applied to each foot and leg.

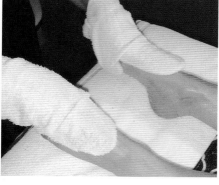

3 Towelling mitts are used to remove the exfoliating service. These have been steamed and are warm when used.

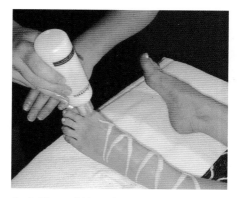

4 A skin-nourishing milk lotion is applied to each foot and leg using a 'drizzling' technique. The milk is particularly beneficial for dry skin.

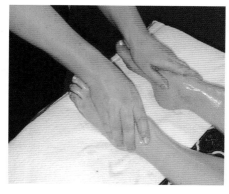

5 Massage movements are applied using *effleurage* and *petrissage* manipulations to introduce the massage medium into the skin.

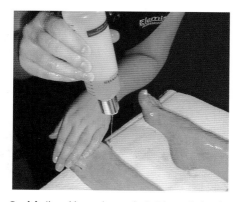

6 A further skin service product oil is applied and massaged into the skin. This will act as a service mask for the skin to soften and condition.

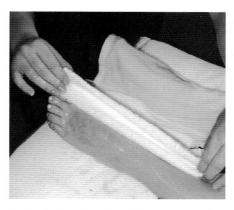 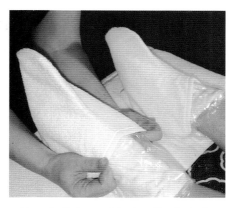

7 The feet are then placed in steamed towels, encased in a plastic bag and dry towelling foot mitten for 10–15 minutes.

Foot and lower leg massage

As with a manicure massage, the pedicure massage is carried out near the end of the service, prior to nail polishing. The pedicure massage includes the foot and the lower leg, and offers the following benefits to the client as follows:

- moisturises the skin with the massage medium, cream, lotion or oil
- increases blood circulation to the lower leg and foot
- helps maintain joint mobility
- eases discomfort from arthritis or rheumatism
- relaxes the client
- muscle tone is improved as the muscles receive an improved supply of oxygenated blood, essential for cell growth
- lymphatic circulation is improved aiding the removal of waste products from the body
- helps remove any dead skin cells (desquamation)

The massage incorporates classic massage movements, each with different effects:

- **Effleurage** – a stroking movement, used to begin the massage as a link manipulation, and to complete the massage sequence.
- **Petrissage** – movements, including **kneading**, where the tissues are lifted away from the underlying structures and compressed. Pressure is intermittent, and should be light yet firm.
- Tapotement, also known as **percussion**, may be included – tapotement movements are performed in a brisk, stimulating manner to increase blood supply and improve tone of the skin and muscles. Movements include clapping and tapping.

The therapist can adapt the massage application according to the needs of the client. Either the *speed of application* or *depth of pressure* can be altered.

Step-by-step: Foot and lower leg massage

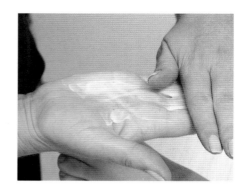
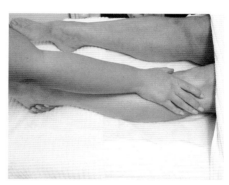

1 Dispense the massage medium into the hands, warm the product over the palms and apply to the client's skin using effleurage technique.

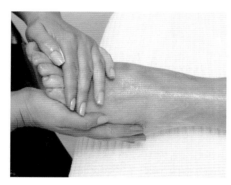
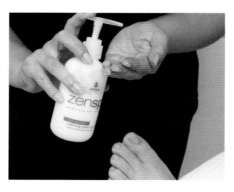
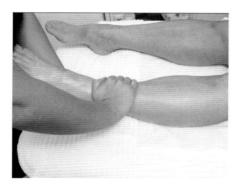

2 **Effleurage from the foot to the knee** Use long sweeping strokes from the toes to the knee, moving on both the back and the front of the leg.

Repeat step 2 a further 5 times.

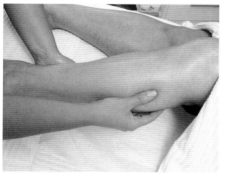
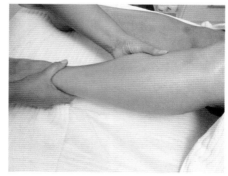
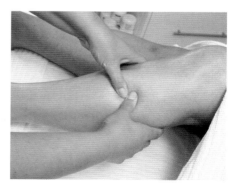

3 Flex the client's knee and using a petrissage movement in an upwards direction pick-up, and gently squeeze the gastrocnemius muscle.

4 Slide the palm down to the ankle and using the thumbs knead gently upwards along the tibialis anterior muscles on the outer shin.

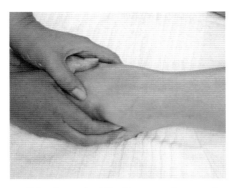

5 Using the pads of the fingers perform small circular kneading movements around the malleolus (ankle) bone. Massage both sides of the ankle bone at the same time.

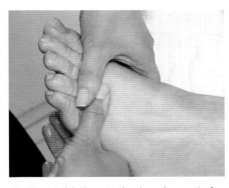

6 **Thumb frictions to the dorsal aspect of the foot** Use the thumbs, one in front of the other, and move backwards and forwards in a gentle sawing action. Move from the toes to the ankle, then slide back down to the toes.

   Repeat step 6 a further 2 times.

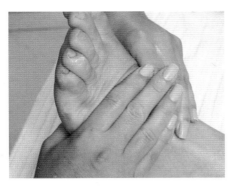

7 **Thumb frictions to the plantar aspect of the foot** Use the same movement as in step 6, but on the sole of the foot, moving from the toes to the heel.

   Repeat step 7 a further 2 times.

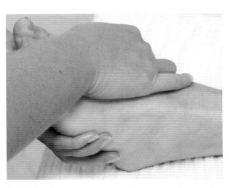

8 **Palm kneading to the plantar surface of the foot** Place the heel of the hand into the arch of the foot and massage with deep circular movements.

   Repeat step 8 a further 5 times.

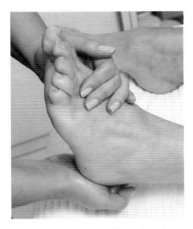
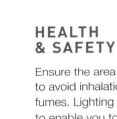

9 Support the foot with one hand and using the palm cup the heel and perform a circular kneading movement.

HEALTH & SAFETY

Ensure the area is well ventilated to avoid inhalation of excessive fumes. Lighting should be good to enable you to avoid eyestrain. It is a good idea to use a table lamp when painting the nails.

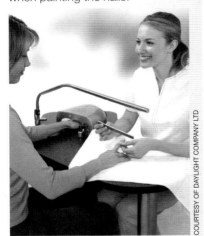

A nail work station with lamp

COURTESY OF DAYLIGHT COMPANY LTD

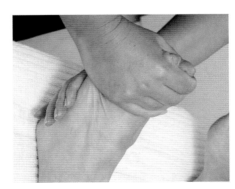

10 Place the hand either side of the toes; gently press together and rotate all the toes three times clockwise and three times anticlockwise.

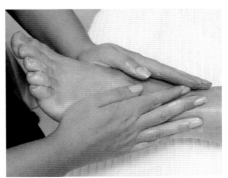

11 Effleurage from the foot to the knee. Use the same movements as in step 2.

   Repeat step 11 a further 5 times.

Nail polish application

Nail polish is applied to coat the nail plate for a numbers of reasons:

- to adorn the nail
- to disguise stained toenails
- to improve the condition and appearance of the nail
- to co-ordinate with clothes
- to create designs and effects called 'nail art'

Types of polish

- **Cream** – this has a matt finish, and requires a top coat application to give a sheen.
- **Pearlized** – this has a frosted, shimmery appearance by the addition of natural fish scales or synthetic ingredients such as bismuth oxychloride.
- **Base coat** – this protects the nail from staining by a strong coloured nail polish; it also gives a good grip to polish, and smoothes out minor surface irregularities.
- **Top coat** – this gives a sheen to cream polish, and adds longer wear as it helps to prevent chipping.

Contra-indication to nail polish Do not apply polish in these circumstances:

- if there are diseases and disorders of the nail plate and surrounding skin
- if the client is allergic to nail polish

How to apply nail polish Before nail polish is applied any jewellery worn in the area may replaced to avoid smudging afterwards.

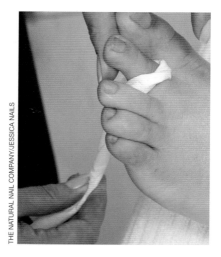

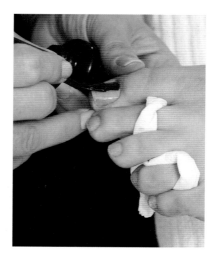

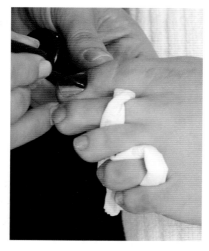

THE NATURAL NAIL COMPANY/JESSICA NAILS

1 Place disposable toe separators or other hygienic equivalent to separate them and facilitate polish application.

2 After ensuring that the nail plate is free from oil, start with the big toe. Apply three to four brush strokes down the length of the nail from the cuticle to the free edge, beginning in the centre, then down either side close to the nail wall.

Take care to avoid touching the cuticle or nail wall. If flooding occurs, remove the polish immediately with an orange stick and nail polish remover.

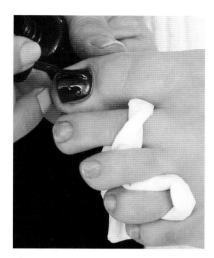

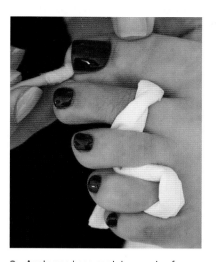

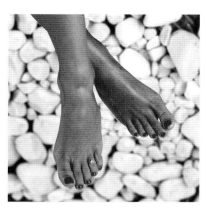

2 Continued.

3 Apply one base coat, two coats of coloured polish and one top coat. Top coat is required only after using cream polish; pearl polish does not need a top coat but a third coat of polish may be applied.

Ready for the holidays

Styles of application

- **Traditional application** – This style is one of the most commonly requested by clients: the entire plate is covered with polish.

- **French application** – This style involves painting the nail plate of the nail pink or pale beige, and the free edge white.

See Chapter 12, pages 396-398 for further information about nail polish application, including tips why it may chip or peel, and how to store.

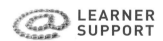

LEARNER SUPPORT

Pedicure true or false?

Outcome 4: Provide aftercare advice

Learn how to provide aftercare advice which supports and meets the needs of your client by:

1 Giving **advice** and recommendations accurately and constructively.

2 Giving your clients suitable **advice** specific to their individual needs.

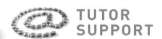

TUTOR SUPPORT

Activity 3: Home care advice handout

Offering aftercare advice at the end of a pedicure service will help the client to look after their feet between salon visits, and is also an ideal opportunity to recommend retail products.

Aftercare advice will differ slightly for each client according to individual needs, but generally it will be as follows:

- Change socks or tights daily.

- Apply moisturising lotion daily to the feet preferably after bathing when the skin is softened.

- Ensure that the feet are thoroughly dry after washing, especially between the toes.

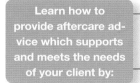

BEST PRACTICE

Advise on further professional services.

If a client has dry skin on her heels, take the opportunity to recommend an **exfoliant** service for her next appointment.

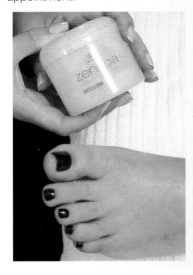

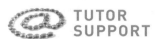

TUTOR SUPPORT

Activity 5: Promote luxury pedicure task

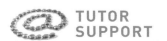

TUTOR SUPPORT

Activity 4: Pedicure wordsearch

- Apply talcum powder or a special foot powder between the toes to help absorb moisture.

- Foot sprays containing peppermint or citrus oil to cleanse and refresh are useful to refresh the feet during the day.

- Go barefoot wherever it is safe and practical to do so.

- Ensure that footwear fits properly. Foot problems such as bunions can be aggravated by incorrect footwear.

- Avoid wearing high heels for long periods of time. They can cause postural problems and increase hard skin callus formation.

- Advise on appropriate nail/skincare products to remedy the problems present, e.g. dry skin, nails, stained nails.

- Advise the client of any other professional services you could recommend.

- Advise the client on a service plan to improve the nail/skin condition and the time intervals recommended between each service.

- When filing the nails, always file straight across in one direction.

- If any pain is felt in the feet visit a chiropodist.

- It is also necessary to advise the client what to do in the event of a contra-action.

Have retail products available for the client to purchase. These include emery boards, coloured nail polishes, nail polish remover and nail/skin service products.

It is a good idea to have available the nail polish colours that you have used. The client can then touch up any accidental chips themselves.

Recommend the use of top coat applied every three to four days to protect the nail polish, increase its durability and impart shine.

Finally, at the end of the pedicure service ensure the clients records are updated, accurate and signed by the client and pedicurist. Ensure the finished result is to the client's satisfaction and meets the agreed treatment plan.

Exercises for the feet and ankles As part of the homecare advice given to a pedicure client **foot exercises** should be mentioned – these can play a very important role in keeping the client's feet healthy. They help:

- to stimulate circulation

- to keep joints mobilized, allowing a greater range of movement in the toes and ankles

- to keep muscles strong, reducing the chance of fallen arches (flat feet)

Here are some examples of exercises:

1 Sitting on a chair with the feet flat on the floor raise the toes upwards and then relax

2 Stand on tiptoes, and relax down again

3 Sitting on a chair with the feet flat on the floor, lift one leg slightly and draw a circle with the toes so that the ankle moves through its full range of movement

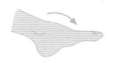 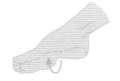 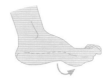

Dorsiflexion   Plantar flexion   Inversion   Eversion

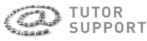

TUTOR SUPPORT

Activity 7: Re-cap, revision and evaluation

4 **Dorsiflexion:** bending the foot backwards towards the body

5 **Plantar flexion:** pointing the foot down towards the ground

6 **Inversion:** moving the foot inwards towards the middle of the body

7 **Eversion:** moving the foot out towards the side of the body

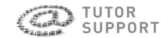

TUTOR SUPPORT

Activity 8: Multiple choice quiz

GLOSSARY OF KEY WORDS

Aftercare advice recommendations given to the client following service to continue the benefits of the service.

Base coat a nail polish product applied to protect the natural nail and prevent staining from coloured nail polish.

Blue nail nail condition where the nail bed has a blue tinge rather than a healthy pink colour due to poor blood circulation in the area.

Bruised nail nail condition where the nail appears blue/black in colour where bleeding has occurred on the nail bed following injury.

Bunion a foot condition. The large joint at the base of the big toe protrudes, forcing the big toe inwards towards the other toes.

Callus foot condition, displaying thick, yellowish hardened skin, usually found on prominent areas of the foot such as the heel.

Chilblains poor blood supply where the toes become red, blue or purple in colour and the area may become painful and itchy; aggravated in cold weather.

Chiropodist a person who is trained and qualified to treat minor foot complaints.

Client groups this term is used in a number of the units and it refers to client diversity. The CRE (Commission for Racial Equality) ethnic group classification is used in the range for these units. These cover white, mixed, Asian, black and Chinese.

Consultation assessment of client's needs using different assessment techniques, including questioning and natural observation.

Contact dermatitis a skin disorder caused by intolerance of the skin to a particular substance, or a group of substances. On exposure to the substance the skin quickly becomes irritated and an allergic reaction occurs.

Contra-action an unwanted reaction occurring during or after service application.

Contra-indication a problematic symptom that indicates that the service may not proceed.

Corn small areas of thickened skin on the foot. Often white in appearance.

Cuticle cream or oil a cosmetic preparation used to condition the skin of the cuticle.

Cuticle knife a metal tool used on the nail to remove excess eponychium and perionychium (the extension of the skin of the cuticle at the base of the nail).

Cuticle nippers a metal tool used to remove excess cuticle and neaten the skin around the cuticle area.

Cuticle remover a cosmetic preparation used to soften and loosen the skin cells and cuticle from the nail.

Diabetes a disease that prevents sufferers breaking down glucose in their cells.

Eczema of the nail inflammation of the skin; different changes to the nail

may occur including ridges, pitting, nail separation and nail thickening.

Effleurage a stroking massage movement, used to begin the massage, as a link manipulation and to complete the massage sequence.

Emery board a nail file used to shape the free edge of the nail.

Exfoliant a mild abrasive cream applied and massaged over the skin's surface to remove dead skin cells and improve the appearance and texture of the skin.

Foot and nail services specialized products and equipment designed to improve the condition and appearance of different nail and skin conditions.

Foot cream/oil a cosmetic mixture of waxes and oils applied to soften the skin of the feet and cuticles.

Foot rasp a pedicure tool used to remove excess dead skin from the foot.

Foot spa a foot bath incorporating massage and water aeration, creating a bubbling effect to cleanse and relax the feet.

Hoof stick a nail tool used to gently push back the cuticles when softened.

Ingrowing toenails nail condition where the side of the nail penetrates the nail wall; redness, inflammation and pus may be present.

Mask a service mask applied to the skin of the feet to treat and improve the condition of the skin; this may include stimulating, rejuvenating or moisturising properties.

Nail finish the product finally applied to the natural nail to enhance its appearance, e.g. choice of polish application.

Nail polish a clear or coloured nail product that adds colour/protection to the nail. Cream polish has a matt finish and requires a top coat application. Pearlized polish produces a frosted, shimmery appearance and top coat is not required.

Nail polish drier an aerosol or oil preparation applied following nail polish application to increase the speed at which the polish hardens.

Nail polish remover a solvent used to remove nail polish and grease from the nails prior to applying polish. Nail polish solvent used to thin nail polish and restore its consistency.

Necessary action the appropriate action to take in the case of a contra-action or contra-indication to ensure the welfare of the client.

Onycholysis nail condition where the nail plate separates from the nail bed.

Orange stick a disposable wooden tool used around the cuticle and free edge of the nail and to apply products to the nail.

Paraffin wax this is heated and applied to the skin of the feet to provide a heating effect. This improves skin functioning, aids the absorption of service products and is beneficial to ease the discomfort of arthritic and rheumatic conditions.

Paronychia bacterial infection where swelling, redness and pus appears in the cuticle area of the nail wall.

Pedicure a service to care for and improve the condition and appearance of the skin and nails of the feet.

Petrissage massage movements, including kneading, where the tissues are lifted away from the underlying structures and compressed. Pressure is intermittent, and should be light yet firm.

Psoriasis of the nail an inflammatory condition where there is an increased production of cells in the upper part of the skin. Pitting occurs on the surface of the nail.

Scissors nail tools used to shorten the length of the nail before filing.

Service plan after the consultation, suitable service objectives are established to treat the client's conditions and needs.

Tapotement, also known as percussion, massage movements performed in a brisk, stimulating manner to increase blood supply and improve tone of the skin and muscles. Movements include clapping and tapping.

Thermal booties electrically heated boots in which the feet are placed following the application of a skin service product such as a mask. The heat aids the absorption of the product and improves skin functioning.

Tinea corporis or body ringworm fungal infection of the skin where small scaly red patches, which spread outwards and then heal from the centre, leave a ring.

Tinea pedis or athlete's foot fungal infection of the foot occurring in the webs of the skin between the toes. Small blisters form, which later burst. The skin in the area can become dry with a scaly appearance.

Tinea unguium fungal infection of the nails. The nail is yellowish-grey in colour.

Top coat nail polish product applied over another nail polish to provide additional strength and durability to the finish.

Verruca or plantar wart a viral infection where small epidermal skin growths appear, either raised or flat depending upon their location, and have a rough surface.

ASSESSMENT OF KNOWLEDGE AND UNDERSTANDING

Having covered the learning objectives for **Provide pedicure services**, test what you need to know and understand answering the following short questions below.

The information covers:

- organizational and legal requirements

- how to work safely and effectively when performing pedicure services

- consult, plan and prepare for the service with clients

- contra-indications and contra-actions

- pedicure services

- aftercare advice for clients

Organizational and legal requirements

For full legislation details, see Chapter 4.

1 What information does the industry Code of Practice for Nails provide?

2 What actions must be taken before a client under 16 years of age receives a pedicure?

3 How can you ensure compliance with the legislation of the Disability Discrimination Act?

4 How can cross-infection be avoided when carrying out pedicure services? State three examples.

5 How should all client records be stored to comply with the Data protection Act (1998)?

6 What is the commercially acceptable service time for a basic pedicure and a specialized pedicure including a foot and nail service?

7 Why is it important for staff to be familiar with the different pedicure pricing structures?

8 What details should be recorded on the client's record card? Why is it important to keep accurate records which are maintained?

9 How can you ensure that the position of the client for pedicure minimizes potential risk of injury to yourself?

How to work safely and effectively when performing pedicure services

1 What personal protective equipment may be used when performing pedicure and explain its purpose?

2 What are the symptoms of the skin disorder Non-glass and how can it be caused when performing pedicure services? What steps could you take to minimize the risk of developing contact dermatitis?

3 What environmental conditions should you check are adequate to work safely and effectively when providing nail services?

4 Taking into account client comfort and modesty, why is it important that the client is correctly prepared for service?

5 What are the methods of disinfecting and sterilizing tools and equipment? Give three examples of tools and equipment that are sterilized and disinfected.

6 Give three effects on the nail and skin of the incorrect use of pedicure tools.

7 Personal presentation and hygiene is important to create a good impression. Give three examples relevant to the Code of Practice for Nails of good personal presentation and hygiene practice.

8 Why is it important to complete your pedicure service in the allocated time?

9 Why is it advisable to dispose of waste in a lined, metal bin with a lid?

10 Why is it good practice to maintain the appearance of your work station and keep it orderly?

Consult, plan and prepare for the service with clients

1 What is the purpose of the client consultation? What communication techniques are important to use in your consultation to gather all the information you require?

2 Why is it important to assess the condition of the client's foot and nail condition before service commences?

3 What should be considered when designing a pedicure service plan for a client?

4 Why would you not diagnose a contra-indication when performing the foot and nails analyzis?

5 What is the legal significance of the record card if a client was unhappy with the service plan?

6 Why should you encourage the client to ask questions related to her pedicure service before it commences?

Contra-indications and contra-actions

1 Name three contra-indications observed at the consultation that would prevent a pedicure being carried out?

2 What conditions, if present, would restrict your pedicure application?

3 Why is diabetes considered a contra-indication to pedicure service?

4 Name three contra-actions that could occur during or following a pedicure service?

5 What advice should be given to a client who develops an allergic reaction to a product following a pedicure service?

Anatomy and physiology

For full anatomy and physiology details, see Chapter 2.

1 How many bones form the foot? Name them.

2 Name the bones of the lower leg.

3 Name the main arteries of the lower leg.

4 Name the two muscles of the foot.

5 Name two muscles of the lower leg.

Pedicure Services

1 What service products would you recommend for dry nails, discoloured nails and overgrown cuticles?

2 When would you choose to include the following foot and nail services in your service plan:

- heat services?

- exfoliation?

3 Why should the toenail be cut and filed straight across and not shaped at the corners?

4 What is the purpose of the soaking medium usually added to the warm water to soak the client's feet?

5 Describe the methods available for removing hard skin from the feet?

6 How should the skin be left following hard skin removal?

7 Name three service products used in pedicure and their effect on the nail, cuticle or skin of the foot as applicable.

8 How may you adapt your pedicure service when treating a male client?

9 How is the quantity and type of massage medium selected for each client?

10 How and why should massage be adapted for each client?

11 State four benefits of foot and leg massage.

12 What are the terms used for the different types of massage applied in a pedicure?

13 Why should grease and debris be removed from the nail plate prior to nail polish application?

14 What is the correct technique for removing polish from the nails?

15 How is the type if base coat selected for a client?

16 How many coats of polish are usually applied with:

- cream polish?

- pearlized polish?

17 Following nail polish application, how should the painted nail and cuticle appear?

18 Why are several services often required and recommended to improve the nail and skin condition?

19 Why should the client's records be up to date following each pedicure service?

Aftercare advice for clients

1 State the general aftercare advice that you would give to a pedicure client.

2 List three retail products that you could recommend to a pedicure client.

3 How often would you recommend a pedicure to maintain the condition and appearance of the nails and feet?

4 What advice would you give to a client about maintaining the length and shape of the toenails?

5 For each of the clients below suggest a service routine. Detail the service plan to include the cause of the condition, aims of the service, products used, services recommended, relevant retail sales and homecare advice:

- a middle-aged retail worker who has very hard, cracked skin on the soles of her feet around both heels

- an elderly male client who has little movement in his ankle joints and slightly distorted joints in his toes

- a pregnant client who has tired, aching feet and swollen ankles

14 Waxing Services (B6)

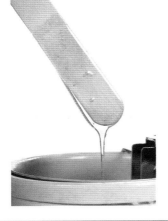

B6 Unit Learning Objectives

This chapter covers **Unit B6 Carry out waxing services**.
This unit is all about how to remove facial and body hair using temporary methods including hot wax and warm wax. The areas to be treated include the eyebrows, face, underarm, legs and bikini areas. Aftercare instruction is an important part of this service to promote skin healing.

There are **four** learning outcomes for Unit B6 which you must achieve competently:

1 Maintain safe and effective methods of working when removing hair by waxing

2 Consult, plan and prepare for the waxing service with clients

3 Remove unwanted hair

4 Provide aftercare advice

Your assessor will observe you on **at least four occasions**, each involving a different client.

From the **range** statement, you must show that you have:

● used all consultation techniques

● taken the **necessary action** where a contra-action, contra-indication or service modification occurs

● removed hair from all the **waxing treatment** areas

● used both hot and warm wax **products**

● used all waxing work techniques

● provided relevant **aftercare advice**

However, you must prove that you have the necessary knowledge, understanding and skills to be able to perform competently across the range.

When providing waxing services it is important to use the skills you have learnt in the following units:

Unit B5 Enhance appearance of eyebrows and eyelashes

(continued on the next page)

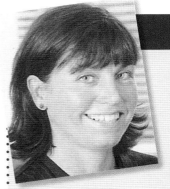

ROLE MODEL

Janice Brown
Director of HOF Beauty
(House of Famuir Ltd)

" My career journey has taken me from working in and later managing a group of salons, through, sales, teaching, training, research and development and I am currently director of HOF Beauty Ltd. Along the way I have specialized in electrolysis and hair removal. I am the co-author of *The Encyclopedia of Hair Removal* along with Gill Morris. I am proud to say that I have been able to make a real difference to people's lives by helping to correct skin, body and hair growth issues. I hope I have also been able to inspire and encourage fellow beauty therapists through the training I have provided. In the course of my career I have been fortunate enough to travel the world and work with wonderful people. Beauty therapy for me is not only a career but is a true passion.

(continued)

Unit G20 Make sure your own actions reduce risks to health and safety

Unit G18 Promote additional products or services to clients

Unit G8 Develop and maintain your effectiveness at work

Essential anatomy and physiology knowledge requirements for this unit, **B6**, are identified on the checklist in Chapter 2, page 16.

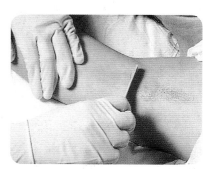

Hair removal

Hair removal methods

Hair removal is a popular service in the beauty salon, where both temporary and permanent methods of removal are usually available. Temporary removal must be repeated regularly, as the removed hair will regrow. With permanent methods, the client needs to visit the salon regularly to have the hair removed; thereafter, the part of the hair responsible for its growth has been destroyed and the hair will not grow again (see the hair growth diagram on page 33).

Temporary methods of hair removal

Depilatory waxing Wax depilation, using a warm, hot or cold wax, involves applying wax to the service area and embedding the hairs in it. When the wax is removed from the area, the hairs are removed also, at their roots so the regrowth is of completely new hairs with soft, fine-tapered tips. They grow again in approximately four weeks.

Plucking Plucking or tweezing uses a pair of tweezers to remove the hair. These grasp the hair near the surface of the skin, and the hair is then plucked in the direction of growth, again removing it at its root. The hair grows again in approximately four weeks.

Due to the sensitive nature of the eye tissue, tweezing is often considered the most suitable choice for temporary hair removal from eyebrows.

Threading Threading involves the use of a thread of twisted cotton, which is rolled over the area from which the hair is to be removed: the hairs catch in the cotton, and are pulled out. This skill is frequently practised by people of Asian or Mediterranean origin. Please see Chapter 17, for more information on this technique.

> **"** Waxing is one of, if not the most popular service on offer for beauty professionals. Clients therefore have a vast choice. By creating the right atmosphere, giving excellent service and paying attention to details you will encourage the client to return to *you* for their waxing service.
>
> **Janice Brown**

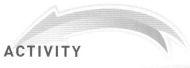

ACTIVITY

Hair removal
Make short notes on the suitability and effectiveness of the different methods of hair removal available.

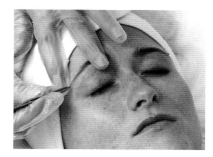

Plucking

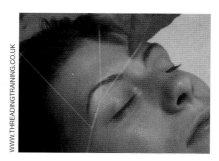

WWW.THREADINGTRAINING.CO.UK

Threading

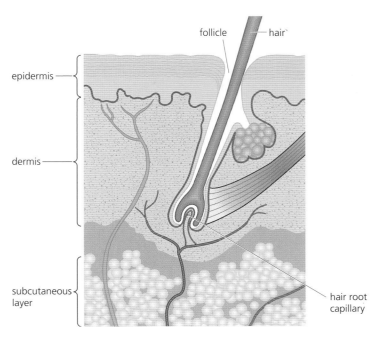

The hair in its follicle

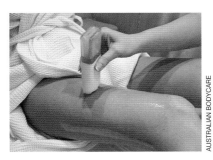

Depilatory waxing

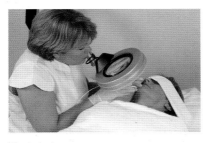

Electrolysis

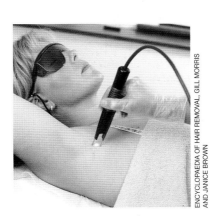

Laser hair removal

Waxing, plucking and threading removes the entire hair, including the visible hair above the skin's surface and the part that cannot be seen in the hair follicle.

Permanent methods of hair removal

Electrical current methods **Galvanic electrolysis, electrical epilation** and the **blend epilation technique** are all techniques that use an electrical current. The current is passed to the hair root via a fine needle inserted into the hair follicle. The current destroys the hair root, preventing hair regrowth.

Laser hair removal Laser energy works by producing light at various wave lengths, energy output and pulse widths. It is passed through the epidermis of the skin, which stops the activity of the hair follicle creating hair growth through a process called photothermolysis. The melanin pigment that provides hair colour absorbs the laser energy that is converted to heat, which at a sufficient temperature destroys the part of the hair follicle where the cells divide to create the hair.

The more melanin, the more destruction occurs. Therefore, generally laser hair removal works best for light-skinned people with dark hair.

A course of laser service is required. Service length will depend on the coarseness of the hair type and the size of the hair follicle. The service is most effective when the hair is in the anagen (growth) stage of the hair growth cycle. Subsequent services therefore target different hairs in their anagen stage of growth until all hairs cease to grow.

The client needs to understand that the hair will never grow back if effectively treated with any of the above permanent methods. This is an important consideration when treating the brow hair, as the desired shape and thickness of the brows change frequently under the influence of fashion.

Intensed Pulsed Light Intensed Pulsed Light (IPL) systems work on the same principle as laser; that of absorption of light energy into melanin in the skin and hair. The

HEALTH & SAFETY

Laser hair removal
Registration with the Care Quality Commission (CQC – www.cqc.org.uk) is a requirement to practise laser hair removal.

Part of their remit is to drive up quality of health care and they have a wide range of enforcement powers.

"For waxing services, it is important to keep your client warm. If your client becomes cold, the hair follicle will tighten around the hair, making the service more uncomfortable and the hair difficult to remove.

If it's a very cold day, at the skin preparation stage briskly rub or massage your client's skin with the preparatory products as this will increase blood supply thereby increasing skin temperature.

Janice Brown

ALWAYS REMEMBER

Waxing service legal requirements
Habia have provided a Code of Practice for Waxing. This should be referred to ensuring that you are complying with your responsibilities under relevant health and safety .

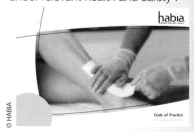

Habia Code of Practice for waxing

light energy is converted to heat energy which causes damage to the specific target area. There are two beams of light, one yellow and one red, which together affect both the existing hair and the follicles where the hair grows. The high-energy light pulses removes the hair.

IPL systems differ to laser in that they can deliver hundreds of wave lengths of light in each burst of light instead of just one wave length, increasing the area of skin that can be treated. Certain filters are used that target these flashes of light so that they can work in a similar way to lasers.

Other methods of hair removal

There are other methods of hair removal that the client may have used at home previously.

- ● *Cutting the hairs with scissors* Scissors are used to trim the hair close to the skin's surface.

- ● *Shaving* A razor blade is stroked over the skin, against the natural hair growth. This removes the hair at the skin's surface.

- ● *Depilatory cream* A strong alkaline chemical cream containing ammonium thioglycollate is applied to the hair, and removed after five to ten minutes: the hair will have been dissolved at the skin's surface.

- ● *Abrasive mitt* An abrasive glove is rubbed against the skin and the hair is broken off at the skin's surface.

Regrowth

Because of the cyclical nature of hair growth and the fact that follicles will be at different stages of their growth cycle when the hair is removed, the hair will not all grow back at the same time. Waxing, along with threading and plucking, can therefore appear to reduce the *quantity* of hair growth. This is not so, however, and the hair will all grow back eventually: waxing is therefore classed as a temporary form of hair removal.

Nevertheless, certain bodily changes (such as ageing), when *combined* with waxing, can result in permanent hair removal. This effect is so erratic and unpredictable, though, that waxing cannot reliably be sold as a permanent method of hair removal.

Outcome 1: Maintain safe and effective methods of working when removing hair by waxing services

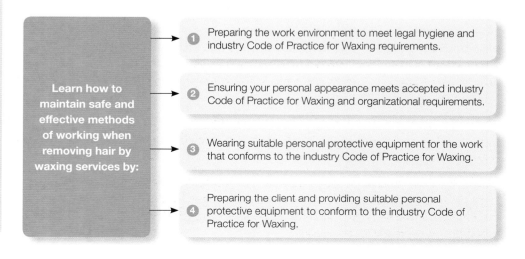

Learn how to maintain safe and effective methods of working when removing hair by waxing services by:

1. Preparing the work environment to meet legal hygiene and industry Code of Practice for Waxing requirements.

2. Ensuring your personal appearance meets accepted industry Code of Practice for Waxing and organizational requirements.

3. Wearing suitable personal protective equipment for the work that conforms to the industry Code of Practice for Waxing.

4. Preparing the client and providing suitable personal protective equipment to conform to the industry Code of Practice for Waxing.

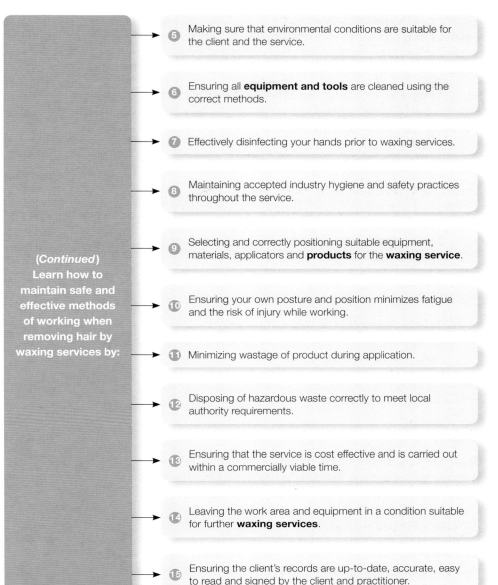

⑤ Making sure that environmental conditions are suitable for the client and the service.

⑥ Ensuring all **equipment and tools** are cleaned using the correct methods.

⑦ Effectively disinfecting your hands prior to waxing services.

⑧ Maintaining accepted industry hygiene and safety practices throughout the service.

(Continued)
Learn how to maintain safe and effective methods of working when removing hair by waxing services by:

⑨ Selecting and correctly positioning suitable equipment, materials, applicators and **products** for the **waxing service**.

⑩ Ensuring your own posture and position minimizes fatigue and the risk of injury while working.

⑪ Minimizing wastage of product during application.

⑫ Disposing of hazardous waste correctly to meet local authority requirements.

⑬ Ensuring that the service is cost effective and is carried out within a commercially viable time.

⑭ Leaving the work area and equipment in a condition suitable for further **waxing services**.

⑮ Ensuring the client's records are up-to-date, accurate, easy to read and signed by the client and practitioner.

HEALTH & SAFETY

Sensitive skin
Increasingly products are being formulated which contain only natural ingredients which can reduce skin irritation. Ingredients include sugar and plants such as chamomile and lavender to sooth the skin.

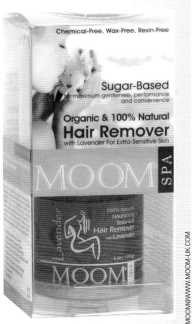

Organic sugar-based hair remover

Preparing the work area

Check the suitability of the environmental conditions.

To enable the hairs to be removed effectively the service area should be well lit and warm as the client must be made as comfortable as possible when performing the service. If the client is cold the follicles will restrict, making hair removal more difficult. Ensure ventilation is adequate to remove odours and remove humid air, providing sufficient air movement to keep the air fresh.

Before the client is shown through, the work area its contents should be checked to ensure that they are clean and tidy. The bins should have been emptied since the previous client.

Check the trolley to ensure that you have all that you need for carrying out the service and that it is suitably positioned to prevent unnecessary stretching or walking which will affect commercial timing and could cause repetitive strain injury. The wax should be of a suitable consistency, i.e. ready for application.

ACTIVITY

Methods of hair removal
As well at the professional use of depilatory waxing, threading and plucking, other methods of temporary hair removal include the home use of plucking, cold wax using ready-waxed strips, sugaring, electrical devices, chemical depilatory creams, shaving and pumice powder. Find out how each method works and assess its effectiveness. Are any of them potentially hazardous?

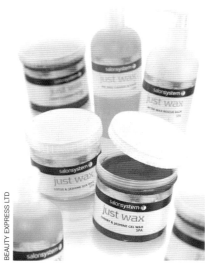

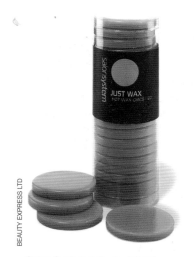

Warm wax

BEAUTY EXPRESS LTD

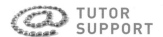

Salon System hot wax (discs)

BEAUTY EXPRESS LTD

@ TUTOR SUPPORT

Activity 1: Hair removal research task

The plastic-covered couch should be clean, having previously been washed with hot soapy water and wiped thoroughly with a disinfectant which is bactericidal, fungicidal and virucidal. The use of an additional heavy-duty plastic sheet is recommended: this is easier to wipe than the couch, and can be replaced if damaged.

All disinfectable surfaces must be disinfected after thorough cleaning between services.

The couch should then be covered and protected with a long strip of paper-tissue bedroll. Place a towel neatly on the couch, ready to protect the client's clothing and to cover them when they have undressed. The tissue should be disposed of after use, and the towel freshly laundered for each client.

The couch should be in the sit-up position, unless the client is only having their bikini line or underarm areas waxed, in which case it should be flat.

Before beginning the waxing service, check that you have the necessary equipment and materials to hand and that they meet legal hygiene and industry requirements for working services.

Equipment and materials list: types of wax

Warm wax This first became available in 1975 and is now the market leader for hair removal. It is clean and easy to use.

Warm wax is used at a low temperature, around 43°C, so there is little risk of skin burning, and in less sensitive areas the wax can be re-applied once or even twice if necessary.

Warm wax does not set but remains soft at body temperature. It adheres efficiently to hairs and is quick to use; service is relatively pain-free. It can remove even very short hairs (2.5mm) from legs, arms, underarms, the bikini line, the torso, the face and the neck.

Warm waxes are frequently made of mixtures of glucose syrup, resin to help the wax stick, zinc oxide to provide an opaque colour, oil to help removal (e.g. almond oil), water and fragrances. Honey (fructose syrup) can be used instead of glucose syrup and this formulation is often called **honey wax**.

Hot wax This takes longer to heat than warm wax, and is relatively slow to use, taking approximately double the time of a warm waxing. This time reduces when skill is attained.

As hot wax is used at quite a high temperature, 50°C, extra care must be taken to avoid accidental **burns**. Because of this risk, hot wax cannot be re-applied to already treated areas.

Hot wax cools on contact with the skin. It contracts around the hair shaft, gripping it firmly. This makes it ideal for use on stronger, short hairs.

Hot waxes for hair removal need to be a blend of waxes and resins so that they stay reasonably flexible when cool. **Beeswax** is a desirable ingredient, and often comprises 25–60 per cent of the finished product.

Cetiol, azulene and vitamin E are often added to wax preparations to soothe the skin and minimize possible skin reactions.

Cold wax This is already applied to a strip. The pre-coated strip is applied firmly to the area of skin for hair removal and then removed quickly against hair growth. The hair sticks to the wax and is removed as the wax strip is removed, against hair growth.

x

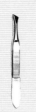

Sugar wax There are two methods of sugar wax hair removal – **sugar paste** and **strip sugar**.

Sugar paste is applied to the skin, using the hands, in the direction of hair growth. The hairs embed in the wax, which is then removed swiftly against hair growth, removing the hairs.

Strip sugar is similar in application and removal to warm wax and requires a wax removal strip to remove the wax, against hair growth. Sugar wax has pure sugar as the main ingredient, plus other natural ingredients such as lemon.

MOOM® WWW.MOOM-UK.COM

ACTIVITY

Wax heaters
Look in current beauty magazines for the different types of wax heater and applicators. Try to see demonstrations of them working. Discuss size, cleaning, safety, hygiene and any other points that you think are important. Which heater would you choose, and why?

BEST PRACTICE

Accommodating disabilities
Hydraulic couches are effective as they enable clients with mobility problems easier access on to the couch.

HEALTH & SAFETY

Wax and related product use
All products used in the waxing service should be used in accordance with the Cosmetic Regulations (2003).

Personal Protective Equipment Act (PPE) at Work Regulations (1992)
Waxing is a service where there is a risk of contamination and cross-infection, therefore protective equipment such as gloves and an apron should be available and worn.

HEALTH & SAFETY

Storage of products
All products should be stored as guided by the material safety data sheets (MSDS) in compliance with COSHH Regulations (2002).

EQUIPMENT AND MATERIALS LIST

ELLISONS

Couch
With sit-up and lie-down positions and an easy-to-clean surface

ELLISONS

Trolley
To hold all the necessary equipment and materials

ELLISONS

Disposable wooden spatulas (a selection of differing sizes)
For use on different body areas

ELLISONS

Wax-removal strips (bonded-fibre)
Thick enough that the wax does not soak through, but flexible enough for ease of work. These strips should be cut to size and placed ready in a container

ELLISONS

Cotton wool pads
For cleaning equipment and applying various skin soothing/cleansing preparations

ELLISONS

Tissues (white)
For blotting skin dry and protecting the client's clothing in the area

Anti-bacterial skin cleanser
(Also known as **pre-wax lotion**) or professional antiseptic wipes

ELLISONS

Wax heater
With a thermostatic control, a lid and a central bar

Tweezers
For removing stray hairs following wax depilation or defining the brow shape following a brow waxing service

Single-use disposable synthetic powder free gloves
To ensure a high standard of hygiene and to reduce the possibility of contamination

Waste container
This should be a lined metal bin with a lid

Hand disinfectant
To clean hands before each waxing service

ELLISONS

YOU WILL ALSO NEED:

Disposable tissue couch roll Disposable consumable placed over the couch cover prior to each treatment to prevent the client sticking to the couch cover and for reasons of hygiene

Protective plastic couch cover A durable covering which can be cleaned with a disinfectant agent before each client service. It is then covered with disposable tissue roll

Talcum powder To absorb body perspiration and to facilitate hair removal

Disposable panties These may be provided when carrying out bikini waxing

Surgical spirit Or a commercial cleaner designed for cleaning waxing equipment

Towels (medium-sized) For draping around the client

Small scissors For trimming over-long hairs

Disinfecting solution In which to immerse small metal tools following sterilization in the autoclave. This must be changed regularly as stated in manufacturers' instructions

Wax A choice to suit skin types and hair types

After-wax lotion With soothing, healing and antiseptic qualities

Mirror (clean) For facial waxing services

Apron To protect work wear from spillages

Client record card Confidential card recording details of each client registered at the salon to record the client's personal details, products used and details of the service

Aftercare leaflets Recommended advice for the client to refer to following service

TOP TIP

After-wax lotion
After-wax lotions reduce redness and promote skin healing. They contain ingredients such as tea tree, aloe vera, azulene and witch-hazel. These are an ideal retail product to recommend to your client to ensure effective skin healing.

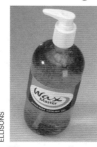

ELLISONS

After-wax cooling gel

> Selling is a vital part of the role of a therapist. It is important that the client gets the right service and products in order to get the results they are after. Clients do not buy our services or products, they buy the benefits and results. It is your job to help them imagine how using the products and services will make them look and feel. Remember that we all hate to be sold to but love to buy; so practice and perfect your selling skills.

Janice Brown

ACTIVITY

Electrical testing
How can you ensure that your wax heater is safe to use?

How can you ensure you comply with the Electricity at Work Regulations (1989)?

What actions must you ensure are taken?

When choosing a wax, select one with the following qualities:

- It should be easy to remove from equipment.

- It should be able to remove short, strong hairs (25mm).

- It should have a pleasant fragrance or no smell.

- It should not stick to the skin, but only to the hair.

Sterilization and disinfection

Disposable waste from waxing may have body fluids on it: potentially it is a health risk. It must be handled, collected and disposed of according to the local environmental health regulations. It is a requirement to wear disposable gloves while carrying out bikini and underarm wax services, to protect yourself from body fluids and the client from contamination.

These should be disposed of after each waxing service.

Wash your hands regularly with anti-bacterial soap, before and after preparing the work area and before application of the disposable gloves. This shows the client that you have a high standard of hygiene.

An apron should be worn to protect work wear from wax spillage.

All metal tools should be sterilized in the autoclave before use. This includes tweezers and scissors.

After the waxing service they must be replaced and resterilized.

Increasingly systems which minimize the risk of cross-infection are being adopted. These include single use pots, cartridges and disposable applicator heads.

Outcome 2: Consult, plan and prepare for waxing service with clients

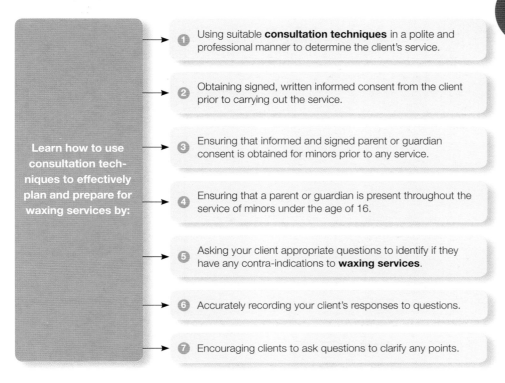

Learn how to use consultation techniques to effectively plan and prepare for waxing services by:

1. Using suitable **consultation techniques** in a polite and professional manner to determine the client's service.

2. Obtaining signed, written informed consent from the client prior to carrying out the service.

3. Ensuring that informed and signed parent or guardian consent is obtained for minors prior to any service.

4. Ensuring that a parent or guardian is present throughout the service of minors under the age of 16.

5. Asking your client appropriate questions to identify if they have any contra-indications to **waxing services**.

6. Accurately recording your client's responses to questions.

7. Encouraging clients to ask questions to clarify any points.

ACTIVITY

Safe storage
How should flammable products used in the waxing service be stored – consider the environmental conditions also.

HEALTH & SAFETY

Avoiding cross-infection
Never filter hot wax after use: it cannot be used again as it will be contaminated with skin cells, tissue fluid, and perhaps even blood.

HEALTH & SAFETY

Contaminated waste
Any wax waste that contains bodily fluids should be bagged separately from other regular waste and special arrangements made for its disposal by a registered waste carrier in an approved incinerator in accordance with the Controlled Waste Regulations (1992).

TOP TIP

See the Habia *Hygiene in Beauty Therapy* booklet for further guidance to hygiene best practice. Also check Habia website for specifications and updates.

ACTIVITY

Maintaining hygiene
Spreading wax on the client and dipping the used spatula back into the tub with the spatula method creates the possibility of cross-infection between clients. How can cross-infection be avoided, with this method and the use of roll-on wax applicators?

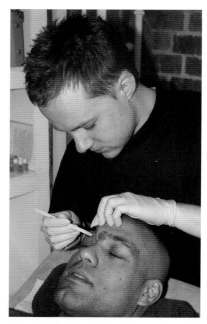

Wear disposable gloves when carrying out waxing services

(Continued) **Learn how to use consultation techniques to effectively plan and prepare for waxing services by:**

8 Ensuring client advice is given without reference to a specific medical condition and without causing undue alarm and concern.

9 Taking the **necessary action** in response to any identified contra-indications and the client's suitability for **waxing service**.

10 Clearly explaining the possible contra-actions to the client prior to agreeing to the **waxing service**.

11 Agreeing the **waxing service** and outcomes that are acceptable to the client and meets their needs.

12 Ensuring the client is in a suitable position for the area to be treated during the **waxing service**.

13 Ensuring your client's clothing, hair and accessories are effectively protected or removed.

HEALTH & SAFETY

Couch covers

If the salon chooses to use stretch-towelling couch covers or additional towels to provide extra comfort, these must be provided clean for each client and laundered in hot soapy water at a temperature of 60° after use.

ALWAYS REMEMBER

Check the salon's insurance guidelines relating to age restrictions for intimate waxing delivery. Check age restrictions in your area (note that in England a minor is under 18, whereas in Scotland it is 16) – refer to current guidance.

Reception

When the client is booking their service they should be asked whether they have had a wax service before in the salon. If they have not, a small area of waxing should be carried out as a skin sensitivity test, to ensure that the client is not sensitive to the technique or allergic to any of the products used. If the **sensitivity test** causes an unwanted reaction within 48 hours, then the service must not be undertaken. Unwanted reactions include excessive redness, irritation and swelling, referred to as contra-actions.

Service	Warm waxing (minutes)	Hot waxing (minutes)
Half leg	20–30	30
Half leg and bikini	30	45
Full leg	50	60
Full leg and bikini	60	60–70
Bikini	15	15–20
Underarm	10–15	15–20
Half arm	10–15	15–20
Full arm	20–30	20–30
Top lip	5	5–10
Chin and throat	10	15–20
Top lip and chin	15	15–20
Eyebrows	10–15	15

Advise the client not to apply any lotions or oils to the area on the day of the service – these could prevent the adhesion of the wax to the hairs being removed. Ask them also to allow at least one week, and preferably two, between any home shaving or other depilatory service and a salon waxing service. This is to let the hairs grow to a length sufficient to be waxed.

When a client makes an appointment for a wax depilation service, the receptionist should advise the client how long the service will take.

It is important to complete service in the time allowed in order to be efficient in service application and to ensure the appointment schedule runs smoothly and clients are not kept waiting.

Allow a four- to six-week interval between successive wax depilation appointments. The times to be allowed for wax services are as shown in the table (opposite). However, repeat bookings vary according to the natural hair regrowth and client requirements.

All staff, especially the staff communicating with clients at reception should be familiar with the different pricing structures for the range of waxing services and products available for retail.

Clients under 16 years of age (minors) must be accompanied by a parent/guardian who will be required to sign a consent form for service to proceed.

TOP TIP

If a client is allergic to plasters she may possibly be allergic to wax as it contains resin a substance that is found in plasters.

Always perform a skin sensitivity test in this case.

ALWAYS REMEMBER

Accurately record your client's answers to necessary questions to be asked at consultation on the record card.

> Consultation is the key to a success-ful service. You may be asking yourself why you need to consult your client, you may feel you already know what they want, or see it as a card filling exercise, so you should just get them on the couch and get started. However, you'd be wrong. Consultation is your opportunity and to gain the information you need to enable you to give a safe effective service. Learn exactly what your client wants and needs, in order to sell them the suitable products and services. It is also your opportunity to impress potential clients with your knowledge and professionalism to ensure they build a trust in you and become a regular customer.
>
> **Janice Brown**

Consultation

A consultation must be performed for all clients who have not received the service before or are new clients to you. Discuss what methods of hair removal have been used before and when they were last used. Discuss the known sensitivity of the client's skin. If necessary a skin sensitivity test should be provided to assess tolerance. A positive reaction where there is redness, irritation or swelling means that the service cannot proceed. A positive reaction means that it can. Maintain client privacy at all times during the consultation. Explain what is involved with the method of hair removal technique to be used, the expected costs, sensations, service reactions and aftercare requirements.

It is a good idea to discuss the hair growth cycle with the client using a visual aid. This will help the client to understand that hairs that grow through following hair removal were at a different stage of the hair growth cycle and were below the skin's surface at the time of the service. It also is beneficial to support the need for regular intervals between waxing appointments as hairs will be at a similar hair growth pattern.

Immediately following hair removal, the skin becomes slightly red around the follicle where the hair has been removed. There may also be slight swelling of the skin in the area. This will soon disappear following service but this will vary according to skin sensitivity and hair strength and the quantity of hair that has been removed.

Invite the client to ask questions. It is important that they understand fully what the service includes.

Advise the client following the consultation and completion of the record card of the most appropriate method of temporary hair removal having considered the type of hair (vellus/terminal) and amount and the sensitivity of the skin.

HEALTH & SAFETY

Diabetes

Clients who have the medical condition diabetes should be treated with care. This is because diabetics generally have poor circulation and are slow to heal. As there is some tissue damage to the skin during wax depilation when the hair is removed from the follicle, secondary infection could occur. Approval to treat should be obtained by the client from their GP before temporary hair removal service.

Contra-indications

When a client attends for a wax depilation service, the therapist should always check that there are no contra-indications that might prevent service.

If the client has any of the following, wax depilation must not be carried out:

- **skin conditions** such as thin and fragile skin
- **skin disorders** such as severe eczema or psoriasis
- **eye disorders** such as conjunctivitis when treating the face
- **swellings** – the cause may be medical
- **diabetes** – a client with this condition is vulnerable to infection as they have slow skin healing
- **defective circulation** – poor skin healing may occur
- **recent scar tissue (under six months old)** – the skin lacks elasticity
- **fractures or sprains** – discomfort may occur
- **phlebitis** – an inflammatory condition of the vein
- **retin-A, Tetracycline medication** as the skin is more sensitive weaker and prone to skin irritation and tearing
- **loss of skin sensation** – the client would be unable to identify if the wax was too hot
- **scar tissue** – under six months old
- **allergies to products** – such as the ingredient resin, an ingredient found in wax

Further contra-indications that prevent waxing service

Name	Description
Bruising 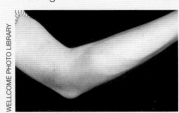	Injury to an area causes blood to leak from damaged blood vessels. Bruises may swell, appearing dark purple or blue at first and then turn, brown, green or yellow as they fade.
Folliculitis 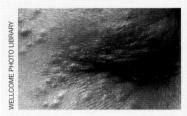	A bacterial infection where pustules develop in the skin tissue around the hair follicle.
Severe varicose veins 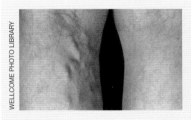	Veins are vessels that carry blood away from the body tissues and back to the heart. Veins have valves to prevent backflow as they carry blood under low blood pressure back towards the heart. If valves become weak and their elasticity is lost, it becomes a *varicose vein*. The area appears knotted, swollen and bluish-purple in colour.

HEALTH & SAFETY

Precaution if there is a restrictive contra-indication present

If there is a hairy mole or small abrasion you may apply petroleum jelly to avoid wax adherence.

BEST PRACTICE

Waxing a client with a recent well-established suntan may cause the loose sun-damaged epidermis to peel and be lost, along with the hair. Inform the client of this at consultation.

Certain contra-indications restrict service application. This may mean that the service has to be adapted for the client. For example, in the case of a small, localized bruise the area could be avoided.

Other contra-indications that restrict service include:

- *Cuts* – secondary infection could occur.
- *Mild skin disorders* such as psoriasis or eczema and skin tags.
- *Abrasions* – secondary infection could occur.
- *Self tan* – waxing will remove the surface skin cells and the chemically tanned skin.
- *Bruises* – client discomfort may be caused and the condition made worse.
- *Sunburn* – the skin is damaged due to acute over-exposure to the sun.
- *Varicose veins* (non-severe) – avoid the area.
- *Moles* – avoid wax application to the area.
- Ingrowing hairs – the area should be avoided as the hair will not be removed. Also, infection commonly occurs at the site of an ingrowing hair, leading to folliculitis.

BEST PRACTICE

If there is any bruising on the client's legs, tactfully draw their attention to these bruises, or they might later think that the service has caused them.

Further contra-indications that restrict waxing service

Name		Description
Heat rash	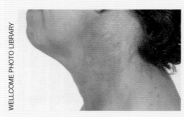	A reaction to heat exposure where the sweat ducts become blocked and sweat escapes into the epidermis. Red pimples occur and the skin becomes itchy.
Warts	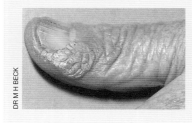	Small epidermal skin growths. Warts may be raised or flat, depending upon their position. Usually they have a rough surface and are raised.
Hairy moles	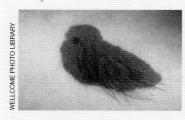	Models exhibiting coarse hairs from their surface. Hair growing from a mole may be cut, not plucked: if plucked, the hairs will become coarser and the growth of the hairs further stimulated.
Skin tags	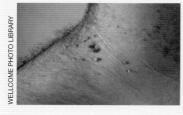	Skin-coloured threads of skin 3–6mm long, projecting from the skin's surface. Skin tags often occur under the arms.

Contra-actions

Inform the client at consultation of any contra-actions that may occur and the action to take.

A contra-action is an unwanted reaction to a waxing service which may occur during or following the service.

Contra-actions which are quite common with waxing include:

- ingrowing hairs
- removal of skin
- burns – both wax and friction burns
- erythema – increased blood flow to the skin, giving a slight redness

HEALTH & SAFETY

Hygiene

When carrying out any of these procedures, wear protective gloves. Both client and therapist must observe hygienic procedure; for example you should wipe over the area with a skin disinfectant before touching it.

HEALTH & SAFETY

If a contra-action, an unwanted reaction during service, occurs discontinue the service and provide appropriate advice.

Ingrowing hairs Ingrowing hairs can arise in three ways:

- *Over-reaction to damage* An excessive reaction by the skin and the follicle to the 'damage' produced by depilation may cause extra cornified cells to be made. These may block the surface of the follicle, causing the newly growing hair to turn around and grow inwards.

- *Overtight clothing* If after the service the client wears clothing that is too tight, this too can block the follicle.

- *Dry skin* Likewise dry skin can cause blockage of the follicle.

Ingrowing hairs can usually be recognized to be one or other of three types:

- *A hair growing along beneath the surface of the skin* Identify the tip (the pointed end); then pierce the tissues over the root end with a sterile needle. Free the tip and leave it in place so that the follicle can heal around it.

- *A coiled ingrowing hair* This looks like a small black spot or dome on the skin. If this is gently squeezed and rolled between the fingertips, using a tissue, it will release the coiled ingrowing hair and some hardened sebum. If the hair does not fall out, it should be left in place (as above).

- *An infected ingrowth* If the trapped sebum or hair starts to decay, either of the two preceding forms can become infected or begin to display an immune response. The area first becomes red (irritation); then an infected white dome-shaped pustule develops. Release the trapped tissue (as above), and cover the affected area – which may bleed, or leak tissue fluid – with a sterile non-allergenic dressing.

Skin removal If the upper, dead, protective cornified layer of the skin is accidentally removed during a service – leaving the granular layer of the living, germinative layer exposed – the skin should be treated as if it has been burnt. Cool the area immediately by applying cold-water compresses for 10 minutes. Dry it carefully; then apply a dry, non-fluffy dressing to protect the area from infection. The dressing should be worn for three to four days, and the area then left open to the air. (Antiseptic cream by itself should be used only when the injury is very minor.) Medical attention should be sought if necessary.

Burns A burn should be treated as 'skin removal'. If blisters form, they should not be broken – they help prevent the entry of infection into the wound. Medical attention should be sought.

Erythema Erythema is a visible redness, accompanied by an increase in warmth on the surface of the skin. It derives from increased blood flow through the capillaries near the surface of the skin, caused by the histamine reaction after waxing. Ask the client to follow the recommended aftercare advice.

Certain waxing ingredients such as rosin, a resin may cause an allergic reaction in some people.

The symptoms of an allergic reaction could be:

- redness of the skin (erythema)
- itching
- swelling
- blisters

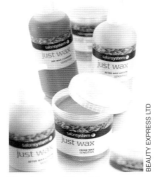

TOP TIP

Sensitive skin
Waxing products designed for sensitive skin are available. It is a good idea to have such products available to accommodate all skin types

Wax for sensitive skin

ALWAYS REMEMBER

Reactions to service
Damage to the skin that occurs during a waxing service causing cells called *mast cells* to burst in the skin releasing a chemical substance called histamine. Histamine is released into the tissues causing the blood capillaries to dilate, giving the redness called erythema. The increased blood flow limits damage and begins repair.

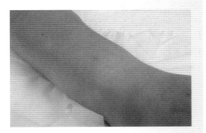

Erythema

While assessing the client's skin for waxing service, you should also be looking for contra-indications to treatment.

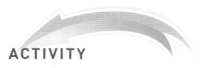

ACTIVITY

Ensuring client comfort

Imagine that you are a client who has never had a waxing service before. You are shown through to a cubicle and left to 'Get yourself ready, please'. How would you feel? What would you do? What clothing would you think it necessary to remove for each area of waxing?

If the client had mobility issues identified at consultation how could you prepare the work area to accommodate this need?

In the case of an allergic reaction, if it occurs during waxing application stop service and remove any remaining product. Apply a cool compress and soothing agent to the area to reduce redness and irritation. Identify the possible cause of the allergic reaction. If symptoms persist, seek medical advice.

Always record any allergies on the client's record card, so that the offending product may be avoided in the future. Try an alternative **waxing products** to assess skin tolerance. In some cases the skin is too sensitive and intolerant to waxing service.

Always date and record any contra-actions on the client record card, with actions taken/ recommendations provided and outcome.

After the record card has been completed, the client should be asked to read the list of contra-indications and sign to state that they are not suffering from any of the problems stated.

The therapist must not carry out a wax service immediately after a heat service, such as a sauna, or steam or ultra-violet services, as the heat-sensitized tissues may be irritated by the wax service.

If you are unsure if service may commence, tactfully refer the client to their General Practitioner for permission to treat. A copy of the GP's letter on receipt should be kept with the client's record card. If the service cannot be carried out for any reason, always explain why, without naming a contra-indication, as you are not qualified to do so. Clients will respect your professional advice.

Following the consultation an appropriate service plan will be confirmed with the client. Their understanding of the service is important to ensure that their needs are met and that they will not be disappointed.

Record all client details accurately on the client record card. A sample record card follows.

ALWAYS REMEMBER

Client records

In accordance with the **Data Protection Act (1998)**, confidential information on clients should only be made available to persons to whom consent has been given. All client records should be stored securely, and be available to refer to at any time as required. They must be kept for up to three years.

Sample client record card

Date	Beauty therapist name	

Client name	Date of birth (Identifying client age group.)

Home address	Postcode

Email address	Landline phone number	Mobile phone number

Name of doctor	Doctor's address and phone number

Related medical history (Conditions that may restrict or prohibit service application.)

Are you taking any medication? (This may affect the sensitivity and skin reaction following service.)

CONTRA-INDICATIONS REQUIRING MEDICAL REFERRAL
(Preventing hair removal service.)

☐ bacterial infection (e.g. impetigo, conjunctivitis)
☐ viral infection (e.g. herpes simplex/warts)
☐ fungal infection (e.g. tinea corporis)
☐ severe skin conditions
☐ diabetes
☐ severe varicose veins
☐ phlebitis

TEST CONDUCTED
☐ self ☐ client

WAX PRODUCTS

☐ hot wax
☐ warm wax – spatula method
☐ warm wax disposable applicator/tube/cartridge system
☐ strip sugar
☐ sugar paste

WORK TECHNIQUES

☐ keep the skin taut during application and removal
☐ speed of product removal
☐ direction and angle of removal
☐ ongoing wax product temperature checks

CONTRA-INDICATIONS WHICH RESTRICT SERVICE
(Service may require adaptation.)

☐ cuts and abrasions
☐ bruising and swelling
☐ self tan
☐ skin disorders
☐ heat rash
☐ sunburn
☐ hairy moles
☐ mild eczema/psoriasis

AREAS TREATED FOR HAIR REMOVAL
(Service may require adaptation.)

☐ eyebrows
☐ face
　☐ upper lip
　☐ chin
☐ legs
　☐ full leg
　☐ half leg
☐ underarm
☐ bikini line

Beauty therapist signature (for reference)

Client signature (confirmation of details)

Sample client record card (continued)

SERVICE ADVICE*

Half leg wax – *allow 30 minutes*

Full leg wax – *allow 50 minutes*

Bikini wax – *allow 15 minutes*

Underarm wax – *allow 15 minutes*

Eyebrow wax – *allow 15 minutes*

Facial wax   top lip or chin – *allow 10 minutes*

top lip and chin – *allow 15 minutes*

*Waxing timings may differ according to the system used. Always allow slightly longer when using hot wax.

SERVICE PLAN

Record relevant details of your service and advice provided for future reference.

Ensure the client's records are up to date, accurate and fully completed following service. Non-compliance may invalidate insurance.

DURING

Monitor:

- client's reaction to service to confirm suitability

Note:

- any adverse reaction, if any occur

AFTER

Record:

- results of service
- any modification to service application that has occurred
- what products have been used in the wax removal service
- the effectiveness of service
- any samples provided (review their success at the next appointment)

Advise on:

- use of aftercare products following wax removal service
- maintenance procedures
- the recommended time intervals between services

RETAIL OPPORTUNITIES

Advise on:

- products that would be suitable for the client to use at home to care for and maintain the service area (these include body exfoliation and moisturising skincare products)
- recommendations for further services
- further products or services that the client may or may not have received before

Note:

- any purchase made by the client

EVALUATION

Record:

- comments on the client's satisfaction with the service
- if poor results are achieved, the reasons why
- how you may alter the service plan to achieve the required service results in the future, if applicable

HEALTH AND SAFETY

Advise on:

- how to care for the area following service to avoid an unwanted reaction
- avoidance of any activities or product application that may cause a contra-action
- appropriate necessary action to be taken in the event of an unwanted skin or eye irritation

Preparing the client

The client should be shown through to the service cubicle, and asked to remove specific items of clothing as necessary so that the service may be carried out. Disposable briefs may be provided if a bikini wax service is to be received.

If it is the first time the client has had the service, explain to them that the service can be uncomfortable, but it is quick and any discomfort experienced is tolerable.

Be efficient and quick, so that the client does not have to wait. Try to get the client talking about something pleasant, such as a holiday, to take their mind off the service. Throughout the service, reassure them, praising them in order to motivate them to continue with the services. Do try to be sympathetic to your client's feelings, and provide support and encouragement when necessary. Waxing, although a necessity for many people, is not a particularly pleasant or relaxing service.

How to prepare the client for service

1 Use a towel to protect the client's remaining clothing.

2 Wipe the area to be waxed with a professional antiseptic pre-wax cleansing lotion on cotton wool. This should be dispensed from a pump or spray bottle or removed with a spatula if in a container. Blot the area dry with tissues before applying the wax. While wiping the skin, look for contra-indications that restrict the service, e.g. varicose veins.

3 Record any bruising on the record card to avoid potential problems later.

4 If the client's skin is very greasy (they may for example have applied oil before coming to the salon), cleanse it using an astringent lotion such as witch-hazel. Talcum powder may be applied lightly to the area to facilitate hair removal.

5 Immediately before starting the service, wash your hands. Apply PPE as required according to the body part being treated.

6 Perform a **thermal sensitivity test**: before applying the wax, check its temperature. Test the wax on yourself first, to ensure that it's not too warm; then try a little on the client on the area to be treated (to check tolerance to the heat) before spreading it on other areas.

Outcome 3: Remove unwanted hair

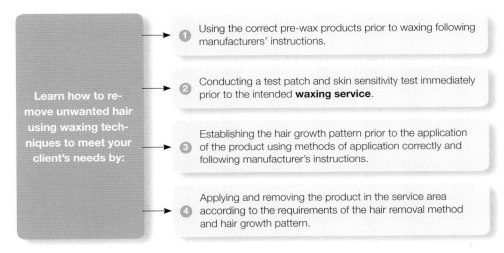

Learn how to remove unwanted hair using waxing techniques to meet your client's needs by:

1 Using the correct pre-wax products prior to waxing following manufacturers' instructions.

2 Conducting a test patch and skin sensitivity test immediately prior to the intended **waxing service**.

3 Establishing the hair growth pattern prior to the application of the product using methods of application correctly and following manufacturer's instructions.

4 Applying and removing the product in the service area according to the requirements of the hair removal method and hair growth pattern.

TOP TIP

Trimming hair

Trim long hair before waxing to avoid unnecessary client discomfort and to enable the hair growth direction to be more easily viewed.

Skin disorders such as skin tags can be hidden if the hair is too long.

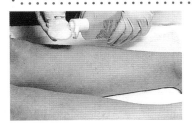

Cleansing the skin of the lower leg

TOP TIP

A woman's pain threshold is at its lowest immediately before and during her period. The hormones which stimulate the regrowth of hair are also at their most active during this period. For these two reasons, avoid wax depilation at this time if possible.

TOP TIP

An angled follicle may cause the hair to be broken off at the angle during waxing, instead of being completely pulled out with its root. If this happens, broken hairs will appear at the skin's surface within a few days.

By causing damage to the follicle and changing its shape, waxing can cause the regrowth of hairs to be frizzy or curled where previously they were straight.

TOP TIP

The thinner the wax, the easier the service is to carry out and the better the result. Also, less wax and fewer strips are used.

HEALTH & SAFETY

It is unhygienic to return a spatula to the wax after it has been in contact with the body part. It is therefore recommended that a new spatula be used for each entry to the wax. This applies to warm, hot and sugar-strip wax.

(5) Maintaining the client's modesty and privacy at all times.

(6) Providing clear instructions to the client on how and when to support their skin during the **waxing service**.

(7) Ensuring your **work techniques** minimize discomfort to the client.

(8) Checking the client's well-being throughout the waxing service.

(9) Stopping the **waxing service** and providing relevant advice if contra-actions occur.

(10) Ensuring the client's treated area is left free of product and hair and treated with a suitable soothing product.

(11) Ensuring that the finished result is to the client's satisfaction.

(Continued) **Learn how to remove unwanted hair using waxing techniques to meet your client's needs by:**

> "Removing the entire hair including the bulb is the aim of waxing, (though many therapists do not always achieve this goal) to ensure you always remove all the hair and so provide a lasting service get two things right:
>
> ● When removing the wax, hold the skin taught this will 'open the follicles' which means you are more likely to remove the entire hair.
>
> ● Master an effective 'flicking' action when removing the wax strip; flick backwards, keeping it parallel to the skin, always against the direction of hair growth. Do not pull upwards as this is more likely to 'snap' off the hairs at the surface of the skin.
>
> **Janice Brown**

Warm wax techniques

Warm waxing has a few basic rules which must be followed to ensure a good result.

Observe the direction of hair growth. Warm wax must always be **applied with** the direction of hair growth, and **removed against** the direction of growth. This ensures both maximum adhesion between the hair, the strip and the wax, and that the hair will be pulled back on itself in the follicle and thus removed complete with its bulb.

Spatula application technique

1 Dip the spatula into the wax. Remove the excess on the sides and tip by wiping the spatula against the metal bar or the sides of the tub. Place the strip under the spatula while transferring it to the client: this will control dripping and improve your technique.

2 Place the spatula onto the skin at a 90° angle, and push the wax along in the direction of the hair growth. Do not allow the spatula to fall forward past 45°. The objective is to coat the area with a very thin film of wax. Quite a large area can be spread with each sweep of the spatula, as warm wax does not set. Do not attempt to smooth out or go over areas on which wax has already been spread, however, as the wax will have become cooler and will not move again, but will drag painfully on the client's skin.

3 Fold back 20mm at the end of a strip and grip the flap with the thumb widthways across the strip. The flap should provide a wax-free handle throughout the service.

4 Place the strip at the bottom end of the wax-covered area, and make a firm bond between the wax and the strip by pressing firmly along the strip's length and width, following the direction of hair growth. If the strip is placed anywhere but at the bottom of a waxed area, the hairs at the **bottom** of the strip will become tangled together and held in the wax on the area below the strip: the removal of the strip will then be far more painful for the client.

5 Using the non-working hand, stretch the skin to minimize discomfort. Gripping the flap tightly, use the working hand to remove the strip against the direction of hair growth. Use a firm, steady pull. Make sure that the strip is pulled back on itself, close to the skin. (To obtain the correct angle of pull, stand at the side of the client, facing them.) Maintain this same horizontal angle of pull until the last bit of the strip has left the skin: *do not pull the strip upwards at the end of the pull* as this would break the hairs at the end of the strip and be very painful.

6 The strip may be used many times; in fact it works best when some wax builds up on its surface. When there is too much wax on the surface it will stop picking up more: throw it away and start with a new one.

7 Do not repeatedly spread and remove wax over one area. In particular, wax should not be spread and removed more than twice on sensitive areas such as the bikini line, the face and the underarms. Any remaining stray hairs must instead be removed using sterilized tweezers.

Alternatively, warm wax may be applied using a disposable cartridge/tube applicator system. This system is discussed on page 459.

Different temperatures Summer heat and winter cold can each give rise to problems with the wax service. In summer, the wax stays too warm on the body, becoming sticky and difficult to work with, and tending to leave a sticky residue on the treated areas. In winter, the client's legs may be cold, causing the wax to set too quickly as you spread it, so that it becomes too thick. This prevents the efficient removal of both the wax and the hair growth.

To some extent these problems can be overcome by using thicker waxes with higher melting points in the summer, and thinner waxes with lower melting points in the winter.

How to provide a half-leg wax service

The areas of the body where warm-wax hair removal is most frequently used are the lower legs. This is often referred to simply as a **half-leg service**. A 'pair of half legs' should take 20–30 minutes to treat, and use no more than two or three strips.

1 Prior to the service, the area to be waxed should be cleansed as previously described.

2 Sit the client on the upraised couch, with both legs straight out in front of her.

3 Spread the wax on the *front* of the leg further away from you. Use three sweeps of the spatula: each sweep should go from just below the knee to the end of hair growth at the ankle.

Repeat this pattern of spreading on the leg nearer to you. (By spreading the further leg first, you will not have to lean over an already waxed area.)

4 Starting with the nearer leg, remove the wax using the strip. Start at the ankle and work upwards towards the knees.

Repeat for the other leg.

5 Ask the client to bend her legs to one side. Beginning again with the further leg, spread wax on one *side* of the leg, from the knee to the ankle, using two sweeps of the spatula.

Repeat for the nearer leg.

TOP TIP

To take the sting out of the removal, immediately place a hand or finger over the depilated area.

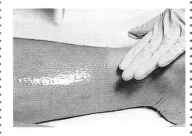

Wax removal

TOP TIP

The faults most commonly seen in warm-wax depilation are these:

- spreading the wax too thickly
- placing the strip in the middle of a wax-spread area, instead of starting at the bottom and working up
- pulling the strip upwards instead of backwards, away from the leg, causing breakage of the hair

" Different brands of wax have a range of melting point temperatures so it is important to follow manufacturers' instructions regarding melting times and advised heats.

Janice Brown

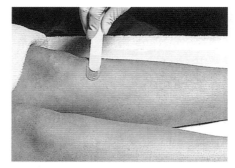

Applying warm wax to the lower leg

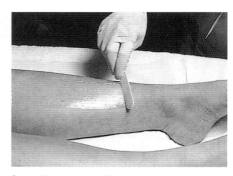

Spreading on wax (with correct spatula angle)

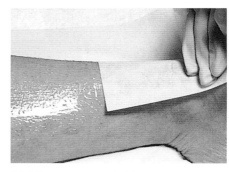

Applying a wax removal strip

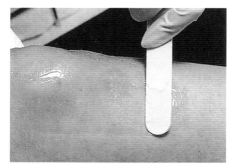

Applying warm wax to the knee

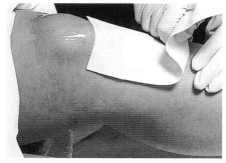

Removing the wax strip from the knee

TOP TIP

Thick lumps of wax stuck to the legs (the winter problem) can be removed by pulling more slowly than normal, or by reversing the direction of pull on the strip. A sticky residue on the legs (the summer problem) must be removed using after-wax lotion.

HEALTH & SAFETY

Contra-action as a result of waxing service

If any contra-action appears to be more than minor, advise the client to see their GP straight away after service.

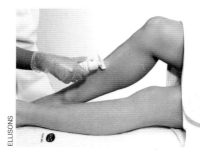

Leg wax application using disposable application warm wax technique

6 Starting with the nearer leg, remove the wax from the bottom upwards.

Repeat for the other leg.

7 Repeat steps **5** and **6** for the other side of the legs.

8 Bend one knee. Spread the wax from just above the knee, downwards.

9 Remove this wax from the bottom upwards, remembering that strips cannot pull around corners effectively. To keep the angle of the pull horizontal, remove wax below the knee first, then that above the knee.

10 Repeat steps **8** and **9** for the other knee.

11 Lower the backrest and ask the client to turn over.

12 On the *back* of the legs, the direction of hair growth is not from the top to the bottom but sweeping at an angle, from the outside to the inside of the calf muscle.

Starting with the further leg, spread wax following the direction of the natural hair growth.

Repeat for the nearer leg.

13 Starting with the nearer leg, remove the wax against the direction of the natural hair growth.

Repeat for the other leg.

14 Finally, apply after-wax lotion to clean cotton wool and apply this to the back of the client's legs. As you apply the lotion, check for hairs left behind: if there are any, remove them using tweezers.

Ask the client to turn over, and repeat application on the front of the legs. Remove any excess using a tissue.

Disposable warm wax application to leg Wax is heated in its container applied through the disposable applicator head directly to the skin area. A wax strip is used to remove the hairs from the area removing the wax strip against hair growth.

Toes Clients frequently request that their toes be waxed in conjunction with a half leg or full-leg service. When doing this, follow the normal guidelines for waxing, but be aware that hair may grow in many directions. Cut strips into small pieces to effectively remove hair.

Full-leg service

A full-leg wax should take 40–50 minutes and four to six strips should be sufficient.

When doing a full-leg wax, follow the same sequence of working as with the half leg. On the thighs, observe the direction of hair growth carefully, as the hair grows in different directions. It is best not to spread wax on too large an area at once, or you may forget the direction of growth. Each direction of hair growth should be treated as a separate area. It is of prime importance that you support the skin on the thighs as you remove the strip – the tissues in this area can bruise very easily. The two essential factors in preventing bruising, pain and hair breakage are:

- the correct angle of pull
- adequate support for the tissues

How to provide a bikini-line service

A **bikini-line service** takes 10–15 minutes, and requires a new strip for each section to ensure effective hair removal from this delicate area.

1   Treat one side at a time. It is best if the client lies flat, as the skin's tissues are then pulled tighter, but the service can be carried out in a semi-reclining position if the client prefers. Bend the client's knee out to the side, and put her foot flat against the knee of the other leg. This is sometimes referred to as the **figure-four position**.

2   Tuck a protective tissue along and under the lower edge of the client's briefs. Raise this edge and agree with the client where she wants the final line to be. Hold the briefs slightly beyond this line, and ask the client to place her hand on top of the protective tissue to hold everything in place. This leaves you with both hands free, one to pull the strip and one to support the skin.

3   Cleanse and dry the areas to be waxed.

4   Using sterilized scissors, trim both the hair to be waxed and the adjacent hairs down to about 5–12mm in length. This is essential to avoid tangling, pulling and pain, and to prevent wax going onto hair that you do not want to remove.

5   Spread and remove the wax in two or three separate and distinct areas, the number depending on the directions of hair growth.

6   Use half of the strip length to remove the wax. Do not cover the whole area and tear it off at once! As soon as an area is completed, apply after-wax lotion. If necessary, use a clean tissue to remove excess lotion.

7   With both legs straight out in front on the couch, place a protective tissue along the top edge of the client's briefs, against the abdomen. Lower the briefs as

ALWAYS REMEMBER

The most common fault seen in half-leg waxing is trying to take too big an area at once over the calf muscle and not supporting the surrounding tissues adequately. This will result in a painful service for the client.

BEST PRACTICE

Wax spills

If you spill wax on the couch cover, immediately place a quarter-width facial-sized piece of strip on top of the spill. This prevents the wax from damaging the client's clothing when they move.

TOP TIP

Intimate waxing

Intimate waxing is a range of waxing techniques which remove pubic and/or anal body hair. This is an advanced waxing service covered in NVQ/SVQ Level 3 and differs from the requirements of a bikini waxing service.

ALWAYS REMEMBER

Bruising

Bruising is neither normal nor acceptable, but a sign of faulty technique.

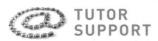

TUTOR SUPPORT

Activity 3: Service treatment times

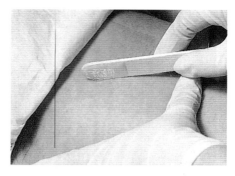

Applying warm wax to the bikini line

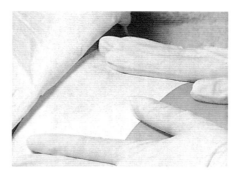

Applying a strip

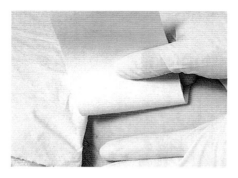

Removing the wax strip

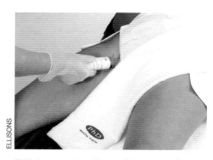

ELLISONS

Bikini wax: using disposable applicator warm wax technique

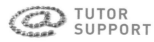

TUTOR SUPPORT

Activity 2: Aftercare leaflet design task

necessary to expose just the hair to be removed – check this with your client. Usually the direction of hair growth here sweeps in from the sides and then up to the navel.

8 Trim the hair as before.

9 Apply and remove the wax in small sections, carefully observing hair growth. On completion, apply after-wax lotion.

Disposable warm wax application to bikini area Wax is applied in small sections through the applicator head to the skin area. A wax strip is used to remove the hairs from the area removing the wax strip against hair growth.

How to provide an underarm service

An underarm service should take 5–15 minutes and two strips, one for each underarm.

1 With her bra still on, ask your client to lie flat on her back with her hands behind her head, elbows flat on the couch.

2 Cleanse both underarms with pre-wax lotion on clean cotton wool; blot with a tissue.

3 Place a protective tissue under the edge of the bra cup on the side away from you. Ask the client to bring her opposite arm down and over, and to pull the breast away from the underarm being waxed and across towards the middle of her chest. This pulls the tissues tight, making the service a lot more comfortable for her; it also leaves you with both hands free, one to pull and one to support.

4 Underarm hair usually grows in two main directions. Observe the directions of hair growth, then apply and remove the wax separately for each small area.

HEALTH & SAFETY

Both bikini-line and underarm waxing can be uncomfortable, especially if the hair growth is thick – always bear this in mind when carrying out the service. Some slight bleeding can be expected as the hairs in this area are very strong and have deep roots. Any waste contaminated by blood must be disposed of hygienically in a sealed bag.

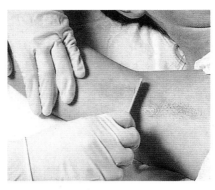

Applying warm wax to the underarm

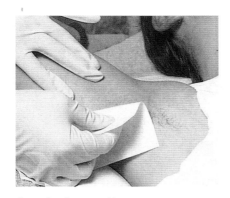

Removing the wax strip

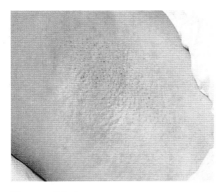

The completed area

5 Apply after-wax lotion to the treated area. Check for stray hairs; remove these with sterile tweezers.

6 Blot any excess cream with a clean tissue.

Disposable warm wax application to underarm Wax is applied in small sections through the applicator head to the skin area. A wax strip is used to remove the hair from the area, removing the wax strip against hair growth.

Step-by-step: Arm service

Depilation in this area should take 10–15 minutes for a **half-arm service** and 20–30 minutes for a **full-arm service**. Half the length of the strip should be used.

Arms are usually waxed with the client in the sitting position, with their general clothing protected with a towel. Sleeve edges can be protected with tucked-in tissues; ideally, though, upper outer clothing should be removed.

The roundness of the arm means that in order to effect a horizontal pull the work must be done in short lengths. Other than this, follow the general rules for waxing.

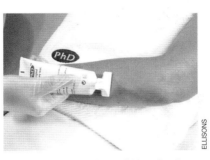

Forearm wax using disposable application warmwax technique

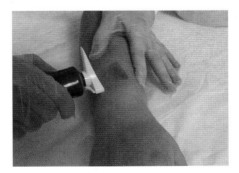

1 Wax applied in the direction of hair growth using disposable applicator warm-wax technique.

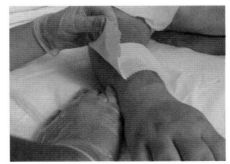

2 Wax is removed against hair growth, ensuring that the skin is held taut to minimize discomfort and ensure effective hair removal.

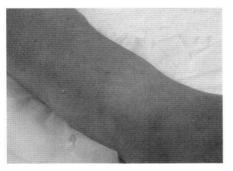

3 Mild erythema of the skin following hair removal. Check the area from all angles to ensure all hairs have been removed.

Step-by-step: Face service

The **face service** must always be approached with extra care as facial skin is more sensitive than skin elsewhere on the body. Faulty technique can result in the top layer of skin being removed. (If this happens, a scab will form after about a day and the mark will take days to heal and fade completely.)

ALWAYS REMEMBER

Previously bleached hair tends when waxed to break off at skin level. Clients should be told not to bleach facial hair if it is to be waxed.

TOP TIP

Dark superfluous facial hair

Avoid obvious lines when removing facial hair. Ensure the outer border of the area treated blends into the adjacent area of skin.

ALWAYS REMEMBER

The lips

The lips are extremely sensitive. To avoid possible irritation, do not allow the wax to come into contact with them.

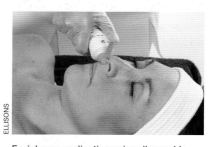

Facial wax application using disposable applicator warm wax technique

HEALTH & SAFETY

When performing an eyebrow wax, eyebrow hair that does not need to be removed may be protected with petroleum jelly.

Cotton wool pads may be placed over the eyes to protect the eye and eyelashes from accidental wax spillage.

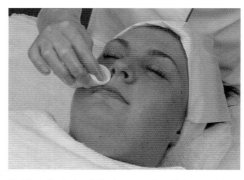
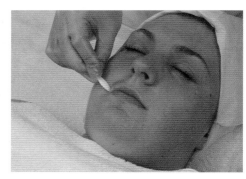

1 The client should be in a semi-reclining position, with her head supported and a clean towel draped across her shoulders to protect her clothing. A clean headband can be used to keep the hair away from the face.

2 Cleanse and wipe over the area using an antiseptic cleansing lotion. Blot it dry with a tissue.

3 Application of warm wax to the upper lip using a disposable applicator, paying close attention to the direction of natural hair growth. Hair removal is only required to the outer upper lip area. You might need to spread one-half of the top lip with wax; remove this in three or four narrow strips; repeat the process on the other half; and finally treat the central section immediately under the nose.

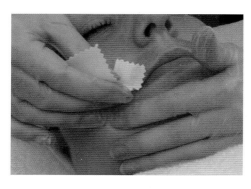
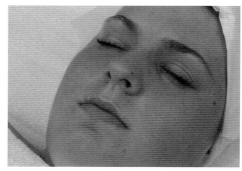

4 Removal of wax against hair growth. The area is held taut to minimize discomfort and ensure effective hair removal.

5 The completed area, free from superfluous hair.

A **top-lip wax** should take approximately 5 minutes, a **chin and throat wax** approximately 10 minutes, and a **lip and chin wax** approximately 15 minutes. A removal strip of no more than one-eighth normal size should be used on the face. Do not allow wax to build up on the facial wax strips – such a build-up could lead to skin removal. Use a new strip for each area.

If the chin is to be treated this area is less sensitive than the upper lip so if treating both areas complete the chin area last. Apply the wax according to the type of wax used. You may find that when treating a female client there may be small groupings of hairs and the wax may be applied to these areas only. If the client has dark superfluous facial hair it may be necessary to treat the sides of the face also.

A disposable warm wax application to facial area

Wax is applied in small sections through the applicator head to the skin area. A wax strip is used to remove the hair from the area removing the wax strip against growth.

How to provide an eyebrow service

Eyebrows, as a part of the face, are treated accordingly (see above). An **eyebrow wax** should take approximately 10–15 minutes.

1 Study the eyebrows and decide upon their final shape and proportions.

2 Brush the eyebrows and separate the unwanted hair from the line of the other hairs.

3 Using a small spatula, apply a thin film of wax to the unwanted hairs in a small area. Remove the wax using a clean strip. Repeat in different areas, using a clean strip each time, until all the unwanted hairs have been removed.

4 Apply a soothing antiseptic cream and use sterile tweezers to remove any stray hairs.

TOP TIP

Other areas of the neck and face can be treated by wax depilation – for example to tidy up a haircut at the neckline, or to remove sideburns – provided that you follow the general guidelines for facial services.

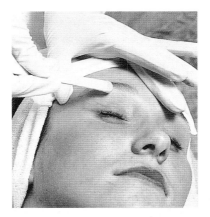

Applying warm wax to an eyebrow

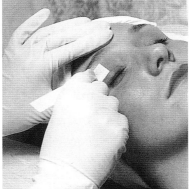
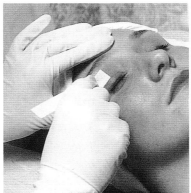

Removing the wax strip

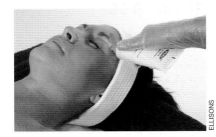

Eyebrow wax application: disposable applicator technique

ELLISONS

HEALTH & SAFETY

Sensitisation

Under no circumstances should wax be applied to facial hair, underarm hair or bikini-line hair more than twice during any one service. If after this any hairs remain, they must be removed with tweezers. The delicate skin in these areas readily becomes sensitized.

A disposable warm wax application to the eyebrow area Wax is applied in small sections through the applicator head to the skin area. A wax strip is used to remove the hair from the area removing the wax strip against growth.

Outcome 4: Provide aftercare advice

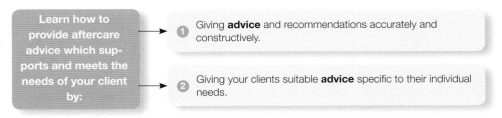

Learn how to provide aftercare advice which supports and meets the needs of your client by:

1 Giving **advice** and recommendations accurately and constructively.

2 Giving your clients suitable **advice** specific to their individual needs.

HEALTH & SAFETY

Aftercare insurance requirements

Many insurance companies require that aftercare instructions are provided in written form as well as verbally following the service. This will ensure that the client understands the necessity and possible consequences of not carrying these instructions out. Check your salon policy regarding this.

Aftercare and advice

The following aftercare and advice should be provided after each waxing service is completed to reconfirm the client's understanding of these important procedures.

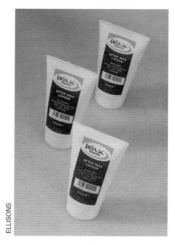

ELLISONS

After-wax products

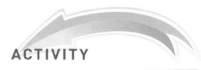

ACTIVITY

Aftercare leaflets

Discuss why aftercare leaflets should be given to clients, as well as giving them the advice verbally.

What could happen if aftercare advice is not given?

Design a suitable aftercare leaflet you could provide for your clients following waxing service.

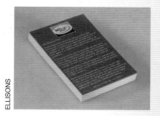

ELLISONS

Aftercare leaflet

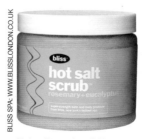

BLISS SPA: WWW.BLISSLONDON.CO.UK

Hot salt scrub exfoliant

An after-wax antiseptic, soothing lotion should be applied, using clean cotton wool, at the end of the service. This breaks down any wax residue, helps to guard against secondary infection and irritation, and takes away any feelings of discomfort. Encourage your client to continue with the use of such a lotion at home for up to three days: it will protect against dryness, discomfort, infection and ingrowing hairs.

BEST PRACTICE

After-wax lotion

Before after-wax lotion is applied ensure that the service area is free of waxing product and hair and check that the finished result is to the client's satisfaction.

Any residue left will cause dirt and materials in the area to stick which could lead to secondary infection.

Products have been formulated to apply to the skin following wax depilation to slow hair re-growth. The product when entering the empty hair follicle aims to weaken the cell's matrix, slowing cell division in this area which is responsible for creating the new hair. These are available for your client to purchase as a retail product.

Advise the client against wearing any tight clothing (such as tights or hosiery) over the waxed areas for the 24 hours following a service. Such clothing could lead to irritation and ingrowing hairs.

If the client suffers from ingrowing hairs, they should **exfoliate** their skin every four to seven days, starting two or three days after the service. Exfoliation prevents the build-up of dead skin cells on the surface of the skin; these would otherwise block the exit from the follicle and cause a growing hair to turn back on itself and grow inwards. Ingrowing hairs should be freed and, if possible, left in place so that the follicle exit will re-form around the hair's shaft. Demonstrate to the client the correct use and benefits of the exfoliant product.

Advise the client that for the 24 hours following their service they should not apply any talcum powders, deodorants, antiperspirants, perfumes, self-tanning products or make-up over the treated areas. Any of these products could block the pores or cause irritation or allergy reactions on the temporarily sensitized area. During this time she must use only plain, unperfumed soap and water on the treated area.

For the same 24-hour period they should preferably avoid exercise, especially swimming, and not apply heat or ultra-violet services – hot baths, for example, or the use of a sun bed or sauna – as these would add to the heat generated in the skin following the service and would probably cause discomfort or irritation. They must also refrain from touching or scratching the area, so as to avoid infecting the open follicles.

Aftercare leaflets should contain this information: as best practice these can be given to the client at the end of the service to remind them what to do at home.

If there is a contra-action following service such as excessive redness and irritation, advise the client to apply a cool compress with soothing antiseptic lotion. If the redness does not disappear she must contact the salon. Advise the client to receive the service as follows: facial waxing 3–4 weeks; body waxing 4–6 weeks. Repeat bookings vary according to the natural hair regrowth and client requirements.

Ensure that the client's records are up to date, accurate and complete following the waxing service and provide written instructions in an aftercare leaflet.

Hot waxing

In **hot waxing**, the wax is applied at a higher temperature than warm wax. The hairs embed in the wax and are gripped tightly as the wax cools and contracts. When the wax is pulled away, it removes the hair from the base of the follicle.

Equipment and materials

The equipment and materials required for hot waxing are the same as for warm waxing (pages 443–444), except that:

- *a wax heater* suitable for hot wax should be selected

- *wax-removal* strips are not necessary

- *pre-wax oil* may be applied to the skin before wax application to make wax removal easier

Some people prefer to apply the hot wax with disposable brushes rather than spatulas, but either can be used.

How to carry out the service

1. Ensure that the area to be waxed is clean and grease-free.

2. Apply a small amount of talc against the direction of hair growth. This will make the hairs stand on end and stick more firmly into the wax.

3. Keep the same order of work as for warm waxing.

4. Apply wax in strips approximately 5cm wide and 10cm long, with about 5cm distance between the strips.

5. Carefully observe the direction of hair growth and the size of the area to be waxed.

6. Test the heat of the wax on the inside of the wrist.

7. Using either a disposable spatula or a brush, apply a layer of wax about 5cm × 10cm *against* the direction of hair growth. Apply a second layer *with* the direction of growth; and a third layer against the direction of growth. (If two or three strips are applied at the same time, you can work faster.) Keep the edges of the wax thicker than the middle, to make it easier to remove. Overlap the lower edge by about 2cm onto a hair-free area: this makes it less painful later, when you lift the edge to make a lip to pull.

   Curl up the lower end of the wax to make a lip, and press and mould the wax firmly onto the skin.

8. Leave the wax for a minute or so to cool. The wax has to cool sufficiently to grip the hairs, but not so much that the wax becomes brittle and breaks on removal. As it sets, it starts to lose its gloss: it should be removed when this happens and while it is still pliable.

9. Support the area below the wax, grasp the lip, and tear the wax off the skin *against* the direction of hair growth in one movement (as with warm-wax removal). Immediately press or firmly stroke the area with your hand: this takes away some of the discomfort.

TOP TIP

When selecting a hot wax, choose one that does not go brittle when cool. Wax sold as small bars is preferable as this melts quickly.

ALWAYS REMEMBER

Wax temperature

If the wax is *not hot enough* when it is applied, it will not contract effectively around the hair and will therefore not grip it properly. This may result in poor depilation and possible hair breakage.

If on the other hand the wax is allowed to *overheat*, it may cause burns. Also, the quality of the wax will deteriorate and the wax will become brittle as it cools.

TOP TIP

If the wax becomes too cool and brittle for removal, fresh hot wax may be applied with care over the area to soften it.

10 Check the area for any remaining wax and any stray hairs. Remove using tweezers. (Second applications are not advisable when using hot wax, because of the risk of burning.)

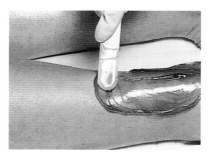

Applying hot wax to the lower leg

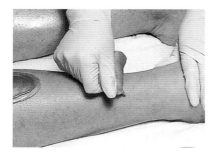

Removing the hot wax

If this general application technique is followed, any area of the body can be depilated – use the same order of work as for warm waxing: observe the direction of hair growth and take into account the body area; use smaller strips in smaller areas; support the skin; and use the correct angle of pull for removal.

Sugaring and strip sugar

Sugaring is an ancient and popular method for hair removal. The superfluous hairs become embedded in a pliable organic paste of sugar, lemon and water. The sugar paste is then removed from the skin's surface, against the hair's growth, leaving the skin hair-free.

Sugaring may be applied using a paste formulation removed with the hands, referred to as sugar paste, or in a formulation similar to warm wax, removed with material strips, referred to as strip sugar. Sugaring is effective on fine hair growth, and as it contains no chemicals or additives this method is unlikely to cause skin allergy.

Reception

Re-book the client for sugaring hair removal every four to six weeks, dependent upon the hair growth rate and area. For effective hair removal, the hairs must be at least 2mm long.

Equipment and materials

The equipment and materials required for sugaring are the same as for warm waxing (pages 443–444), except for the following differences.

Sugar paste

- **Wax beater (with a thermostatic control) or microwave** – to heat the paste.
- **Sugaring paste** – either soft or hard, depending on your personal preference and the temperature of the working environment: hard paste is a better choice in warmer temperatures and when working on coarser hair.

ALWAYS REMEMBER

Talcum powder

Talc aids the sugaring service technique, by reducing stickiness when working with the paste, and by absorbing perspiration (particularly in areas such as the underarms).

- *Talc (purified)* **to reduce stickiness and absorb perspiration** – to prevent the sugar sticking to the skin.

- *Bowl of clean water* – to remove the sugar paste from the hands, reducing stickiness.

Strip sugar

- *Wax heater (with a thermostatic control)* – to heat the strip sugar.

- *Strip sugar*.

- *Talc (purified)* **to reduce stickiness and absorb perspiration** – to prevent the sugar sticking to the skin.

- *Disposable wooden spatulas* – a selection of differing sizes, for use on different body areas.

- *Wax-removal strips (bonded-fibre)* – thick enough that the wax does not soak through, but flexible enough for easy working.

- *Disposable gloves*.

Sterilization and disinfection As sugar paste is water-soluble, it is easily cleaned from any surface. However, the wax heater containing the sugar wax must be regularly disinfected.

Step-by-step: Preparing the client

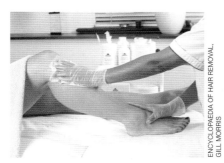

Cleanse the area to be treated, using an antiseptic cleansing tissue. Blot the skin dry.

ENCYCLOPAEDIA OF HAIR REMOVAL, GILL MORRIS

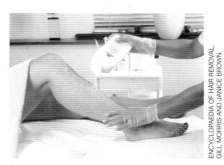

Apply talc to cover the area: this prevents the sugar from sticking to the skin.

ENCYCLOPAEDIA OF HAIR REMOVAL, GILL MORRIS AND JANICE BROWN

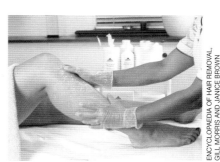

Rubbing in the talc

ENCYCLOPAEDIA OF HAIR REMOVAL, GILL MORRIS AND JANICE BROWN

How to provide a sugar paste service

The sugar paste adheres to the hair and not to the skin, which allows the sugar to be reapplied to a service area. Technique is important and it takes practice and experience to become skilled.

1 Heat the sugar gently, to soften it.

2 Apply talc to the area.

3 Apply the sugar paste to the skin by hand. Select the amount used according to the service area. Draw the paste over the area *in the direction* of the hair growth, embedding the hair in the paste. This can be termed 'rubbing' s it collects and embeds the hair in the wax as rubbed over skin's surface.

TOP TIP

Sugar wax – both strip and paste – may be heated in a microwave to soften it. Check guidelines set by the microwave manufacturer on power and timing.

However, also check with your salon policy as there may be potentially an increased risk of burning and the insurance may be invalid in such cases.

4 Remove it quickly *against* the hair growth.

5 If necessary, reapply the paste to the area to remove further hairs. Continue this process until no hair remains.

6 After use, discard the paste as it will be contaminated with excess hair and dead skin cells: this affects the ease of paste removal, and presents a risk of cross-infection.

7 To complete the service, a cooling spray may be applied to the area, followed by a soothing cream.

8 Record details of the service on the client's record card.

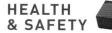

HEALTH & SAFETY

Temperature – thermal test
Ensure that the temperature is correct – neither too hot, which may cause burning, nor too cool, which may make working uncomfortable and inefficient.

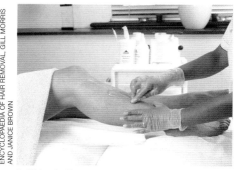

Applying sugar paste

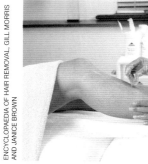

Rubbing in the sugar paste

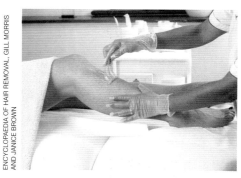

Removing the sugar paste

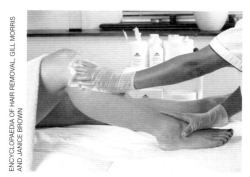

Applying antiseptic products

How to provide a strip sugar service

This is similar in application and removal to warm wax.

1 The wax is gently heated until it is fluid.

2 Apply the wax using a spatula *in the direction of* the hair growth to cover the service area.

3 Remove the wax *against* the hair growth using a clean strip.

4 To complete the service, a cooling spray may be applied to the area, followed by a soothing cream.

5 Record details of the service on the client's record card.

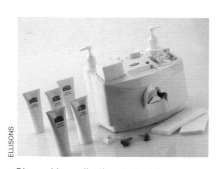

Disposable application starter kit

Disposable applicator roller waxing systems

Using a roller wax system is a hygienic method, using disposable applicators that are new for each client. A disposable applicator head screws onto the wax applicator tube in place of a cap. This reduces the possible risk of contamination through cross-infection. The method is less messy, as the wax is contained in the tube or cartridge and is not exposed until application.

Each tube/cartridge of wax as needed is heated to working temperature, which minimizes the risk of burning.

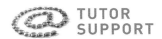

TUTOR SUPPORT

Activity 4: Wordsearch

Step-by-step: Waxing the legs using disposable applicator

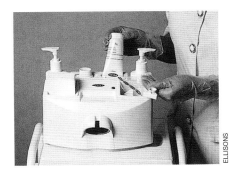

1 Remove the disposable applicator from the right-hand heating and storage compartment.

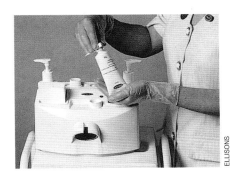

2 Remove the cap from the tube of wax. Attach the applicator head to the tube.

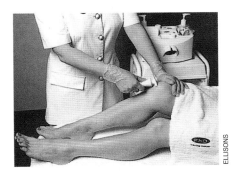

3 Release the applicator by lifting the lever upwards. Squeeze until a small amount of wax appears on the front of the applicator, then apply the wax. Hold the applicator at a 45° angle to the leg, and glide it smoothly down the leg.

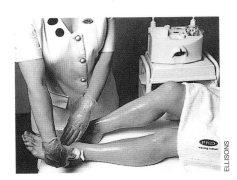

4 Apply a thin film of wax to the front of both legs, then press down the closing device on the applicator to stop wax flow.

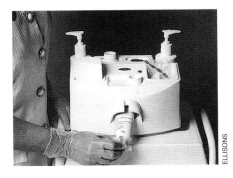

5 Wipe any wax residue from the front of the applicator and return the tube to heat.

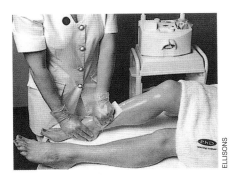

6 Remove wax from the leg, starting at the ankle and working towards the knee. Support the skin with one hand, and firmly stretch it against the removal of the wax. Continue application and removal to the sides and back of the legs.

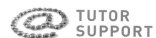

TUTOR SUPPORT

Activity 5: Re-cap, revision and evaluation

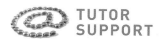

TUTOR SUPPORT

Activity 6: Multiple choice quiz

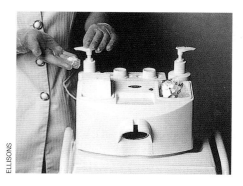

7   When service is complete, apply antiseptic soothing lotion (shown). Record details of the service on the client's record card.

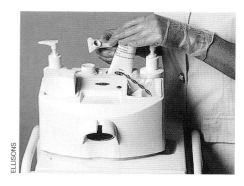

8   Remove the applicator from the tube, replacing the cap and returning the tube to the heater. Dispose of the applicator head.

GLOSSARY OF KEY WORDS

Aftercare advice recommendations given to the client following service to continue and enhance the benefits of the service.

After-wax lotion a product applied to the skin following hair removal to reduce redness and promote skin healing.

Allergic reaction reaction to ingredients in a product producing symptoms including erythema, swelling, itching and bruising.

Anagen the active stage of the hair growth cycle.

Burn injury to the skin caused by excess heat; the skin appears red and may blister.

Client groups this term is used in a number of the units and it refers to client diversity. The CRE (Commission for Racial Equality) ethnic group classification is used in the range for these units. These cover white, mixed, Asian, black and Chinese.

Cold wax a wax already applied to a strip and ready for use. The pre-coated strip is applied firmly to the skin and then removed quickly against hair growth, removing the hair in the area.

Consultation assessment of client's needs using different assessment techniques, including questioning and natural observation.

Contra-action an unwanted reaction occurring during or after service application.

Contra-indication a problematic symptom which indicates that the service may not proceed.

Disposable applicator used to apply wax hygienically to the area of hair removal without contaminating the wax flowing back into the tube following application. The applicator head is disposed of after each service.

Equipment and tools used within a waxing service that enable the service to be completed competently, e.g. magnifying light, wax heater and tweezers.

Erythema reddening of the skin, caused by increased blood circulation to the area.

Folliculitis a bacterial infection where pustules develop in the skin tissue around the hair follicle.

Hair a long slender structure that grows out of, and is part of, the skin. Each hair is made up of dead skin cells, which contain the protein called keratin.

Hair follicle an appendage (structure) in the skin formed from epidermal tissue. Cells move up the hair follicle from the bottom (the hair bulb), changing in structure to form the hair.

Hair growth cycle the cyclical pattern of hair growth, which can be divided into three phases: anagen, catagen and telogen.

Hairy moles moles exhibiting coarse hairs from their surface.

Heat rash a reaction to heat exposure where the sweat ducts become blocked and sweat escapes into the epidermis. Red pimples occur and the skin becomes itchy.

Histamine a chemical released when the skin comes into contact with a substance that it is allergic to. Cells called 'mast cells' burst, releasing histamine into the tissues. This causes the blood capillaries to dilate, which increases blood flow to limit skin damage and begin repair.

Hot wax a system of wax depilation used to remove hair from the skin. Hot wax cools and sets on contact with the skin. They are a blend of waxes, such as beeswax and resins, which keep the wax flexible. Soothing ingredients are often included to avoid skin irritation.

Ingrowing hair a build-up of skin occurs over the hair follicle, causing the hair to grow under the skin.

Laser hair removal a technique of permanent hair removal. Laser energy is passed through the skin which stops the activity of the hair follicle creating hair growth through a process called photothermolysis.

Melanin a pigment in the skin and the hair that contributes to the skin/hair colour.

Minor a person classed as a child who requires by law to have a guardian or parent present.

Necessary action the action taken to deal safely with a contra-action or contra-indication.

Photothermolysis an effect created when using a laser for hair removal. The melanin pigment that provides hair colour absorbs the laser energy, which is converted to heat, and at a sufficient temperature destroys the part of the hair follicle where the cells divide to create the hair.

Pre-wax lotion an antibacterial skin cleanser to clean the skin before wax application.

Roller wax a warm wax used to remove hair from the skin. The wax is contained in a cartridge container with a disposable applicator, which rolls the wax onto the skin's surface. The applicator is renewed for each client.

Service plan after the consultation, suitable service objectives are established to treat the client's conditions and needs.

Skin removal accidental removal of the upper, dead, protective cornified layer of the skin, leaving the granular layer exposed.

Skin tags skin-coloured threads of skin 3mm to 6mm long, projecting from the skin's surface.

Strip sugar a system of wax depilation similar to the warm-wax technique, used to remove hair from the skin. Made from sugar, lemons and water, the sugar wax is applied to the skin, and is then removed using a wax removal strip.

Sugar paste a system of wax depilation. An organic paste made from sugar, lemons and water is used to embed the hair, which is then removed by the paste from the skin.

Sugaring an ancient popular method of hair removal using organic substances, sugar and lemon.

Thermal sensitivity test a test performed before wax application to check that the temperature of the wax is not too warm. The wax is tested by the therapist on themselves, usually on the inner wrist, and then on the client on a small visible area such as the inside of the ankle.

Varicose veins veins whose valves have become weak and lost their elasticity. The area appears knotted, swollen and bluish/purple in colour.

Warm wax a system of wax depilation. Warm wax remains soft at body temperatures. It is frequently made of mixtures of glucose syrup and zinc oxide. Honey can be used instead of glucose syrup; this is referred to as honey wax.

Wax depilation the temporary removal of excess hair from a body part using wax.

Waxing products cosmetic preparations used with a waxing service which have specific benefits to cleanse the skin, assist in hair removal care and improve the appearance and healing properties of the skin following hair removal.

Work techniques the methods you use to carry out waxing services.

ASSESSMENT OF KNOWLEDGE AND UNDERSTANDING

Having covered the learning objectives for **Carry out waxing services**, test what you need to know and understand answering the following short questions below.

The information covers:
- organizational and legal requirements
- how to work safely and effectively when providing waxing services
- consult, plan and prepare for services with clients
- anatomy and physiology
- contra-indications and contra-actions
- equipment and products for waxing
- waxing services
- aftercare advice for clients

Organizational and legal requirements

For full legislation details, see Chapter 4.

1 What are your responsibilities under the relevant local and national health and safety legislation when carrying out waxing services? Give three examples.

2 What actions must be taken before a client under 16 years of age receives a waxing service?

3 Give an example of how you may need to modify your service to treat a client with a particular disability, e.g. mobility, visual or hearing impairment.

4 Why must a client's signature be obtained before commencing waxing service?

5 How would you prepare yourself for service to comply with Personal Protective Equipment (PPE) legislation requirements?

6 How should all clients' records be stored to comply with the Data protection Act (1998)?

7 How long would you allow to complete a full leg and bikini wax service?

8 Why is it important for staff to be familiar with the waxing pricing structures?

9 What details should have been recorded on the client's record card by the end of the service and why is it important to gain the client's signature?

10 What is contaminated waste and how should this be disposed of following waxing service?

How to work safely and effectively when providing waxing services

1 Why is it important to wear PPE?

2 How can you minimize the risk of acquiring the skin condition contact dermatitis when performing waxing services?

3 Give three examples of when both sterilization and disinfection methods are used to comply with hygiene regulations when performing a waxing service.

4 What is the Code of Practice for Waxing Service? Why is it best practice to be familiar with its content and any Habia updates?

5 What is the recommended temperature of wax when using:
- hot wax?
- warm wax spatula method?
- warm wax roller/disposable applicator method?
- strip sugar?

6 Why is it important to disinfect your hands before each service even though disposable gloves are to be worn?

7 What are the necessary environmental conditions required for waxing? Consider lighting, heating and ventilation in your answer.

8 How can cross-infection be prevented when carrying out waxing service? Provide three examples.

9 Poor posture could lead to muscle fatigue, poor removal techniques and repetitive strain injury. Explain how you can avoid personal injury by positioning equipment, materials and the client for the service.

Consult, plan and prepare for services with clients

1 To reassure the client, how would you explain to them the waxing service sensation and expected post service skin reaction?

2 It is necessary to check the hair growth before hair removal. How long should hair growth be before wax depilation can be carried out?

3 A client complains that on their previous service (which was their first), stubbly hairs appeared the following week. What could have been the cause?

4 How would you position the client for wax depilation for:
- a bikini wax?
- an underarm wax?
- a chin wax?

5 Why would you refer to the menstrual cycle when performing a waxing service on a female client?

6 What is a patch test and a skin sensitivity test? When and why would you perform each?

7 How should the area to be treated for wax depilation be prepared to ensure effective hair removal?

8 Why is it necessary to explain contra-actions that may occur with the client at the consultation?

9 It is necessary to consider the direction of hair growth for the hair removal technique chosen. Why is this?

10 Why is it important to consider the client's privacy and modesty?

Anatomy and physiology

For full anatomy and physiology details, see Chapter 2.

1 How many layers form the epidermis of the skin? Name them.

2 What is the name of the structure that the hair grows from in the skin?

3 What is the difference between a sebaceous and sudoriferous gland?

4 What are the three stages of the hair cycle? Briefly explain what happens to the hair at each stage.

5 If the client was too cold or too warm when receiving waxing service how would this affect the hair and surrounding skin being treated?

6 What are the main functions of the skin?

7 What are the three main parts if you looked at a cross section of the hair?

8 What is the name given to coarse pigmented hair and where is it mainly found on the body?

Contra-indications and contra-actions

1 What would be three undesirable post-service skin reactions? How would these be avoided?

2 Which contra-indications restrict service, meaning that the service may proceed, but the area contra-indicated must be avoided?

3 When observing the area for hair removal you identify what you think to be a contra-indication requiring referral. What action would you take?

4 Why is diabetes normally regarded initially as a contra-indication to waxing service?

Equipment and products for waxing

1 Certain ingredients may cause an allergic reaction; therefore it is important that you know what the product contains. What are the main ingredients in:
- warm wax?
- hot wax?

2 What is the purpose of pre-wax lotion when used in a waxing service?

3 What should be applied to the skin following wax depilation? What action does this product have on the treated area?

4 When might you apply talc to the skin in a waxing service?

Waxing service

1 It is important to select the most suitable method to remove the hair type. From the following temporary hair removal methods – warm wax, hot wax and strip sugar – identify which you would select for:
- the face
- the underarm
- the bikini

2 How do hot wax and warm wax (spatula/roller/disposable applicator head) differ in relation to:
- application?
- removal?

3 How does warm wax applied with a roller/disposable applicator head differ from that applied with a spatula to ensure hygiene compliance?

4 Give an example of the precautions you would need to take when performing waxing service around an area where this is a contra-indication that restricts service. State what your contra-indication is.

5 Explain three other temporary methods of hair removal and three permanent methods of hair removal. If a client had received these services previously how would this affect the service plan for waxing?

6 How should the skin be supported during the waxing service by the beauty therapist and the client?

7 What is the normal skin reaction to waxing service that should be explained to the client at the consultation?

8 What additional precautions should be taken to ensure that the wax is used at a comfortable temperature for the client?

Aftercare advice for clients

1 What activities should be avoided immediately following the waxing service and for how long should they be avoided?

2 In what forms should aftercare instructions be provided to the client following waxing service to ensure compliance with insurance requirements?

3 If your client suffers from ingrowing hairs, what advice would you give them that could possibly prevent them recurring?

4 When would you book a client to return for the following repeat depilation services, and how long would you allow for treatment of the:
- eyebrow?
- full leg?
- bikini?
- underarm?
- face?

5 What contra-actions could occur following waxing service? What advice should you provide regarding actions to take?

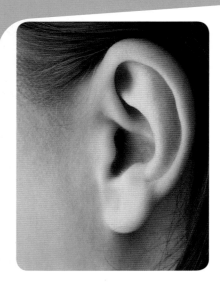

15 Ear-Piercing (B7)

B7 Unit Learning Objectives

This chapter covers **Unit B7 Carry out ear-piercing**.

This unit is all about providing the service skin piercing of the earlobe safely to ensure the correct placement and healing of the skin tissue avoiding any contra-action complications.

There are **four** learning outcomes for Unit B7 which you must achieve competently:

1 **Maintain safe and effective methods of working when piercing ears**

2 **Consult, plan and prepare for earlobe piercing with clients**

3 **Pierce the earlobes**

4 **Provide** aftercare advice

Your assessor will observe you on **at least two occasions with two different clients**.

From the **range** statement, you must show that you:

● have used all **consultation techniques**

● taken the **necessary action** where a contra-action, contra-indication or service modification occurs

● used all ear-piercing **equipment, materials and products**

● provided relevant **aftercare advice**

However, you must prove that you have the necessary knowledge, understanding and skills to be able to perform competently across the range.

When providing ear-piercing services it is important to use the skills you have learnt in the following units:

Unit G20 Make sure your own actions reduce risks to health and safety

(continued on the next page)

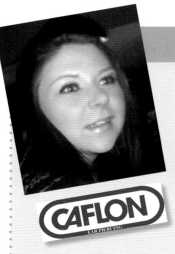

Jade Rogers

Sales Technician

" My job is to represent Caflon Ltd within the UK. Currently 70 per cent of my time is spent training people in how to pierce ears and the remainder of the time I visit our customers throughout the UK and Ireland ensuring that they have adequate stock and answering any queries.

The role is very challenging, dealing with many differing types of people. Our customers come from the world of hair and beauty, others from the medical field and a core of clients from the jewellery industry.

Attending training in colleges, conducting seminars for our wholesale customers and one-to-one training, means that many miles are travelled throughout the year, along with exhibiting at trade shows both home and abroad.

Although it can be lonely, working at Caflon is very rewarding and I have been lucky to enjoy the ten years spent with this international organization.

I have shared important tips for my role as a sales technician, a career you may consider on qualifying.

(continued)

Unit G18 Promote additional products or services to clients

Unit G8 Develop and maintain your effectiveness at work

Ear-piercing is the perforation of the skin and underlying tissue of the ear to create a hole in the skin where jewellery is inserted. It is a quick, profitable and popular salon service, which also has the potential to generate further custom. This may be the client's first visit to a beauty salon, and the service they receive may encourage them to return for further services.

The ears

The structure and function of the earlobe

The external ear collects sound waves and directs these to the inner ear. The part of the ear that is commonly seen pierced is called the **pinna**, which comprizes the **helix** and **lobule**. The helix is composed of cartilage, which does not heal quickly, can be painful and can form lumpy scar tissue; it is therefore considered unsuitable for piercing. The lobule, in contrast, consists of fibrous and fatty tissue with no cartilage, and is therefore suitable for piercing.

Earlobe piercing

Outcome 1: Maintain safe and effective methods of working when piercing earlobes

TOP TIP

Cosmetic piercing
Skin piercing of the ear-lobe and cosmetic body piercing are classified in the single term cosmetic piercing.

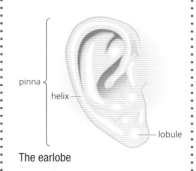

pinna
helix
lobule

The earlobe

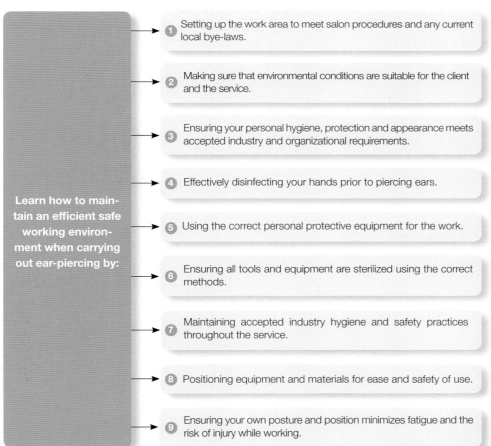

Learn how to maintain an efficient safe working environment when carrying out ear-piercing by:

1. Setting up the work area to meet salon procedures and any current local bye-laws.

2. Making sure that environmental conditions are suitable for the client and the service.

3. Ensuring your personal hygiene, protection and appearance meets accepted industry and organizational requirements.

4. Effectively disinfecting your hands prior to piercing ears.

5. Using the correct personal protective equipment for the work.

6. Ensuring all tools and equipment are sterilized using the correct methods.

7. Maintaining accepted industry hygiene and safety practices throughout the service.

8. Positioning equipment and materials for ease and safety of use.

9. Ensuring your own posture and position minimizes fatigue and the risk of injury while working.

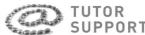 **TUTOR SUPPORT**

Activity 1: Label the ear structure

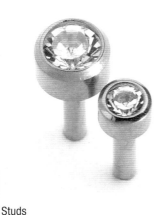

CAFLON

Studs

10 Disposing of waste materials safely and correctly.

(Continued)
Learn how to maintain an efficient safe working environment when carrying out ear-piercing by:

11 Ensuring that the service is cost effective and is carried out within a commercially viable time.

12 Leaving the work area in a condition suitable for further services.

13 Ensuring the client's records are up to date, accurate, easy to read and signed by the client and practitioner.

Preparing the work area

Ear-piercing can be carried out either in a private cubicle or at reception. Use your discretion to decide which would be more appropriate.

Good ventilation and lighting is important – some clients may feel faint following the service. The client should sit on a chair at a comfortable height for you.

All furniture and fittings in the service area should be kept clean and in good repair so that they can be cleaned effectively.

The surface that the ear-piercing equipment is to be placed on should be cleaned immediately prior to service with detergent and disinfectant. It should then be covered with disposable tissue roll, which is disposed of immediately following service. All work surfaces must be kept clean at all times and covered with a smooth, impervious surface.

Check where the client will be positioned when performing the service. The earlobe should be easily accessible without risk of injury to the client. Remember awkward positioning for the beauty therapist can lead to repetitive strain injury and must be avoided.

Before carrying out the ear-piercing check that you have the necessary equipment and materials to hand and that they meet legal hygiene and industry requirements for ear-piercing.

You will need the following equipment and materials:

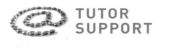

@ TUTOR SUPPORT

Activity 3: Equipment wordsearch

EQUIPMENT AND MATERIALS LIST

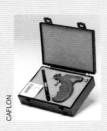

CAFLON

Ear-piercing gun
Ear-piercing gun one that complies with current health and safety legislation

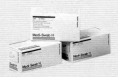

Pre-packed alcohol-based sterile tissues (2) or manufacturer's cleansing solution
Used to cleanse the ear area

YOU WILL ALSO NEED:

Studs A variety of styles and designs to accommodate differing client preferences. These must be manufactured from hypo-allergenic metal to minimize allergic reactions in people with metal allergies, e.g. nickel

Non-toxic surgical skin-marker pen To mark where the piercing will be. This is usually in gentian violet ink

Disinfectant (70 per cent alcohol) e.g. surgical spirit for cleaning the gun after use

Clean cotton wool To apply lotions/cleaning products

Single use disposable synthetic powder-free gloves To ensure a high standard of hygiene and to reduce the possibility of contamination

Disposable tissue roll Such as bedroll

Waste container (with yellow coloured waste liner to collect contaminated waste) This should be a lined metal bin with a lid to collect waste

Sharps box To dispose of studs

Headband (clean) or clip To hold the hair away from the ear during ear-piercing

Hand mirror (clean) To show the client the proposed placement of the earrings, after marking and after the ear-piercing

Client record card To record the client's personal details, products and equipment used and details of the service

Aftercare solution Either to offer for sale or to include as part of the cost of the service

Aftercare instruction leaflet Instructions for the client to keep to minimize healing times and reduce the risk of secondary infection

Ultra-violet light cabinet To store the ear-piercing gun between piercing services; helps avoid the risk of contamination

Hand disinfectant Usually containing chlorhexidine to cleanse and disinfect hands

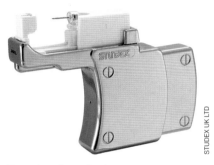

STUDEX UK LTD

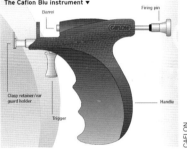

The Caflon Blu instrument ▼

Barrel — Firing pin

Clasp retainer/ear guard holder — Handle

Trigger

CAFLON

SURGICAL MARKER PEN

WWW.CARESSMANUFACTURING.CO.UK

Examples of ear-piercing guns

Be aware the manufacturers' systems may vary depending on the type of ear-piercing gun you are using.

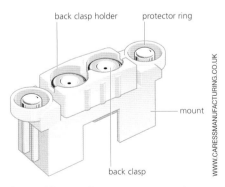

back clasp holder protector ring

mount

back clasp

WWW.CARESSMANUFACTURING.CO.UK

Disposable cassette

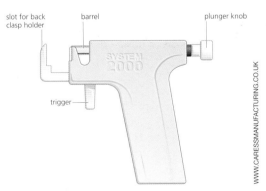

slot for back clasp holder barrel plunger knob

trigger

SYSTEM 2000

WWW.CARESSMANUFACTURING.CO.UK

Ear-piercing gun

HEALTH & SAFETY

Marker pens
Keep the marker pen in a safe hygienic place – if left out, somebody might mistake it for an ordinary felt-tip pen!

HEALTH & SAFETY

See the Habia *Hygiene in Beauty Therapy* booklet for more details. It is available as a download from the Habia website.

Sterilization and disinfection The premises should be kept clean and hygienic. The floor covering should be such that the surface can be cleaned with a disinfectant and hot soapy water; work surfaces likewise should be washed regularly with detergent and water and wiped with a disinfectant. Hypochlorite solutions (bleach) are recommended for disinfecting work surfaces. Potential hazards include cross infection due to poor hygiene practice to both client and beauty therapist.

HEALTH & SAFETY

Cross-infection

If you have any cuts on your hands or fingers, these should be covered with a clean dressing before you treat the client. It is essential to wear disposable gloves.

Also, if you have an acute cold, i.e. respiratory infection, do not perform ear-piercing service to prevent airborne transfer of infection.

HEALTH & SAFETY

The Control of Substances Hazardous to Health (COSHH) Regulations (2002) – including biological agents

The Control of Substances Hazardous to Health (COSHH) Regulations (2002) require employers and the self employed to prevent or control the exposure of employees and clients to hazardous substances. This includes exposure to biological agents such as bacteria, fungi and viruses and chemical cleaning/sterilizing agents. Records of the COSHH assessment must be available for inspection.

A COSHH essential information document is available for cosmetic piercers at www.coshh-essentials.org.uk.

TOP TIP

Disposable ear-piercing gun

Available for ear-piercing is a sterile disposable ear gun. This ensures a sterile gun with preloaded ear studs and clasp.

Some salons that offer the ear-piercing service also sell earrings. Those designed for pierced ears should not be tried on by a client, in the interest of health and hygiene. (Although there have been no reported cases of transmission of hepatitis B or HIV in this way, all possible risks should be avoided.) Such earrings may instead be attached to a special clear acrylic slide that can be held against the ear to assist in selection.

The gun approved for ear-piercing is designed so that it does not come into contact with the client's skin, and is used with pre-sterilized ear studs and ear clasps.

The studs are provided in sterile packs. Many give a date after which their sterility can no longer be assumed; others have a seal that changes colour when the expiry date has been reached. Only use studs that come from a sealed package.

The Local Government (Miscellaneous Provisions) Act (1982) requires that salons offering any form of skin-piercing be registered with the local health authority. This registration includes both the operators who will be carrying out the service and the salon premises where the service will be carried out.

The Local Government Act (2003) (section 120 and schedule 6) has amended the 1982 Act to enable each local authority to regulate businesses providing cosmetic body piercing. Each local authority can introduce its own bye-laws to set the standards as required for cosmetic piercing.

Premises are inspected by a local authority enforcement officer, who checks that relevant local bye-laws are being followed. (The bye-laws are to ensure that service is carried out in a healthy, safe and hygienic manner.)

If the inspector is satisfied, the salon will be issued with a certificate of registration; this should be displayed in the reception area at all times. Any breach of the Act or the bye-laws could result in a fine, and permission to carry out the service could be withdrawn.

The Greater London Council (General Powers) Act (1982) covers the London boroughs and relates to cosmetic piercing. It provides that no person can carry out cosmetic piercing unless they and the business are registered. Records are required to be kept. This is essential for a business with five employees or more. A business with fewer than five employees requires minimal records but it is best practice to have the following available for inspection relating to cosmetic piercing:

- COSHH assessment records
- dated client service plan records
- sterilization methods and records

The London Local Authorities Act (1991 and 2007) states that no person shall carry out cosmetic piercing at an establishment without obtaining a licence from a participating council. Conditions can be attached to the licence such as hygiene practices, age limits, etc.

Outcome 2: Consult, plan and prepare for earlobe-piercing with clients

Learn how to use consultation techniques to effectively plan and prepare for carrying out ear-piercing by:	**1** Using **consultation techniques** in a polite and friendly manner to determine the client's service.
	2 Obtaining signed, written informed consent from the client prior to carrying out the service.

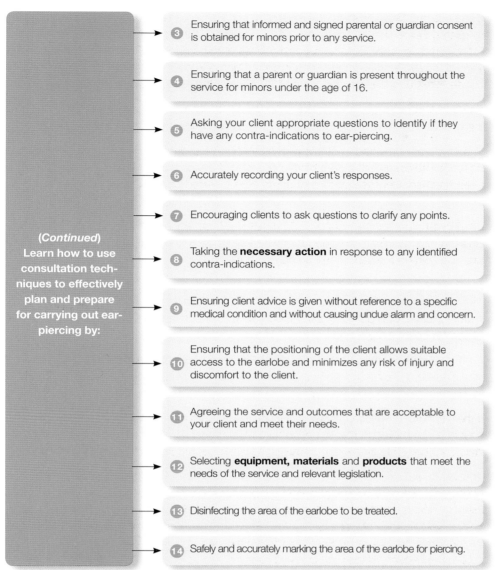

(Continued)
Learn how to use consultation techniques to effectively plan and prepare for carrying out ear-piercing by:

③ Ensuring that informed and signed parental or guardian consent is obtained for minors prior to any service.

④ Ensuring that a parent or guardian is present throughout the service for minors under the age of 16.

⑤ Asking your client appropriate questions to identify if they have any contra-indications to ear-piercing.

⑥ Accurately recording your client's responses.

⑦ Encouraging clients to ask questions to clarify any points.

⑧ Taking the **necessary action** in response to any identified contra-indications.

⑨ Ensuring client advice is given without reference to a specific medical condition and without causing undue alarm and concern.

⑩ Ensuring that the positioning of the client allows suitable access to the earlobe and minimizes any risk of injury and discomfort to the client.

⑪ Agreeing the service and outcomes that are acceptable to your client and meet their needs.

⑫ Selecting **equipment, materials** and **products** that meet the needs of the service and relevant legislation.

⑬ Disinfecting the area of the earlobe to be treated.

⑭ Safely and accurately marking the area of the earlobe for piercing.

HEALTH & SAFETY

Ear-piercing guidelines
The Chartered Institute of Environmental Health has developed useful best practice guidance for those employed as operators in body art, cosmetic therapies and other special services.

HEALTH & SAFETY

If only one stud of a pair is used in an ear-piercing, the other stud should be discarded as it is no longer in a sterile state.

ACTIVITY

Personal cleanliness
Personal cleanliness is a fundamental requirement of the Local Government (Miscellaneous Provisions) Act (1982) and its amendments. Discuss how a high standard of personal cleanliness can be guaranteed. It is important to check any updates to the Act on a regular basis to ensure compliance.

ACTIVITY

Research ear-piercing service in three local salons. These may include hairdressing salons as it is a popular service to perform in the hair salon.

What is the cost of this service?

Reception

When making an appointment for this service, allow 15 minutes. Although ear-piercing is completed quickly, time must be allowed to complete the client's record card, determine the client's service plan and give clear concise aftercare instructions. Good communication is important. Speak clearly, establish what the client's requirements are and listen to ensure communication is effective and that a professional relationship is developed with the client, gaining client confidence.

A record card should be prepared for the client, recording just the information that is relevant to the ear-piercing service. Record-keeping protects both the beauty therapist and client. While completing the record card you will be able to ascertain whether the client is suited to this service – if the client is under 16 years of age (a minor), for example, it is necessary for a parent or guardian to accompany them and sign a **consent form** containing a disclaimer in the event of **contra-indications**. These should be kept for a period of three years for inspection, enabling checks to be made on clients' ages.

Contra-indications to ear-piercing should be checked for. If the area for piercing is unsuitable, politely explain to the client why this is so.

ALWAYS REMEMBER

Examples of ear-piercing service modification include:

- if a second piercing is requested, ensure the first stud is placed to accommodate leaving a 9mm distance for the second piercing
- if the client has fat lobes, adjust the tightness following piercing
- if 6mm or more thickness, the lobe requires a 'long post' stud

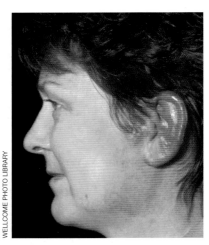

Inflammation of the ear

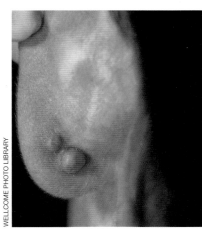

Keloid scarring of the ear

Contra-indications

In certain circumstances you should not carry out the ear-piercing service. Use your professional judgement to assess the suitability of each client. The **consultation** will draw any contra-indications to your attention.

- *If a client is particularly nervous* it would be inadvisable to pierce their ears – they might faint or jump while the service was being carried out, causing incorrect placement of the earring.

- *Do not pierce the ears of a client who may have allergies* to the metal used for the jewellery stud.

If any of the following are present, do not proceed with ear-piercing:

- *Diabetes* – the skin is very slow to heal, so infection of the area would be a strong possibility.

- *Epilepsy* – the stress before the service and the possible shock incurred during it might induce a fit.

- *Skin disease or disorder*.

- *Hepatitis B or HIV (Human Immunodeficiency Syndrome)* – though the client may not know that they are a carrier, or may choose not to disclose the fact if they do (hygienic practice is vital, for this reason).

- *Inflammation of the ear*.

- *Open wounds, cuts or abrasions* in the area.

- *Moles or warts* in the area.

- *Circulatory disorders* such as high or low blood pressure.

- *A predisposition to keloid scarring* – lumpy scar tissue (black skin often forms keloid scar tissue following skin healing).

- *Following an operation* – piercing must not be carried out at the site of a recent operation.

- *Anti-coagulant drugs* – individuals are likely to bleed persistently.

- *Inflammation of the ear* – the skin in the area appears red, swollen and pus, a sign of infection, may be present.

- *Keloid scarring* – **keloids** occur following skin injury and are overgrown abnormal scar tissue which spreads, characterized by excess deposits of collagen. The skin tends to be red, raised and ridged at the site of the wound.

Where there is any contra-indication to ear-piercing, the client must seek written permission from their GP before service can be carried out.

Feel the area to be pierced to check for cysts or keloids wearing disposable gloves for protection. Do not pierce through cysts or keloids or infection could occur.

Inform the client of possible contra-actions that could occur. Especially if the correct aftercare procedures are not followed.

Contra-actions

- **Infection** – redness, swelling, inflammation and the exudation (oozing/weeping) of serum all signify that the ear is infected. If this occurs, the client should contact the salon. Depending on what they describe, it may be possible to give them adequate instructions over the telephone, or it may be necessary to make an appointment for the therapist to look at the ear. If, following action by the therapist, the infection persists, the client should be advised to contact their GP. Infection usually results from incorrect aftercare, removing the studs too early, or wearing cheap earrings.

  Closed holes are caused by removing the studs too early, or by not continuing to wear earrings after the removal of the original studs.

  Infections of the ear can be painful, and if ignored lead to scarring and at worst the skin tissue can die leading to disfigurement of the area.

- **Jewellery embedding** – this occurs when the ear jewellery descends beneath the skin's surface. This is usually a sign of infection, rejection or allergy to the ear jewellery. The client should contact the salon for advice. If, following action by the therapist, the jewellery remains embedded, the client should be advised to visit their GP.

- **Keloids** – overgrowths of scar tissue – sometimes occur at the site of ear-piercing. If a client suffers from keloids, advise them not to have their ears pierced more than once – further keloid tissue could develop, giving an unsightly appearance.

- **Dizziness and fainting** – may occur if the client was particularly nervous beforehand. The shock of the ear-piercing service may cause a short period of unconsciousness due to insufficient blood flow to the brain. If a client faints, loosen any restrictive clothing. Reassure the client, and position them lying flat with their feet raised higher than their head, or sat with their head bent forwards between their knees. Instruct them to breathe deeply and slowly. Increase ventilation in the area.

- **Allergy to the aftercare lotion** – The client may be allergic to the aftercare lotion. Check for known allergies to products at the client consultation.

All details recorded on the client record card are confidential and should be stored in a secure area following service. Access to this information will require written consent from the client. This is enforced through the Data Protection Act (1998) – legislation designed to protect the client's privacy and confidentiality. These records should be kept for at least three years, and be available for inspection as required. This may be by an authorized officer from the local health authority.

Explain the simple service procedure. Most clients will be interested to know what to expect – usually the client's first question is "Will it hurt?".

Discuss aftercare. It is important to check that the client does not have any known allergies that may be contained in products to be used in the service, e.g. the aftercare lotion. Also, clients are more likely to pay attention at this stage.

Prepare the equipment required for ear-piercing, and show the client the range of studs available. The stud's post has a larger diameter than regular earring posts to allow for shrinkage during the healing process, explain this to the client.

Some salon receptionists are trained to carry out this service. This is practical: many clients will be acting on impulse in deciding to have their ears pierced, and will not have made an appointment.

HEALTH & SAFETY

Secondary infection

If the client's ears become slightly red, indicating a possible infection, they should cleanse the area more frequently.

TUTOR SUPPORT

Activity 2: Aftercare leaflet design

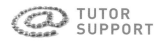

> With a diary schedule often booked eight months in advance, I have learnt how important it is to be organized and independent.
>
> **Jade Rogers**

> I always try to remember that no matter how often I have made my training presentation, this is the first time my group have heard it, therefore it's important to keep it fresh and professional.
>
> **Jade Rogers**

ALWAYS REMEMBER

Accurately record your client's answers to necessary questions to be asked at consultation on the record card.

A sample client record card

Date	Beauty therapist name	
Client name	Date of birth (Identifying client age group.)	
Home address	Postcode	
Email address	Landline phone number	Mobile phone number
Name of doctor	Doctor's address and phone number	
Related medical history (Conditions that may restrict or prohibit service application.)		
Are you taking any medication? (E.g. anti-coagulant drugs may affect the sensitivity of the skin and reaction to the service.)		

CONTRA-INDICATIONS REQUIRING MEDICAL REFERRAL
(Preventing ear-piercing service.)

- ☐ bacterial infection
- ☐ viral infection
- ☐ fungal infection
- ☐ severe skin conditions
- ☐ diabetes
- ☐ ear infections
- ☐ cardiovascular problems
- ☐ dysfunction of the nervous system
- ☐ allergies to metals
- ☐ epilepsy
- ☐ anti-coagulant drugs

EQUIPMENT, MATERIALS AND PRODUCTS

- ☐ ear-piercing gun
- ☐ surgical skin marker pen
- ☐ sterile pre-packed alcohol skin-cleansing wipes
- ☐ personal protective equipment
- ☐ sterile pre-packed ear studs (metal type identified)
- ☐ consumables
- ☐ aftercare products
- ☐ mirror
- ☐ sharps disposal box (for use in the event of disposing of a contaminated ear stud)
- ☐ waste bin (with disposable liner)

CONTRA-INDICATIONS WHICH RESTRICT SERVICE
(Service may require adaptation.)

- ☐ cuts and abrasions
- ☐ bruising and swelling
- ☐ recent scar tissue
- ☐ skin disorders
- ☐ moles
- ☐ skin inflammation
- ☐ keloid scar tissue (piercing around the keloid permitted)

AREA TREATED

- ☐ earlobe

Beauty therapist signature (for reference)
Client signature (confirmation of details)

A sample client record card (continued)

SERVICE ADVICE
Ear-piercing – *allow 15 minutes*

SERVICE PLAN
Record relevant details of your service and advice provided for future reference.
Ensure the client's records are up to date, accurate and fully completed following service. Non-compliance may invalidate insurance.

DURING
Discuss:
- details that may influence the client's ear-piercing service (e.g., thickness of earlobes)

Note:
- any adverse reaction, if any occur

AFTER
Record:
- results of service
- any modification to service application that has occurred
- what type of ear studs have been used in the ear-piercing service
- the effectiveness of service

Advise on:
- use of specialized aftercare products following ear-piercing service for homecare use to promote skin healing and prevent contra-actions from occurring
- aftercare product application in order to gain maximum benefit from their use
- general ear-piercing and maintenance advice
- the recommended time interval before removal of the stud
- the recommended time interval between ear-piercing services

Provide:
- an aftercare ear-piercing leaflet

RETAIL OPPORTUNITIES
Note:
- any purchases made by the client

EVALUATION
Record:
- comments on the client's satisfaction with the service
- if poor results are achieved, the reasons why
- how you may alter the service plan to achieve the required service results in the future, if applicable

HEALTH AND SAFETY
Advise on:
- how and when to turn the ear stud
- how and when to remove the ear stud
- recommended replacement of the ear stud used for piercing
- appropriate action to be taken in the event of an unwanted reaction to the service

HEALTH & SAFETY

Recommended metals for ear-piercing

Certain metals may cause an allergy. These include nickel, poor quality gold-plated metals and 9ct gold. The use of nickel-containing jewellery is subject to the Dangerous Substances and Preparations (Nickel) (Safety) Regulations (2005).

Recommended metals are surgical stainless steel, titanium (6AL4V) and 14ct gold.

Check what metal is used for your ear jewellery with your supplier, and that it complies with the Regulations.

> There is a real buzz when after a presentation the people you have taught feel confident enough that they wish to purchase a starter kit.
>
> **Jade Rogers**

HEALTH & SAFETY

Piercing ears

Never perform multiple piercing in each ear. The ears will swell, causing discomfort and possible infection.

When more than one hole is required in the same ear (or a hole already exists), the piercing must be at least 9mm apart.

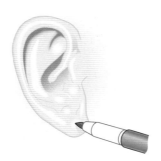

Marking the ear prior to piercing

Preparation of the beauty therapist and client

If the position of the stud has not already been marked, do this now with the surgical skin-marker pen.

1 Wash your hands using a hand disinfectant that contains chlorhexidine as an active ingredient and apply a fresh pair of disposable gloves.

2 Secure the client's hair away from the treatment area. Place paper tissue roll over client's shoulder.

3 Thoroughly cleanse the back and the front of the client's earlobes. Allow the skin to dry. (If moisture is present, the mark will blur.)

4 Holding a mirror in front of the client, discuss with them where the stud should be placed. Mark the position using the sterile pen.

Remember that the ears are not at the same level on each side of the head, and may protrude at different angles. Take time when marking the position of the studs, to ensure that the final appearance is balanced.

HEALTH & SAFETY

Secondary infection

As you cleanse the client's earlobes, you may notice that their skin, ear or hair is dirty. You may proceed, but when giving her the aftercare instructions politely and tactfully point out the importance of cleanliness in preventing secondary infection.

Ear studs

Studs are preferable to hooped earrings or sleepers, as dirt is less likely to cling to the stud and infect the ear. Select studs that are manufactured from hypo-allergenic material.

ALWAYS REMEMBER

If the client has fat lobes explain that the studs may feel a little tight.

Adjust tightness of stud in each ear using a clean tissue to hold the stud. Fresh disposable gloves must be worn if adjustment is necessary. Lobes more than 6mm thick need special care and may require a long post stud.

Piercing the ears

Outcome 3: Pierce the earlobes

Learn how to carry out piercing the earlobes to meet your client's needs by:

1 Piercing the earlobe accurately and safely in the marked position.

2 Minimizing discomfort to the client by ensuring a quick and effective service.

3 Maintaining hygienic conditions and client safety throughout your work.

4 Using **equipment, materials** and **products** according to manufacturers' instructions.

5 Ensuring that the finished result is to the client's satisfaction.

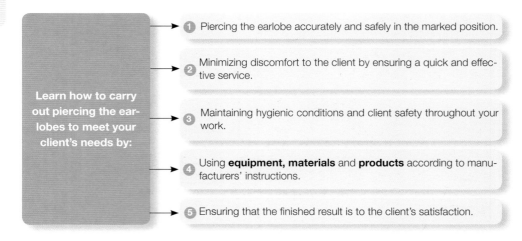

HEALTH & SAFETY

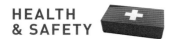

Hazards caused by poor practice

Medical complications can occur where conditions that are contra-indicated are not diagnosed or treated. Poor technique due to poor anatomy and physiology knowledge and understanding can cause damage to blood vessels, nerves and skin tissue, e.g. keloid scarring.

Step-by-step: Piercing the ears

The following procedure illustrates the general technique, with the beauty therapist wearing powder-free vinyl gloves. The details differ according to the ear-piercing gun you are using. Always follow the manufacturers' instructions.

Ensure the service is cost effective and completed in a commercial time, 15 minutes.

ALWAYS REMEMBER

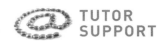

Placement

Try to aim for a central position on the earlobe – this will achieve the best result.

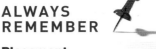

TUTOR SUPPORT

Activity 5: Client record card task

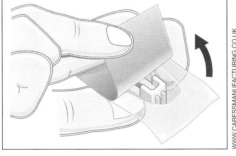

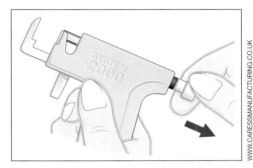

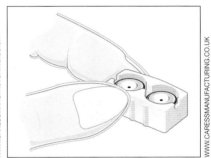

1 Holding the stud pack firmly, remove the backing paper. Take care not to drop the cartridge on the floor! (If you do drop it you will have to throw it away.)

2 Pull back the plunger knob on the back of the gun, until it is fully extended – you will hear it click.

3 Remove the plastic cartridge from the package, holding it by the plastic mount. To avoid contamination, make sure that you do not touch the stud or backing clasp.

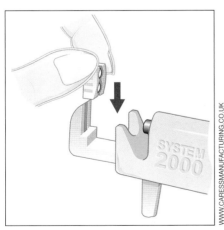

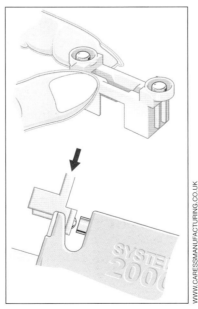

4 There are two parts, which must be separated. One part holds the back clasps: this is positioned in the slot. Push the cartridge down until it will go no further. The second holds the studs: position this against the stud barrel of the gun, which places a protective plastic ring around the barrel of the gun and stud.

5 Gently pull the holder upwards, away from the barrel: this will deposit the stud in the barrel.

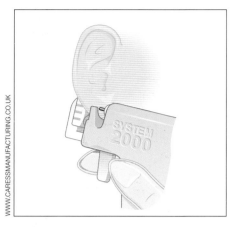

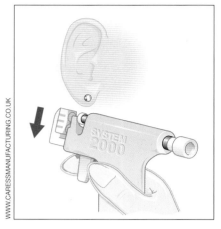

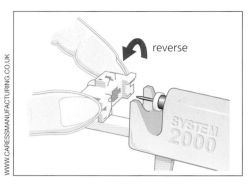

6 Holding the gun horizontally, position the stem of the stud at right angles to the ear so that it is accurately placed over the mark on the earlobe.

Gently squeeze the trigger until it stops. Check that the point of the stud is still in the correct position. If it is, squeeze the trigger again. The ear will be pierced, with the back clasp placed onto the back of the stud.

Check that the earring and back clasp are securely connected.

7 Gently, move the gun down from the lobe. Hold the gun upside down and discard the plastic ring into the waste bin. Pull back the plunger knob and insert the next stud and protective ring.

8 Holding the gun in one hand, grip the back-clasp holder (using the mount in the other hand) and remove the holder from the gun. Invert the holder and place it back into the gun, with the remaining clasp in the top position.

9 Now pierce the second ear, repeating stage **6**. If only one piercing is required where double packs of studs are used, the other stud should be discarded.

10 Using the hand mirror, show the client her pierced ears and check that the result is to the client's satisfaction.

> " Never become complacent with your customers, or over-familiar; we are at work and it is a business.
>
> **Jade Rogers**

HEALTH & SAFETY

Do not handle studs with your bare hands
Follow the manufacturer's instructions for correct loading. There should not be a need to touch the studs or stud-holding devices.

ALWAYS REMEMBER

Technique
Always hold the gun either horizontally or upwards. Never point the gun downwards once it has been loaded – if you do, the studs will fall out.

ALWAYS REMEMBER

Gun malfunction
If the piercing is successful but the clasp fails to attach to the post, firmly attach this manually without causing the client unnecessary distress.

If the ear stud needs adjustment following piercing, rewash your hands and apply a fresh pair of gloves before touching the pierced ear.

BEST PRACTICE

Technique
To avoid anxiety to the client, pierce the second ear without hesitation, yet safely.

BEST PRACTICE

Client comfort
Allow the client to sit still for a few minutes following the service. Offer them tea or coffee. Some clients may be very anxious and need time to relax.

How to complete the service

1 Discuss the aftercare instructions with the client (see page 488).

2 When the service has been completed, invert the gun, eject the protective ring, and remove the empty back-clasp holder. Dispose of the plastic cartridges into the waste bin.

3 Clean the gun using clean cotton wool and surgical spirit, and place it in the ultra-violet sterilizing cabinet. Always refer to manufacturers' instructions for guidance on hygiene maintenance of the gun.

4 Dispose of all used products in the covered lined waste bin.

HEALTH & SAFETY

Disposal of waste

Waste from skin-piercing procedures is classed as clinical waste.

All consumable materials used during the ear-piercing service should be placed in a covered, lined waste bin, and disposed of in a sealed bag.

Waste materials that have come into contact with body fluids must be collected and disposed of by special arrangement.

The disposal of clinical waste is controlled by the Environment Agency. *The Environment Protection Act (1990): Waste Management: The Duty of Care, A Code of Practice* (ISBN 011 752577 X) provides further information on this subject.

5 Any article that has been used on a client must be sterilized before use on another client to prevent *secondary infection*, or *cross-infection*.

Any article that has penetrated the skin must be disposed of hygienically immediately in a sharps box and should be disposed of safely in compliance with clinical waste procedures.

BEST PRACTICE

Technique

The gun should not point down or up when piercing. If the angle of piercing is incorrect, the earring will hang forward, sideways or backwards. Hold at a right angle to the ear.

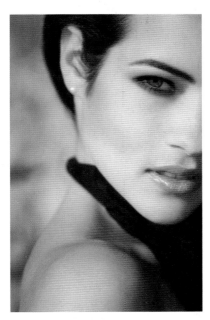

Studs can add to the glamour

ACTIVITY

Differing procedures

The procedure for loading the different ear-piercing guns varies. The procedure given above is one example. Referring to the literature you have collected on the different guns, note ways in which the various service procedures differ.

Outcome 4: Provide aftercare advice

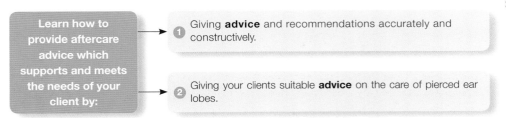

Learn how to provide aftercare advice which supports and meets the needs of your client by:

① Giving **advice** and recommendations accurately and constructively.

② Giving your clients suitable **advice** on the care of pierced ear lobes.

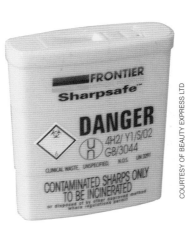

Sharps box

COURTESY OF BEAUTY EXPRESS LTD

Aftercare advice

After the ear-piercing, complete details of the service on the client's record card. It is normal to experience minor pain and redness on the area following the service, explain this to the client. The client should be given clear instructions on how to care for their ears to prevent secondary infection and promote skin healing. The studs must not be removed for five to six weeks to enable effective skin healing and prevent infection. Invite the client to return to the salon after this period for you to remove the studs.

Remind the client always to wash their hands before cleaning the ear area. (If someone else is going to clean the ears, they also must wash their hands with soap and warm water before touching the client's ears.) The ears should be cleaned twice daily, using an aftercare lotion. The lotion must be applied as directed by the manufacturer. It should be applied to clean cotton wool, and the cotton wool squeezed to allow the lotion to run around the stud, at the front of the ear and then at the back. While the ears are being bathed with the cleansing solution, the stud should be rotated by holding it firmly at the front.

Even if the client cleanses their ears effectively, infection could still occur in other ways. These include the following:

- Long nails harbour germs. Infection of the ear can occur while the client is turning the stud.

- The client may touch the stud and ear at times other than when cleaning the ear.

- Shampoo and dirty water may collect around the ear while shampooing the hair. Remind the client to rinse the ear thoroughly with clean water after shampooing.

- The area can get wet e.g. after showering. Dry the area with a clean tissue if so.

- The client should protect their ears when applying hair lacquer or perfume, to avoid sensitizing the ear.

- Following the removal of the studs, the client should only wear gold earrings. Cheap fashion earrings should be worn only for short periods of time, or allergic reactions and ear infections may occur. Earrings must be worn to ensure the pierced hole doesn't heal following removal of the stud posts.

After oral instructions have been given, the client should be provided with an aftercare leaflet containing these instructions.

Body piercing

You may advance your piercing skills further to perform body piercing. **Body piercing** is currently very fashionable. Common areas for piercing include the nipples, the eyebrows, the nose and the navel. Note that body piercing is inappropriate for clients under 17 years of age, as the body is still growing.

Beauty therapy salons that offer ear-piercing are often also asked for body piercing. Body piercing should be undertaken only if you have had thorough training, however, and only if you have the necessary specialized equipment and appropriate insurance cover.

Equipment

The equipment for piercing is either a **body-piercing** gun, which inserts a hollow reed, or the **needle and clamp** method. With the latter, the clamp reduces circulation in the area, thereby anaesthetizing it, and the needle is inserted into the skin. The opening made by the needle is then filled with a ring of high-quality non-reactive surgical steel or gold (above 16 carat).

Aftercare and advice

Special care should be taken of the area for one month following piercing. Ideally the jewellery must not be changed for four to six months to avoid tissue damage and possible infection. If infection occurs, causing excessive redness, swelling or a discharge, the client should return to the salon.

HEALTH & SAFETY

Body piercing
Before performing body piercing, approval is required from your local environmental health authority and registration is required.

Age and consent issues can be confirmed with your local authority who may have used licensing powers to impose licensing conditions relating to the age of the client.

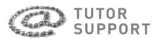

TUTOR SUPPORT

Activity 4: Re-cap, revision and evaluation

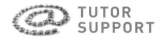

TUTOR SUPPORT

Activity 6: Multiple choice quiz

GLOSSARY OF KEY WORDS

Aftercare advice recommendations given to the client following service to continue the benefits of the service.

Certificate of registration awarded when the premises have been successfully inspected to ensure that the local bye-laws are being followed in relation to cosmetic piercing.

Client groups this term is used in a number of the units and it refers to client diversity. The CRE (Commission for Racial Equality) ethnic group classification is used in the range for these units. These cover white, mixed, Asian, black and Chinese.

Clinical waste waste from ear-piercing is classed as clinical waste. The disposal of clinical waste is controlled by the Environment Agency. Waste materials that have come into contact with body fluids must be collected and disposed of by special arrangements. *The Environment Protection Act (1990): Waste Management: The Duty of Care, A Code of Practice* (ISBN 011 752577 X) provides further information on this subject.

Consent form written permission obtained from a parent or guardian to perform a service on a client under 16 years of age.

Consultation assessment of client's needs using different assessment techniques, including questioning and natural observation.

Contra-action an unwanted reaction occurring during or after service application.

Contra-indication a problematic symptom that indicates that the service may not proceed.

Control of Substances Hazardous to Health (COSHH) Regulations (2002) (Including Biological Agents) Regulations legislation that requires employers and the self-employed to prevent or control the exposure of employees and clients to hazardous substances. This includes exposure to biological agents such as bacteria, fungi and viruses and chemical cleaning/sterilizing agents. Records of the COSHH assessment must be available for inspection.

Dangerous Substances and Preparations (Nickel) (Safety) Regulations (2005) the use of nickel has been found to cause allergies. Check what metal is used for your supplier's ear-piercing jewellery and that it complies with the regulations.

Ear-piercing the perforation of the skin and underlying tissue of the earlobe to create a hole in the skin where jewellery is inserted.

Greater London Council (General Powers) Act (1981) this act covers the London boroughs and relates to cosmetic piercing. It provides that no person can carry out cosmetic piercing unless

they and the business are registered. It also states what records are required to be kept.

Keloids overgrowths of scar tissue, occurring at the site of the ear-piercing.

Local Government Act (2003) (section 120 and schedule 6) has amended the Local Government (Miscellaneous Provisions) Act (1982) to enable each authority to regulate businesses providing cosmetic body piercing. Each local authority can introduce its own bye-laws to set the standards for cosmetic piercing.

Local Government (Miscellaneous Provisions) Act (1982) requires that salons offering any form of skin piercing be registered with the local health authority. This registration includes the operators who will be carrying out the service and the salon premises where the service will be carried out.

London Local Authorities Act (1991 and 2007) this act states that no person shall carry out cosmetic piercing at an establishment without obtaining a licence from a participating council. Conditions can be attached to the licence, such as hygiene practices, age restrictions, etc.

Service plan after the consultation, suitable service objectives are established to treat the client's conditions and needs.

ASSESSMENT OF KNOWLEDGE AND UNDERSTANDING

Having covered the learning objectives for **Carry out ear-piercing**, test what you need to know and understand answering the following short questions below. The information covers:

- organizational and legal requirements
- how to work safely and effectively when piercing earlobes
- consult, plan and prepare for earlobe piercing
- anatomy and physiology
- contra-indications and contra-actions
- equipment, materials and products
- earlobe piercing
- aftercare advice for clients

Organizational and legal requirements

1   Why is it necessary to obtain parental/guardian consent for children under the age of 16 years?

2   How long should be allowed when booking for this service?

3   Taking into account health and safety hygiene requirements, how would you prepare yourself for ear-piercing service?

4   What does the Local Government (Miscellaneous Provisions) Act (1982) and its amendments require of those performing ear-piercing?

5   Which external government body monitors the implementation of the Miscellaneous Provisions Act (1982) and its amendments?

6   What information should be recorded on the client's record card following the ear-piercing service, and why is this important?

7   Why is it important for staff to be familiar with the ear-piercing pricing structures?

How to work safely and effectively when piercing earlobes

1   What personal protective equipment must be worn when carrying out the ear-piercing service?

2   Why is it essential to wear personal protective equipment during ear-piercing?

3   How is the ear-piercing gun cleaned following the ear-piercing service?

4   How should the client be positioned for ear-piercing service? Why is this important?

5   How can you prevent infection when carrying out the ear-piercing service?

6   How should waste be disposed of safely and correctly?

7   What salon environmental factors should be considered to ensure that the piercing is carried out competently?

8   How can you ensure that you and the client are correctly positioned for the ear-piercing service to be performed safely and to avoid discomfort?

Consult, plan and prepare for earlobe piercing

1   How can you ensure that the position of the ear stud will be correct?

2   How would you describe the procedure of ear-piercing to ensure a client was confident both about the procedure and your expertise?

3   If a second piercing to the lobe was requested, when would you recommend this takes place?

4   What advice and recommendations would you give when piercing the earlobes of:
   - a client who has previously suffered from keloid scarring?
   - a particularly nervous client?
   - a client with fat earlobes?
   - a client with diabetes?
   - a client who is allergic to nickel?
   - a client who has had their earlobes previously and this is a second piercing?

5   Why should you record your client's responses to questions asked at consultation?

6   Contra-indications are not always visible. How can you ensure the clients suitability for ear-piercing service?

Anatomy and physiology

1   Which part of the ear is recommended for ear-piercing?

2   Which parts of the earlobe are considered unsuitable to pierce and what dangers may result if piercing took place?

Contra-indications and contra-actions

1   State three conditions that would contra-indicate an ear-piercing service.

2   Sate three conditions that would restrict ear-piercing service.

3   If you suspected a client had a contagious contra-indication what actions would you take for the welfare of the client, yourself and others?

Equipment, materials and products

1   If the ear-piercing gun malfunctions, what action should be taken?

2   What should be checked to ensure that the ear-piercing system is a recommended method and complies with local authority bye-laws?

3   What equipment, materials and products are required in addition to the ear-piercing gun?

4   Why is it necessary to provide aftercare retail products and aftercare guidance literature?

Earlobe piercing

1   Why should only one pair of studs be fitted at once?

2   How is the ear cleaned before ear-piercing service?

3   What is the normal reaction following ear-piercing service? Why must this be discussed with the client?

4   If the client failed to follow the aftercare instructions, what complications could occur?

5   How would infection of the earlobe be recognized?

6   What is the healing period for earlobe piercing? Why should the piercing studs not be removed during the healing period?

Aftercare advice for clients

1   What aftercare instructions should be given to the client following ear-piercing service?

2   If an infection of the earlobe were to occur, what action should a client take?

3   Daily, how often should the ear studs be rotated during the healing period?

4   How should this be performed by the client to prevent secondary infection?

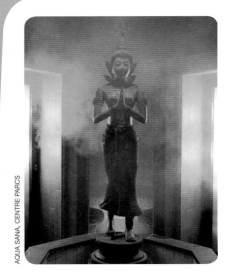

AQUA SANA, CENTRE PARCS

16 Spa Operations (S1)

S1 Unit Learning Objectives

This chapter covers **Unit S1 Assist with Spa Operations**.

This unit is all about how to assist with spa operations. This will require that you can check the quality and maintain the general condition of spa work areas. This will include cleaning, replenishing consumables, setting up and shutting down work areas.

There are four learning outcomes for Unit S1 which you must achieve competently:

1   Maintain safe and effective methods of working when assisting with spa

2   Clean and set up spa work areas

3   Check and maintain the spa work areas

4   Shut down work areas

Your assessor will observe you on **at least four separate occasions** which must include wet areas and changing rooms.

From the **range** statement, you must show that you:

●   have performed all operations competently in all work areas:

○   wet areas

○   service areas

○   changing rooms

○   relaxation areas

○   service areas

However, you must prove that you have the necessary knowledge, understanding and skills to be able to perform competently across the range.

(continued on the next page)

(continued on the next page)

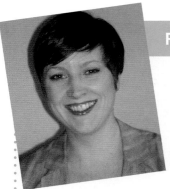

ROLE MODEL

Sally Biles
Senior Spa Trainer
The Sanctuary, London

" I have worked in the beauty industry for over 18 years, after graduating from The London College of Fashion in 1991 with a BTEC ND. I then continued my studies, attaining a BTEC HNC, City & Guilds 7307 Teaching Certificate and a Certificate in Education. Over the years, I have worked as a therapist, spa manager, college lecturer and trainer, gaining experience and knowledge. I currently work at The Sanctuary in Covent Garden and am responsible for training and service development.

(continued)

When assisting with spa operations it is important to use the skills you have learnt in the following units:

Unit G20 Make sure your own actions reduce risks to health and safety

Unit G18 Promote additional products or services to clients

Unit G8 Develop and maintain your effectiveness at work

Essential anatomy and physiology knowledge requirements for this unit, **S1**, are identified on the checklist chart in Chapter 2, page 16.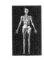

Introduction to spa services

Spa services are used for their beneficial effects upon the whole body. The spa environment and spa services induce a physical and mental sense of well-being.

The term 'spa' is said to be derived from a village near Liege, in Belgium called *Spau*. It had mineral hot springs that people would visit to improve their health and ailments.

The choice of spa services offered in the workplace will depend on the space available and the nature of other service services offered. Health farms commonly offer a comprehensive range of spa services whereas leisure centres and gyms popularly offer heat services such as sauna, steam and spa pools.

Spa services include:

- Sauna – a dry heat service where air is heated.

- Relaxation room – sometimes referred to by the Latin name *tepidarium*, a room of ambient temperature (close to body temperature).

- Steam service – a wet heat service where water is heated.

- Hydrotherapy – where water is used for its therapeutic effect.

- Flotation – the body is suspended (wet flotation), or supported (dry flotation), inducing relaxation.

- Body wrapping – the body is wrapped in bandages, plastic sheets or thermal blankets for different therapeutic effects. Ingredients such as marine minerals or clay are applied to the bandages or directly to the skin to achieve different results.

General effects of spa therapy services

Spa heat services and therapeutic skin-conditioning services have the following effects:

- Relaxation is induced through services that raise the body temperature, increasing the blood circulation generally, which soothes sensory nerve endings and causes muscle relaxation. Heat therapy is a popular de-stressing service.

- Blood pressure falls as the superficial capillaries and vessels dilate.

TOP TIP

Before adding spa services to your services available, consider client usage and profitability. If you do not have a shower facility you will be limited in the range of spa services you can offer.

ALWAYS REMEMBER

Spa services as a preparatory service

Spa services are beneficial when applied before other body services as they make the body tissues and systems more receptive.

Spa services as a rehabilitation service

Water is used for the service of medical conditions such as rheumatism and rehabilitation after injury.

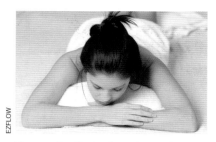

EZFLOW

Therapeutic effects of spa therapy improve physical and mental well-being

ALWAYS REMEMBER

History of spa services

The therapeutic effects of spa services including steam, sauna and spa pools have been recognized throughout the ages.

During the Roman Empire baths were used for their healing health benefits and as a social meeting place. Examples of these original bath houses can still be seen today in the city of Bath, England.

For thousands of years people from all cultures including Europe, Russia, the Middle East and India have used steam baths, and the medical benefits of the Turkish or Middle Eastern *hamman* steam baths date back to 200 BC. Hippocrates, the founder of Western medicine more than 2000 years ago said, '*Give me the power to create a fever and I will cure any disease*'.

Water is still used in medicine today for the service of sport injuries, rehabilitation and rheumatic disease.

HEALTH & SAFETY

Sweat loss during heat services

The amount of sweat lost during heat services can vary from 0.15 to 1.5 litres.

It is important that the client is given water during and after heat service as necessary to rehydrate and avoid the contra-action dehydration.

● Heart rate and pulse rate increase.

● Blood circulation is improved. Vasodilation occurs, which increases the blood flow through the area, supplying oxygen and nutrients to the cells.

● Lymphatic circulation is increased, assisting with the elimination of toxins and waste materials.

● Desquamation – the removal of surface dead skin cells from the stratum corneum is increased.

● Increased activity of the sebaceous and sudoriferous glands improves skin condition. This also creates a deep-cleaning action.

● Metabolism may be increased or decreased depending upon the service received.

● Flotation service causes a fall in heart and pulse rate due to its relaxation effect.

● Body wrapping services cause a rise in pulse rate due to an increase in body temperature.

Anatomy and physiology

Heat services: sauna, steam and relaxation room

When heat services are applied, there is an increase in body temperature generally of about 1–2°C. Vasodilation of the blood capillaries occurs, lowering the body temperature by increasing heat loss. This vasodilation effect causes erythema, where the skin becomes reddened. This effect soon subsides after application.

The increase in body temperature causes a corresponding increase in the heart and pulse rates. There is a fall in blood pressure as the resistance of the capillary walls is reduced when the capillaries dilate.

The dilation of the blood capillaries enables the blood to transport increased nutrients to the skin, enhancing its function and appearance.

The maximum temperature that the body can tolerate varies according to the type of service – dry or wet. Dry air holds less heat than water vapour, and body sweat is able to evaporate in dry heat, thus cooling the skin. This enables the body to tolerate a higher temperature.

Air that is saturated with water vapour is able to hold more heat, and body sweat is unable to evaporate so the body cannot cool itself. The body therefore cannot tolerate very high temperatures in wet heat.

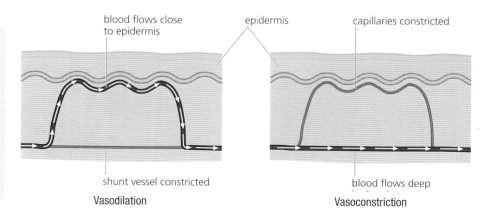

Vasodilation Vasoconstriction

Hydrotherapy service

Hydrotherapy uses water to induce physical and mental well-being.

Hydrotherapy services include:

- spa pools
- hydro baths and foam baths

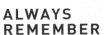

ALWAYS REMEMBER

Metabolism
Metabolism is a series of chemical reactions which utilizes the nutrients required for growth and body repair.

Spa pool Also known as a whirlpool or jacuzzi bath, a spa pool will increase blood and lymphatic circulation due to the thermal and mechanical stimulating effect of the water. The rise in body temperature causes the pulse to increase.

Air is forced by a compressor through the water, passed through small openings in the bath. Water jets striking the skin's surface create a skin toning effect. Muscular pain and fatigue is reduced as accumulated toxins and waste are dispersed in the improved lymphatic circulation.

Hydro bath The hydro bath is fitted with air and water jets that massage the tissues of the body as an air compressor aerates the water. These can be pressure controlled to achieve different effects. A hose may also be used to manually direct air over the body. This can be used to improve the skin tone in specific areas and can relieve muscular aches and pains by the heating effect and improved circulation.

Body temperature is increased which causes muscles to be relaxed due to increased blood circulation. Metabolism is increased.

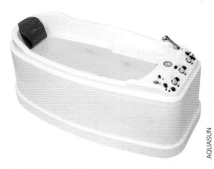

Hydrotherapy bath

Foam bath In a foam bath an air compressor creates foam when air is passed through a shallow bath of water containing a foaming agent. The foam surrounds the body of the client and has a thermal effect, insulating the body and keeping it warm. The heating effect on the body induces perspiration but this cannot evaporate as the surrounding air is saturated with water vapour.

Increased perspiration aids elimination of waste products and toxins from the skin. Muscles are relaxed due to the rise in body temperature and increased blood circulation.

Flotation services During flotation service total relaxation occurs and this affects the autonomic nervous system which has two divisions: the *parasympathetic* and the *sympathetic*.

- The parasympathetic division is stimulated in periods of relaxation.
- The sympathetic division is stimulated in periods of stress.

During flotation service, the sympathetic system is deactivated and the parasympathetic division is stimulated. A calming effect on the body occurs as pulse rate slows, metabolism reduces, and muscles relax.

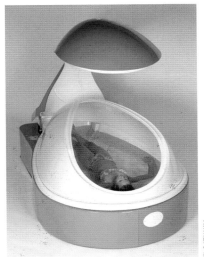

Wet flotation service

Body wrapping Body wrapping results in an increase in body temperature, blood circulation generally and pulse rate.

The dilation of the blood capillaries enables the blood to transport increased nutrients to the skin, enhancing its function and appearance. As the skin warms, therapeutic ingredients are absorbed by the skin and have a skin-conditioning effect. They are absorbed through the pores, hair follicles and the epidermis (stratum corneum).

The increase in body temperature also increases perspiration and waste elimination. Ingredients such as clay are used to help to draw out toxins.

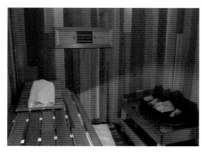

Sauna (traditional wood)

The lymphatic circulation increases, which aids the elimination of excess fluid and toxins in the improved circulation.

Where heating is an effect of the body wrap, this helps to relax tense muscles.

Spa operation

Sauna – dry heat service

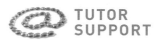

TUTOR SUPPORT

Activity 4: Compare heat treatments task

Sauna is a dry heat service. There are alternative methods of sauna including traditional Finnish or Tyrolean sauna, and the Laconium sauna.

Finnish or Tyrolean sauna The sauna is usually a timber construction, often made from pine, which is a porous wood. This allows the condensation created to be absorbed and the internal furnishing walls to breathe. The sauna air is usually heated by an electric stove to between 70°–110°C.

The sauna is heated by a stove that contains rocks. These rocks are often made up of Peridotite, a dense coarse, grained rock. The coals get very hot and steam is created by pouring water onto them. An air inlet is situated at floor level and an outlet is found near the top of the cabin.

This high temperature is tolerable because the heat is reduced on contact with the skin and the sweat induced rapidly reduces the skin temperature.

Laconium sauna This sauna creates an evenly distributed mild dry heat. The temperature in the Laconium sauna is approximately 55°C, generated by under floor heating as opposed to heat created from a stove.

Laconium is suitable for gently heating the skin for the purpose of cleansing and purifying. Some clients will prefer this sauna type as the heat is less intense.

Electricity is used to produce the heat and a sauna is operated by the mains supply because of the high power rating used.

ALWAYS REMEMBER

Sauna history
Saunas were used in Scandinavia as part of ancient historical religious ceremonies to cleanse physically, mentally and spiritually.

Additional therapeutic effects of dry heat:

- elimination of metabolic waste is increased
- skin cleansing occurs as the pores dilate, secreting sweat onto the skin's surface, thereby eliminating waste products
- respiratory congestion can be relieved
- increased sweating can cause temporary weight loss. However, this loss is quickly replaced with fluids consumed following service
- muscles are relaxed due to the rise in body temperature and increased blood circulation

TOP TIP

Infrared sauna

An infrared sauna heats the body directly, rather than heating the air which in turn heats the body. Infrared radiators penetrate the body tissues to a depth of 45mm and this stimulates the cardiovascular system which improves cellular metabolism and improves muscular fatigue and tension.

The positive effect of colour as a therapy – called *phototherapy* – can be combined with this service.

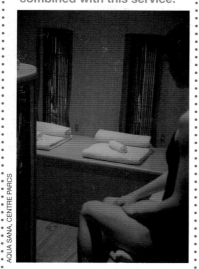

AQUA SANA, CENTRE PARCS

Infrared sauna

Relaxation room The relaxation room enables the client to rest between experiencing different spa services, allowing the body temperature and blood pressure to lower. The air is ambient, the same as the body's temperature. The air in the room is dry to enhance the body's immune system and relieve stress. It is important that this area is very quiet to induce relaxation. Heated couches warmed by a heat-conducting hot mortar may be found in this room. These are ideal for clients unsuitable to receive heat service, which significantly increases blood circulation, e.g. sauna service.

Additional therapeutic effects of the relaxation room:

- heating effect soothes the sensory nerve endings
- relieves muscular aches and pains
- increases blood flow and removes waste products
- the relaxing environment reduces stress and tension

Electricity is used to produce the heat. The room is operated by the mains supply because of the high power rating used.

Steam – a wet heat service

Steam service can be received individually in a steam bath, or communally in a steam room. To produce steam, water is heated to 100°C. This then mixes with air to produce water vapour.

Steam bath This is constructed from fibreglass. A hinged door allows access and encloses the client; an opening at the top of the bath exposes the client's head. The client sits on a seat inside the bath that is adjustable for the height of each client and for their comfort.

Water is heated in a small tank inside the bath, situated underneath the seat. On boiling, the water produces steam. The steam mixes with the air in the bath and produces water vapour, which circulates inside the cabinet. The temperature inside the cabinet is most comfortable at 45°–50°C.

Steam room To provide steam for a room, the water is heated in a boiler. The steam created is passed through tubes and the water vapour created circulates inside the room.

The *calidarium* is a steam room that uses natural herbal essences to create an aromatic steam room.

The *hamman* is a communal steam bath with a hot, moist aromatic atmosphere to purify and detox. The hamman bath traditionally has a dome-shaped central chamber with further chambers, of differing temperatures, leading from it. The hottest room is heated from the floor.

HEALTH & SAFETY

Temperature in the steam room
The air in the steam bath/room is saturated with water vapour (that is, it is unable to hold more water) and sweat on the skin's surface is unable to evaporate to create the skin-cooling effect. For this reason, the temperature for steam service is lower than that for sauna to avoid the body overheating.

HEALTH & SAFETY

Sauna temperature
High temperatures are only recommended in larger saunas where there is a greater volume of air.

Humidity in the sauna
Water can be sprinkled onto the rocks in the sauna to raise moisture content (humidity).

ALWAYS REMEMBER

Steam cubicles
These are filled with steam and offer an alternative to the steam bath. The air is gently heated to 45°C and usually infused with herbal aromatic oils for their therapeutic effect.

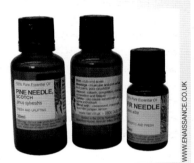

Sauna pine oils

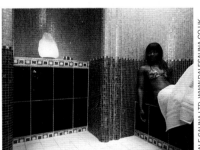

Calidarium

ALWAYS REMEMBER

Bath houses have been used for thousands of years – the ancient Romans had hot rooms.

WWW.ENAISSANCE.CO.UK

DALE SAUNA LTD. WWW.DALESAUNA.CO.UK

TOP TIP

Hydrotherapy

Hydrotherapy bath water may have seaweed, sea salt or essential oils added to enhance its therapeutic effect.

ALWAYS REMEMBER

Hydrotherapy pool – weighing less

When in water the human body weighs 10 times less than normal.

ALWAYS REMEMBER

Natural spas

Natural spas are swimming pools filled with mineral water and are considered to have therapeutic effects.

TOP TIP

Hydro-oxygen baths

This is a bath-type cabinet. A compressor aerates hot water which strikes the body; the cabinet is also diffused with oxygen which is extremely stimulating to the skin. It is important for the client to relax following service.

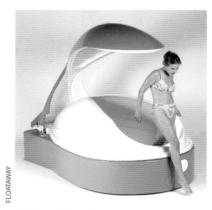

FLOATAWAY

Flotation bath: wet

Additional therapeutic effects of steam heat:

- muscles are relaxed due to the rise in body temperature and increased blood circulation

Hydrotherapy

In hydrotherapy, water is used for its therapeutic effect.

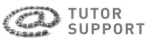

TUTOR SUPPORT

Activity 2: Effect of heat treatment task

Spa pool A spa pool is full of heated warm water in which the client sits. It is constructed from shaped, durable acrylic, or tiled concrete. Provided with an electric power supply, air is forced through small openings and jets of air pass through the water, creating bubbles. These bubbles massage the surface of the skin from all directions, which has a stimulating effect.

The pool may incorporate features such as jets placed to massage different body parts, for example the lower back, and water fountains which can massage the neck with the power of the water flow.

Hydro baths and foam baths The hydro bath is usually made of acrylic and is filled with warm water. Operated by electricity, an air compressor provides underwater massage through high-powered jets. The air is forced through perforations in a duckboard or through outlet holes in the bath. A hose can also be used to manually direct water to stimulate circulation in specific areas.

The bath may be used to maintain wellbeing or as a rehabilitation service. Features include preset massage programmes to achieve different effects.

Foam baths are usually made of acrylic. A plastic duckboard perforated with small holes is located at the bottom of the bath. Operated by electricity, an air compressor forces air through the holes which mixes with water and a foam agent to create the foam bath.

Additional therapeutic effects of hydrotherapy service:

- relaxation – the body weight is supported by the warm water and gently massaged
- skin cleansing – as the water massages the skin's surface, desquamation is increased
- skin toning – when using jets of water to massage the body tissues
- muscle fatigue and joint pain – can be relieved by the increased blood and lymph circulation and increased cellular metabolism

Flotation, wet and dry

The body is suspended, floats or is supported, inducing physical and mental relaxation.

Wet flotation in a bath or tank Flotation baths or tanks are commonly capsule-shaped and constructed from fibreglass. The inside is lined with plastic resin.

Flotation pools are also available.

The service uses Epsom salts diluted in water at high concentration which enables the body to float, and be suspended in the water. Approximately 280 kgs of Epsom salts are diluted in 500 litres of water, which is maintained at body temperature. This is approximately 570g of Epsom salts to 1 litre of water.

Due to the high salt content, the skin does not lose body salts, and does not wrinkle, as would commonly occur when exposed to warm water for long periods of time.

Dry flotation Here the client lies on a warmed tank of water, protected by a polymer flexible membrane covering protected by paper roll. The client lies on a bench that is lowered by the therapist so that the client is suspended by the water but has no direct contact with it.

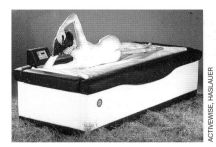

Flotation bath: dry

ACTIVEWISE, HASLAUER

The client may have specific therapeutic skincare products applied to the skin to nourish or purify and detoxify. The body is then wrapped to maintain heat and absorb the products.

Additional therapeutic effects of flotation service:

- stress is reduced as blood pressure is lowered
- skin conditioning occurs as circulation is increased, or in dry flotation the skin benefits from the therapeutic skin products applied
- beneficial to those with back injuries, as the water supports the body and takes pressure off the back
- rheumatic conditions are relieved as there is improved blood circulation between the affected joints and relief of muscular tension
- slower brain wave patterns, known as theta waves, occur in wet flotation

Equipment
When using a dry flotation bed always explain the sensations and noises the float will make to your client at the consultation stage of the service. This will ensure the client knows what to expect and what is normal.

Sally Biles

Body wrapping

A manual service. There are various service techniques used in body wrapping according to the effect to be achieved or the service product used. Always refer to manufacturer's instructions.

The skin may be prepared for service by applying an exfoliating service or by body brushing, which stimulates both blood and lymphatic circulation.

The body may be wrapped in hot linen bandages that have been soaked in therapeutic ingredients.

Alternatively service products using ingredients such as marine minerals or clay may be applied to the skin to achieve different skin conditioning results, including detoxification.

The body can then be wrapped in a thermal blanket, foil, plastic or bandages to maintain and increase body heat which increases lymphatic circulation and fluid loss, achieving a slimming effect.

Therapeutic effects of body wrapping service:

- cellular regeneration is increased
- waste products and toxins are eliminated
- temporary weight loss through increased sweating and increased loss of body fluids
- the therapeutic effect of body products helps balance the skin and body by skin stimulation caused by the cleansing, heating action

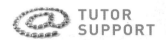

TUTOR SUPPORT

Activity 7: Spa well-being poster task

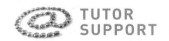

TUTOR SUPPORT

Activity 3: Body wraps handout

BEST PRACTICE

Your work role

Your role is to assist with spa services and you must work within your job responsibilities. However, it is important to respond courteously to requests for assistance from colleagues and anticipate their needs to ensure the smooth running of the spa.

Outcome 1: Maintain safe and effective methods of working when assisting with spa operations

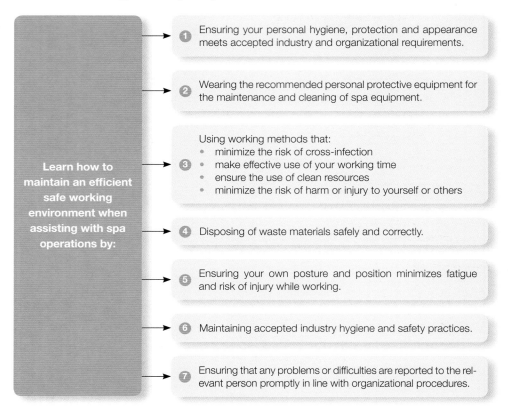

Learn how to maintain an efficient safe working environment when assisting with spa operations by:

1. Ensuring your personal hygiene, protection and appearance meets accepted industry and organizational requirements.

2. Wearing the recommended personal protective equipment for the maintenance and cleaning of spa equipment.

3. Using working methods that:
   - minimize the risk of cross-infection
   - make effective use of your working time
   - ensure the use of clean resources
   - minimize the risk of harm or injury to yourself or others

4. Disposing of waste materials safely and correctly.

5. Ensuring your own posture and position minimizes fatigue and risk of injury while working.

6. Maintaining accepted industry hygiene and safety practices.

7. Ensuring that any problems or difficulties are reported to the relevant person promptly in line with organizational procedures.

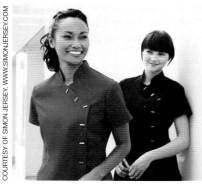

Personal presentation and uniform

HEALTH & SAFETY

Hygiene guidance is available for the swimming pool, jacuzzi and spa pool as follows:

- Health Protection Agency (HPA)
- The Swimming Pool and Allied Trades Association (SPATA)
- HSE Managing Health and Safety in Swimming Pools
- Local Environmental Health Agency

Personal presentation

It is important that within your work role you wear the necessary personal protective equipment provided as some tasks will involve working with hazardous substances. In addition to your work wear this will involve a face and eye protection shield, eye goggles, PVC gloves, protective boots, apron and, as necessary, overalls when carrying out operations in the plant room. A work wear uniform is usually provided and the trousers are typically a shorter length to accommodate working in a wet environment. A protective apron may be worn for cleaning tasks to prevent marking and contaminating the work wear. Hair if long should be secured for reasons of hygiene. Footwear should have a sole with a non-slip surface. Jewellery should be minimal to avoid moisture remaining in contact with the skin which could lead to contact dermatitis, a skin disorder caused by intolerance of the skin to a particular substance, or a group of substances. On exposure to the substance the skin quickly becomes irritated and an allergic reaction occurs.

Employers have a responsibility to provide a safe working environment for their employees and clients and must comply with the **Management of Health and Safety at Work Regulations (MHSWR) (1999)**, managing any risks associated with spa operations.

The spa will have a set of operational procedures which should be checked at the start of the working day, during and on completion. The regularity of ongoing quality and health and safety checks will also be scheduled. It is necessary that these checks are dated and signed when completed and are available as an auditable document. An authorized officer from the Environmental Health Department may request to inspect both client records and related health and safety periodical checks. Procedures must comply with the requirements of Section 3 of the **Health and Safety at Work Act (1974)** that, as far as is reasonably practicable, the public is not exposed to risks of health and safety. It is important that you comply with the work policy operational procedures for cleaning, preparing, maintaining and shutting down the spa areas. The spa work area should be clean and hygienic at all times. Manufacturers' guidelines should be followed on the correct and safe use of cleaning and disinfection materials. All spa staff should be trained and competent in cleaning and disinfection procedures within their area of responsibility infection control; health and safety and emergency action plan procedures.

If you encounter any risk or hazard that is outside your responsibility you should inform the relevant qualified person immediately of the concern.

Avoid risk of injury at all times by observing your posture when performing any activity.

If moving goods around the work place remember to use safe lifting and handling techniques, see Chapter 3, pages 73 and 74.

Reception

Heat services can be offered as individual services, but are also beneficial when given before other body services to increase their therapeutic effects. If you offer communal sauna, steam or other spa services, there will be a recommended number of clients who can use these facilities at once. Make sure you are aware of this to avoid overbooking.

For the client's first heat service, service time is shorter to monitor their physiological and psychological response to service.

Service type	Service details
Sauna	Service may be received 2–3 times per week. Service duration 15–20 minutes.
Relaxation room	Service may be received 2–3 times per week. Service duration 30 minutes.
Steam room	Service may be received 2–3 times per week. Service duration 10–15 minutes.
Steam bath	Service may be received 2–3 times per week. Service duration 10–20 minutes.
Hydrotherapy spa pool	Service may be received daily. Service duration 10–15 minutes.
Hydrotherapy/foam bath	Service may be received 2–3 times per week. Service duration 15–20 minutes.
Flotation	Service may be received 1–2 times per week. Wet flotation service duration 20–60 minutes. Dry flotation service duration 40 minutes.
Body wrap	Service may be received 2–3 times per week. Service time 45–60 minutes, depending on the technique used.

ALWAYS REMEMBER

Data Protection Act (1998)
Remember client records should be stored securely and viewed only by those authorized to do so.

HEALTH & SAFETY

Health and Safety at Work Act (HASAWA) (1974)
This Act is the main legislation covering employers' responsibilities to a variety of healthy, safe working practices and associated regulations.

Chemicals used in the spa and to clean and maintain the spa must be stored, handles and used correctly – see the **Control of Substances Hazardous to Health Regulations (COSHH) (2002)**.
If necessary protective clothing may have to be worn – see the **Personal Protective Equipment (PPE) at Work Regulations (1992)**.

> **The importance of linked products (to the success of the business)**
>
> Linked selling is important where products are promoted to support the service aim. Linking product sales increases your spa/salon's 'spend per client' and should also ensure the effectiveness of your client's service e.g. using an exfoliator with a moisturiser to improve a dry skin condition.
>
> **Sally Biles**

HEALTH & SAFETY

Skin sensitivity test for allergies

If a client has allergies or hypersensitive skin, assess skin tolerance by applying a small amount of the service product to the skin behind the ear or at the inner elbow.

Skin allergy will be recognized by skin irritation itching, redness and swelling.

Record this on the client's record card and do not perform the service.

HEALTH & SAFETY

Preventing cross-infection

Disposable paper slippers may be worn to prevent cross-infection for spa therapy services such as body wrapping. Ensure these are available if provided.

Verruca socks may be worn for hydrotherapy services.

Reception staff must be aware that a client consultation is necessary before use of the spa facilities to check suitability.

Advise the client that a bathing costume may be worn if preferred for heat services. Inform the client beforehand that jewellery should not be worn during heat services and may have to be removed for body wrapping. They may prefer to not wear it for the appointment for reasons of security.

If the client is attending for a body wrap that contains iodine, check that the client does not have an allergy to it. If unsure the client may receive a skin sensitivity test to assess skin reaction before service.

Heat and hydrotherapy services generally may be received two to three times per week.

Allow time for client questions when booking or advising on any spa service. It is important that the client has a thorough understanding of the service plan.

Question the client to check for contra-indications.

Contra-indications

If a client is found to have any of the following, heat service must not be received:

- Severe skin conditions, e.g. acute eczema.
- Systemic medical conditions:
  - High/low blood pressure.
  - Thrombosis, a clot in the blood vessel or heart.
- Phlebitis, inflammation of the vein.
- Lymphatic disorders such as medical oedema.
- Epilepsy, a disorder of the nervous system.
- Respiratory conditions e.g. bronchitis/asthma.
- Diabetes, a decreased insulin secretion which causes excess glucose (sugar) to accumulate in the bloodstream. Increased urination occurs to excrete the excess glucose.
- Liver, kidney or pancreatic conditions.
- Viral, bacterial or fungal skin disorders such as verrucas and athlete's foot.
- Disorders requiring medication.
- Allergy to iodine, found in seaweed-based skin preparations: this must be checked when performing body wraps.
- Severe varicose veins (avoid heat service, massage and body wrapping on the lower limbs).
- Claustrophobia – unsuitable services for clients with a fear of being in a confined area include flotation service and heat services such as the sauna and steam room.

Other contra-indications may be temporary and include:

- Pregnancy.
- Menstruation, first days.

- Not having eaten for several hours – fainting may occur.

- A recent heavy meal within one and a half hours.

- Recent active exercise – wait approximately 20–30 minutes.

- Recent alcohol consumption.

- Recent drug use.

- Recent over-exposure to UV light.

- Recent wax depilation, electrical epilation service (24–48 hours before a spa service) to avoid skin sensitivity and possible secondary infection.

- A wound.

- A migraine.

- Severe bruising.

- High body temperature with infections such as influenza.

All clients must complete a medical questionnaire to identify if they have any contra-indications.

If the client is a minor under the age of 16, it is necessary to obtain parent/guardian permission for service. The parent/guardian will also have to be present when the service is received. Certain spa services however are prohibited for minors aged 8 years and under, check your operational guidance procedures.

Outcome 2: Clean and set up spa work areas

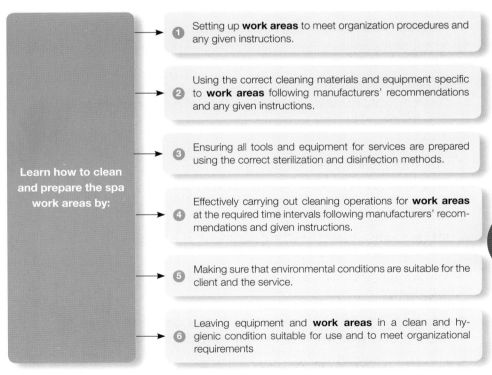

Learn how to clean and prepare the spa work areas by:

1. Setting up **work areas** to meet organization procedures and any given instructions.

2. Using the correct cleaning materials and equipment specific to **work areas** following manufacturers' recommendations and any given instructions.

3. Ensuring all tools and equipment for services are prepared using the correct sterilization and disinfection methods.

4. Effectively carrying out cleaning operations for **work areas** at the required time intervals following manufacturers' recommendations and given instructions.

5. Making sure that environmental conditions are suitable for the client and the service.

6. Leaving equipment and **work areas** in a clean and hygienic condition suitable for use and to meet organizational requirements

Follow organizational and legal requirements to set up the spa work areas. The spa work areas listed provide a checklist of associated resource requirements which should be prepared for use and available at all times.

HEALTH & SAFETY

Treating a client with a contra-indication

Certain contra-indications, if mild or under GP control, may be treated. A GP's permission must be sought before a contra-indicated service can be given.

Client's well-being should be monitored at regular intervals according to organizational policy.

HEALTH & SAFETY

Flotation service and skin disorders

Some skin disorders can become aggravated by the salt used in wet flotation service. Alternatively, if available, dry flotation service may be offered.

HEALTH & SAFETY

Increase in pulse

The heart works much faster during heat services. It needs to pump the blood to the surface of the skin to regulate body temperature and can increase from 72 beats per minute to 150 beats per minute.

Because there is an increase in pulse rate with a body wrap it is necessary to gain a GP's permission to treat if the client has high or low blood pressure.

TOP TIP

Claustrophobia

To enable clients to become accustomed to the enclosed environment of the flotation bath, some models have a door which may be kept open during service. Make clients aware of this feature if less confident.

Equipment and materials

Sauna service

- **Sauna** – with adequate space for the air to circulate around the sauna.

- **Client guidance instructions** – clearly sited.

- **Appropriate ventilation.**

- **Shower** – to cleanse the skin and regulate body temperature

- **Body and hair shampoos** – may be provided

- **Protective footwear** – to avoid cross-infection, e.g. disposable paper slippers.

- **Clean towels for each client** – to drape the body after showering and to protect the hair.

- **A wooden pail containing purified water to ladle over the coals** – the water boils when poured onto the heated coals which increases the humidity (water vapour content of the air), cooling the air and making breathing more comfortable. This raising of humidity also makes the sauna feel hotter.

HEALTH & SAFETY

For safety the relative humidity of the air should be between 50–70 per cent

$$\text{Relative humidity (per cent)} = \frac{\text{Actual water vapour content of the air}}{\text{Maximum it can hold at the temperature}}$$

- **Temperature gauge** – to record the heat of the sauna, 70°C for a mild sauna, 110°C for a hot sauna.

- **An electric stove** – which heats the stones or coals, protected by a guard.

- **Hygrometer** – an instrument to measure relative humidity – generally the reading should be between 50–70 per cent.

- **Drinking water** – to rehydrate following service.

- **Relaxation area** – to use following service.

Steam service

- **Steam bath or steam room**.

- **Distilled water** – to fill the water tank.

- **Essence** – to introduce into the steam room, e.g. pine.

- **Appropriate ventilation**.

- **Client guidance instructions** – clearly sited.

- **Shower** – to cleanse the skin and regulate body temperature.

- **Body and hair shampoos** – may be provided.

- **Protective footwear** – to avoid cross-infection e.g. disposable paper slippers.

- **Clean towels for each client** – to drape over the seat and over the floor to protect the back of the client's legs from scalding by the steam, to provide modesty, dry the body after showering and to protect the hair. Also a small towel may be draped around the opening of the cabinet during service to prevent moist heat escaping.
- **Drinking water** – to rehydrate following service.
- **Relaxation area** – to use following service.

Spa pool

- **Spa pool** – with filtration system to maintain water quality; the floor area must be reinforced to withstand the weight of the water.
- **Plant room** – within five metres of the pool with appropriate power supply and ventilation.
- **A heavy-duty control panel** – all fittings should be strong, safe and reliable.
- **Water testing equipment** – the pH should read 7.2–7.8.
- **Water temperature should be 37–40°C.**
- **Client guidance instructions** – clearly sited.
- **Shower** – to cleanse the skin and regulate body temperature.
- **Body and hair shampoos** – may be provided.
- **Protective footwear** – to avoid cross-infection, e.g. disposable paper slippers.
- **Drinking water** – to rehydrate following service.
- **Clean towels** – for each client to dry the body after showering.
- **Relaxation area** – to use following service.

Hydro bath

- **Water temperature should be 34–38°C.**
- **Position duckboard** (if used).
- **Shower** – to cleanse the skin and regulate body temperature.
- **Body and hair shampoos** – may be provided.
- **Protective footwear** – to avoid cross-infection, e.g. disposable paper slippers.
- **Client towels** – for each client to dry the body after showering.
- **Drinking water** – to rehydrate following service.
- **Relaxation area** – to use following service.

Foam bath

- **Water temperature should be 37–40°C.**
- **Foam agent** – to add to the water.
- **Position duckboard.**
- **Shower** – to cleanse the skin and regulate body temperature.

HEALTH & SAFETY

Steam room

The relative humidity in a steam room is probably 95 per cent as the air is saturated with water vapour. The temperature for steam service must therefore be lower than that for sauna service.

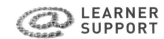

LEARNER SUPPORT

Spa true or false?

ALWAYS REMEMBER

Body temperature

The temperature of the skin's surface is 37°C.

Temperatures above 37°C heat the body – the *hyperthermal effect*. Temperatures below 33°C reduce body temperature – the *hypothermal effect*.

- **Body and hair shampoos** – may be provided.

- **Protective footwear** – to avoid cross-infection, e.g. disposable paper slippers.

- **Clean towels** – for each client to dry the body after showering.

- **Drinking water** – to rehydrate following service.

- **Relaxation area** – to use following service.

Flotation – wet

- **Flotation tank/pool.**

- **Epsom salts** – (common name for magnesium sulphate).

- **Chemicals** – to maintain water cleanliness.

- **Client guidance instructions** – clearly sited.

- **Water temperature preheated to 35°C.**

- **Shower** – to cleanse the skin.

- **Petroleum jelly** – to cover any small abrasions.

- **Ear plugs** – to prevent water entering the ears.

- **Neck support** – if required.

- **Clean towels** – for each client to dry the body after showering.

- **Service gown** – for client modesty.

- **Protective footwear** – to avoid cross-infection, e.g. disposable slippers.

- **Shower facility** – to use following service.

- **Drinking water** – to rehydrate following service.

- **Relaxation area** – to use following service.

BEST PRACTICE

Flotation service environment

The service may be received in silence or meditation/relaxation tapes may be played according to client choice.

Check client preferences.

Flotation – dry

- **Flotation bed.**

- **Paper roll** – to cover the polymer membrane covering.

- **Service product** – to apply to the skin during dry flotation if required.

- **Clean towels** – for the client to dry the body after showering to cleanse the skin.

- **Client guidance instructions** – clearly sited.

- **Clean towels** – for each client to dry the body after showering.

- **Service gown** – for client modesty.

- **Protective footwear** – to avoid cross-infection, e.g. disposable slippers.

- **Shower facility** – to remove service product.

- **Steamed towels** – should be used to cleanse the skin if there is no shower.

- **Drinking water** – to rehydrate following service.

- **Relaxation area** – to use following service.

Body wrapping

- **Service couch**.

- **Paper briefs** – for the client to wear.

- **Service gown** – for client modesty.

- **Headband** – to protect the hair.

- **Clean bandages, plastic, metallic spa sheet** – (dependent upon system used). There must be sufficient bandages available for demand.

- **Bowls** – to mix products as applicable.

- **Water** – used to mix with powder mask ingredients (as applicable).

- **Service products** – herbal; essential oils; sea clay; marine algae; seaweed.

- **Spatulas/brushes** – to apply service products.

- **Thermal blankets** – to maintain heat (if required).

- **Tape measure** – to measure the client before and after service if performing a slimming body wrap.

- **Shower facility** – to cleanse the skin before service and remove service products following service.

- **Hot, steamed towels** – may be used to remove product if the workplace does not have a shower facility.

Relaxation room

- **Neutral, calm decor.**

- **Seating** – to allow the client to sit or lie down.

- **Service gown** – for client modesty and to maintain warmth.

- **Drinking water** – to rehydrate.

ALWAYS REMEMBER

Spa products
Seaweed is particularly high in minerals and is a key ingredient of many spa products. Sea water can be used on its own or mixed with seaweeds, muds and essential oils. Marine minerals include sodium, copper, magnesium, zinc, potassium and iron.

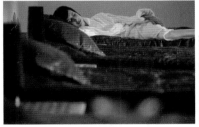

AQUA SANA, CENTRE PARCS

Relaxation room

Sterilization and disinfection

Where the spa services are communal and involve heat and moisture they provide ideal breeding conditions for harmful microorganisms. Infections that can be spread if health and safety procedures are inadequate include:

- **E-coli (Escherichia coli) bacteria**, found in the intestines of animals and humans. There are different types some of which are harmful. The bacteria are found in faeces and can survive in the environment. It can be transferred to humans by ingesting contaminated water. The symptoms include severe stomach cramps and blood loss through the stools. In those with a weakened immune system it can prove fatal.

- **Legionnaires disease**, bacteria that live in water systems associated with the workplace. Exposing the lungs to the bacteria can lead to Legionnaires disease, a fatal form of pneumonia.

- **Pseudomonas aeruginosa** a bacteria which can be passed on due to contact with contaminated water. In pool areas this can lead to pseudo folliculitis, infection of the hair follicles, eye and ear infections. The above are effectively controlled with effective monitoring, service and control of water quality.

- **Athlete's foot (tinea pedis)** can be caught through direct contact with skin debris on flooring. It is recognized by small blisters which appear on the skin between the toes. The skin becomes itchy, dry and scaling can occur. It is highly contagious and clients with this condition are contra-indicated to spa bathing.

- **Impetigo** a bacterial infection of the top layers of the skin. The skin becomes itchy and red and blisters form which later crust. Direct contact with the fluid from the blisters or from towels, etc. that have been in contact can cause cross-infection. It is highly contagious and clients with this condition are contra-indicated to spa bathing until treated.

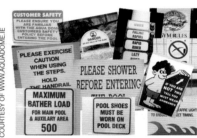

Safety signs

It is important that all furnishings are regularly cleaned and disinfected as recommended by the manufacturers' instructions. This will also avoid stale smells occurring.

A plentiful supply of towels and robes is required. Towels should be boil washed at 60°C to ensure effective laundering and prevent cross-infection.

Written instructions should be displayed in the service area and hygiene practice brought to the attention of the client, e.g. showering thoroughly before using the spa pool, etc.

This practice complies with the **Health and Safety (Safety Signs and Signals) Regulations (1996)**. The purpose of the Regulations is to encourage the standardization of safety signs throughout the Member States of the European Union (EU) so that safety signs, wherever they are seen, have the same meaning. The Regulations cover various means of communicating health and safety information. They require employers to provide specific safety signs whenever there is a risk that has not been avoided or controlled by other means. Where a safety sign would not help to reduce that risk, or where the risk is not significant, there is no need to provide a sign.

Regular safety checks should be made to ensure that the facilities are clean, safe and hygienic. The correct cleaning materials and equipment should be used according to the work area. These checks may need to be made on a daily, weekly or monthly basis. Sample checklist records follow.

HEALTH & SAFETY

- All chemical storage areas should be clearly identified and accessible to authorized persons.
- Keep all chemicals stored as directed by manufacturers' instructions.
- Handle the chemicals wearing protective clothing to avoid skin contact and potential injury. Protective eye goggles which conform to the relevant British Safety Standard may also be a requirement.
- Follow manufacturers' instructions when carrying out sterilization and disinfection procedures.
- Emergency first aid procedures must be operative and adequate.
- First aid resources must be readily available in a designated place.
- Fire alarm systems may be available depending upon legal requirements and fire-fighting equipment should be available. Regular training is important to ensure staff are familiar with evacuation procedures.

Pre-opening Checks

Check	Monday		Tuesday		Wednesday		Thursday		Friday		Saturday		Sunday		Remarks
	OK	Initials	OK	Initials	OK	Initials	OK	Initials	OK	Initials	OK	Initials	OK	Initials	
Emergency alarm/call buttons working/tested															
First aid kits are properly stocked															
Hairdryers and electric cables are in safe condition															
Emergency telephone operating correctly															
Safe use guidance displayed gym equipment, sauna, steam room, swimming pool and spa pool															
Pool/spa pool water test carried out															
Pool/spa pool water clarity satisfactory, bottom free of debris															
Pool/spa pool water temperature satisfactory															
Life buoys with throw ropes available for use															
Sauna/steam room temperature set to appropriate level															
Stairs/steps and handrails are secure															
Evacuation routes/fire exits clear and freely opening															
No slip/trip hazards															

Steam Room Daily Checks

Check	Monday		Tuesday		Wednesday		Thursday		Friday		Saturday		Sunday		Remarks
	OK	Initials	OK	Initials	OK	Initials	OK	Initials	OK	Initials	OK	Initials	OK	Initials	
Earth leakage circuit breaker operating correctly															
Door and door catch working correctly															
Cabin clean, free of debris															
Steam room vent is open															
Light fittings working and in safe condition															
Level of steam room essence adequate															
Steam operation and cover plate satisfactory															
Steam outlet cover secure															
No damage/protrusions to floor/wall															
Seating safe and secure															

CHAPTER 16 (S1) SPA OPERATIONS

INTERCONTINENTAL HOTEL GROUP, HOLIDAY INN HOTEL, NEWTON-LE-WILLOWS, SPIRIT HEALTH CLUB

INTERCONTINENTAL HOTEL GROUP, HOLIDAY INN HOTEL, NEWTON-LE-WILLOWS, SPIRIT HEALTH CLUB

Changing Area – Daily Checks

Check	Monday		Tuesday		Wednesday		Thursday		Friday		Saturday		Sunday		Remarks
	OK	Initials	OK	Initials	OK	Initials	OK	Initials	OK	Initials	OK	Initials	OK	Initials	
No slip/trip hazards															
No damaged floor surfaces															
All mirrors in safe condition															
No damaged to fixtures/fittings/benches															
Storerooms locked															
No hazardous substances left out/unattended															
Waste bins emptied regularly and frequently															
All lights secure in the ceiling and working															
All areas clean and free of debris															

Fitness Room (Gym) Daily Checks

Check	Monday		Tuesday		Wednesday		Thursday		Friday		Saturday		Sunday		Remarks
	OK	Initials	OK	Initials	OK	Initials	OK	Initials	OK	Initials	OK	Initials	OK	Initials	
All equipment and stop buttons operating correctly															
No obvious damage to electric cables on equipment															
Adequate space between equipment															
Air conditioning working and air temperature 17°C–18°C															
No trip hazards from trailing cables/floor boxes															
No damage/trip/slip hazards to floor surfaces															
All mirrors in safe condition															
Television secure on wall and in working condition															
All glazing in safe condition															
Water units stable and not leaking water															
No hazardous substances left out															
Waste bins emptied regularly and frequently															
Evacuation routes/fire exits clear and freely opening															
Wall surfaces in safe condition															
Ceilings free from leaks and damage															
Light fittings secure and working															

Swimming Pool Daily Checks

Check	Monday		Tuesday		Wednesday		Thursday		Friday		Saturday		Sunday		Remarks
	OK	Initials	OK	Initials	OK	Initials	OK	Initials	OK	Initials	OK	Initials	OK	Initials	
All fixtures and fittings secure															
Pool surround and overflow channel grating secure															
Pool tank free from obvious signs of damage/debris															
Reach poles available for use															
Evacuation routes/fire exits clear and freely opening															
Pool plant room															
Pool pumps operating correctly															
Pool dosing controls working and set to correct levels															
Chemical dosing tanks full															
Chemical injectors operating correctly															
Hazardous substances stored in correct areas															
No leaks evident															
PPE available															

Sauna Daily Checks

Check	Monday		Tuesday		Wednesday		Thursday		Friday		Saturday		Sunday		Remarks
	OK	Initials	OK	Initials	OK	Initials	OK	Initials	OK	Initials	OK	Initials	OK	Initials	
Earth leakage circuit breaker operating correctly															
Door and door catch operating smoothly															
Cabin clean, free of debris															
No dangerous timbers, protrusions, splinters in cabin															
Light fittings working and in safe condition															
Heater guard secure															
Check and record settings of thermostat															
Check and record operating temperature															
Air vent open															

Spa Pool Daily Checks

Check	Monday		Tuesday		Wednesday		Thursday		Friday		Saturday		Sunday		Remarks
	OK	Initials	OK	Initials	OK	Initials	OK	Initials	OK	Initials	OK	Initials	OK	Initials	
Test earth leakage circuit breaker															
Calibrate sensor probes (if required)															
Top up spa pool chemicals															
Record filter pressures															
Fixtures and fittings secure															
Spa surround and overflow channel grating secure															

INTERCONTINENTAL HOTEL GROUP, HOLIDAY INN HOTEL, NEWTON-LE-WILLOWS, SPIRIT HEALTH CLUB

Closing Checks

Check	Monday		Tuesday		Wednesday		Thursday		Friday		Saturday		Sunday		Remarks
	OK	Initials	OK	Initials	OK	Initials	OK	Initials	OK	Initials	OK	Initials	OK	Initials	
Pool Closing Checks															
Disinfectant levels adequate															
Carry out pool water test															
Area free of customers															
Changing Area Closing Checks															
Area free of customers															
Cleanliness satisfactory															
All switches to "off"															
Sauna Closing Checks															
Area free of customers															
Cabin cleanliness satisfactory															
All switches to "off"															
Door left open															
Steam Room Closing Checks															
Area free of customers															
Internal cabin cleanliness satisfactory															
All switches to "off"															
Door left open															
Spa Pool Closing Checks															
Drain spa completely															
Refill spa pool															
Disinfectant levels adequate															
Spa pool water test															
Backwash the filter															
Area free of customers															

INTERCONTINENTAL HOTEL GROUP, HOLIDAY INN HOTEL, NEWTON-LE-WILLOWS, SPIRIT HEALTH CLUB

Sauna

- Clean the sauna furnishings and floor regularly with a suitable disinfectant.

- Check that the internal shelving is smooth to avoid splinters entering the skin and also harbouring germs.

- Empty the wooden bucket of water when not in use to avoid mould formation.

- Floor mats should be regularly cleaned.

- When not in use, keep the sauna door open to allow fresh air to enter.

- Complete disinfecting shut-down organizational procedure at the end of the day.

Steam cabinet/room

- Clean the steam cabinet/room internal walls and floor furnishings regularly with a suitable disinfectant that removes surface grease. This also prevents unpleasant smells created by stale body odours.

- Complete disinfecting shut-down organizational procedure at the end of the day.

Hydro baths and foam baths

- These should be drained and cleaned after each client use.

- Specialized cleaning agents should be used as directed by the manufacturer. These will help prevent discolouration, algae formation and lime scale build-up.

- The surrounding floor should be dry.

- Dirty towels in the area should be removed.

- All waste should be disposed of in a covered, lined waste bin.

- Complete disinfecting shut-down organizational procedure at the end of the day.

Flotation – wet

- The water should be checked to see that it looks clear; hair, etc. should be removed.

- The surface of the flotation tank should be cleaned regularly to remove body oils and dead skin cells, which would otherwise form a scum. Use sodium hypochlorite solution mixed as per manufacturer's instructions.

- Chemicals are added to maintain water cleanliness.

- The pH of the water is tested daily – a pH of 7.2–7.4 is normal.

- The water is filtered between each session.

- All waste should be disposed of in a covered, lined waste bin.

- The water depth should be 25cm.

- Epsom salts need to be added regularly to maintain water density. Add these as guided by the manufacturer.

- Complete disinfecting shut-down organizational procedure at the end of the day.

> " Your initial NVQ course is just the start of your learning. You should continue improving your skills by attending other training, trade exhibitions, and by giving and receiving services. Your learning never stops!
>
> **Sally Biles**

Flotation – dry

- Wipe the vinyl surface of the flotation bed with a proprietary disinfectant cleaner following the manufacturer's instructions.

- Ensure the vinyl surface is kept smooth and wrinkle free.

- Ensure the floor area is clean and dry.

- All waste should be disposed of in a covered, lined waste bin.

- Complete disinfecting shut-down organizational procedure at the end of the day.

Body wrapping

- Wipe the surface of the service touch with a proprietary disinfectant cleaner following manufacturer's instructions.

- Boil wash the bandages at 60°C using a detergent or as directed by manufacturer's instructions.

- Thoroughly clean bowls used to mix service products.

- Brushes used to apply products should be washed in warm soapy water, rinsed, dried and disinfected, e.g. placed in the ultra-violet cabinet.

- All waste should be disposed of in a covered, lined waste bin.

Relaxation room

- Seating should be cleaned regularly.

- Used towels should be collected.

- Ensure there are no spillages from drinks, etc.

- Replenish drinking cups and maintain water facility to rehydrate.

- Empty waste bins.

Shower

- Clean regularly with a suitable disinfectant cleaner.

- Check after each client use, clean to remove residue body skin service products such as marine clay, etc.

- Ensure there are adequate consumables, body shampoo, etc.

- Shower heads should be cleaned according to operational requirements.

Hydrotherapy spa pool

- The spa is not drained and filled after every use, but relies on the water being continually filtered and chemically treated.

- Carry out water testing procedure every two hours.

- The edge of the spa pool should be cleaned daily to remove body oils and dead skin cells, which would otherwise form a scum.

- Remove excess water around the spa pool regularly.

ALWAYS REMEMBER

Electrical equipment

All electrical equipment must be protected from contact with water. There should be sufficient drainage around the spa to avoid flooding, so monitor this.

In many cases the spa services such as sauna, steam and hydrotherapy and relaxation room will be used on a continuous basis.

Ensure the area is hygienically maintained, any waste such as disposable paper drinking cups removed, floor areas cleaned regularly and any water spillage dealt with to prevent slippage and accidents.

There are checks to be made on a daily, weekly and monthly basis. These ensure that the condition of the spa meets legal and organizational requirements.

Everyday consumables should be checked and replenished daily. Shortages should be reported to the supervisor.

Preparing for spa operations

Ensure that all equipment and materials are regularly maintained. Prepare equipment and materials for specific services as required, e.g. foam baths, body wrapping. Ensure operating temperatures of heat and flotation services are correct.

Preparing the spa work areas

Sauna

- Turn the system on at the mains as per manufacturers' instructions.

- Heat the sauna adequately before use to allow the heat to evenly penetrate the timber surfaces. This will be between 1 hour and 1 hour 30 minutes depending on the size of the sauna.

- Select the preferred temperature: 70–110°C for a Finnish/Tyrolean sauna, 55°C for a Laconium sauna.

- Ensure air vents are open and clear from obstruction.

- Ensure lighting is operational.

- Ensure that there is no metal exposed, which would burn the client's skin on contact.

- Fill the wooden bucket with water (if used). Water poured on the sauna coals raises the humidity of the sauna atmosphere. Position ladle for pouring water onto the coals.

- Clean towels may be provided for the client to place over the seating.

- Position floor mats.

Steam bath

- Drape clean towels over the seat of the bath and the floor.

- Fill the tank with water to cover the heating element. There should be at least 5cm of water above the heating element.

- Cover the opening of the bath with a clean towel to prevent heat loss.

- Switch the machine on at the mains.

- Set the temperature of the bath with the temperature dial and set the control for 15 minutes to preheat the cabinet.

HEALTH & SAFETY

All equipment should be serviced as recommended by the manufacturers. A trained member of staff should regularly check all electrical equipment for safety, usually on a weekly basis, although daily safety checks occur.

This will follow compliance with the **Electricity at Work Regulation (1989)**.

TOP TIP

The steam bath is less claustrophobic for clients than a steam room, as the head remains exposed. It also offers a more private service and the temperature may be adjusted to suit the client.

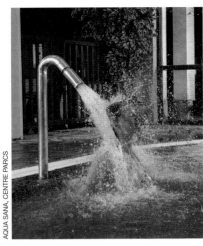

AQUA SANA, CENTRE PARCS

Water jets in hydrotherapy pool

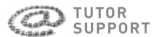

TUTOR SUPPORT

Activity 6: Spa treatment wordsearch

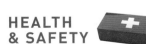

HEALTH & SAFETY

Underwater massage
The hose attachment, when used, should be kept under water at all times to prevent injury and unnecessary water spillage.

Steam room

- Turn the system on as per manufacturers' instructions.
- The preheating time will depend on the size of the steam room.
- The recommended temperature is 40°C.
- Provide water for the clients to pour over their skin in the hamman steam room.

Hydrotherapy spa pool

- Turn the system on as per manufacturers' instructions.
- The water in the spa should be regularly tested to ensure that it has a balanced pH of 7.2–7.8.
- The operating temperature is usually 36–40°C, again this should be regularly checked.
- Check the water levels at the beginning of each day and regularly throughout the day.

Hydrobath

- Rinse and clean the jets at the start of each day.
- Fill the bath with warm water; ensure the water level covers all jets before operation but will be no higher than the client's shoulders.
- Add ingredients to the bath for their therapeutic properties as the bath is filling.
- The operating temperature is usually 36–40°C.
- Switch the compressor on after the client has got into the bath. Air aerates the bath water creating bubbles through the duckboards' perforated holes, or jets situated in the bath.

Foam bath

- Cover the duckboard with hot water, approximately 38–43°C, to a depth of approximately 10–15cm.
- Add a foam ingredient to the water in the quantity directed by the cosmetic manufacturer.
- Switch on the compressor, which aerates the water causing the foam to rise. When near the top of the bath, approximately 15cm, the compressor is switched off.

Flotation – wet

- The water should be filtered between each use and the level checked daily.
- The temperature should be checked and maintained at surface body temperature (34.5–35.5°C).
- The condition of the water should be regularly monitored and should be clear at all times.
- The water should be regularly tested to ensure it has a balanced pH of 7.2–7.4.
- Test the alkalinity and free chlorine as per manufacturer's guidelines for usage.

- Ensure the lighting is working in the room.
- Gentle meditation music may be played.
- Check the panic alarm is working.

Flotation – dry

- Heat the water to the correct temperature as advised by the manufacturer.
- Atmospheric mood music may be played to relax the client.
- Raise the board to the top of the tank. Protect the polymer membrane covering with paper roll.
- Ensure the floor is protected adequately to avoid marking from the skin service product mask if used.

Body wrapping

- Ensure the room is warm, clean and aromatic to enhance the sensory experience.
- Atmospheric mood music may be played to relax the client.
- Prepare the bandages, if used, as appropriate. This may include soaking the bandages in the service product.
- Ensure there are sufficient bandages to cover the body service area adequately.

Relaxation room

- Ensure the room is at an ambient temperature (close to body temperature) of 30–40°C.
- Ensure that any waste is removed on a regular basis.

TOP TIP

Music
Music selection is important for inducing the relaxation atmosphere of the spa. Meditational, peaceful background music is an appropriate choice.

TOP TIP

Fibre-optic lighting
Colour influences the senses through the autonomic nervous system. This can affect the client's mental and physical state. Importantly it reinforces the effects of the spa service, inducing relaxation and a feeling of well-being.

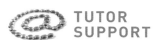 **TUTOR SUPPORT**

Activity 5: Spa destination research

Outcome 3: Check and maintain the spa work areas

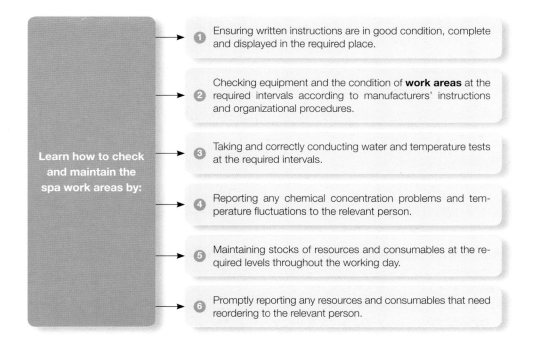

Learn how to check and maintain the spa work areas by:

1. Ensuring written instructions are in good condition, complete and displayed in the required place.

2. Checking equipment and the condition of **work areas** at the required intervals according to manufacturers' instructions and organizational procedures.

3. Taking and correctly conducting water and temperature tests at the required intervals.

4. Reporting any chemical concentration problems and temperature fluctuations to the relevant person.

5. Maintaining stocks of resources and consumables at the required levels throughout the working day.

6. Promptly reporting any resources and consumables that need reordering to the relevant person.

HEALTH & SAFETY

Legionnaires' disease

Legionnaires' disease is a potentially fatal form of pneumonia. If suffering from a weakened immune system life threatening symptoms may occur.

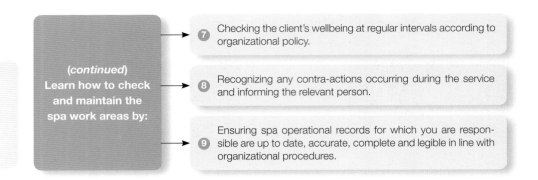

(continued)
Learn how to check and maintain the spa work areas by:

7 Checking the client's wellbeing at regular intervals according to organizational policy.

8 Recognizing any contra-actions occurring during the service and informing the relevant person.

9 Ensuring spa operational records for which you are responsible are up to date, accurate, complete and legible in line with organizational procedures.

> **Best practice**
> The client's comfort is always paramount so it is important that you check this when necessary. Ensure the temperature of the room/couch, massage pressure, music, supports and covers are all to your client's liking.
>
> **Sally Biles**

HEALTH & SAFETY

Wash hands before water testing to prevent contamination which could lead to false readings.

TOP TIP

Backwashing requirement

An electronic meter is available which shows the total dissolved particles in the water. A reading of over 1500 requires a backwash of the water.

HEALTH & SAFETY

COSHH

Only trained staff should handle chemicals.

HSDA sheets should be available to refer to.

Checking spa work areas Check equipment and condition of work areas at the required intervals.

Water testing

It is essential in the spa to ensure that this damp and warm environment is as free from contamination as possible. Diseases such as Legionellosis (Legionnaires' disease) could prove fatal. This is controlled by following stringent cleaning and water tests to check for water balance.

Backwashing is important to filter out harmful organisms not killed by disinfectant.

An integral strainer removes hair and other debris such as skin flakes and plasters from the water and this should be routinely cleaned to maintain its efficiency.

Water is kept free from potential hazard by the use of chemical disinfectants such as sodium and calcium hypochlorite. The normal operating range of the chemical will depend upon the disinfectants used. The water is tested according to the chemical disinfectant selected to ensure it is safe, effective and balanced. This will also assess the water to prevent water corrosion, staining and scaling.

Water is regularly tested for the following:

- pH (acidity/alkalinity)
- hardness (calcium salt content)
- temperature

Regular testing of water and maintenance of records is an essential part of spa operation. This should occur every two hours for free chlorine, combined chlorine, total chlorine, pH level and temperature.

Weekly tests occur for total alkalinity, total dissolved solids (TDS) and calcium hardness.

These measurements are known as **Langalier index** or **Palintest balanced water index**. Water samples are compared against acceptable operating levels. The quantity of disinfectant agents required will depend upon the hydrotherapy pool usage and the results of the water testing.

The amount of available free chlorine (that available to neutralize contaminants in the water) and the pH value need to be controlled and the amount and the effectiveness of the sterilizing agent determined. Further chemicals may also need to be added to raise or lower alkalinity or calcium levels. Chemicals used to control the pH of water include sodium bicarbonate and carbon dioxide (CO_2).

Step-by-step: Water testing

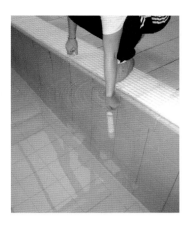

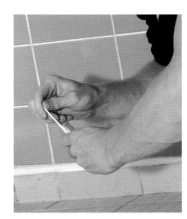

1 Using a thermometer to check the temperature of the water.

Pool temperature should read 28–31°C.

Spa pool temperature should read 37–41°C.

2 A spa pool water sample is taken. A phenol red tablet is added to the water which develops in colour according to the chemical content. The resulting colour is compared against the colour metric system to identify the reading for pH. This indicates pH chemical level, which should read between 7.2–7.8.

A pool/spa water sample is taken in a 100ml test tube.

3 Test chlorine level

A pool water sample is taken from the area furthest from the filters and should always be taken from the same place. This is dispensed as follows, fill one test tube to the word Palintest. Pour the top of the water into a second test tube leaving 10 ml in the first test tube.

Add a DPD1 tablet to the test tube with the least amount of water and allow to dissolve. Top up with water to the 10 ml line.

Calculate the free chlorine level, which should read between **1–3**. Free chlorine is the chlorine available to bind to bacteria.

Place tube in photometer. Following directions obtain the **free chlorine reading** which should be between 1 and 3.

Add the DPD3 tablet to the same sample and dissolve.

Replace the tube in photometer, positioned as directed. Activate the reading to show the **total chlorine reading**.

The difference between the first and second reading is the **combined chlorine reading**. To calculate the combined chlorine level subtract the reading using the DPD 1 tablet from the reading obtained from the DPD3 tablet. The combined chlorine should be no more than one third of the total chlorine.

The combined chlorine should be no more than one third of the total chlorine.

A combined chlorine low level reading is preferred as this indicates a low level of bacteria.

All equipment should be rinsed in clean water after use in preparation for future use.

Any irregular readings should be immediately reported to the relevant qualified person to take appropriate action.

Test pH level

Take the second sample of pool water collected.

Calculate the **pH chemical level**, which should read between **7.2–7.8**.

Fill a test tube with 10ml of pool water.

Add a phenol red tablet and dissolve.

Place tube in photometer, following directions to obtain the pH reading.

HEALTH & SAFETY

Chemicals
Because of lower water levels in the spa pool it is important to avoid introducing high chemical levels. The pH of water will be affected by any substance introduced into it. Above pH 7 skin and eye irritation occurs.

HEALTH & SAFETY

Bather load
Ensure the bather load (number of bathers) levels are adhered to for both pool and spa pool areas. Negative effect of pool client capacity excess is that the bottom of the pool cannot be seen and the filters cannot maintain pool/spa cleanliness.

Bather load will differ according to the size of the pool.

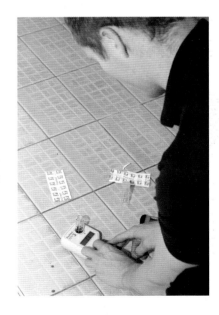

TOP TIP

Photometer
Current water-measuring equipment passes a beam of light through a coloured water sample and provides a digital reading which calculates the result automatically. The results can be printed out as record.

HEALTH & SAFETY

pH levels
Where pH values are above the recommended range solids are less effectively removed and bacteria levels increase.

HEALTH & SAFETY

Chlorine
When chlorine oxidises contaminants (chloramines) form. High levels of chloramines will produce an unpleasant smell and cause irritated eyes, making those using the bather think chlorine levels are high. In fact, there is sufficient free chlorine available.

ALWAYS REMEMBER

Ozone water treatment
Ozone systems may be used as a water treatment for the maintenance of the spa, destroying harmful bacteria and viruses.

HEALTH & SAFETY

The Environmental Health Authority
Heat services for use by the public are subject to inspection by the Environmental Health Authority. In spa service, the water is checked for safe bacterial levels and the presence of *E. Coli* and coliform organisms.

---

4 When performing water testing ensure your hands are clean and always avoid touching the tablets.

Shoes worn beside the pool must have protective coverings placed over them.

A record of tests carried out by an authorized person must be kept for inspection by the local health authority. Failure to carry out this legally required duty by a responsible staff member can result in disciplinary action being taken. The Environmental Health Officer (EHO) will make regular checks to ensure that effective maintenance/hygiene is being enforced and will check standards.

Training will be provided on daily checks required for the pool plant room. These checks include checking:

- the pool pumps are operating correctly
- display to see that pool dosing controls are at the correct levels
- chemical dosing tanks are full
- chemical injectors are operating correctly

Pool and spa pool temperature This is controlled by a thermostat. A valve is opened to allow warm water into the pool and is closed when the correct temperature is achieved which is 30°C.

Test for total dissolve solids (TSD) The quantity of chemical substances dissolved in pool water is measured by an electronic device which when immersed in the water passes an electric current between two points. The conductivity of water is measured and provides the TSD reading. Guidance is provided on the acceptable TSD measure.

Ventilation

The spa pool will create heat, humidity and chemical smells. Adequate **ventilation** is necessary. High levels of humidity can cause discomfort because the body cannot cool and becomes overheated but on contact with colder surfaces condensation occurs. This may result in a corrosive action as chemicals are deposited in the air. A relative humidity of 50–70 per cent is recommended. Air must be transported into the area through fan units fitted with filters and then heated.

HEALTH & SAFETY

pH levels in the water affect the efficiency of disinfection. The pH should always be at a level which renders the water safe. Risks to bathers from chemicals used in disinfection include sore eyes and skin irritation. All bathers must be instructed to have a thorough pre-pool shower to cleanse the skin and avoid water contamination which will affect the pH level.

Overseeing client's well-being and correct usage of spa services

Also check the client's well-being and that spa services are being used as per organizational procedures.

A consultation will have been completed which explains the service thoroughly. This will enable the client to gain maximum relaxation from the service. Before a client receives a service you must explain:

- The service procedure to the client, its effects and use of equipment as applicable.

- The expected skin sensations, service effects and contra-actions that they must inform you of as necessary.

- That all outside clothing must be removed in a private changing area.

- That personal possessions and clothing should be stored in a secure area.

- That contact lenses, glasses and jewellery should be removed.

You must also:

- Provide the client with clean towels and disposable slippers and required.

- Encourage the client to ask questions to confirm understanding of procedures.

- Instruct the client to shower before service to remove any cosmetics from the skin's surface. Shower facilities are essential in the spa to cleanse before, during and after spa therapy services to remove exfoliating products and body masks from the skin such as those with a mud, marine algae or seaweed base.

- Ensure that the shower is at a comfortable temperature and instruct on shower operation. A non-slip mat must be placed in the shower to prevent the client slipping.

Pre-service, the client may receive an exfoliating service such as a salt, herb or enzyme scrub. This removes dead skin cells, increases blood and lymph circulation and increases cellular metabolism.

Sauna

1 Before the client enters the sauna:

- check the temperature of the sauna by reading the thermometer

- check the relative humidity by reading the hygrometer

2 The client then enters the sauna. New clients should be advised to sit on the lower benches where the air temperature is cooler. Existing clients may move to higher positions.

3 Check client well-being at regular intervals.

4 After a 10–12 minute period the client should take a shower to cool the skin.

5 The client may return to the sauna for a further 10 minutes. During this time water may be poured onto the coals. The client then takes a final shower.

6 Service time is approximately 30 minutes.

7 Provide the client with water for hydration.

8 The client should rest after the final shower to allow the blood pressure to return to normal.

Steam bath/room

1 Service time is normally 15–20 minutes.

2 Before the client enters the steam cabinet/room, check the temperature in the steam cabinet.

HEALTH & SAFETY

Monitoring clients
Jewellery will become hot during a heat service such as sauna, as will any exposed metal. It is important that the client's skin is not in contact with any metal as this could cause burns.

TOP TIP

Therapeutic showers
Showers may be offered as a therapeutic service in itself.

Multi-sensory showers offer different experiences in temperature and sensation where the shower simulates rain. Certain showers provide water massage therapy. These may be used after each spa experience to revitalize the body.

Client communication
Your consultation is key to a successful service as this is when you can find out your client's needs and then ensure you adapt the service to meet those needs.

Ask open-ended questions, observe your client, use your sense of touch, actively listen, and learn to read between the lines!

Sally Biles

HEALTH & SAFETY

Sauna safety
The sauna door has a glass window that enables you to check the client without opening the door. This attention will reassure the client if it is their first sauna session. Check the temperature of the sauna on a regular basis: it may be necessary to record these temperatures.

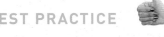
3 In the steam bath, adjust the seating height for the height of the client. Close the hinged door.

4 Replace the towel around the neck of the steam bath to avoid loss of steam.

5 Supervise the client at all times in the steam bath.

6 Provide the client with water for hydration.

7 A shower should be taken at the end of the service to cleanse and cool the skin.

Hydrotherapy spa pool

1 A bathing time of 15–20 minutes is recommended.

2 Monitor the client during service.

3 A shower should be taken at the end of the service.

4 Provide the client with water for rehydration.

5 Allow the client to rest following service.

Hydrobaths

1 The client may be advised to hold onto the handles for balance and support during the underwater massage.

2 At conclusion of service – 15–20 minutes – switch the compressor off.

3 Provide the client with water for rehydration.

4 Allow the client to rest following service.

Foam bath

1 The client should lie in the shallow water with their head exposed and their body covered with foam.

2 The client should be allowed to relax but be monitored regularly.

3 Service time is approximately 15–20 minutes.

4 A shower should be taken at the end of the service.

5 Provide the client with water for rehydration.

6 Allow the client to relax.

Flotation – wet

1 The client should take a cleansing shower and make-up, if used, should have been removed, as it will contaminate the water.

2 Advise the client on how long they will be in the flotation room.

3 Explain how to operate the door, demonstrate this and then observe them to confirm understanding.

4 Explain how to alter the lighting level, adjust the audio level, operate the panic alarm.

5 Explain how they should position themselves in the water. These procedures will facilitate relaxation.

6 The client may then apply the earplugs to prevent water entering the ears.

7 A neck cushion may be provided to support the client's neck.

8 Check on the client during service as necessary. If the client is enclosed in a room or capsule this may be through the intercom system. This is an important feature to reassure a highly nervous/anxious client.

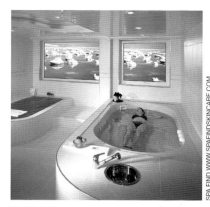

Wet flotation

Flotation – dry

1 The client should take a cleansing shower and make-up, if used, should have been removed.

2 Advise the client on how long the flotation service will take. Often a body wrap is received in conjunction with the dry floatation service.

3 Provide the client with water for rehydration.

4 The lighting level may be lowered to induce relaxation.

5 The client should take time to relax following service. A suitable area should be provided for this purpose.

Body wrapping Ensure the room is warm, clean and aromatic to enhance the sensory experience. Atmospheric mood music may be played to relax the client.

Service will vary depending upon the body wrapping system used. The client may receive a pre-service before the body wrap such as a heat service, shower and exfoliation or dry body brush.

Provide the client with water for rehydration following service.

Relaxation room

1 Guide the client on facilities and use of the room.

2 Explain the importance of drinking water to rehydrate.

3 Check on the client's well-being at regular intervals.

After the spa service

Confirm the client's well-being at the end of the spa service, further recommendations may be provided.

TOP TIP

Body wraps

Body wraps may be applied to specific body parts only such as the foot and lower leg.

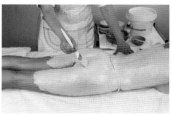

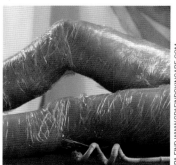

Therapeutic product application stage of a body wrap service

- Heat services and body wraps cause a loss of body fluids through perspiration. Clients must be provided with still water or fruit juices to rehydrate following service. Water imbalances of only 1–2 per cent can lead to ill health. Increased water consumption aids toxin elimination. Ensure refreshments are available.

- Following heat services and those that induce relaxation, such as flotation service, the client should rest for 20–30 minutes. In the case of heat services this is to allow body temperatures and blood pressure to return to normal. Sudden movements can cause dizziness and fainting. Monitor the client's reactions during the rest period to check for any contra-action that may occur.

- Advise the client about other services that can be given. Provide literature or a service plan for the client to refer to.

- The client may be encouraged to recreate the benefits of spa mineral services at home through the sale of retail products. These contain ingredients such as seaweed, sea salts, algae and mud.

Contra-actions to services

In the case of any contra-action to service it is important that the spa service is discontinued. You should take the appropriate remedial action if qualified or authorized to do so, or contact the relevant member of staff trained to deal with the situation.

Aftercare advice should always be given to the client in the case of a contra-action occurring following the service.

Contra-actions include:

Service duration too long.

- Low blood pressure and loss of water from the body. Dehydration will occur, causing the cells to absorb fluid from other organs in the body. This may also cause the client to feel faint.

Sauna services – relative humidity too low.

- Excessive water loss may occur, leading to dehydration. Also, breathing difficulties may be experienced due to lack of moisture in the air. The temperature of the air will also be higher, causing discomfort when breathing.

- Nausea and dizziness caused by heat exhaustion. This can also be caused by the heat and motion in the spa pool.

Action

- The client should lie down and rest. Raise the legs to avoid fainting.

- Water should be given to rehydrate.

- Seek medical attention if necessary.

Heat exhaustion caused by loss of fluids and sodium chloride (body salt).

This results in symptoms such as dizziness, sickness, headaches and fainting.

Action

- The client should lie down and rest, raise legs to avoid fainting.

- Fruit juices or sports drinks may be taken.

ALWAYS REMEMBER

Spa cosmetic products

Always check to ensure that you are storing spa products correctly and that the use by date is clearly identified.

ACTIVITY

Retail sales

Following a heat service what products could you recommend for the client to maintain and enhance the skin condition? For each product listed explain why.

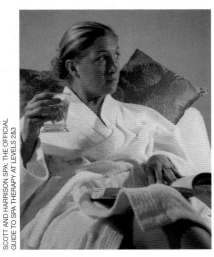

SCOTT AND HARRISON SPA: THE OFFICIAL GUIDE TO SPA THERAPY AT LEVELS 2&3

Client resting

- Seek medical attention if necessary.
- Salt tablets may be recommended by the GP to replace lost salts.

Cramp caused by excessive perspiration.

Action

- Stretch the muscle and massage the area.
- Encourage the client to drink water. Salts may be added to replace lost body salts.

Burning/scalding the skin.

- Through not ladling the water over the coals in the sauna with an outstretched arm, causing the skin to come into contact with the rising steam.
- Skin contact with the heated metal in the sauna.

Action

- Cool the area with cold water immediately.
- Apply a dry dressing, which will not stick to the skin injury. This will protect the skin against infection.
- Medical service may be advisable dependent upon the severity of the burn.

Nosebleed due to irritation of the mucous membranes and the effect of the high temperature upon the circulatory system.

Action

- Bend the head forwards. The client should breathe through their mouth.
- The nose should be gently but firmly pinched for about ten minutes.
- If the bleeding does not cease after 30 minutes seek medical attention.

Skin reaction.

- Skin irritation due to chemicals in the spa pool.
- Skin irritation due to high temperatures in the steam or sauna room and irritant effect of the dry heat in the sauna room.

Action

- The client should take a cool shower to remove the products/chemicals from the skin or lower skin temperature.
- Apply a soothing cream to reduce irritation.
- Medical treatment may be advisable if skin irritation continues.

Respiratory disorders may be aggravated due to the heat of the sauna or steam room.

Clients with respiratory disorders should avoid heat services where they have to breathe hot air directly.

Action

- Sit the client down, and if they have medication with them, allow them to use it.
- Seek medical assistance if necessary.

HEALTH & SAFETY

Client safety

If at any time during a heat service the client feels light-headed, faint or nauseous, the therapist must be informed. Advise the client of this at consultation and monitor their reaction during the service. The client should never be left unattended, to avoid over-exposure to the effects of heating which could lead to fainting, etc.

HEALTH & SAFETY

Notices providing information on the safe use of the spa equipment/pool area must be clearly displayed by each system.

HEALTH & SAFETY

Heat therapy should not be taken together with ultraviolet service to avoid further stimulation of blood in the area.

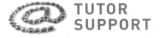

TUTOR SUPPORT

Activity 1: Contra-actions to spa treatment

Outcome 4: Shut down work areas

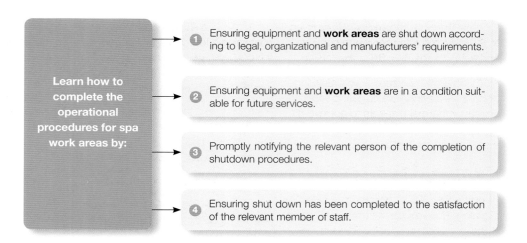

Learn how to complete the operational procedures for spa work areas by:

1. Ensuring equipment and **work areas** are shut down according to legal, organizational and manufacturers' requirements.

2. Ensuring equipment and **work areas** are in a condition suitable for future services.

3. Promptly notifying the relevant person of the completion of shutdown procedures.

4. Ensuring shut down has been completed to the satisfaction of the relevant member of staff.

When you have been using the spa for services it is important that it is prepared for subsequent services.

Hygiene and cleaning of the spa areas should occur following legal and organizational procedures.

Service areas should be shut down in accordance with manufacturers' instructions and legal and organizational procedures.

Refer to the checklists provided in **Outcome 3: Check and maintain the spa work area**, page 517.

Following services such as a hydrotherapy bath or foam bath, equipment, water supplies and electricity at the mains should be switched off.

Following flotation service and heat therapy services switch off the equipments at the mains.

The spa boosters that create the aeration of the spa pool are switched off at the end of the working day (the switch is located in the plant room). The pump which circulates the water is left on. A backwash, which reverses the flow of water through the filter removing waste particles and debris, may occur.

A final water test is recommended before pool shutdown in order that any problems with water quality can be rectified before the next working day. Regular testing and the maintenance of records is an essential part of spa plant operation and health and safety maintenance.

All waste and used towels must be removed in accordance with workplace policy at the designated collection point. The spa and all areas of the working environment should be left clean and tidy ready for the next working day. Remember many spas have early opening times so the spa on opening must be ready for use.

It is important to work within your responsibilities when operating shutdown of the spa area.

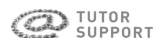

TUTOR SUPPORT

Activity 8: Re-cap, revision and evaluation

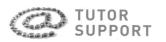

TUTOR SUPPORT

Activity 9: Multiple choice quiz

GLOSSARY OF KEY WORDS

Aftercare advice recommendations given to the client following service to continue and enhance the benefits of the service.

Body wrapping a service where the body is wrapped in bandages, plastic sheets or thermal blankets to achieve different therapeutic effects including skin toning and weight loss.

Client groups this term is used in a number of the units and it refers to client diversity. The CRE (Commission for Racial Equality) ethnic group classification is used in the range for these units. These cover white, mixed, Asian, black and Chinese.

Consultation assessment of client's needs using different assessment techniques, including questioning and natural observation.

Contra-action an unwanted reaction occurring during or after service application.

Contra-indication a problematic symptom that indicates that the service may not proceed or may restrict service application. Further contra-indications identified for spa services are discussed in more detail in Chapter 3.

Flotation a spa service where the body is suspended in water (wet flotation) or supported on water (dry flotation), inducing relaxation.

Foam bath a shallow bath of water containing a foaming agent surrounds the body, achieving a thermal effect. Increased perspiration caused by this effect aids the elimination of wastes and toxins.

Heat services these include sauna, steam and the relaxation room. When heat services are applied, there is an increase in body temperature of about 1–2°C.

Humidity moisture content of the air.

Hydrotherapy spa services where water is used for its therapeutic effect.

Langalier index or Palintest balanced water index the method of regular testing and maintenance of water quality in the spa whirlpools/swimming pool.

Minor a person classed as a child who requires by law to have a parent or guardian present.

pH the degree of acidity or alkalinity measured on a pH scale. This scale goes from 0–14. In the range of 0–6.9 the lower the pH value, the greater the acidity. Above 7, the greater the pH value, the greater the alkalinity. A pH of 7 is neutral – it is neither acid or alkaline. Spa pool water is regularly tested for its pH.

Relaxation room a room of ambient temperature (close to the body's own temperature) and often referred to by the Latin name tepidarium.

Sauna a service room of timber construction where the air inside is heated to produce a therapeutic effect on the body.

Service plan after the consultation, suitable service objectives are established to treat the client's conditions and needs.

Spa pool a pool of warm water in which the client sits with jets of air passing through to create bubbles which massage the skin.

Spa services services used to induce a physical and mental sense of wellbeing. The term 'spa' is said to be derived from a village near Liege in Belgium called Spau. It had mineral hot springs which people could visit to improve their health and ailments.

Steam service water is heated to create steam, which is applied to the body for its therapeutic purposes.

Systemic medical condition a medical condition caused by a defect in one of the body's organs, e.g. the heart.

Thermometer equipment used to measure temperature.

Ventilation the transport of fresh air into an area. The spa pool will create heat, humidity and chemical smells. Adequate ventilation is necessary.

ASSESSMENT OF KNOWLEDGE AND UNDERSTANDING

Having covered the learning objectives for **Assist with spa operations**, test what you need to know and understand answering the following short questions below.

The information covers:

- organizational and legal requirements
- how to work safely and effectively when assisting with spa operations
- cleaning, setting up and checking equipment and spa work areas
- client care

Organizational and legal requirements

1 Who enforces and monitor local bye-laws with regard to water, temperature and quality of spa services?

2 What health and safety legislation should be complied with in the spa environment?

3 Why should maintenance records be available and kept updated?

4 Whom would you contact to check waste disposal requirements for spa operations?

5 What Health and Safety legislation states how chemicals required for spa services should be stored and used?

6 Research what must be considered in choice of work wear and personal appearance for spa industry requirements.

7 Your workplace will have a schedule for cleaning, maintenance, checking and shutdown of spa work areas. Give **three** examples of what should be completed on a daily basis in terms of cleaning, maintenance checks and the shutdown operation of the spa work area.

8 Provide **three** examples of how the required ambience for the spa area can be created.

9 Who should problems that arise in the spa workplace be reported to?

10 Your workplace will have operational records to ensure the safety and quality of the spa is maintained and at a consistent standard. How should these checks be carried out and recorded?

How to work safely and effectively when assisting with spa operations

1 What type of personal protective equipment should be available and worn when working in the spa and assisting with spa operations?

2 How can the skin condition contact dermatitis be avoided when maintaining the spa work environment?

3 How can cross-infection be avoided in the spa area? State three examples of cross-infections and what can be done to avoid them.

4 Why must you check a client regularly when they are receiving spa services?

5 How can the effects of dehydration be avoided when a client is receiving spa services?

Cleaning, setting up and checking equipment and spa work areas

1 What are the recommended operating temperatures of a:

- spa pool?
- hydrotherapy bath?
- wet flotation?
- mild sauna?
- steam cabinet service?

2 How is humidity measured in the sauna room?

3 Where and why should written instructions about spa service usage be displayed?

4 How are water and chemical concentrations checked for in the spa pool?

5 For each of the following spa services explain how you would ensure the spa equipment was safe, clean and hygienic for each client:

- wet flotation?
- sauna?
- steam room?

6 What is the recommended pH level for a:

- spa pool?
- wet flotation pool?

7 What dangers can occur if the chemical pH concentrations in the spa pool are not checked regularly?

8 Why should a client shower before entering the spa area?

9 How often may heat service be received per week?

10 How long should be allowed for a:

- spa pool service?
- wet flotation service?
- hydrotherapy bath?

11 What contra-actions can occur if recommended services times are exceeded?

12 How are the following spa services shut down at the end of the working day:

- spa pool?
- steam room?
- sauna?

Client care

1 Why should up to date records be kept for clients receiving spa services?

2 How would you deal with the following contra-actions:

- fainting
- allergic reactions
- breathing difficulties

3 Why is it important for the client to relax following spa service?

4 How can you ensure that the client's modesty and privacy is respected when receiving spa services?

17 Threading Services (B34)

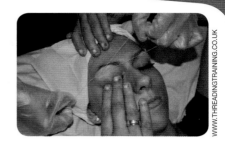

B34 Unit Learning Objectives

This chapter covers **Unit B34 Provide threading services**.

This unit is about removing hair from areas of the face using a variety of threading techniques. It will also include reference to shaping and maintenance of different eyebrow shapes. For brow shaping using the manual tweezer technique please see Chapter 8.

You will need to be able to consult with the client, prepare for the threading service and produce a service plan. You will also need to provide service advice to the client including future service needs and aftercare advice.

To carry out this unit, you must maintain effective health, safety and hygienic procedures and show a professional and ethical approach throughout this service.

There are **four** learning outcomes for Unit B34 which you must achieve competently:

1   Maintain safe and effective methods of working when providing threading services

2   Consult, plan and prepare for threading services with clients

3   Remove unwanted hair

4   Provide aftercare advice

Your assessor will observe your performance **on at least four occasions**, each involving a different client, two of which must include total reshape of the brows.

From the **range** statement you must show that you have:

● used all **consultation techniques**

● taken all **necessary action** where contra-indication, modification or contra-action occur

● treated all treatment areas

● used all three instructional techniques

(continued on the next page)

ROLE MODEL

Lorraine Onorato
Director
National School of Threading and Principal of The Surrey School of Beauty & Complementary Health

> Following a career in nursing I entered the beauty industry in 1995.

After many years as a therapist and salon owner I decided to follow my passion for education and began to lecture at a further education college in Surrey.

I gained further professional skills and qualifications including writing examination questions for CIBTAC (Confederation of International Beauty Therapy and Cosmetology), achieving the Cert.Ed. teaching qualification and becoming a beauty therapy examiner.

I set up my first training company, The National School of Threading, and have since given many demonstrations and lectures.

I have been privileged to work alongside high profile businesses including Nails Inc - trade testing, training and launching their 'Get Lashed' brand, and GMTTEC Training Education Consultancy. Since 2007 I have been working closely with the ASA (Asian Style Awards) to assist the regulation of South Asian treatments and training, in particular threading, with a view to raising standards.

More recently I have been working with Habia to develop threading standards for a new industry qualification in threading.

My plan for 2010 is to begin recruiting students at my new school established in September 2009 in Surrey – The Surrey school of Beauty & Complementary Health – and to expand my threading expertise into Europe where the skill is still relatively unknown.

(continued)

● applied instruction to cover brow re-shapes and brow maintenance

● applied instruction on aftercare and homecare advice

However, you must prove that you have the necessary knowledge, understanding and skills to be able to perform competently across the range.

When providing threading services it is important to use the skills you have learnt in the following units:

Unit G20 Make sure your own actions reduce risks to health and safety

Unit G18 Promote additional products or services to clients

Unit G8 Develop and maintain your effectiveness at work

Unit B6 Carry out waxing service

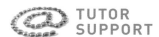

TUTOR SUPPORT

Activity 17.1: Promote threading services

TOP TIP

Threading has less effect on the skin than other hair removal services, e.g. waxing which can cause irritation from heat, allergic reactions and possible skin removal.

BEST PRACTICE

Some specialist threading thread has an anti-bacterial coating added to it during the manufacture process to give protection to the skin while performing the service and so reduce the risk of infection.

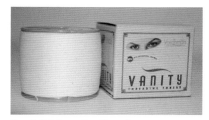

Specialist threading thread

Introduction

History

Threading has been used for many centuries. Its origin is a little uncertain but it is believed that it was originally used in Arabia, Turkey and India.

Threading is an ancient manual method of temporary hair removal, similar to tweezing. It involves the use of a loop of twisted cotton thread which is passed across the skin to trap the hairs and so 'pluck' them from their follicles. There are three main methods of threading, the mouth technique, neck technique and hand technique which are discussed later in the chapter.

Benefits of threading

Threading is a simple, inexpensive and an efficient way of removing unwanted hair with minimal pain and skin irritation. Neat results are achieved with hair regrowth approximately two to four weeks. An advantage is that very short hair can be removed with little irritation to the area making it possible to go over the area more than once. Hair can be removed individually or in 'lines' to create a perfect shape and can be removed from both above and below the eyebrow giving the threaded eyebrow its characteristic groomed appearance. Threading is also good for individuals that have undergone strong acne treatments, e.g. roaccutane, retin A where the skin becomes very delicate or those that have other contra-indications to waxing.

What type of thread is used for threading?

A specialist 100 per cent cotton thread is used for threading. This thread allows strength but resilience during the service which is important in order to perform threading to a high standard.

What body areas can be threaded?

Threading is mainly performed on the face, e.g. eyebrows, upper lip, chin, sides of face, nose, ears, neck and forehead but can be used all over the body if desired.

Advantages	Disadvantages
● Only removes hair not skin.	● Some clients may find side effects following the service.
● Good for short hairs.	● The area may be uncomfortable for a short while.
● Can isolate one hair at a time.	● Itching may occur following hair removal.
● Can go over an area more than once without causing skin irritation.	● In-growing hair may occur when the hair re-grows or as a result of poor technique.
● Sharp, defined shape can be achieved.	● It is good practice to use specialist threading thread to perform the service as this thread will be the correct strength and thickness to facilitate accurate technique and results. It should be placed back into its box or a sealed container when not in use to avoid contamination.
● Inexpensive to perform.	
● Fast results.	
● Ideal for eyebrows and facial hair.	● Infections may occur i.e. folliculitis if homecare advice is not followed as the follicle will remain open for up to 24 hours following the service.
● Minimal skin irritation – good for delicate, sensitive skin types.	● Excessive skin reddening (erythema).
	● Short term puffiness of tissues treated can occur.

Like tweezing, threading can be combined with other eye services to enhance the service. A good example would be to tint the eyebrows and lashes (ensure skin sensitivity test has been completed 48 hours in advance of the service with a negative result obtained) before performing the threading service.

To further enhance the eye area, eyelash extensions may be applied also.

For male grooming an eyebrow service can combined with a barbering service. Hair can also be removed from the tops of the cheeks, nose and ears.

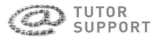

TUTOR SUPPORT

Activity 17.2: Research threading services

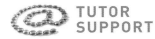

TUTOR SUPPORT

Activity 17.3: Comparing hair removal techniques

> " It is good practice to use specialist threading thread to perform the service as this thread will be the correct strength and thickness to facilitate accurate technique and results. It should be placed back into its box or a sealed container when not in use to avoid contamination.
>
> **Lorraine Onorato**

Outcome 1: Maintain safe and effective methods of working when providing threading services

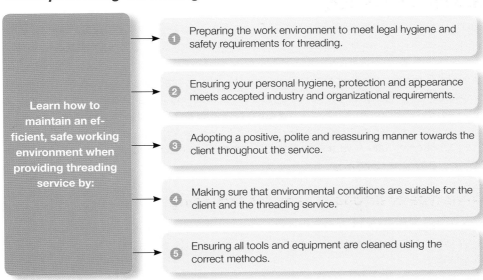

Learn how to maintain an efficient, safe working environment when providing threading service by:

1. Preparing the work environment to meet legal hygiene and safety requirements for threading.

2. Ensuring your personal hygiene, protection and appearance meets accepted industry and organizational requirements.

3. Adopting a positive, polite and reassuring manner towards the client throughout the service.

4. Making sure that environmental conditions are suitable for the client and the threading service.

5. Ensuring all tools and equipment are cleaned using the correct methods.

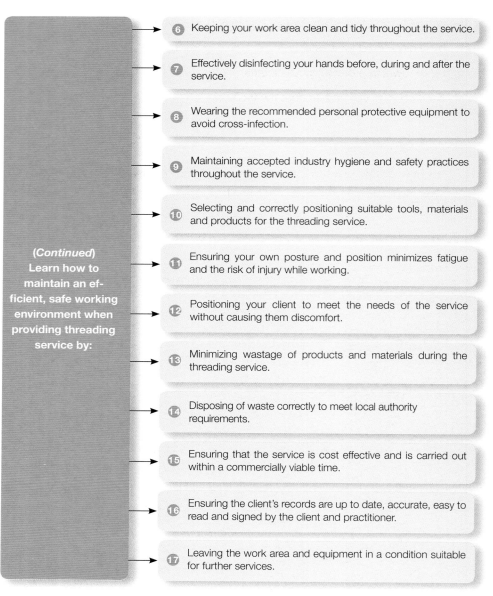

6 Keeping your work area clean and tidy throughout the service.

7 Effectively disinfecting your hands before, during and after the service.

8 Wearing the recommended personal protective equipment to avoid cross-infection.

9 Maintaining accepted industry hygiene and safety practices throughout the service.

10 Selecting and correctly positioning suitable tools, materials and products for the threading service.

11 Ensuring your own posture and position minimizes fatigue and the risk of injury while working.

12 Positioning your client to meet the needs of the service without causing them discomfort.

13 Minimizing wastage of products and materials during the threading service.

14 Disposing of waste correctly to meet local authority requirements.

15 Ensuring that the service is cost effective and is carried out within a commercially viable time.

16 Ensuring the client's records are up to date, accurate, easy to read and signed by the client and practitioner.

17 Leaving the work area and equipment in a condition suitable for further services.

(Continued) Learn how to maintain an efficient, safe working environment when providing threading service by:

HEALTH & SAFETY

Contaminated waste must be disposed of in accordance with the environmental health department of the local council.

TOP TIP

Cornflour is traditionally used as an alternative to talc, to dry the skin and lift the hair before the service. Some threading specialists use the powder to ensure the smooth gliding of the thread on the skin's surface.

Equipment and materials

Standard equipment is necessary as for other hair removal services, e.g. couch or chair with neck and foot support, trolley, lamp, etc. with the addition of the following:

- hand disinfectant
- cotton wool in covered container
- tissues
- specialist threading thread
- powder – purified talc or other specialist powder supplied by the manufacturer for this purpose
- disinfecting solution to store sterilized tweezers
- specialist eyebrow trimming scissors
- eyebrow brush

- antiseptic soothing lotion for use before and after service
- lined bin with lid for waste
- clean towel to protect client's clothes
- head band to secure hair from the face
- bedroll
- disposable gloves
- mirror to discuss the hair removal requirements at consultation and show the client the finished result

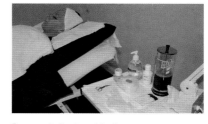

Prepared client and trolley

Outcome 2: Consult, prepare and plan for threading services

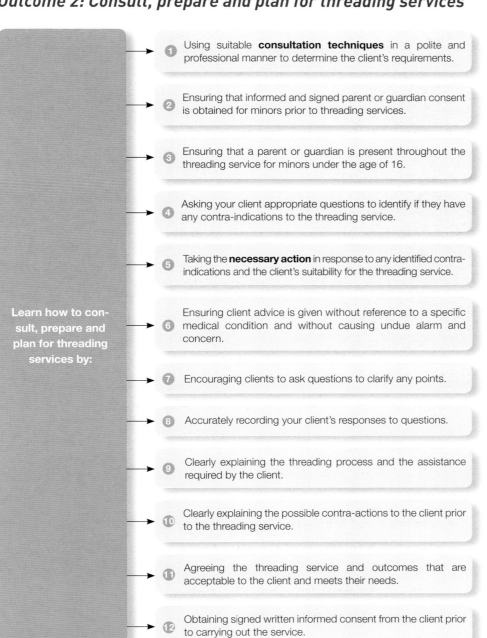

Learn how to consult, prepare and plan for threading services by:

1. Using suitable **consultation techniques** in a polite and professional manner to determine the client's requirements.

2. Ensuring that informed and signed parent or guardian consent is obtained for minors prior to threading services.

3. Ensuring that a parent or guardian is present throughout the threading service for minors under the age of 16.

4. Asking your client appropriate questions to identify if they have any contra-indications to the threading service.

5. Taking the **necessary action** in response to any identified contra-indications and the client's suitability for the threading service.

6. Ensuring client advice is given without reference to a specific medical condition and without causing undue alarm and concern.

7. Encouraging clients to ask questions to clarify any points.

8. Accurately recording your client's responses to questions.

9. Clearly explaining the threading process and the assistance required by the client.

10. Clearly explaining the possible contra-actions to the client prior to the threading service.

11. Agreeing the threading service and outcomes that are acceptable to the client and meets their needs.

12. Obtaining signed written informed consent from the client prior to carrying out the service.

TOP TIP

Disposable mascara wands can be used to brush the eyebrows as an alternative to a brow brush – which can then be hygienically disposed of.

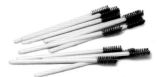

Disposable mascara wands

ACTIVITY

Collect magazines, look at images of eyebrows and see if you can identify which eyebrows have been threaded. You will need to look for a sharp and defined angular eyebrow.

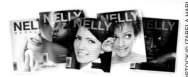

ISTOCK/© IZABELA HABUR

TOP TIP

A contra-action is what may occur as a result of the service. This must be discussed at consultation and must be indicated on the client's record card where appropriate with action taken recorded.

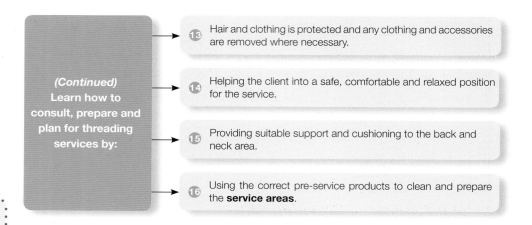

13   Hair and clothing is protected and any clothing and accessories are removed where necessary.

(Continued)
Learn how to consult, prepare and plan for threading services by:

14   Helping the client into a safe, comfortable and relaxed position for the service.

15   Providing suitable support and cushioning to the back and neck area.

16   Using the correct pre-service products to clean and prepare the **service areas**.

> Keep up to date with current developments in industry and be aware of changing fashion – we need to be ahead of our clients!
>
> **Lorraine Onorato**

Consultation

As with all services consultation is essential and should be carried out in a comfortable and quiet area where the client is able to ask any questions and clarify points if necessary. All details should be recorded and signatures obtained.

Consult with the client ensuring there is a clear understanding of the area to be treated and what is realistically achievable both short- and long-term. Encourage clients to ask questions to clarify any points.

Check client suitability, certain contra-indications will prevent threading.

Contra-indications

HEALTH & SAFETY

Contact lenses must be removed as clients will be required to support the eye area during the threading service.

BEST PRACTICE

Before beginning a new client wash your hands at the hand basin with antibacterial cleanser.

Although threading is considered to be more suitable for individuals with skin sensitivities resulting from conditions like psoriasis, eczema, dermatitis and diabetes, as with all hair removal techniques contra-indications will apply and will be the same as other hair removal techniques e.g. waxing and tweezing. There is also the possibility that contra-actions may arise. This can be avoided by ensuring a thorough consultation prior to the service to assess clients' suitability for the service and giving clear aftercare instructions on completion of the service.

Examples of possible contra-actions:

- **folliculitis**
- **erythema**
- ingrowing hairs
- blood spots
- broken hair
- histamine (allergic reaction)
- excessive erythema

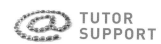

TUTOR SUPPORT

Activity 17.4: Threading wordsearch

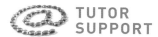

TUTOR SUPPORT

Activity 17.5: Threading wordsearch 2

> An eyebrow threading specialist must use their initiative to create the perfect eyebrow shape for each individual client. It may be necessary for the client to leave some areas of the eyebrow to grow in order to achieve a good result and this should be discussed and agreed during the consultation.
>
> **Lorraine Onorato**

Complete the record card ensuring that signatures are obtained. Any additional details are to be recorded on the reverse of the card. Existing clients will need to indicate whether there have been any changes since their last service, which must also be noted down on the record card.

Please refer to the sample client record card in Chapter 8, pages 247–248.

Service preparation

Preparation for the service is as important as the preparation of the beauty therapist (see Chapter 8, page 233) and must be carried out thoroughly and professionally:

1 Escort the client to the service area and assist with removal of clothing/accessories e.g. jewellery, scarves etc. and help the client onto the couch where necessary.

2 Confirm required shape discussed at consultation and advise where necessary.

3 Disinfect your hands and apply disposable gloves.

Outcome 3: Remove unwanted hair

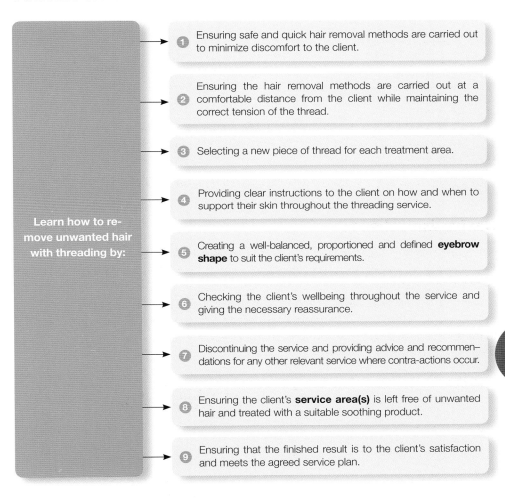

Learn how to remove unwanted hair with threading by:

1 Ensuring safe and quick hair removal methods are carried out to minimize discomfort to the client.

2 Ensuring the hair removal methods are carried out at a comfortable distance from the client while maintaining the correct tension of the thread.

3 Selecting a new piece of thread for each treatment area.

4 Providing clear instructions to the client on how and when to support their skin throughout the threading service.

5 Creating a well-balanced, proportioned and defined **eyebrow shape** to suit the client's requirements.

6 Checking the client's wellbeing throughout the service and giving the necessary reassurance.

7 Discontinuing the service and providing advice and recommen–dations for any other relevant service where contra-actions occur.

8 Ensuring the client's **service area(s)** is left free of unwanted hair and treated with a suitable soothing product.

9 Ensuring that the finished result is to the client's satisfaction and meets the agreed service plan.

Service procedure

1 First remove any facial creams or cosmetic products from the area to be treated by using some cotton wool and a disinfecting product, e.g. witch hazel, and then blot dry with a clean tissue disposing of both in a lined waste bin.

2 Brush the eyebrows in an upwards and then downwards direction to ensure the hairs are laying flat and trim any long hairs that may spoil the finished result. Brush eyebrows back into place.

HEALTH & SAFETY

PPE should ideally be worn.

HEALTH & SAFETY

Ensure barbicide (or similar) is diluted as per the manufacturers' guidelines and wear disposable gloves when handling it as it is an irritant.

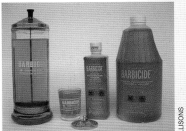

Barbicide

ELLISONS

TOP TIP

Long hairs are trimmed by first brushing the eyebrow hair in an upwards direction. The point of the scissors should be angled towards the bridge of the nose with the shank laying flat to the skins surface. The long hair is then trimmed to match to length of the other eyebrow hair. This process is then repeated underneath the eyebrow by brushing the hair in a downwards direction.

ALWAYS REMEMBER

Avoid invading your client's space during the service by working at approximately arms length distance of the area.

3 With a clean piece of cotton wool, apply a light dusting of powder (optional) to the area – this will enable the thread to glide over the skin and is particularly good when the skin is hot and moist.

4 Decide the method of threading to be used (examples below) and prepare the cotton.

5 The client must now support the area to be treated – for eyebrows one hand should be over the eye and one over the top of the eyebrow (see image below). The area should be supported firmly in order to avoid the skin being pinched or cut by the thread.

6 The hairs are removed against the direction of hair growth with the thread firmly placed onto the skin ensuring even tension throughout the service. This will enable effective and accurate removal of the hair from the root, avoiding snapping while reducing any discomfort to the client.

7 Remove all hairs as necessary using the thread to brush away any loose ones dropping onto the skin during the service. Keep checking the threaded area to ensure symmetry of both eyebrows.

8 On completion of the service apply soothing aftercare lotion to the area using cotton wool to remove loose hairs and soothe the area and then dispose of in a lined bin.

9 Brush the eyebrows into shape and show client the finished result.

10 Assist client from couch and give appropriate homecare advice.

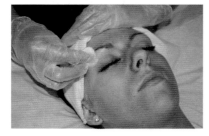

Cleanse the area to be treated

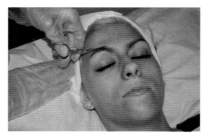

Trim long hairs if necessary

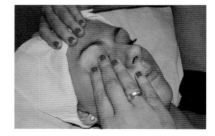

Client to support the area to be treated

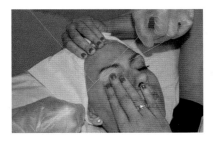

Thread against hair growth

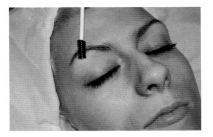

Brush eyebrow and show client finished result

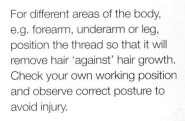

Wipe over area to remove loose hair and apply aftercare product

BEST PRACTICE

To avoid client dissatisfaction, especially when re-shaping a thick eyebrow shape it is advisable to show the client the shape as it is developing.

ACTIVITY

For different areas of the body, e.g. forearm, underarm or leg, position the thread so that it will remove hair 'against' hair growth. Check your own working position and observe correct posture to avoid injury.

TOP TIP

On completion of the service you could recommend a retail product or further eye service e.g. a soothing massage to the eye area with a suitable aftercare cream to enhance the service.

ALWAYS REMEMBER

Avoid skin tags and removal of hair from moles.

HEALTH & SAFETY

To avoid cross-contamination ensure all disposables and waste are put immediately into the bin and not left on the trolley.

> In order to enhance your chances of employment you should be able to perform an eyebrow thread to a high standard in 15mins. To achieve this you must be committed to practicing your skill at every opportunity.
>
> **Lorraine Onorato**

Threading techniques

There are three techniques that are commonly used:

1 **Mouth technique** – Hair removal using thread where one part of the thread is anchored in the mouth and the other part is looped in the hands. This is the most commonly used technique, originating from the Far East and is also know as the Asian or single looped method.

2 **Neck technique** – A substitute for the mouth technique where one part of the thread is anchored around the neck and the other part is looped in the hands. This technique originates from the Middle East and is also known as the Arabian or single looped method.

BEST PRACTICE

Ensure that you are removing hair against direction of hair growth.

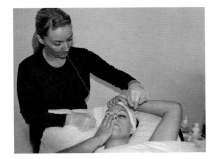

The Mouth Technique

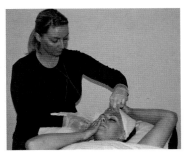

The Neck Technique

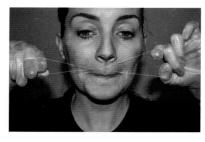

The Hand technique (self-threading)

3 **Hand technique** – Hair removal using thread held and looped between both hands. Commonly used by practitioners on themselves. This technique is also known as cats cradle, doubled looped or self technique.

Outcome 4: Provide aftercare advice

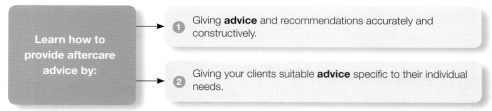

Learn how to provide aftercare advice by:

1 Giving **advice** and recommendations accurately and constructively.

2 Giving your clients suitable **advice** specific to their individual needs.

> "Ensure you have related products to retail following the service for the client to maintain and enhance her eyebrows between appointments e.g. brow make-up kits, brow setting mousse and tweezers.
>
> **Lorraine Onorato**

ALWAYS REMEMBER

To schedule the client's next appointment as part of the aftercare advice.

Aftercare advice

Aftercare advice and homecare advice are essential not only to avoid contra-actions but in order to maintain the service results. It is important to give general as well as specific advice.

For the next 12–24 hours it is important to avoid:

● swimming

● heat services, e.g. hot water, sauna, steam or sun bed

● perfumed products applied the area treated

● facial services/exfoliation

● touching the area

● excessive sweating

● applying make-up to the area

To avoid in-growing hairs it is important to **gently exfoliate** the area after three days and twice weekly thereafter.

If needed the area can be soothed with either a recommended product or a soothing and calming product, e.g. aloe vera gel.

If there is a contra-action following service advise the client what action should be taken. Advise the client to receive the service in the specified time according to her hair growth cycle. Repeat bookings vary according to the natural hair regrowth and client requirements.

Ensure that the client's records are up-to-date, accurate and complete following the threading service. Provide written instructions in an aftercare leaflet.

GLOSSARY OF KEY WORDS

Client groups this term is used in a number of the units and it refers to client diversity. The CRE (Commission for Racial Equality) ethnic group classification is used in the range for these units. These cover white, mixed, Asian, black and Chinese.

Contra-actions an unwanted reaction occurring during or after service application.

Contra-indication a problematic symptom that indicates that the service may not proceed or may restrict service application. Further contra-indications identified for spa services are discussed in more detail in Chapter 3.

Cross contamination transfer of an infection directly from one person to another or indirectly from one person to a second person via a fomite.

Erythema reddening of the skin cause by increased blood circulation to the area.

Folliculitis a bacterial infection where pustules develop in the skin tissue around the hair follicle.

ASSESSMENT OF KNOWLEDGE AND UNDERSTANDING

Having covered the learning objectives for **Provide threading services,** test what you need to know and understand answering the following short questions below. The information covers:

- organizational and legal requirements
- working safely and effectively
- consult, plan and prepare for threading
- anatomy and physiology
- contra-indications and contra-actions
- threading tools, materials and equipment
- service specific knowledge
- aftercare advice for the clients

Organizational and legal requirements

For full legislation details, see Chapter 4.

1 Which 'act' relates to the importance of not discriminating against clients with illnesses and disabilities?

2 What is the purpose of insurance for the beauty therapist?

3 Why is important to maintain hygiene standards before, during and after services?

4 Why is it important to have a parent/guardian present when treating minors?

5 Where and how must client's record cards be stored Why?

Working safely and effectively

1 What is repetitive strain injury? Give **three** examples of how it can be avoided.

2 When should the thread be changed during the service?

3 Why is it important to record client's responses during the consultation?

4 How would you prepare yourself for a threading service?

5 What is the best method of disinfecting the hands prior to the service?

Consult, plan and prepare for threading

1 Why is it important to clearly explain the threading service to the client?

2 Why is it important to allow time for the client to ask questions?

3 What is a contra-action?

4 Why should you explain the possible contra-actions to the client?

5 Why is it important to agree a service plan with your client?

Anatomy and physiology

For full anatomy and physiology details, see Chapter 2.

1 What is the indentation in the skin that the hair grows from?

2 What is the portion of the hair that we see on the skin's surface called?

3 What is hair composed of?

4 Hair growth is under the influence of which of the body's systems?

5 List **three** characteristics of terminal hair.

6   How would you recognize an ingrowing hair? What would you advise the client to do to avoid further problems?

7   List **three** causes of hair growth.

8   How many layers of the epidermis are there?

9   Where are hair germs cells produced from?

10 In which phase of hair growth is a hair resting?

Contra-indications and contra-actions

1   What is a contra-indication?

2   List **five** contra-indications that would prevent service.

3   List **five** contra-indications that would restrict service.

4   Why should the therapist not name specific contra-indications when encouraging a client to seek medical advice?

5   How would you recognize and deal with a histamine reaction to a threading service?

Threading tools, materials and equipment

1   List the tools necessary to carry out a threading service.

2   Why is it important to use specialist threading thread?

3   Give two examples of products that can be used pre- and post-service.

4   Why is it important to have the correct equipment for a threading service?

5   What is the best method of sterilization for threading scissors?

Service-specific knowledge

1   Threading is an ancient manual technique of hair removal popular in which countries?

2   In which area is threading mainly used?

3   List **three** benefits of threading.

4   Why is it important to measure the eyebrows prior to an eyebrow threading service?

5   List **three** disadvantages of threading?

6   What other services can be combined with a threading service?

7   How would you adapt the threading technique for a male client with strong hair?

8   Why is it important for the client to support the skin during the service?

Aftercare advice for the clients

1   Give **three** reasons why aftercare advice is important.

2   List the general aftercare advice for an eyebrow threading service.

3   Why is exfoliation of the area important?

4   What is the recommended interval between services?

5   Why is it important that you receive a signature for aftercare advice given?

6   What can the client use to soothe any irritation following the service?

7   How long should the client avoid applying make-up to the area for?

Glossary

Accident book a written record of any accident in the workplace. Incidents in the accident book should be reviewed to see where improvements to safe working practice could be made.

Accident form a detailed report form to be completed following any accident in the workplace.

Acid mantle the combination of sweat and sebum on the skin's surface, creating an acid film. The acid mantle is protective and discourages the growth of bacteria and fungi. The pH scale is used to measure the acidity or alkalinity of a substance using a numbered scale. The skin's pH is acid at 5.5-5.6.

Additional products and services products and services offered by your salon that a client may receive or purchase to enhance their service benefits.

Adhesive specialized glue used to attach artificial lashes to the natural lashes. This glue differs in formulation according to the lash type strip or individual flare lashes.

Aftercare advice recommendations given to the client following service to maintain the finished result and enable the benefits to be continued at home.

After-wax lotion a product applied to the skin following hair removal to reduce redness and promote skin healing.

Age groups the different classification of age groups to be covered: 16–30, 31–50 and over 50 years.

Allergic reaction reaction to ingredients in a product producing symptoms including erythema, swelling, itching and bruising.

Anagen the active growth stage of the hair growth cycle.

Antioxidant properties of some foods that maintain the health of the skin, fighting the damaging effects of free radicals (unstable molecules which can cause skin cells to degenerate) in the body. Antioxidant ingredients are increasingly being included in skincare preparations to neutralize free radicals or repel them from the skin.

Antiseptic a chemical agent that prevents the multiplication of microorganisms. It has limited action and does not kill all microorganisms.

Apocrine gland sweat gland found in the armpit, nipple and groin area. Larger than the eccrine sweat gland and attached to the hair follicle. These sweat glands are controlled by hormones and become active at puberty.

Appointment arrangement made for a client to receive a service on a particular date and time.

Appraisal a process whereby a supervisor, referred to as an appraiser, identifies and discusses with an individual their performance and achievements in their job role, against previously set targets.

Arrector pili muscle a small muscle attached to the hair follicle and base of the epidermis. When the muscle contracts (shortens) it causes the hair to stand upright in the hair follicle.

Artificial lashes threads of nylon fibre which are attached to the natural hair. These are referred to as strip lashes, individual artificial lashes and single lash extensions.

Aseptic The methods used to eliminate bacteria when performing treatment procedures from British standards. Glossary of terms relating to disinfectants.

Assistance providing help or support.

Autoclave an effective method of sterilization, suitable for small metal objects and beauty therapy tools. Water is boiled under increased pressure and reaches temperatures of 121–134°C.

Bacteria minute, single-celled organisms of various shapes. Large numbers live on the skin's surface and are not harmful (they are non-pathogenic); others, however, are harmful (pathogenic) and can cause disease.

Base coat a nail polish product applied to protect the natural nail and prevent staining from coloured nail polish.

Bevelling a nail filing technique used at the free edge of the nail to ensure it is smooth.

Blepharitis inflammation of the eyelid caused by an infection or an allergic reaction.

Blood nutritive liquid circulating through the blood vessels. It transports essential nutrients to the cells and removes waste products. It also transports other important substances such as oxygen and hormones.

Blood vessel transports blood through the body in either an artery or a vein. An artery transports blood away from the heart at high pressure, the vein returns blood to the heart at low pressure.

Blue nail nail condition where the nail bed has a blue tinge rather than a healthy pink colour due to poor blood circulation in the area.

Blusher cosmetic applied to add warmth to the face and emphasize the facial contours.

Body language communication involving the body.

Body wrapping a service where the body is wrapped in bandages, plastic sheets or thermal blankets to achieve different therapeutic effects including skin toning and weight loss.

Bone the hardest structure in the body. It protects the underlying structures, gives shape to the body and provides an attachment point for muscles.

Bones of foot and lower leg a type of connective tissue that provides a surface for muscle attachment. These include in the foot the tarsals, metatarsal and phalanxes. In the lower leg the tibia and fibula.

Bones of lower arm and hand a type of connective tissue that provide a surface for muscle attachment. These include in the lower arm the radius and ulna. In the hand the carpals, metacarpals and phalanges.

Bones of the chest a type of connective tissue that protects the inner organs, and provides a surface for muscle attachment that allows movement and includes the sternum.

Bones of the neck a type of connective tissue that supports the skull and includes the cervical vertebrae.

Bronzing products make-up product applied to create a healthy, natural or subtle tanned look. They are formulated to create a matt or shimmer effect and are also suitable as a highlighting contouring product.

Bruised nail nail condition where the nail appears blue/black in colour where bleeding has occurred on the nail bed following injury.

Buffer a manicure tool with a handle made of plastic and a pad with a replaceable cover, used on the nail to give a sheen, increase blood supply to the area and, if used with the gritty cream buffing paste, to help smooth out nail surface irregularities.

Bunion a foot condition. The large joint at the base of the big toe protrudes, forcing the big toe inwards towards the other toes.

Burn injury to the skin caused by excess heat; the skin appears red and may blister.

Callus foot condition, displaying thick, yellowish hardened skin, usually found on prominent areas of the foot such as the heel.

Camouflage needs identifying the area and skin imperfection requiring camouflage, e.g. tattoos, hyperpigmentation, hypopigmentation and erythema (redness).

Camouflage products cosmetic make-up products designed to conceal skin imperfections including creams, powders and setting products for the face and body.

Catagen the stage of the hair growth cycle where the hair becomes detached from its source of nourishment, the dermal papilla, and stops growing.

Cell basic units of life which specialize in carrying out particular functions in the body. Groups of cells which share function, shape, size or structure are called tissues. The human body consists of trillions of cells.

Certificate of registration awarded when the premises have been successfully inspected to ensure that the local bye-laws are being followed in relation to cosmetic piercing.

Charge card an alternative form of payment where the complete amount of credit spent must be repaid by the cardholder each month to the card company.

Cheque an alternative form of payment to that of using cash. A cheque must be accompanied by a cheque guarantee card.

Chilblains poor blood supply where the toes become red, blue or purple in colour and the area may become painful and itchy; aggravated in cold weather.

Chiropodist a person who is trained and qualified to treat minor foot complaints.

Circulatory system transports material around the body.

Cleanser a skincare preparation that removes dead skin cells, excess sweat and sebum, make-up and dirt from the skin's surface to maintain a healthy skin complexion. These are formulated to treat the different skin types, skin characteristics and facial areas.

Cleanser a skincare preparation that removes dead skin cells, excess sweat and sebum, make-up and dirt from the skin's surface to maintain a healthy skin complexion. These are formulated to treat the different skin types, skin characteristics and facial areas.

Client groups this term is used in a number of the units and it refers to client diversity. The CRE (Commission for Racial Equality) ethnic group classification is used in the range for these units. These cover white, mixed, Asian, black and Chinese.

Clinical waste waste from ear-piercing is classed as clinical waste. The disposal of clinical waste is controlled by the Environment Agency. Waste materials that have come into contact with body fluids must be collected and disposed of by special arrangements. The Environment Protection Act (1990): Waste Management: The Duty of Care, A Code of Practice (ISBN 011 752577 X) provides further information on this subject.

Code of conduct workplace service standards with regard to appearance and behaviour while in the working environment.

Code of practice the expected standards and behaviour for the professional beauty therapist to follow, which will uphold the reputation of the industry and ensure best working practice for the industry and protect members of the public. Beauty therapy professional bodies produce codes of practice for their members. A business may have its own code of practice.

Cold wax a wax already applied to a strip and ready for use. The pre-coated strip is applied firmly to the skin and then removed quickly against hair growth, removing the hair in the area.

Collagen protein fibre found in the dermis of the skin that gives the skin its strength.

Colour corrector make-up product applied to target problem areas. It contains pigments which balance skin tone.

Colour theory the colour wheel places the three primary colours with the secondary colours in-between. These result from mixing the two adjacent primary colours. In-between these are the tertiary colours achieved by mixing the primary and secondary colours. Colour is reduced or removed by mixing colours that are directly opposite each other in the colour wheel.

Colouring characteristics the client's natural hair colouring, i.e. fair, red, dark and white.

Comedone removal facial techniques used to extract comedones (blackheads) from the skin. A small tool called a comedone extractor is used for this purpose.

Communication the exchange of information and the establishment of understanding between people.

Complaints procedure a formal, standardized approach adopted by the organization to handle any complaints.

Concealer cosmetic product used to disguise minor skin imperfections such as blemishes, uneven skin colour or shadows.

Conjunctivitis a bacterial infection. Inflammation of the mucous membrane that covers the eye and lines the eyelid. The skin of the inner conjunctiva of the eye becomes inflamed, the eye becomes very red, itchy and sore, and pus may exude from the eye area.

Consent form written permission obtained from a parent or guardian to perform a service on a client under 16 years of age.

Consultation techniques methods used to identify the client's needs using differing assessment techniques, including questioning, manual and natural observation.

Consultation assessment of client needs using different assessment techniques including questioning and natural observation.

Consumer Protection (Distance Selling) Regulations (2000) these Regulations, (as amended by the Consumer Protection (Distance Selling) (Amendment) Regulations (2005), are derived from a European Union directive and cover the supply of goods/services made between suppliers acting in a commercial capacity and consumers. They are concerned with purchases made by telephone, fax, internet, digital television and mail order.

Consumer Protection Act (1987) this act follows European Union directives to protect the customer from unsafe, defective services and products that do not reach safety standards.

Consumer Safety Act (1978) this act aims to reduce risks to consumers from potentially dangerous products.

Contact dermatitis a skin disorder caused by intolerance of the skin to a particular substance, or a group of substances.

On exposure to the substance the skin quickly becomes irritated and an allergic reaction occurs.

Continuous Professional Development (CPD) activities undertaken to develop technical skill and expertise to ensure current, professional experience in the beauty industry is maintained.

Contour cosmetics applied to cosmetically change and enhance the shape of the face and facial features.

Contra-action an unwanted reaction occurring during or after service application.

Contra-indication a problematic symptom that indicates that the service may not proceed or may restrict service application. Further contra-indications identified for spa services are discussed in more detail in Chapter 3.

Control of Risk the means by which risks identified are removed or reduced to acceptable levels.

Control of Substances Hazardous to Health (COSHH) Regulations (2002) (Including Biological Agents) Regulations legislation that requires employers and the self-employed to prevent or control the exposure of employees and clients to hazardous substances. This includes exposure to biological agents such as bacteria, fungi and viruses and chemical cleaning/sterilizing agents. Records of the COSHH assessment must be available for inspection.

Controlled Waste Regulations (1992) categorizes waste types. The Local Authority provides advice on how to dispose of waste types in compliance with the law.

Corn small areas of thickened skin on the foot. Often white in appearance.

Cortex the thickest layer of the hair structure.

Cosmetic Products (Safety) Regulations (2008) part of consumer protection legislation that requires that cosmetics and toiletries are safe in their formulation and are safe for use for their intended purpose as a cosmetic and comply with labelling requirements.

Credit card an alternative form of payment to that of using cash. These cards are held by those who have a credit account, where there is a pre-arranged borrowing limit. These can only be used if your business has an arrangement to deal with the relevant credit card company.

Cross contamination transfer of an infection directly from one person to another or indirectly from one person to a second person via a fomite.

Cross-infection the transfer of contagious microorganisms.

Customer care statement defined customer service standards that are expected.

Cuticle cream or oil a cosmetic preparation used to condition the skin of the cuticle.

Cuticle knife a metal tool used on the nail to remove excess eponychium and perionychium (the extension of the skin of the cuticle at the base of the nail).

Cuticle nippers a metal tool used to remove excess cuticle and neaten the skin around the cuticle area.

Cuticle remover a cosmetic preparation used to soften and loosen the skin cells and cuticle from the nail.

Cyclical pattern of growth the hair growth cycle, which can be divided into three phases: anagen, catagen and telegen.

Cyst localized pocket of sebum that forms in the hair follicle or under the sebaceous glands in the skin. Semi-globular in shape, either raised or flat, and hard or soft. Cysts are the same colour as the skin, or red if bacterial infection occurs.

Dangerous Substances and Preparations (Nickel) (Safety) Regulations (2005) the use of nickel has been found to cause allergies. Check what metal is used for your supplier's ear-piercing jewellery and that it complies with the regulations.

Data Protection Act (1998) legislation designed to protect client privacy and confidentiality.

Debit card alternative method of payment where the card authorizes immediate debit of the cash amount from the client's account.

Dermal papilla an organ that provides the hair with blood, necessary for hair growth.

Dermis the inner portion of skin situated underneath the epidermis.

Diabetes a disease that prevents sufferers breaking down glucose in their cells.

Disability Discrimination Act (1996) implemented to prevent disabled persons being discriminated against. Employers have a responsibility to remove physical barriers and to adjust working conditions to prevent discrimination on the basis of having a disability.

Discrepancy a disagreement over amounts of money etc. This is referred to in instances where a client disagrees with what they are being asked to pay or the amount of change received.

Disinfectant a chemical agent that destroys most microorganisms.

Disposable applicator used to apply wax hygienically to the area of hair removal without contaminating the wax flowing back into the tube following application. The applicator head is disposed of after each service.

Ear-piercing the perforation of the skin and underlying tissue of the earlobe to create a hole in the skin where jewellery is inserted.

Eccrine gland simple sweat producing gland responsive to heat, appearing as tiny tubes which are straight in the epidermis, and coiled in the dermis. Its function is to maintain the body temperature by sweating.

Eczema of the nail inflammation of the skin, causing changes to the nail including ridges, pitting, nail separation and nail thickening.

Effleurage a stroking massage manipulation used to begin the massage, as a link manipulation, and to complete the massage sequence. Applied in a rhythmic, continuous manner, it induces relaxation.

Eggshell nail nail condition where thin, fragile white nails curve under at the free edge.

Elastin protein fibre found in the dermis of the skin which gives the skin its elasticity.

Electricity at Work Regulations (1989) these regulations state that electrical equipment in the workplace should be tested every 12 months, by a qualified electrician. The employer must keep records of the equipment tested and the date it was checked.

Emery board a nail file used to shape the free edge of the nail.

Employers' Liability (Compulsory Insurance) Act (1969) this provides financial compensation to an employee should they be injured as a result of an accident in the workplace. A certificate indicating that a policy of insurance has been purchased should be displayed.

Enquiries questions presented by clients or business contacts to find out more information.

Environmental conditions this includes heating, lighting, ventilation and general comfort requirements for the workplace or service.

Epidermis the outer layer of the skin.

Equal opportunity non-discrimination on the basis of sex, race, disability, age, etc.

Equipment and tools used within a service that enable the service to be completed competently.

Erythema reddening of the skin cause by increased blood circulation to the area.

Evaluation method used which measures the value of the instructional activity.

Exfoliant a service used to remove excess dead skin cells from the surface of the skin, which has a skin cleansing, cell rejuvenating action. This process can be achieved using a specialized cosmetic, or mechanically by using facial equipment where a brush is rotated over the skin's surface.

External ear structure funnels sound waves into the ear to enable hearing. It comprises the pinna, lobe, cartilage and cartilaginous tissue.

Eye shadow cosmetic applied to the eye to complement the natural eye colour, to give definition to the eye area and enhance the natural shape of the eye.

Eyebrow colour cosmetic applied to emphasize the eyebrows, alter their shape, and which can make sparse eyebrows look thicker.

Eyebrow shaping involves the removal of eyebrow hair to create a new shape (reshape) or to remove stray hairs to maintain the existing brow shape (maintenance). Small metal tools, called tweezers, are use to remove the hairs.

Eyelash adhesive used to apply strips and individual eyelashes

Eyelash and eyebrow tinting definition of the brow and lash hair, achieved by the application of a permanent dye especially formulated for use around the delicate eye area.

Eyeliner cosmetic applied to define and emphasize the eye area.

Face shape the size and shape of the facial bone structure. Face shapes include oval, round, square, heart, diamond, oblong and pear.

Facial bones a type of connective tissue forming a hard structure that forms the face and forms an attachment point for muscles. These include the zygomatic, mandible, maxilla, nasal, vomer, turbinate, lacrimal and palatine.

Facial features the size of a person's nose, eyes, forehead, chin, neck, etc. When applying make-up products, make-up application can emphasize or minimize the appearance of facial features.

Facial products skincare used with a facial service which have specific benefits to care for and improve the function and appearance of the skin.

Facial a service to improve the appearance, condition and functioning of the skin and underlying structures.

False eyelashes threads of nylon fibre or real hair attached to the natural eyelash hair. There are two main types: individual or strip.

Fire Precautions Act (1971) legislation that states that all staff must be familiar with, and trained in fire, and emergency evacuation procedures for their workplace.

Fitzpatrick Classification System a scale developed to assess the amount of melanin pigment in the skin providing your skin colour and how your skin will react to sun without protection (photo-sensitivity). There are six skin type classifications from Caucasian (skin type I) to African-Caribbean (skin type VI).

Flotation a spa service where the body is suspended in water (wet flotation) or supported on water (dry flotation), inducing relaxation.

Foam bath a shallow bath of water containing a foaming agent surrounds the body, achieving a thermal effect. Increased perspiration caused by this effect aids the elimination of wastes and toxins.

Folliculitis a bacterial infection where pustules develop in the skin tissue around the hair follicle.

Foot and nail services specialized products and equipment designed to improve the condition and appearance of different nail and skin conditions.

Foot cream/oil a cosmetic mixture of waxes and oils applied to soften the skin of the feet and cuticles.

Foot rasp a pedicure tool used to remove excess dead skin from the foot.

Foot spa a foot bath incorporating massage and water aeration, creating a bubbling effect to cleanse and relax the feet.

Foundation a make-up product applied to produce an even skin tone, to disguise minor skin blemishes and as a contour cosmetic.

Fungi microscopic plants. Fungal diseases of the skin feed off the waste products of the skin. They are found on the skin's surface or they can attack deeper tissues.

Gift voucher a pre-payment method for beauty therapy services or retail sales.

Greater London Council (General Powers) Act (1981) this act covers the London boroughs and relates to cosmetic piercing. It provides that no person can carry out cosmetic piercing unless they and the business are registered. It also states what records are required to be kept.

Grievance a cause for concern or complaint.

Hair follicle an appendage (structure) in the skin formed from epidermal tissue. Cells move up the hair follicle from the bottom (the hair bulb), changing in structure, to form the hair.

Hair growth cycle the cyclical pattern of hair growth, which can be divided into three phases: anagen, catagen and telogen.

Hair a long slender structure that grows out of, and is part of the skin. Each hair is made up of dead skin cells, which contain the protein called keratin.

(Hair) Shaft the part of the hair that can be seen above the skin's surface, extending from the hair follicle.

Hairy moles moles exhibiting coarse hairs from their surface.

Hand and nail treatments specialized products and equipment designed to improve the condition and appearance of different nail and skin conditions.

Hand cream/oil a cosmetic mixture of waxes and oils applied to soften the skin of the hands and cuticles.

Hangnail nail condition where small pieces of epidermal skin protrude between the nail plate and nail wall, accompanying a dry cuticle condition.

Hazard a hazard is something with potential to cause harm.

Health and Safety (Display Screen Equipment) Regulations (1992) these regulations cover the use of visual display units (VDUs) and computer screens. They specify acceptable levels of radiation emissions from the screen and identify correct working posture, seating position, permitted working heights and rest periods.

Health and Safety (First Aid) Regulations (1981) legislation that states that workplaces must have appropriate and adequate first aid provision.

Health and Safety at Work Act (1974) legislation that lays down the minimum standards of health safety and welfare requirements in all workplaces.

Health and Safety policy each employer of more than five employees must have a written health and safety policy issued to their employees outlining their health and safety responsibilities.

Heat rash a reaction to heat exposure where the sweat ducts become blocked and sweat escapes into the epidermis. Red pimples occur and the skin becomes itchy.

Heat services these include sauna, steam and the relaxation room. When heat services are applied, there is an increase in body temperature of about 1–2°C.

Highlighter a make-up product that draws attention to and emphasizes features.

Histamine a chemical released when the skin comes into contact with a substance that it is allergic to. Cells called 'mast cells' burst, releasing histamine into the tissues. This causes the blood capillaries to dilate, which increases blood flow to limit skin damage and begin repair.

Hoof stick a nail tool used to gently push back the softened cuticles.

Hospitality this covers welcoming the client, being helpful and offering refreshments and magazines, and ensuring the client is comfortable while at reception.

Hot wax a system of wax depilation used to remove hair from the skin. Hot wax cools and sets on contact with the skin. They are a blend of waxes, such as beeswax and resins, which keep the wax flexible. Soothing ingredients are often included to avoid skin irritation.

Humidity moisture content of the air.

Hydrogen peroxide (H_2O_2) an oxidant, a chemical that contains available oxygen atoms and encourages chemical reactions.

Hydrotherapy spa services where water is used for its therapeutic effect.

Hygiene requirements the expected standards as required by law, industry codes of practice or written procedures specified by the workplace.

Hyperpigmentation increased pigment production.

Hypopigmentation loss of pigmentation.

Induction an introductory activity delivered when you start or progress into a new job role. Its aim is to provide you with general and essential information related to the work environment, welfare and your job roles and responsibilities.

Infestation a condition where animal parasites live off and invade a host.

Ingrowing hair a build-up of skin occurs over the hair follicle, causing the hair to grow under the skin.

Ingrowing toenails nail condition where the side of the nail penetrates the nail wall; redness, inflammation and pus may be present.

Instructional activity the method used to teach a skill or develop a person's knowledge and understanding in a new area of learning.

Instructional techniques educational methods to teach a person a skill or develop their knowledge and understanding in a new area of learning. These include demonstration, use of instructional diagrams, verbal explanation and use of written instructions.

Job description written details of a person's specific work role, duties and responsibilities.

Keloids overgrowths of scar tissue, occurring at the site of the ear-piercing.

Keratin a protein produced by cells in the epidermis called keratinocytes. Keratin makes the skin tough and reduces the passage of substances into our bodies. Each hair and nail contains keratin.

Langalier index or Palintest balanced water index the method of regular testing and maintenance of water quality in the spa whirlpools/swimming pool.

Laser hair removal a technique of permanent hair removal. Laser energy is passed through the skin which stops the activity of the hair follicle creating hair growth through a process called photothermolysis.

Legislation laws affecting the beauty therapy business relating to products and services, the business premises and environmental conditions, working practices and those employed.

Leuconychia nail condition where white spots or marks appear on the nail plate.

Limits of own authority the extent of your responsibility as determined by your own job description and workplace policies.

Lip balm a lip moisturiser which may contain pigment.

Lip gloss cosmetic applied to the lips to provide a moist, shiny look.

Lip liner cosmetic used to define the lips, creating a perfectly symmetrical outline.

Lip stain make-up product which adds intense colour to the lips.

Lipstick cosmetic applied to the lips to add colour and keep the lips soft and supple.

Local Government (Miscellaneous Provisions) Act (1982) legislation that requires that salons offering any form of skin piercing be registered with the local health authority. This registration includes both the operators who will be carrying out the service and the salon premises where the service will be carried out.

Local Government Act (2003) (section 120 and schedule 6) has amended the Local Government (Miscellaneous Provisions) Act (1982) to enable each authority to regulate businesses providing cosmetic body piercing. Each local authority can introduce its own bye-laws to set the standards for cosmetic piercing.

London Local Authorities Act (1991 and 2007) this act states that no person shall carry out cosmetic piercing at an establishment without obtaining a licence from a participating council. Conditions can be attached to the licence, such as hygiene practices, age restrictions, etc.

Longitudinal ridges nail condition where grooves appear in the nail plate, running along the length of the nail from the cuticle to the free edge.

Lymph vessel referred to as lymphatics. They transport lymph a watery fluid that flows through the lymphatic system from the tissues to the blood.

Lymph a clear, straw-coloured liquid circulating in the lymph vessels and lymphatics of the body, filtered out of the blood plasma.

Lymphatic system closely connected to the blood system. Its primary function is defensive: to remove bacteria and foreign materials to prevent infection.

Make-up cosmetics applied to the skin of the face to enhance and accentuate, or to minimize facial features. Make-up products create balance in the face.

Make-up occasion the context the make-up is to be applied for, i.e. day, evening and special occasion.

Make-up products different cosmetics available to suit skin type, colour and condition, i.e. sensitive or mature. Make-up products include concealing and contour cosmetics, foundations, translucent powders, eye shadows, eyeliners, brow liners, mascaras, lipsticks, lip glosses, lip liners, etc.

Management of Health and Safety at Work Regulations (1999) this legislation provides the employer with an approved code of practice for maintaining a safe, secure working environment.

Manicure a service to care for and improve the condition and appearance of the hands and nails.

Manual Handling Operations Regulations (1992) legislation that requires the employer to carry out a risk assessment of all activities undertaken which involve manual handling (lifting and moving objects).

Mascara cosmetic that enhances the natural eyelashes, making them appear longer, changed in colour and/or thicker.

Mask a service mask applied to the skin of the feet to treat and improve the condition of the skin; this may include stimulating, rejuvenating or moisturising properties.

Massage manipulations movements which are selected and applied according to the desired effect, and which may be stimulating, relaxing or toning. Massage manipulations include effleurage, petrissage, percussion (also known as tapotement) and vibrations.

Massage manipulation of the soft tissues of the body, producing heat and stimulating the muscular, circulatory and nervous systems.

Massage medium a skincare product which acts as a lubricant to allow sufficient slip over the skin's, surface while performing facial massage.

Melanin a pigment in the skin and the hair that contributes to the skin/hair colour.

Melanocytes cells that produce the skin pigment melanin that contributes to skin colour.

Messages communication of information to another person in written, electronic or verbal form.

Method of payment different forms of payment that may be accepted to pay for a product or service including cash, cash equivalents, cheque and payment cards.

Milium extraction skincare technique used to extract milia (whiteheads) from the skin. A small tool called a milia extractor is used for this purpose, which superficially pierces the epidermis, allowing effective removal of the milia.

Mineral make-up is created from finely ground minerals (a process called micronization). It is used in the formulation of different make-up products.

Minor a person classed as a child who requires by law to have a guardian or parent present.

Moisturiser a skincare preparation whose formulation of oil and water helps maintain the skin's natural moisture by locking moisture into the skin, offering protection and hydration. The formulation is selected to suit the skin type, facial characteristics and facial area.

Muscle contractile tissue responsible for movement of the body.

Muscle tone the normal degree of tension in healthy muscle.

Muscles of facial expression muscles which when contracted, pull the facial skin in a particular way and create facial expressions. These include the frontalis, corrugators, temporalis, orbicularis oculi, levator labii, orbicularis oris, buccinators, risorius, mentalis, zygomaticus, masseter, depressor labii.

Muscles of foot and lower leg the muscles of the foot work together to help move the body. The foot is moved by muscles in the lower leg which pull on tendons that attach the muscle to the bone.

Muscles of lower arm and hand the hands and fingers are moved by muscles and tendons. The muscles that bend the wrist in towards the forearm are flexors; the extensors straighten the wrist and hand.

Muscles of the upper body these move the arm and include pectoralis and deltoid.

Muscles that move the neck these include sternocleido mastoid, platysma, trapezius.

Nail finish the product finally applied to the natural nail to enhance its appearance, i.e. buffed nail or nail polish application.

Nail growth cells divide in the matrix and the nails grow forward over the nail bed until they reach the end of the finger. The nail cells harden as they grow through a process called keratinization.

Nail polish a clear or coloured nail product that adds colour/protection to the nail. Cream polish has a matt finish and requires a top coat application. Pearlized polish produces a frosted, shimmery appearance and top coat is not required.

Nail polish drier an aerosol or oil preparation applied following nail polish application to increase the speed at which the polish hardens.

Nail polish remover a solvent used to remove nail polish and grease from the nails prior to applying polish. Nail polish solvent used to thin nail polish and restore its consistency.

Nail polish solvent used to thin nail polish and restore its consistency.

Nail strengthener a nail polish product that strengthens the nail plate, which has a tendency to split.

Nail structure composed for protection the nail is made up of the following parts: nail plate, nail bed, matrix, cuticle, lunula, hyponychium, eponychium, nail wall, free edge, lateral nail fold.

Nails hard, horny, epidermal cells that protect the living nail bed of the fingers and toes.

National Occupational Standards for Beauty Therapy standards that set the relevant performance objectives, range statements and knowledge specifications to support performance. These can be obtained from the Hairdressing and Beauty Industry Authority (Habia) website: www.habia.org.uk.

Necessary action the action taken or service modification required to deal safely with a contra-action or contra-indication.

Negative skin sensitivity test a test where result produces no skin reaction. in this case you may proceed with the service.

Nerve a collection of single neurones surrounded by a protective sheath through which impulses are transmitted between the brain or spinal cord and another part of the body.

Nervous system co-ordinates the activities of the body by responding to stimuli received by sense organs.

Neurones nerve cells which make up nervous tissue.

Non-verbal communication communicating using body language, i.e. using your eyes, face and body to transmit your feelings.

Nutrition the nourishment derived from food, required for the body's growth, energy, repair and production.

Oedema extra fluid in an area, causing swelling.

Onycholysis nail condition where the nail plate separates from the nail bed.

Onychophagy nail condition where a person bites their nails excessively.

Onychorrhexis nail condition where the person has split, flaking nails.

Orange stick a disposable wooden tool used around the cuticle and free edge of the nail and to apply products to the nail.

Paraffin wax this is heated and applied to the skin of the feet to provide a heating effect. This improves skin functioning, aids the absorption of service products and is beneficial to ease the discomfort of arthritic and rheumatic conditions.

Paronychia bacterial infection where swelling, redness and pus appears in the cuticle area of the nail wall.

Pedicure a service to care for and improve the condition and appearance of the skin and nails of the feet.

Personal Protective Equipment (PPE) at Work Regulations (1992) this legislation requires employers to identify through risk assessment those activities that require special protective equipment to be worn.

Petrissage a massage manipulation in which the tissues are lifted away from the underlying structures and compressed. Petrissage improves muscle tone by the compression and relaxation of the muscle fibres.

pH the degree of acidity or alkalinity measured on a pH scale. This scale goes from 0–14. In the range of 0–6.9 the lower the pH value, the greater the acidity. Above 7, the greater the pH value, the greater the alkalinity. A pH of 7 is neutral – it is neither acid or alkaline. Spa pool water is regularly tested for its pH.

Photothermolysis an effect created when using a laser for hair removal. The melanin pigment that provides hair colour absorbs the laser energy, which is converted to heat, and at a sufficient temperature destroys the part of the hair follicle where the cells divide to create the hair.

Pigment the colour of skin and hair, called melanin. The amount of pigment varies for each client, resulting in different skin and hair colour.

Positive skin sensitivity test an allergic reaction to the skin test. The skin appears red, swollen and feels itchy.

Posture the position of the body, which varies from person to person. Good posture is when the body is in alignment. Correct posture enables you to work longer without becoming tired; it prevents muscle fatigue and stiff joints.

Powder cosmetic applied to set the foundation, disguise minor skin blemishes and make the skin appear smoother and oil-free.

Pre-wax lotion an antibacterial skin cleanser to clean the skin before wax application.

Prices Act (1974) this act states that the price of products has to be displayed in order to prevent the buyer being misguided.

Primer provides a base for make-up and acts as a barrier preventing absorption of the make-up products into the skin.

Promotion ways of communicating products or services to clients to increase sales.

Provision and Use of Work Equipment Regulations (PUWER) (1998) this regulation lays down important health and safety controls on the provision and use of equipment.

Psoriasis of the nail an inflammatory condition where there is an increased production of cells in the upper part of the skin. Pitting occurs on the surface of the nail.

Pterygium nail condition where the cuticle is thickened and overgrown.

Public Liability Insurance protects employers and employees against the consequences of death or injury to a third party while on the premises.

Punctual arriving at the correct time.

Reception the area where clients are received.

Receptionist person responsible for maintaining the reception area, scheduling appointments and handling payments.

Record cards confidential cards recording the personal details of each client registered at the business. This information may be stored electronically on the salon's computer.

Regulatory Reform (Fire Safety) Order (2005) this legislation requires that the employer or designated 'responsible person' must carry out a risk assessment for the premises in relation to fire evacuation practice and procedures.

Relaxation room a room of ambient temperature (close to the body's own temperature) and often referred to by the Latin name tepidarium.

Reporting of Injuries, Diseases and Dangerous Occurrences Regulations (RIDDOR) (1995) these regulations require the employer to notify the local enforcement officer in writing, in cases where employees or trainees suffer personal injury at work.

Resale Prices Acts (1964 and 1976) this act states that the manufacturer can supply a recommended price (MRRP), but the seller is not obliged to sell at the recommended price.

Resources the different products, equipment and other things needed to complete an activity.

Responsible persons this term is used in the Health and Safety unit to mean the person or persons at work to whom you should report any issues, problems or hazards. This could be a supervisor, line manager or your employer.

Ridge-filler a nail product used on ridged nails that improves the nail's appearance and provides a more even surface.

Risk the likelihood of a hazard's potential being recognized.

Roller wax a warm wax used to remove hair from the skin. The wax is contained in a cartridge container with a disposable applicator, which rolls the wax onto the skin's surface. The applicator is renewed for each client.

Sale and Supply of Goods Act (1994) goods must be as described, of merchantable, satisfactory quality and fit for their intended purpose.

Salon services covers all the services offered in your workplace.

Sauna a service room of timber construction where the air inside is heated to produce a therapeutic effect on the body.

Scissors nail tools used to shorten the length of the nail before filing.

Sebaceous gland a minute sac-like organ usually associated with the hair follicle. The cells of the gland decompose and produce the skin's natural oil sebum. Found all over the body, except for the soles of the feet and the palms of the hands.

Sebum the skin's natural oil which keeps the skin supple.

Secondary infection bacterial penetration into the skin causing infection.

Sensory nerve endings these nerves receive information and relay this to the brain. They are found near the skin's surface and respond to touch, pressure, temperature and pain.

Service plan after the consultation, suitable service objectives are established to treat the client's conditions and needs.

Shader a make-up product that draws attention away from and minimizes certain facial features.

Shoulder girdle bones a type of connective tissue that provides attachment for the muscles which move the arms, and includes the clavicle and scapula.

Skin allergy if the skin is sensitive to a particular substance, an allergic skin reaction will occur. This is recognized by irritation, swelling and inflammation.

Skin analysis assessment of the client's skin type and condition.

Skin appendages structures within the skin including sweat glands (that excrete sweat), hair follicles (that produce hair), sebaceous glands (produce the skin's natural oil, sebum) and nails (a horny substance that protects the ends of the fingers/toes).

Skin characteristics while looking at the skin type, additional characteristics may be seen. These include skin that may be sensitive, dehydrated, moist or oedematous (puffy), in addition to dry, oily or combination.

Skin condition while looking at the skin type, additional characteristics may be seen that indicate its condition. These include skin that may be sensitive, dehydrated or mature.

Skin removal accidental removal of the upper, dead, protective cornified layer of the skin, leaving the granular layer exposed.

Skin sensitivity test method used to assess skin tolerance/sensitivity to a particular substance or service.

Skin tags skin-coloured threads of skin 3mm to 6mm long, projecting from the skin's surface.

Skin tone the strength and elasticity of the skin.

Skin type the different physiological functioning of each person's skin dictates their skin type. There are four main skin types: normal (balanced), dry (lacking in oil), oily (excessive oil) and combination (a mixture of two skin types, e.g., dry and oily).

Skull bones a type of connective tissue forming a hard structure. It surrounds and protects the brain and forms an attachment point for muscles. These include the occipital, frontal, parietal, temporal, sphenoid and ethmoid.

Solvent a product designed to remove and clean artificial lashes without causing eye irritation.

Spa pool a pool of warm water in which the client sits with jets of air passing through to create bubbles which massage the skin.

Spa services services used to induce a physical and mental sense of wellbeing. The term 'spa' is said to be derived from a village near Liege in Belgium called Spau. It had mineral hot springs which people could visit to improve their health and ailments.

Specialist skincare service products additional skincare preparations available to target improvement. These products include eye gels, throat creams and ampoule services.

Steam service a warming effect created by boiling water, which is then vaporized and used on the skin to achieve both cleansing and stimulation.

Sterilization the total destruction of all microorganisms in metal tools and equipment.

Strip sugar a system of wax depilation similar to the warm-wax technique, used to remove hair from the skin. Made from sugar, lemons and water, the sugar wax is applied to the skin, and is then removed using a wax removal strip.

Stye bacterial infection. Infection of the sebaceous glands of the eyelash hair follicles. Small lumps appear on the inner rim of the eyelid and contain pus.

Subcutaneous layer a layer of fatty tissue situated below the epidermis and dermis.

Sugar paste a system of wax depilation. An organic paste made from sugar, lemons and water is used to embed the hair, which is then removed by the paste from the skin.

Sugaring an ancient popular method of hair removal using organic substances, sugar and lemon.

Sweat gland or sudoriferous glands are composed of a specialized lining tissue called epithelial tissue. Their function is to control body temperature through the evaporation of sweat from the surface of the skin.

Systemic medical condition a medical condition caused by a defect in one of the body's organs, e.g. the heart.

Tapotement, also known as percussion, massage movements performed in a brisk, stimulating manner to increase blood supply and improve tone of the skin and muscles. Movements include clapping and tapping.

Targets goals or objectives to achieve, usually set within a timescale.

Teamwork supportive work by a team.

Telogen the resting stage of the hair growth cycle, when the hair is finally shed.

Terminal hair deep-rooted, thick, course, pigmented hair found on the scalp, underarms, pubic region, eyelash and brow areas.

Thermal booties electrically heated boots in which the feet are placed following the application of a skin service product such as a mask. The heat aids the absorption of the product and improves skin functioning.

Thermal mitts electrically heated gloves in which the hands are placed following the application of a skin service product such as a mask. The heat aids the absorption of the product and improves skin functioning.

Thermal sensitivity test a test performed before wax application to check that the temperature of the wax is not too warm. The wax is tested by the therapist on themselves, usually on the inner wrist, and then on the client on a small visible area such as the inside of the ankle.

Thermometer equipment used to measure temperature.

Tinea corporis or body ringworm fungal infection of the skin where small scaly red patches, which spread outwards and then heal from the centre, leave a ring.

Tinea pedis or athlete's foot fungal infection of the foot occurring in the webs of the skin between the toes. Small blisters form, which later burst. The skin in the area can become dry with a scaly appearance.

Tinea unguium fungal infection of the nails. The nail is yellowish-grey in colour.

Tissues cells in the body which specialize in carrying out particular functions. These include epithelial, connective, muscular and nervous tissue.

Toluenediamine small molecules of permanent dye used in tinting service.

Toning lotion a skincare preparation formulated to treat the different skin types and facial characteristics. It is applied to remove all traces of cleanser from the skin. It produces a cooling effect on the skin and has a skin-tightening effect.

Top coat a nail polish product applied over another nail polish to provide additional strength and durability to the finish.

Towel steaming an alternative to facial steaming using an electrical vapour unit. Small, clean facial towels are heated in a bowl of warm water or specialized heater before application to the face to warm, cleanse and stimulate the skin.

Trade Descriptions Acts (1968 and 1972) legislation that states that information when selling products both in written and verbal form should be accurate.

Transverse furrows nail condition where grooves appear on the nail, running from side to side.

Travellers' cheques alternative form of payment used when travelling abroad and must be compared with the client's passport.

Tweezers small metal tools used to remove body hair by pulling it from the bottom of the hair follicle (small opening in the skin where the hair grows from). There are two types: automatic – designed to remove the bulk of the hair and manual – designed to remove the stray hairs.

Vapour unit an electrical appliance that heats water to produce steam which is applied to the skin of the face and neck, to warm, cleanse and stimulate the skin.

Varicose veins veins whose valves have become weak and lost their elasticity. The area appears knotted, swollen and bluish/purple in colour.

Vellus hair fine, downy and soft hair – found on the face and body.

Ventilation the transport of fresh air into an area. The spa pool will create heat, humidity and chemical smells. Adequate ventilation is necessary.

Verbal communication occurs when you talk directly to another person either face to face or over the telephone.

Verruca or plantar wart a viral infection where small epidermal skin growths appear, either raised or flat depending upon their location, and have a rough surface.

Vibrations massage manipulations applied on the nerve centre. They stimulate the nerves to induce a feeling of wellbeing and to provide gentle stimulation of the skin.

Viruses the smallest living bodies, too small to see under an ordinary microscope. Viruses invade healthy body cells and multiply within the cell. Eventually the cell walls break down and the virus particles are freed to attack further cells.

Vitamin D a fatty substance in the skin converted to vitamin D with UV light from the sun. This circulates in the blood and with the mineral salts calcium and phosphorus helps the formation and maintenance of the health of the body's bones.

Warm wax a system of wax depilation. Warm wax remains soft at body temperatures. It is frequently made of mixtures of glucose syrup and zinc oxide. Honey can be used instead of glucose syrup; this is referred to as honey wax.

Warm-oil service involves gently heating a small amount of oil and soaking the nails and cuticles in it to nourish the nails and soften the cuticles and surrounding skin.

Watery eye over-secretion of tears from the eyes, which would normally drain into the nasal cavity.

Wax depilation the temporary removal of excess hair from a body part using wax.

Waxing products cosmetic preparations used with a waxing service which have specific benefits to cleanse the skin, assist in hair removal care and improve the appearance and healing properties of the skin following hair removal.

Work techniques the methods you use to carry out waxing services.

Workplace (Health Safety and Welfare) Regulations (1992) these regulations provide the employer with an approved code of practice for maintaining a safe, secure working environment.

Workplace policies this covers the documentation prepared by your employer on the procedures to be followed in your workplace. Examples are your employer's safety policy statement, or general health and safety statements and written safety procedures covering aspects of the workplace that should be drawn to the employees' (and "other persons'") attention, pricing policies and customer service policies.

Workplace practices any activities, procedures, use of materials or equipment and working techniques used in carrying out your job. Lifting techniques and maintaining good posture whilst working are also included.

Index